Diagnosis and Management of Hypertrophic Cardiomyopathy

Diagnosis and Management of Hypertrophic Cardiomyopathy

Edited by

Barry J. Maron, MD

Director
The Hypertrophic Cardiomyopathy Center
Minneapolis Heart Institute Foundation
Minneapolis, Minnesota

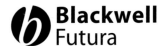

© 2004 by Futura, an imprint of Blackwell Publishing

Blackwell Publishing, Inc., 350 Main Street, Malden, Massachusetts 02148-5020, USA
Blackwell Publishing Ltd, 9600 Garsington Road, Oxford OX4 2DQ, UK
Blackwell Science Asia Pty Ltd, 550 Swanston Street, Carlton, Victoria 3053, Australia

04 05 06 07 5 4 3 2 1

ISBN: 1-4051-1732-X

Catalogue records for this title are available from the British Library and the US Library of Congress

Acquisitions: Jacques Strauss
Production: Julie Elliott
Typesetter: Sparks, in 9.5/12 pt Palatino
Printed and bound by MPG Books Limited, Bodmin, Cornwall, UK

For further information on Blackwell Publishing, visit our website:
www.blackwellfutura.com

Notice: The indications and dosages of all drugs in this book have been recommended in the medical literature and conform to the practices of the general community. The medications described do not necessarily have specific approval by the Food and Drug Administration for use in the diseases and dosages for which they are recommended. The package insert for each drug should be consulted for use and dosage as approved by the FDA. Because standards for usage change, it is advisable to keep abreast of revised recommendations, particularly those concerning new drugs.

Contents

Foreword

I am delighted to have the opportunity to write the foreword for this unique treatise on the complex subject of hypertrophic cardiomyopathy. This multi-authored book provides state-of-the-art discussions on all aspects of the disease. Each chapter is a contribution from experts in the field.

The subject matter is presented in a highly organized fashion. It includes the clinical (phenotypic) expression of hypertrophic cardiomyopathy, genetic aspects, outflow obstruction, diastolic function, the impact of atrial fibrillation, risk factors for sudden death and other prognostic markers, pharmacologic treatment, septal myectomy surgery and non-surgical septal ablation, and the role of implantable defibrillators in the prevention of sudden death. These topics are expertly discussed by knowledgeable investigators. The manuscripts are, in general, balanced and comprehensive. There is much that is contemporary, and aspects that are likely to be controversial by the nature of their novelty are also included.

The editor has included additional, related topics of interest, such as the athlete's heart, arrhythmogenic right ventricular cardiomyopathy, sudden death due to chest blows (commotio cordis) and naturally occurring animal models of cardiovascular disease. An important chapter on the role of the Internet and support groups for patients with hypertrophic cardiomyopathy should be particularly useful to patients, primary clinicians and cardiologists.

This outstanding monograph, edited by Dr Barry Maron, an internationally recognized authority on the subject, provides a comprehensive discussion of the ever-changing spectrum of hypertrophic cardiomyopathy. It should serve as an excellent reference book on the subject for many years to come.

Pravin M. Shah, MD, MACC
Medical Director
Hoag Heart and Vascular Institute
Newport Beach, CA

Dedication and Acknowledgments

This informative, comprehensive, and contemporary multi-authored book—largely devoted to the diagnosis, pathophysiology, clinical course and management of hypertrophic cardiomyopathy—is formally dedicated to the many thousands of patients afflicted with this disease throughout the world.

In addition, I would like to personally acknowledge the longstanding and continued support of my family for this and other related projects, including my wife Donna and all of the other young Maron doctors—Martin, Bradley and Jill—as well as my staff at the Hypertrophic Cardiomyopathy Center of the Minneapolis Heart Institute Foundation, particularly Terri Hanson and Sue Casey. Without their efforts, neither this book nor the substantial amount of data generated from our center over the last 10 years (ultimately important to the care of patients with hypertrophic cardiomyopathy) would have been possible.

Barry J. Maron, MD
Director, Hypertrophic Cardiomyopathy Center
Minneapolis Heart Institute Foundation
Minneapolis, Minnesota

Contributors

Camillo Autore, MD
Dipartimento di Scienze Cardiovascolari e
Respiratorie
Università la Sapienza
Rome, Italy

Ivan Barac, MD
Hypertrophic Cardiomyopathy Program
Division of Cardiology
St Luke's-Roosevelt Hospital Center
Columbia University
College of Physicians and Surgeons
New York, NY

Cristina Basso, MD, PhD
Department of Pathology
University of Padua Medical School
Padua, Italy

Sandro Betocchi, MD
Department of Clinical Medicine
Cardiovascular & Immunological Sciences
Federico II University of Naples
Naples, Italy

Ross Campbell, BSc
Department of Cardiology
Wales Heart Research Institute
University of Wales College of Medicine
Heath Park
Cardiff, United Kingdom

Lucie Carrier, PhD
INSERM U-523
Institut de Myologie
Hôpital de la Salpêtrière
Paris, France

Franco Cecchi, MD
Department of Cardiology
Regional Referral Center for Myocardial Diseases
University Hospital of Careggi
Florence, Italy

Domenico Corrado, MD
Department of Cardiology
University of Padua Medical School
Padua, Italy

Gordon K. Danielson, MD
Division of Cardiovascular Surgery
Mayo Clinic
Rochester, MN

Joseph A. Dearani, MD
Division of Cardiovascular Surgery
Mayo Clinic
Rochester, MN

Michel Desnos, MD
Department of Cardiology 1
Hôpital Européen Georges Pompidou and
INSERM EMI-0016 Faculté de Médecine Necker-
Enfants Malades
Paris V University
Paris, France

Yoshinori Doi, MD, PhD
Professor of Medicine
Chairman, Department of Medicine and Geriatrics
Kochi Medical School
Kochi, Japan

Perry M. Elliott MBBS, MD, MRCP
The Heart Hospital
University College London
London, United Kingdom

Maria Eriksson, MD, PhD
Division of Cardiology
Department of Medicine
Toronto General Hospital
University Health Network and University of
Toronto
Toronto, Canada

N.A. Mark Estes III, MD
Director, Cardiac Arrhythmia Service
New England Medical Center Hospital;
Professor of Medicine
Tufts University School of Medicine
Boston, MA

Lothar Faber, MD
Department of Cardiology
Heart Center NRW
Bad Oeynhausen, Germany

David Focsaneanu
Division of Cardiology
Department of Medicine
Toronto General Hospital
University Health Network and University of Toronto
Toronto, Canada

Philip R. Fox, DVM
Caspary Institute of the Animal Medical Center
New York, NY

Michael P. Frenneaux, FRCP, FRACP
Department of Cardiology
Wales Heart Research Institute
University of Wales College of Medicine
Heath Park
Cardiff, United Kingdom

Takashi Furuno, MD
Lecturer in Medicine
Department of Medicine and Geriatrics
Kochi Medical School
Kochi, Japan

Frank H. Gietzen, MD
Department of Cardiology and Internal Intensive Care
Bielefeld Klinikum
Academic Teaching Hospital of the University of Münster
Bielefeld, Germany

Albert A. Hagège, MD, PhD
Department of Cardiology 1
Hôpital Européen Georges Pompidou and INSERM EMI-0016 Faculté de Médecine Necker-Enfants Malades
Paris V University
Paris, France

Mohammad S. Hamid, MB, MRCP
Cardiology Department
Medway Maritime Hospital
Gillingham, Kent, United Kingdom

Nobuhiko Hitomi, MD
Research Assistant
Department of Medicine and Geriatrics
Kochi Medical School
Kochi, Japan

Carolyn Y. Ho, MD
Cardiovascular Division
Brigham and Women's Hospital
Boston, MA

Munther K. Homoud, MD
Center for the Cardiovascular Evaluation of Athletes
New England Cardiac Arrhythmia Center;
Division of Cardiology/Department of Medicine
Tufts University School of Medicine
Boston, MA

Xavier Jeanrenaud, MD
Division of Cardiology
Department of Medicine
University Hospital
Lausanne, Switzerland

Lukas Kappenberger, MD
Division of Cardiology
Department of Medicine
University Hospital
Lausanne, Switzerland

Hiroaki Kitaoka, MD
Lecturer in Cardiology
Department of Medicine and Geriatrics
Kochi Medical School
Kochi, Japan

Horst Kuhn, MD
Professor of Medicine
Chief of the Department of Cardiology and Internal Intensive Care
Bielefeld Klinikum
Academic Teaching Hospital of the University of Münster
Bielefeld, Germany

Thorsten Lawrenz, MD
Department of Cardiology and Internal Intensive Care
Bielefeld Klinikum
Academic Teaching Hospital of the University of Münster
Bielefeld, Germany

Christian H. Leuner, MD
Bielefeld Klinikum
Department of Cardiology and Internal Intensive Care
Academic Teaching Hospital of the University of Münster
Bielefeld, Germany

Harry M. Lever, MD
Staff Physician
Department of Cardiovascular Medicine
Cleveland Clinic Foundation
Cleveland, OH

Frank Lieder, MD
Department of Cardiology and Internal Intensive
Care
Bielefeld Klinikum
Academic Teaching Hospital of the University of
Münster
Bielefeld, Germany

Mark S. Link, MD
The Center for the Cardiovascular Evaluation of
Athletes
The New England Cardiac Arrhythmia Center;
Division of Cardiology/Department of Medicine
Tufts University School of Medicine
Boston, MA

Raffaella Lombardi, MD
Department of Clinical Medicine
Cardiovascular & Immunological Sciences
Federico II University of Naples
Naples, Italy

Barry J. Maron, MD
Director, Hypertrophic Cardiomyopathy Center
Minneapolis Heart Institute Foundation
Minneapolis, MN;
Adjunct Professor of Medicine
Tufts-New England Medical Center
Boston, MA

Martin S. Maron, MD
Hypertrophic Cardiomyopathy Center
Tufts-New England Medical Center
Boston, MA

Yoshihisa Matsumura, MD
Lecturer in Cardiology
Department of Medicine and Geriatrics
Kochi Medical School
Kochi, Japan

William J. McKenna, MD, FRCP
The Heart Hospital
University College London
London, United Kingdom

Jayne A. Morris-Thurgood, PhD
Department of Cardiology
Wales Heart Research Institute
University of Wales College of Medicine
Heath Park
Cardiff, United Kingdom

Rick A. Nishimura, MD
Division of Cardiovascular Diseases and Internal
Medicine
Mayo Clinic and Mayo Foundation
Rochester, MN

Ludger Obergassel, MD
Department of Cardiology and Internal Intensive
Care
Bielefeld Klinikum
Academic Teaching Hospital of the University of
Münster
Bielefeld, Germany

Iacopo Olivotto, MD
Department of Cardiology
Regional Referral Center for Myocardial Diseases
University Hospital of Careggi
Florence, Italy

Steve R. Ommen, MD
Division of Cardiovascular Diseases and Internal
Medicine
Mayo Clinic and Mayo Foundation
Rochester, MN

Antonio Pelliccia, MD
Department of Medicine
Institute of Sport Science
Rome, Italy

Marco Piccininno, MD
Divisione di Cardiologia
Ente Ospedaliero Ospedali Galliera
Genoa, Italy

†Asifa Quraishi MB, MRCP
Department of Cardiological Sciences
St George's Hospital Medical School
London, United Kingdom

Harry Rakowski, MD
Division of Cardiology
Department of Medicine
Toronto General Hospital
University Health Network and University of
Toronto
Toronto, Canada

Paul Rakowski
Division of Cardiology
Department of Medicine
Toronto General Hospital
University Health Network and University of
Toronto
Toronto, Canada

Angelos Rigopoulos, MD
Department of Cardiology
University of Athens
Athens, Greece

---

†Deceased.

Bhavesh Sachdev, MBBS, MRCP
Cardiology Department
Royal Brompton Hospital
London, United Kingdom

Lisa Salberg
President
Hypertrophic Cardiomyopathy Association
(HCMA)
Hibernia, NJ
www.4HCM.org

Maurizio Schiavon, MD
Center of Sport Medicine
Padua, Italy

Ketty Schwartz, PhD
INSERM U-523
Institut de Myologie
Hôpital de la Salpêtrière
Paris, France

Hubert Seggewiss, MD Prof
Medizinische Klinik 1
Leopoldina-Krankenhaus
Schweinfurt, Germany

Christine E. Seidman, MD
Cardiovascular Division
Brigham and Women's Hospital; Howard Hughes
Medical Institute and Department of Genetics
Harvard Medical School
Boston, MA

Sanjay Sharma, MRCP, MD
Department of Cardiology
University Hospital Lewisham
London, United Kingdom

Win-Kuang Shen, MD
Department of Cardiovascular Disease
Mayo Clinic
Rochester, MN

Mark V. Sherrid, MD
Hypertrophic Cardiomyopathy Program
Division of Cardiology
St Luke's-Roosevelt Hospital Center
Columbia University
College of Physicians and Surgeons
New York, NY

Cairrine Sloggett, RN
Division of Cardiology
Department of Medicine
Toronto General Hospital
University Health Network and University of
Toronto
Toronto, Canada

Paul Sorajja, MD
Division of Cardiovascular Diseases and Internal
Medicine
Mayo Clinic and Mayo Foundation
Rochester, MN

Paolo Spirito, MD
Divisione di Cardiologia
Ente Ospedaliero Ospedali Galliera
Genoa, Italy

Berit Stolle, MD
Department of Cardiology and Internal Intensive
Care
Bielefeld Klinikum
Academic Teaching Hospital of the University of
Münster
Bielefeld, Germany

Claudia Strunk-Muller, MD
Department of Cardiology and Internal Intensive
Care
Bielefeld Klinikum
Academic Teaching Hospital of the University of
Münster
Bielefeld, Germany

Rajesh Thaman, MBBS, MRCP
Research Fellow in Cardiology
The Heart Hospital
University College London
London, United Kingdom

Gaetano Thiene, MD
Department of Pathology
University of Padua Medical School
Padua, Italy

Paul J. Wang, MD
Director
Cardiac Arrhythmia Service
Professor of Medicine
Stanford University School of Medicine
Palo Alto, CA

E. Douglas Wigle MD
Division of Cardiology
Department of Medicine
Toronto General Hospital
University Health Network and University of
Toronto
Toronto, Canada

Anna Woo, MD
Division of Cardiology
Department of Medicine
Toronto General Hospital
University Health Network and University of
Toronto
Toronto, Canada

Naohito Yamasaki, MD
Staff Physician
Department of Medicine and Geriatrics
Kochi Medical School
Kochi, Japan

Peer Ziemssen, MD
Medizinische Klinik 1
Leopoldina-Krankenhaus
Schweinfurt, Germany

CHAPTER 1

Phenotypic Expression and Clinical Course of Hypertrophic Cardiomyopathy

Barry J. Maron, MD

Hypertrophic cardiomyopathy (HCM) is a complex and relatively common genetic cardiac disease and has been the subject of intense scrutiny and investigation for over 40 years.[1-50] HCM is an important cause of disability and death in patients of all ages and is the most common cause of sudden cardiac death in young people, including trained athletes.[51-60] Because of marked heterogeneity in clinical and phenotypic expression, natural history and prognosis,[51-66] HCM often represents a dilemma even to cardiovascular specialists, including those for whom this disease is a focus of their investigative efforts. This chapter is designed to place in perspective and clarify the rapidly evolving concepts predominantly related to the prevalence, phenotypic expression, and clinical course of HCM.

Prevalence

Epidemiologic investigations using echocardiography and with diverse study designs have produced similar estimates for the prevalence of phenotypically expressed HCM in general adult populations: about 0.2% (or 1: 500) (Fig 1.1).[20,39,67-69] These include population surveys of young adults in the USA, echocardiographic screening for cardiovascular disease in rural Minnesota, and other investigations using population samples in Japan and China. Therefore, HCM is not rare; in fact, it is the most common of the genetic cardiovascular diseases, with reports from many countries throughout the world, including most prominently the USA, Canada, Western Europe, South America, Australia, Japan, and China. Taken together, these reports from diverse geographic regions and cultures have suggested a similar clinical presentation and course. Nevertheless, a substantial proportion of individuals harboring a mutant gene for HCM are probably undetected clinically, as evidenced by the uncommon occurrence of HCM in routine cardiology practice, constituting about 1% of an outpatient population.[70] This limited exposure to HCM by practicing clinicians outside of major centers understandably accounts for the uncertainty that prevails regarding this disease and its management.

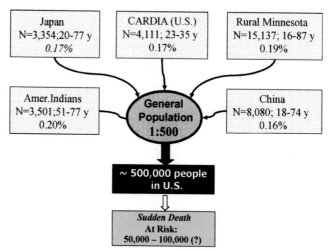

Fig. 1.1 Evidence of the worldwide prevalence of hypertrophic cardiomyopathy and its clinical implications. y = years of age; Amer. = American. Population prevalence data presented are cited in references 20, 39, 67, and 69.

Nomenclature

Since the first modern description in 1958,[1] HCM has been known by a vast and confusing array of names, reflecting its clinical heterogeneity and the skewed experience of early investigators (Fig. 1.2). 'Hypertrophic cardiomyopathy'[71] has become established as the preferred name because it describes the overall disease spectrum without introducing the misleading inference that left ventricular (LV) outflow tract obstruction is an invariable clinical feature (such as hypertrophic obstructive cardiomyopathy; or idiopathic hypertrophic subaortic stenosis). Indeed, under resting (basal) conditions HCM presents as a predominantly nonobstructive disease in which only about 25% of patients demonstrate a sizeable outflow gradient.[2,3,7,25,27,34,37]

Genetics

HCM is inherited as a Mendelian autosomal dominant trait caused by mutations in any one of 10 genes, each encoding proteins of the cardiac sarcomere (components of thick or thin filaments with contractile, structural or regulatory functions).[3,9,35,43,45,46,48–50,59,72] The physical similarity of these proteins represents a unifying principle that makes it possible to regard the diverse HCM spectrum as a single disease entity and a primary disorder of the sarcomere. Recently, missense mutations in the gene that encodes the γ-2 regulatory subunit of the AMP-activated protein kinase (*PRKAG2*) have been reported to cause familial Wolff–Parkinson–White syndrome and LV hypertrophy (due to glycogen accumulation in myocytes).[3,73] This syndrome is a metabolic storage disease distinct from typical HCM, and is caused by mutations in genes

TERMS USED TO DESCRIBE HYPERTROPHIC CARDIOMYOPATHY

Acquired aortic subvalvular stenosis
Apical asymmetric septal hypertrophy
Apical hypertrophic cardiomyopathy
Apical hypertrophic nonobstructive
  cardiomyopathy
Apical hypertrophy
Asymmetric left ventricular hypertrophy
Asymmetric septal hypertrophy
Asymmetrical apical hypertrophy
Asymmetrical hypertrophic cardiomyopathy
Asymmetrical hypertrophy of the heart
Brock's disease
Diffuse muscular subaortic stenosis
Diffuse subvalvular aortic stenosis
Dynamic hypertrophic subaortic stenosis
Dynamic muscular subaortic stenosis
Familial hypertrophic subaortic stenosis
Familial muscular subaortic stenosis
Familial myocardial disease
Functional aortic stenosis
Functional aortic subvalvar stenosis
Functional hypertrophic subaortic stenosis
Functional obstructive cardiomyopathy
Functional obstruction of the left ventricle
Functional obstructive subvalvular
  aortic stenosis
Functional subaortic stenosis
Hereditary cardiovascular dysplasia
Hypertrophic apical cardiomyopathy
HYPERTROPHIC CARDIOMYOPATHY
Hypertrophic constrictive cardiomyopathy
Hypertrophic disease
Hypertrophic hyperkinetic cardiomyopathy
Hypertrophic infundibular aortic stenosis
Hypertrophic nonobstructive apical
  cardiomyopathy
Hypertrophic nonobstructive cardiomyopathy
Hypertrophic nonobstructive cardiomyopathy
  with giant negative T waves
Hypertrophic obstructive cardiomyopathy
Hypertrophic obstructive cardiomyopathy
  of left ventricle
Hypertrophic restrictive cardiomyopathy
Hypertrophic stenosing cardiomyopathy

Hypertrophic subaortic stenosis
Idiopathic hypertrophic cardiomyopathy
Idiopathic hypertrophic obstructive cardiomyopathy
Idiopathic hypertrophic subaortic stenosis
Idiopathic hypertrophic subvalvular stenosis
Idiopathic muscular hypertrophic subaortic stenosis
Idiopathic muscular stenosis of the left ventricle
Idiopathic myocardial hypertrophy
Idiopathic ventricular septal hypertrophy
Irregular hypertrophic cardiomyopathy
Left ventricular muscular stenosis
Low subvalvular aortic stenosis
Mid-ventricular hypertrophic cardiomyopathy
Mid-ventricular hypertrophic obstructive
  cardiomyopathy
Mid-ventricular obstruction
Muscular aortic stenosis
Muscular hypertrophic stenosis of the left ventricle
Muscular stenosis of the left ventricle
Muscular subaortic stenosis
Muscular subvalvular aortic stenosis
Non-dilated cardiomyopathy
Nonobstructive hypertrophic cardiomyopathy
Obstructive cardiomyopathy
Obstructive hypertrophic aortic stenosis
Obstructive hypertrophic cardiomyopathy
Obstructive hypertrophic myocardiopathy
Obstructive myocardiopathy
Pseudoaortic stenosis
Stenosing hypertrophy of the left ventricle
Stenosis of the ejection chamber of left ventricle
Subaortic hypertrophic obstructive cardiomyopathy
Subaortic hypertrophic stenosis
Subaortic idiopathic stenosis
Subaortic muscular stenosis
Subvalvular aortic stenosis
Subvalvular aortic stenosis of the muscular type
Teare's disease
Typical hypertrophic obstructive cardiomyopathy

Fig. 1.2 Terms which have been used to describe hypertrophic cardiomyopathy. From Maron and Epstein. Hypertrophic cardiomyopathy: A discussion of nomenclature. *Am J Cardiol* 1979; **43**: 1242–4, reproduced with permission of the *American Journal of Cardiology.*

encoding proteins of the cardiac sarcomere; future studies are likely to ascribe other HCM subgroups to metabolic disorders (e.g. glycogen storage diseases).

At present, three of the HCM-causing mutant genes predominate: β-myosin heavy chain (the first identified), cardiac troponin T, and myosin-binding protein C. The other genes each account for a minority of HCM cases—cardiac troponin-I, regulatory and essential myosin light chains, titin, α-tropomyosin, α-actin, and α-myosin heavy chain. This diversity is compounded by intragenic heterogeneity, with more than 150 mutations identified, most of which are missense with a single amino acid residue substituted for another (see Chapter 2 for details). The molecular defects responsible for HCM are usually different in unrelated individuals, and many other sarcomeric genes and mutations (each accounting for a small proportion of familial HCM) remain to be identified. The mechanisms by which disease-causing sarcomere mutations cause LV hypertrophy and the HCM disease state are presently unresolved, although several hypotheses abound.[74]

Contemporary molecular genetic studies over the past decade have provided important insights into the considerable clinical heterogeneity of HCM, including the preclinical diagnosis of affected individuals without evidence of the disease phenotype (e.g. LV hypertrophy by echocardiography or ECG).[3,11,35,43,49,75–78] While DNA analysis for mutant genes is the definitive method of establishing the diagnosis of HCM, it is not yet a routine clinical strategy.[72] Because the techniques are complex, time-consuming and expensive, genotyping is confined to research-oriented investigations of highly selected pedigrees. The development of rapid, automated screening for genetic abnormalities will permit more widespread access to the power of molecular biology for resolving diagnostic ambiguities.

Diagnosis

Conventionally, the clinical diagnosis of HCM is established most easily and reliably with two-dimensional echocardiography, by imaging the hypertrophied but nondilated LV chamber, in the absence of another cardiac or systemic disease capable of producing that magnitude of hypertrophy (e.g. systemic hypertension or aortic stenosis) (Fig. 1.3).[2,3,12,15,21,34,37] Initially, the clinical suspicion of HCM may be raised by a heart murmur (occasionally during preparticipation sports examinations), a positive family history, new symptoms or cardiac events, or abnormal ECG.[20,25,79] The physical examination may not be a reliable method for clinical identification, unless a murmur is elicited in the standing position or with the Valsalva maneuver, given that most HCM patients do not have outflow obstruction or loud murmurs in the supine position under resting (basal) conditions.[79]

With regard to pedigree assessment, it is obligatory for the proband and family members to be informed of the genetic nature and autosomal dominant transmission of HCM. Screening of first-degree relatives with history and physical examinations, two-dimensional echocardiography and ECG should be strongly encouraged, particularly if adverse HCM-related events have occurred in the family.

In clinically diagnosed patients, increased LV wall thicknesses range widely from mild (13–15 mm) to massive (≥30 mm; normal ≤12 mm),[2,3,6,10,12,15,52,53,55] and include the most substantial in any cardiac disease—up to 60 mm (Figs 1.4–1.7).[19,80] In trained athletes, modest segmental wall thickening (13–15 mm) occurs occasionally,[81] raising the differential diagnosis between extreme physiologic LV hypertrophy (i.e. athlete's heart) and mild morphologic expressions

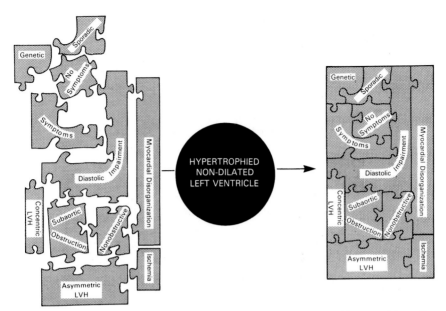

Fig. 1.3 Diagrammatic representation of the basic morphologic definition of hypertrophic cardiomyopathy (in dark circle), as it unifies the clinical and morphologic heterogeneity characteristic of the disease spectrum.

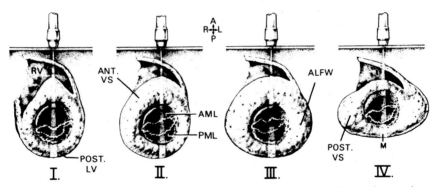

Fig. 1.4 Morphologic variability in hypertrophic cardiomyopathy, based on observations made from two-dimensional echocardiography (Maron classification). All images appear in the short-axis cross-sectional plane at mitral valve level. **I**, Relatively mild left ventricular hypertrophy confined to anterior portion of ventricular septum (VS); **II**, hypertrophy of anterior and posterior septum in the absence of free wall thickening; **III**, diffuse hypertrophy of substantial portions of both the ventricular septum and the anterolateral free wall (ALFW); **IV**, includes more unusual patterns of hypertrophy in which the anterior septum is spared from the hypertrophic process and the thickened portions of the left ventricle are in the posterior septum or anterolateral free wall (as shown here), or the apex. AML = anterior mitral leaflet; A or ANT = anterior; L = (patient's) left; LVFW = LV free wall; P or POST = posterior; PML = posterior mitral leaflet; R = (patient's) right; RV = right ventricle. From Maron *et al.* Patterns and significance of distribution of left ventricular hypertrophy in hypertrophic cardiomyopathy: A wide-angle, two-dimensional echocardiographic study of 125 patients. *Am J Cardiol* 1981; **48**: 418–28, reproduced with permission of the *American Journal of Cardiology*.

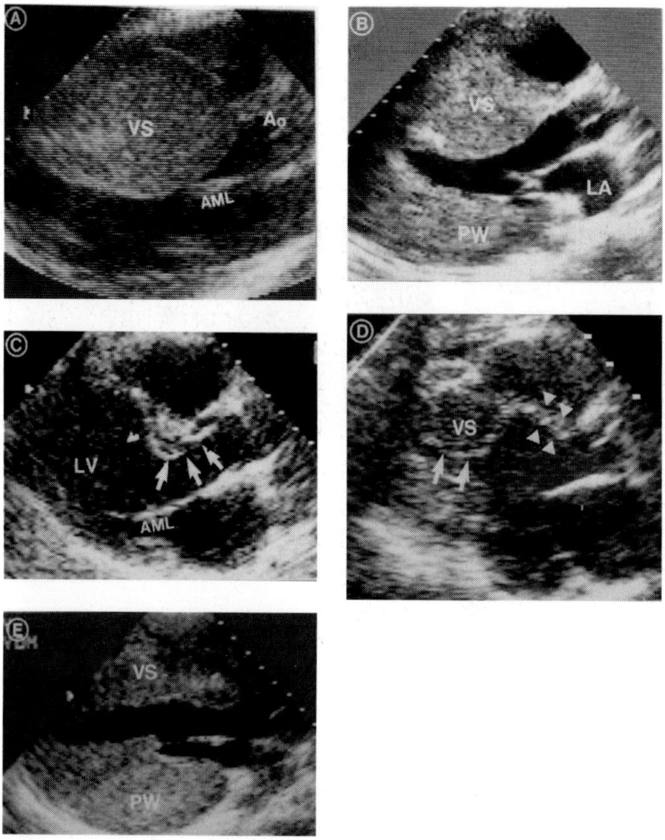

Fig. 1.5 Distribution and extent of ventricular septal thickening as shown in a composite of parasternal long-axis stop-frame images obtained in diastole. (**A**) Massive asymmetric hypertrophy of ventricular septum (VS) with wall thickness exceeding 50 mm. (**B**) Heterogeneous pattern of septal thickening, with distal portion substantially thicker than the proximal region at mitral valve level. (**C**) Hypertrophy sharply confined to the basal (proximal) septum just below the aortic valve (arrows). (**D**) Distal septal thickening (arrows) and particularly abrupt transition to thin proximal septum (<10 mm) (arrowheads). (**E**) 'Inverted' pattern of hypertrophy in which the distal anterior ventricular septum is only mildly thickened but the posterior free wall (PW) is substantially thickened and the posterior free wall (PW) is substantially thickened (to 40 mm). Calibration dots are 1 cm apart. Ao = aorta; AML = anterior mitral leaflet; LA = left atrium; LV = left ventricle. From Klues *et al.* Phenotypic spectrum and patterns of left ventricular hypertrophy in hypertrophic cardiomyopathy: Morphologic observations and significance as assessed by two-dimensional echocardiography in 600 patients. *J Am Coll Cardiol* 1995; **26**: 1699–708, reproduced with permission of the American College of Cardiology.

of HCM,[48] which usually can be resolved with noninvasive testing.[82] Magnetic resonance imaging may be of diagnostic value when echocardiographic studies are technically inadequate or in identifying segmental LV hypertrophy that is undetectable by echocardiography.[83]

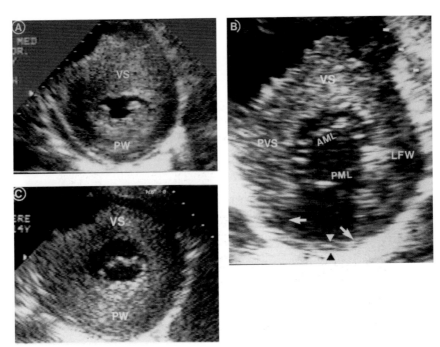

Fig. 1.6 Variability of patterns of left ventricular hypertrophy in patients with hypertrophic cardio-myopathy, shown in a composite of diastolic stop-frame images in the parasternal short-axis plane. (**A, B** and **D**) Wall thickening is diffuse, involving substantial portions of the ventricular septum and free wall. At the papillary muscle level (**A**), all segments of the left ventricle are hypertrophied, including the posterior free wall (PW), but the pattern of thickening is asymmetric with the anterior portion of the ventricular septum (VS) massive (50 mm). (**B**) Hypertrophy is diffuse, involving three segments of the left ventricle but with the posterior wall spared and thin (<10 mm) (arrowheads) and with particularly abrupt changes in wall thickness evident (arrows). (**C**) Marked hypertrophy in a pattern distinctly different from that in **A**, **B** and **D**, in which the thickening of the posterior wall is predominant and the ventricular septum is of nearly normal thickness. (**D**) Diffuse distribution of hypertrophy involving three segments of the left ventricle similar to that in **B** but without sharp changes in the contour of the wall. (**E**) Hypertrophy predominantly of the lateral free wall and only a small portion of contiguous anterior septum (arrows). (**F**) Hypertrophy predominantly of the posterior ventricular septum (PVS) and, to a lesser extent, the contiguous portion of the anterior septum. (**G**) Thickening of anterior and posterior septum to a similar degree but with sparing of the free wall. Calibration dots are 1 cm apart. AML = anterior mitral leaflet; LFW = lateral free wall; PML = posterior mitral leaflet. From Klues *et al. Phenotypic spectrum and patterns of left ventricular hypertrophy in hypertrophic cardiomyopathy: Morphologic observations and significance as assessed by two-dimensional echocardiography in 600 patients. J Am Coll Cardiol* 1995; **26**: 1699–708, reproduced with permission of the American College of Cardiology. (*Continued.*)

The 12-lead ECG is abnormal in 75–95% of HCM patients depending on the particular selection of patients; the ECG typically demonstrates a wide variety of patterns, often bizarre in appearance, although none are character-istic of most patients with HCM.[84,85] The ECG abnormalities most commonly described are LV hypertrophy, ST segment alterations and T wave inversion, left atrial enlargement, abnormal Q waves, and diminished or absent R waves

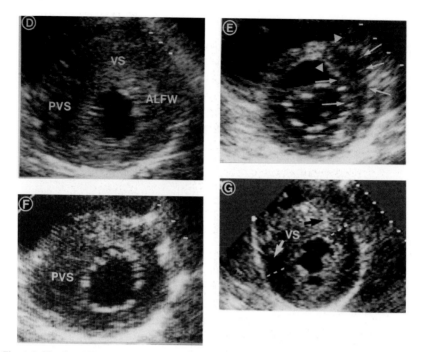

Fig. 1.6 (*Continued.*)

in the lateral precordial leads. Infants and young children with HCM often have the paradoxic finding of right ventricular hypertrophy, which may reflect obstruction to right ventricular outflow. Normal ECGs are most commonly encountered in family members identified as part of pedigree screening and/or when associated with mild localized LV hypertrophy.[43,75–77]

Only a modest relation between ECG voltages and the magnitude of LV hypertrophy assessed by echocardiography is evident, and no particular ECG pattern reliably discriminates patients with or without obstruction to LV outflow or those at risk of sudden death. All of this limits the usefulness of the 12-lead ECG as a routine clinical test.[86] Nevertheless, the 12-lead ECG has been shown to have diagnostic efficacy in raising the suspicion of HCM in family members known to carry a disease-causing mutant gene but without LV hypertrophy, as well as in targeting athletes for diagnostic echocardiography as part of preparticipation sports screening.[43,75–77,85,87] Also, non-preload-dependent measures of diastolic dysfunction with tissue Doppler echocardiography may precede the appearance of LV hypertrophy, providing clues to the impending appearance of the HCM phenotype.[78]

However, not all individuals harboring a genetic defect will at all times express the clinical features of HCM, such as LV hypertrophy by echocardiography, abnormal ECG, or cardiac symptoms.[2,3,21,35,37,43,72,85] Molecular genetic studies have demonstrated that there is no minimum wall thickness obligatory for the diagnosis of HCM at any given time in life; indeed, it is not unusual for

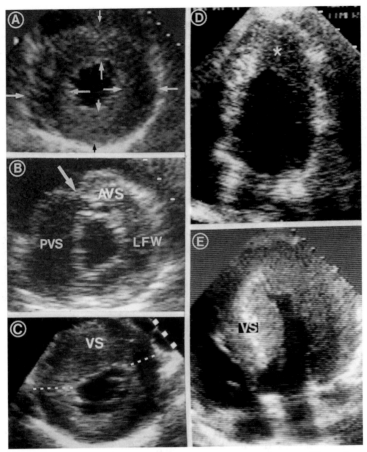

Fig. 1.7 Patterns of left ventricular hypertrophy in five patients with hypertrophic cardiomyopathy. (**A, B** and **C**) Diastolic stop-frame images obtained in the parasternal short-axis plane. (**D** and **E**) Apical four-chamber views. In **A**, relatively mild hypertrophy in a concentric (symmetric) pattern, each segment of septum and free wall having similar or identical thickness (paired arrows). (**B**) 'Butterfly' pattern with prominent indentation (arrow) and localized area of thinning interpositioned at the 11 o'clock position between adjacent thicker areas of the ventricular septum. (**C**) Hypertrophy of the entire ventricular septum (VS) and sparing of most of the left ventricular free wall. (**D**) Myocardial hypertrophy confined to the left ventricular apex (asterisk). (**E**) Image from another patient with hypertrophy of the left ventricular apex but also diffusely involving the ventricular septum and free wall. Calibration marks are 1 cm apart. AVS = anterior ventricular septum; LA = left atrium; LFW = lateral free wall; LV = left ventricle; PVS = posterior ventricular septum. From Klues *et al*. Phenotypic spectrum and patterns of left ventricular hypertrophy in hypertrophic cardiomyopathy: Morphologic observations and significance as assessed by two-dimensional echocardiography in 600 patients. *J Am Coll Cardiol* 1995; **26**: 1699–708, reproduced with permission of the American College of Cardiology.

children under 13 years to carry a mutant HCM gene without demonstrating hypertrophy. This underscores the potential limitation of echocardiographic screening for this disease in pre-adolescents.[2,3,21,35,37,43,49,72,75–77,85]

Substantial LV remodeling with the spontaneous appearance of hypertrophy typically occurs with the accelerated body growth occurring during adolescence, and this morphologic expression is believed to be complete in most instances at the time of physical maturity (about 17–18 years of age) (Fig. 1.8).[2,3,21]

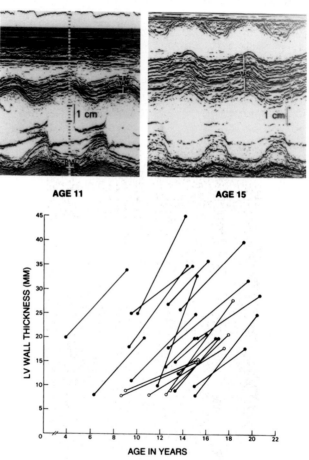

Fig. 1.8 Development and progression of left ventricular hypertrophy in children with hypertrophic cardiomyopathy. (Top) Dynamic, striking changes in left ventricular wall thickness with age in 22 children; each patient is represented by the left ventricular segment that showed greatest change in wall thickness. Open symbols denote five patients who had no evidence of hypertrophy in any segment of the left ventricle at initial evaluation but subsequently developed *de novo* hypertrophy typical of hypertrophic cardiomyopathy. (Bottom) Development of marked hypertrophy of the anterior basal ventricular septum (VS). M-mode echocardiograms were obtained at the same cross-sectional level in girl with a family history of hypertrophic cardiomyopathy. At age 11, ventricular septal thickness was at the upper limit of normal (10 mm); at age 15, septal thickness had increased markedly (to 33 mm). Appearance of the echocardiogram is typical of hypertrophic cardiomyopathy. The patient remained asymptomatic throughout this period but died suddenly and unexpectedly at age 17. PW = posterior left ventricular free wall. From Maron *et al.* Hypertrophic cardiomyopathy: Interrelation of clinical manifestations, pathophysiology, and therapy. *N Engl J Med* 1987; **316**: 780–9 and 844–52, reproduced with permission of the Massachusetts Medical Society.

Recently, novel diagnostic criteria for HCM, based on genotype–phenotype studies, have demonstrated incomplete disease expression with the absence of LV hypertrophy in adult individuals, due most commonly to cardiac myosin-binding protein-C or troponin-T mutations.[2,3,11,43,49] Mutations in the myosin-binding protein C gene have also been associated, in both cross-sectional and serial echocardiographic studies, with age-related penetrance of the HCM phenotype, in which delayed and late *de novo* onset of LV hypertrophy occurs in mid-life and even beyond (Fig. 1.9).[2,3,11,43,88] Such adult morphologic conversions dictate that it is no longer possible to issue definitive reassurance to asymptomatic family members at maturity (or even in middle age) that they are free of a disease-causing mutant HCM gene solely based on clinical findings and a normal echocardiogram. This probably necessitates a strategy of subsequent

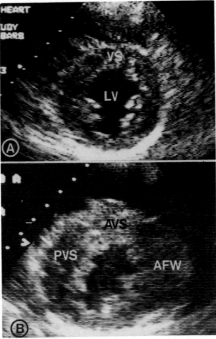

Fig. 1.9 Development of the hypertrophic cardiomyopathy phenotype in adulthood. Stop-frame two-dimensional echocardiograms at end-diastole, at the papillary muscle level in the parasternal short-axis plane, from a woman with familial hypertrophic cardiomyopathy at age 27 years, when genotyping was initiated (**A**) and at age 33 years, after the myosin-binding protein C mutation was known (**B**). (**A**) Left ventricular (LV) thickness is normal (≤ 12 mm) in all segments of the wall, including the ventricular septum (VS). (**B**) Six years later, at age 33, wall thickness was abnormally increased (19–20 mm) in the anterior ventricular septum (AVS) and posterior septum (PVS) as well as the anterolateral free wall (AFW). Mild mitral valve systolic anterior motion (without septal contact or outflow gradient) appeared at this time, although it is not shown here. Calibration marks are 10 mm apart. From Maron *et al.* Clinical course of hypertrophic cardiomyopathy with survival to advanced age. *J Am Coll Cardiol* 2003; **42**: 882–8, reproduced with permission of the *Journal of the American College of Cardiology.*

echocardiographic examinations every 5 years.[72] Otherwise, the recommended strategy for screening relatives in most HCM families calls for such evaluations at intervals of 12–18 months, usually beginning at age 12.

Paradoxically, a small, distinctive subset of HCM patients (2%) evolve to the end-stage (or 'burned-out') phase, characterized by LV wall thinning, ventricular cavity enlargement and systolic dysfunction. This often resembles the dilated form of cardiomyopathy and produces relentlessly progressive and irreversible heart failure (Fig. 1.10).[2,3,66,89,90] Such disease progression is probably due to extensive myocardial scarring on the basis of ischemia related to 'small vessel disease,' but is not associated with atherosclerotic coronary artery disease. This profound remodeling process, progressing from a thick-walled,

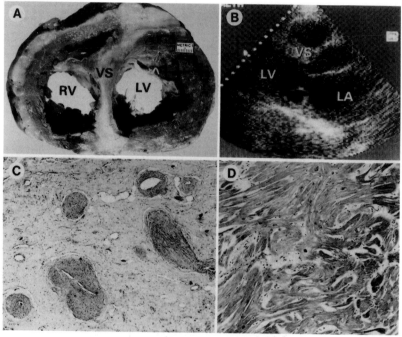

Fig. 1.10 End-stage hypertrophic cardiomyopathy in a 46-year-old man. (**A**) Transverse section of the heart obtained after heart transplantation, showing extensive scarring and thinning of the ventricular septum (VS), which extends into the anterior and posterior free wall. The left ventricular (LV) cavity appears enlarged. RV = right ventricle. (**B**) Stop-frame echocardiogram in parasternal long-axis view (obtained 2 weeks before heart transplantation, showing relatively mild (13 mm) wall thickening confined to the basal anterior ventricular septum. The left atrium (LA) is enlarged (65 mm). (**C** and **D**) Photomicrographs of the left ventricular myocardium. (**C**) Several abnormal coronary arteries with markedly thickened walls and a narrowed lumen, dispersed in an area of replacement fibrosis. Hematoxylin–eosin stain; magnification ×45. (**D**) Bundles of hypertrophied cardiac muscle cells arranged in a chaotic pattern, with adjacent cells oriented at oblique and perpendicular angles to each other. Hematoxylin–eosin stain; magnification ×30. From Hecht *et al.* Coexistence of sudden cardiac death and end-stage heart failure in familial hypertrophic cardiomyopathy. *J Am Coll Cardiol* 1993; **22**: 489–97, reproduced with permission of the American College of Cardiology.

nondilated LV with normal or increased ejection fraction to a thinned and dilated LV with impaired contractility, can develop abruptly or evolve over several years, and may present at any age. Furthermore, end-stage patients and patients with HCM-related sudden cardiac death may coexist in the same family (and therefore share the same genetic substrate); individual patients have even experienced aborted sudden death and subsequently died in the end-stage phase of their disease, all within their lifetime.[60]

Therapeutic options are considerably limited for drug-refractory, severely symptomatic patients with the nonobstructive end-stage form of HCM.[2,3] Only this subset of patients, among the broad HCM clinical spectrum, may become candidates for heart transplantation.[2,3] Other adults, most commonly women,[91] may experience more gradual and subtle LV remodeling, with regression in wall thickness associated with aging (but not linked to systolic dysfunction or clinical deterioration).[2,37,91] Therefore, LV hypertrophy is not a static manifestation of HCM, can appear at virtually any age, and can also increase or decrease dynamically throughout life.[89]

Left ventricular outflow obstruction

LV outflow tract gradients are produced by systolic anterior motion of the mitral valve, and apposition with the ventricular septum (due predominantly to a drag effect[92] or possibly also the Venturi phenomenon)[2,3] has been the most recognizable feature of HCM from its initial clinical description.[93-95] Although previously subject to periodic controversy, there is now widespread recognition that the subaortic gradient and the associated elevation in intracavity LV pressure reflect true mechanical impedance to outflow and are of pathophysiologic and prognostic importance to patients with HCM.[7] Indeed, outflow obstruction under basal (resting) conditions (gradient $\geq$30 mm Hg) is a strong, independent predictor of HCM-related progression to severe limiting symptoms of New York Heart Association (NYHA) classes III and IV, and of death due specifically to heart failure and stroke (relative risk >4.0).[7] However, the likelihood of severe symptoms and death due to outflow tract obstruction was greater when the magnitude of the gradient was increased above the threshold of 30 mm Hg.[7] Over time, disease consequences due to chronic outflow gradients (and concomitant mitral regurgitation) are likely to be related to the resulting increase in LV wall stress, myocardial ischemia, and eventually cell death and replacement fibrosis.[96,97] Indeed, longer durations of obstruction appear to confer a more unfavorable clinical course, leading frequently to heart failure-related disease progression and death.[7]

It is important to underscore that a variety of interventions have been traditionally employed to elicit latent (inducible) gradients in echocardiography, cardiac catheterization, and exercise laboratories (e.g. amyl nitrite inhalation, Valsalva maneuver, post-premature ventricular contraction response, isoproterenol or dobutamine infusion, standing posture, and physiologic exercise). However, rigorous standardization for these maneuvers has been lacking, and many have come to be regarded as nonphysiologic. To define latent gradients

during and/or immediately after exercise for the purpose of major management decisions, treadmill or bicycle exercise testing in association with
Doppler echocardiography is probably the most physiologic, meaningful,
and preferred provocative maneuver, given that HCM-related symptoms are
typically elicited with exertion. Intravenous administration of dobutamine is
undesirable, because subaortic gradients provoked with this agent are widely
regarded as nonphysiologic.[3] Therefore, the presence of LV outflow obstruction justifies intervention with septal myectomy (or alcohol septal ablation in
selected patients) to reduce or abolish clinically relevant subaortic gradients
(≥50 mm Hg at rest or with physiologic exercise)[98] in severely symptomatic
patients who are refractory to maximum medical management.[3] Outflow gradients associated with atrial fibrillation are particularly deleterious in HCM
patients.[99]

HCM phenotype and morphologic features

Left ventricular hypertrophy

Structural heterogeneity in HCM is considerable, no single pattern of LV hypertrophy being regarded as typical (Figs 1.4–1.11).[2,3,15] While many patients
show diffusely distributed LV hypertrophy, almost one-third have mild wall
thickening localized to a single segment,[15] including the apical form,[17,18,65,88]
which appears to be most common in Japanese patients (Fig. 1.7).[65,100] Apical
HCM refers to a nonobstructive form of hypertrophy confined to the most
distal portion of LV, and may (or may not) be associated with giant negative
T-waves on ECG. Also, very rarely, patients with HCM may develop apical
aneurysms of various sizes, associated with mid-ventricular LV hypertrophy
and repetitive monomorphic ventricular tachycardia, for which the prognosis
appears to be particularly unfavorable.[6,101]

   LV hypertrophy in HCM is characteristically asymmetric (with the anterior septum usually the predominant area of thickening) (Figs 1.4–1.9, 1.11),
although an occasional patient may show a symmetric (concentric) pattern in
which wall thicknesses are virtually identical in all LV segments (Fig. 1.7).[15]
The distribution of LV wall thickening shows no direct link to clinical outcome, although distal located hypertrophy is always associated with the absence of LV outflow obstruction. Other relatively common echocardiographic
hallmarks of HCM which *per se* are not prerequisites for diagnosis, include a
hyperdynamic LV and mild systolic anterior motion of the mitral valve.

   Young children may present with LV hypertrophy clinically resembling
HCM as part of other disease states (e.g. Noonan's syndrome, mitochondrial
myopathies, metabolic disorders) but unrelated to HCM-causing sarcomere
protein mutations. The fact that disproportionate thickening of the ventricular
septum is also a characteristic anatomic feature of the normal embryonic and
fetal human heart (Fig. 1.12) suggests the possibility that, in some instances,

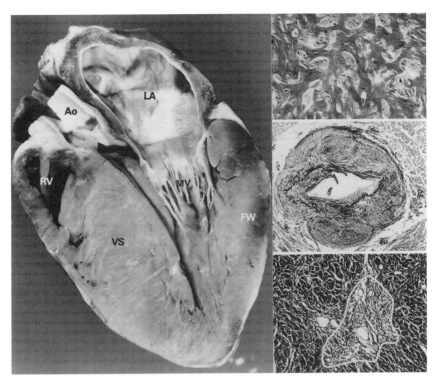

Fig. 1.11 Morphologic features of the myocardial substrate for sudden death in hypertrophic car-diomyopathy. (**Left**) Gross heart specimen from a 13-year-old male competitive athlete showing disproportionate thickening of the ventricular septum (VS) with respect to the left ventricular free wall (LV). RV = right ventricular wall. (**Top right**) Marked disarray of cardiac muscle cells in the disproportionately thickened ventricular septum with adjacent hypertrophied cells arranged in a chaotic pattern at oblique and perpendicular angles, forming the typical disorganized archi-tecture of hypertrophic cardiomyopathy. (**Middle right**) Abnormal intramural coronary artery with markedly thickened walls and narrowed lumen. (**Lower right**) Replacement fibrosis, the consequence of bursts of myocardial ischemia, cell death, and small vessel disease. Hema-toxylin–eosin stains. Adapted from Maron BJ. Hypertrophic cardiomyopathy. *Curr Probl Cardiol* 1993; **18**: 637–704, reproduced with permission of Mosby, Inc.

asymmetric LV hypertrophy in young infants with HCM represents postnatal persistence of a normal anatomic feature of the developing heart.[102]

Histopathologic components

The cardiomyopathic substrate in HCM is defined anatomically by several histologic features.[22,62,63,102–106] Based largely on autopsy observations, LV myo-cardial architecture is disorganized and comprises hypertrophied cardiac muscle cells (myocytes) with bizarre shapes and multiple intercellular con-nections, often arranged in chaotic alignment at oblique and perpendicular angles (Fig. 1.10).[62,63,106] Cellular disarray may be widely distributed, occupying substantial portions of the LV wall (on average, 33% of the septal myocardium

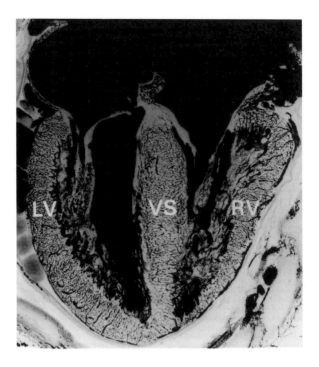

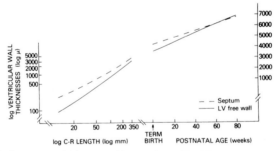

Fig. 1.12 Ventricular anatomy in the normal human fetus. (Top) Frontally sectioned heart of a fetus at 10 weeks of gestation, showing a ventricular septum (VS) that is disproportionately thicker than the left ventricular free wall (LV). Ventricular cavities are filled with India ink that was injected into the umbilical vein at the time of preparation for the specimen. RV = right ventricle. (Bottom) Changes in ventricular septum, left ventricular free wall, and right ventricular wall thickness before and after birth. From Maron *et al.* Disproportionate ventricular septal thickening in the developing normal human heart. *Circulation* 1978; **57**: 520–6, reproduced with permission of the American Heart Association.

and 25% of the free wall),[62,107] and is more extensive in young patients who die of their disease.[62] Disarray is not, however, limited to thickened regions of the left ventricle, and abnormal cellular arrangement may be present in both hypertrophied and nonhypertrophied segments.[106]

Abnormal small intramural coronary arteries, characterized by thickened walls with increased intimal and medial collagen and narrowed lumen, may be regarded as a form of small vessel disease (Fig. 1.11).[108,109] Such architectural alterations of the microvasculature (as well as a mismatch between myocardial mass and coronary circulation) are likely responsible for impaired coronary vasodilator reserve[109,110] and bursts of myocardial ischemia[104,111] leading to myocyte death and repair in the form of patchy or even transmural replacement scarring (Fig. 1.11);[104,105,107] these are identifiable at autopsy or as thallium-201 myocardial perfusion defects.[111] The presence of myocardial scarring supports the clinical evidence that ischemia occurs in HCM and may serve as the substrate for premature heart failure-related death. It is also evident that the cardiomyopathic process in HCM is not confined to areas of gross wall thickening, because nonhypertrophied regions also contribute to ischemia or impaired diastolic function.[2,3]

Disorganized cellular architecture,[62,63,106] myocardial scarring,[104,105,107,108] and the expanded interstitial (matrix) collagen connective tissue compartment[22] probably also serve as an arrhythmogenic substrate predisposing to life-threatening electrical instability by impairing the transmission of normal electrophysiologic impulses, and thereby predisposing to disordered patterns of electrical depolarization and repolarization (Fig. 1.11). This substrate is likely to be the source of primary re-entrant arrhythmias with ventricular tachycardia/fibrillation (VT/VF), the predominant mechanism of sudden death,[23] either primarily or in association with triggers that are intrinsic to the disease process, such as myocardial ischemia, systemic hypotension, supraventricular tachyarrhythmias, or environmental variables (e.g. intense physical exertion). It is also likely that this pathologic architecture of the left ventricle in HCM is responsible for (or contributes substantially to) increased ventricular chamber stiffness and impaired relaxation.[112–115]

Penetrance and variability of phenotypic expression are undoubtedly influenced by factors other than disease-causing mutant genes, such as modifier genes (e.g. the *ACE* genotype), coexistent hypertension, lifestyle, or other environmental factors.[2,3] Indeed, several phenotypic manifestations of HCM do not primarily involve sarcomeric proteins, including increased interstitial collagen,[22] abnormal intramural coronary arteries,[107,108] and mitral valve malformations, such as elongated leaflets[14,61] and papillary muscle insertion directly into mitral valve.[13]

Indeed, a constellation of structural malformations of the mitral valve and apparatus demonstrates that the pathologic process in HCM is not confined to cardiac muscle, thereby expanding the morphologic definition of this disease.[13,14,116,117] In morphometric analysis of mitral valves removed at operation or at necropsy from patients with HCM, about two-thirds showed alterations in size, shape and morphology (Fig. 1.13).[14] These abnormalities included increased overall mitral valve area, ranging up to more than twice the normal size, and due primarily to elongation of the leaflets (but without evidence of myxomatous mitral valve degeneration) (Fig. 1.13). The enlarged and elon-

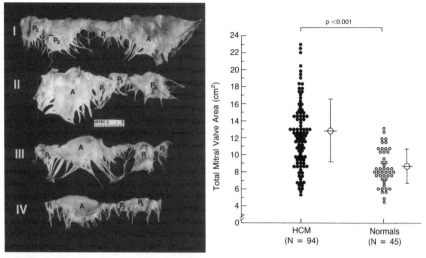

Fig. 1.13 Enlarged and elongated mitral valve in hypertrophic cardiomyopathy. (Left) Photographs of mitral valves from three patients with obstructive hypertrophic cardiomyopathy aged 31, 29 and 60 years (**I**, **II**, and **III**) and from a normal control patient without cardiovascular disease (**IV**), showing variation in valvular size and structure. Valves have been opened with the circumference displayed in a horizontal orientation, exposing the atrial surface. (**I**) Large valve (area = 22 cm^2) in which both the anterior (A) and posterior (P) leaflets are greatly elongated and increased in area. (**II**) Large valve in which increased valve size (area = 18 cm^2) is due primarily to elongation and enlargement of the anterior leaflet. (**III**) Segmental elongation and increased area confined to a lateral scallop of posterior mitral leaflet, which has virtually the same length as the normal-sized anterior leaflet. (**IV**) Valve is normal in area (11 cm^2), length and thickness. (Right) Scatterplot of total mitral valve leaflet area in patients with hypertrophic cardiomyopathy and normal controls. From Klues *et al.* Diversity of structural mitral valve alterations in hypertrophic cardiomyopathy. *Circulation* 1992; **85**: 1651–60, reproduced with permission of the American Heart Association.

gated mitral valves, found primarily in younger patients with HCM (i.e. those under age 50), show considerable variability with regard to structure, including elongation of both anterior and posterior leaflets or asymmetric and segmental enlargement of either the anterior leaflet or the mid-scallop of the posterior leaflet. Compared with more normal-sized mitral valves in HCM, the enlarged and elongated valves are situated more posteriorly in a larger LV outflow tract and also have greater flexibility and systolic excursion, usually with a distinctive sharp-angled bend of the anterior leaflet making localized systolic contact with ventricular septum. This striking pattern of valvular motion is possible because the central and distal portions of the leaflet are relatively free of fibrous thickening.

In addition, some other patients with a virtually normal-sized mitral valve show anomalous insertion of the papillary muscle directly into the anterior mitral leaflet (without interposition of chordae tendineae) (Fig. 1.14), the predominant cause of muscular mid-cavitary outflow obstruction.[13] This is a congenital abnormality resulting from an arrest during embryonic development

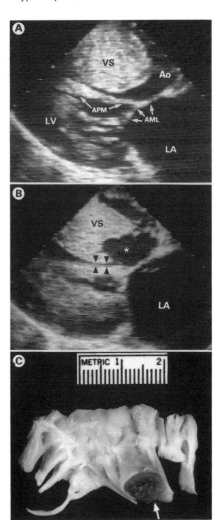

Fig. 1.14 Anomalous papillary muscle (APM) insertion directly into the anterior mitral leaflet in a patient with hypertrophic cardiomyopathy, producing muscular mid-cavity left ventricular outflow obstruction. (**A**) Before myotomy–myectomy. AML in direct continuity with the anterolateral papillary muscle (APM), which is displaced anteriorly within the left ventricular cavity, producing a long area of midcavity contact with the ventricular septum (VS) and outflow obstruction (arrowheads); tips of mitral leaflets coapt in the usual position and typical systolic anterior motion is absent (small arrows). (**B**) After myotomy–myectomy. Extensive muscular resection (*) extends from the base of the septum beyond the distal margins of the anterior mitral leaflet; nevertheless, a large area of direct contact between the papillary muscle and the ventricular septum remains (arrowheads), which is responsible for persistent obstruction of left ventricular outflow. (C) Mitral valve specimen excised at operation. A massively hypertrophied APM (arrows) inserts directly into the body of anterior leaflet. Ao = aorta; LA = left atrium; LV = left ventricle. From Klues *et al.* Anomalous insertion of papillary muscle directly into anterior mitral leaflet in hypertrophic cardiomyopathy: Significance in producing left ventricular outflow obstruction. *Circulation* 1991; **84**: 1188–97, reproduced with permission of the American Heart Association.

in which the chordae tendineae fail to develop, or do so in only a rudimentary fashion, and it is important to recognize it prior to major interventions, such as septal myectomy.

Clinical course

Overall HCM population

HCM is unique among cardiovascular diseases by virtue of its potential for clinical presentation during any phase of life from infancy to old age (>90 years).[2–6,20,25,30,31,36,38,42,64,91,118] While adverse clinical consequences have been recognized for many years (sudden cardiac death in particular, but also progressive heart failure disability), a more balanced perspective regarding prognosis has evolved recently. Historically, misperceptions regarding the clinical significance of HCM have prevailed because of the obstacles of relatively low prevalence,[67] extreme heterogeneity[2,3] and skewed patterns of patient referral creating important patient selection biases.[119] Indeed, much of the data assembled over 40 years was disproportionately generated by a few tertiary centers, and relates largely to patients preferentially referred because of high-risk status or severe symptoms requiring specialized care (such as surgery).[2,3,119] For example, while considerable data have been reported over more than four decades from highly selected patient cohorts, such as the National Institutes of Health, the latter program has recently been terminated permanently. Hence, the older HCM literature was dominated by the most adverse consequences of the disease, while clinically stable, asymptomatic and elderly patients were largely under-represented. Nevertheless, it is now recognized that HCM occurs in both genders and many races, including under-served minorities.[91,120,121] However, while HCM is underdiagnosed in women and minorities, there is no evidence that the disease is expressed differently (either morphologically or clinically) in such subgroups.

The risks of HCM would appear to have been overestimated by dependence on frequently cited, ominous mortality rates of 3–6% per year.[119] These figures, based on skewed tertiary center experience, have contributed importantly to the misguided perception that HCM is a generally unfavorable disorder. Recent reports over the last 8 years from less selected regional or community-based HCM patient cohorts cite mortality rates that are in a much lower range, of about 1% (or less),[25,26,29,30,37] and are not dissimilar to that of the general adult US population (Fig. 1.15).[25]

Such data provide a more balanced view, in which HCM may be associated with important symptoms and premature death, but more frequently with

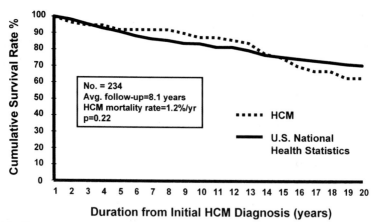

Fig. 1.15 Total mortality (death from any cause) for adult patients with hypertrophic cardiomyopathy in a community-based cohort does not differ with respect to the expected survival in the US general population after adjustment for age, sex, and race. The annual mortality is only about 1%. From Maron *et al*. Clinical course of hypertrophic cardiomyopathy in a regional United States cohort. *JAMA* 1999; **281**; 650–5, reproduced with permission of the American Medical Association.

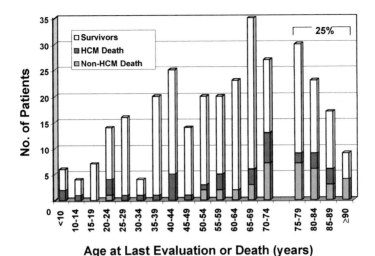

Age at Last Evaluation or Death (years)

Fig. 1.16 Distribution of ages (at last evaluation or death) in a community-based cohort of patients with hypertrophic cardiomyopathy, showing that 25% of the patients survived to an estimated life expectancy of 75 years. From Maron *et al.* Clinical course of hypertrophic cardiomyopathy with survival to advanced age. *J Am Coll Cardiol* 2003; **42**: 882–8, reproduced with permission of the American College of Cardiology.

no or relatively mild disability, and is compatible with normal life expectancy.[25,42]

Of note, HCM is compatible with survival to advanced age, some patients being identified for the first time in their 70s or 80s, or even over 90 years of age.[24,42,64] Elderly HCM patients achieving normal longevity (≥75 years) may constitute as much as 25% of an unselected HCM cohort, only a minority showing overt and severe manifestations of heart failure (Fig. 1.16).[25,42] Indeed, patients with HCM diagnosed ≥50 years of age experience subsequent survival that does not differ from that of the general population (Fig. 1.17).[42] Outflow obstruction is not uncommonly evident in patients of advanced age, suggesting that a subaortic gradient may either be well tolerated for long periods of time without major adverse consequences, or develop later in life. HCM in patients of advanced age can be a genetic disorder caused by dominant sarcomere protein mutations. Most such cases appear to be caused by mutations in cardiac myosin-binding protein C and troponin-I.[50]

Profiles of prognosis

The clinical course and disease consequences for individual HCM patients are most appropriately viewed in terms of specific subgroups that may incur different disease complications rather than by regarding all patients in a similar fashion, by virtue of their being in the overall HCM disease spectrum (Fig. 1.18). Therefore, patients may progress along certain relatively discrete and adverse pathways (Fig. 1.18): (1) high risk for sudden death (Figs 1.19 and 1.20);[2,3,23,27,51–60,122–126] (2) symptoms of heart failure with exertional dyspnea and

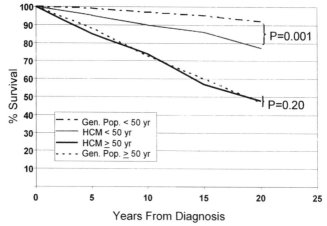

Fig. 1.17 Actuarial curves showing survival probabilities with hypertrophic cardiomyopathy with respect to all-cause mortality, from the time of initial diagnosis. Shown separately for patients with hypertrophic cardiomyopathy diagnosis <50 and ≥50 years and compared with expected survival probabilities of an age- and gender-matched cohort from the US general population (Gen. Pop.). From Maron *et al*. Clinical course of hypertrophic cardiomyopathy in a regional United States cohort. *JAMA* 1999; **281**: 650–5, reproduced with permission of the American Medical Association.

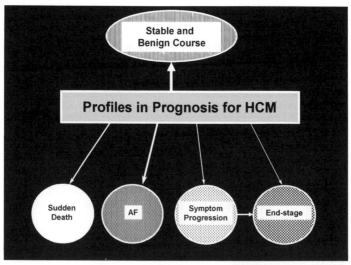

Fig. 1.18 The principal pathways of prognosis, including disease progression, in the broad clinical spectrum of hypertrophic cardiomyopathy. Widths of the respective arrows approximate the frequency with which the pathway occurs in hypertrophic cardiomyopathy. AF = atrial fibrillation. From Maron *et al*. American College of Cardiology/European Society of Cardiology Clinical Expert Consensus Document on Hypertrophic Cardiomyopathy. A Report of the American College of Cardiology Task Force on Clinical Expert Consensus Documents and the European Society of Cardiology Committee for Practice Guidelines and Policy Conferences. *J Am Coll Cardiol* 2003; **42**: 1687–713, reproduced with permission of the American College of Cardiology.

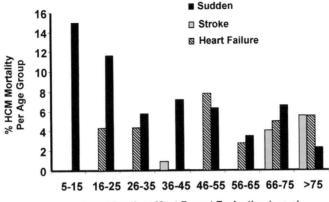

Fig. 1.19 Distribution of ages at the time of hypertrophic cardiomyopathy-related death, displayed as the percentage of hypertrophic cardiomyopathy mortality by age group. For each age group, percentage hypertrophic cardiomyopathy mortality was calculated by dividing the total number of hypertrophic cardiomyopathy deaths by the total number of patients at the end of follow-up. Note that sudden death is most common in adolescents and young adults. From Maron *et al*. Epidemiology of hypertrophic cardiomyopathy-related death: Revisited in a large non-referral-based patient population. *Circulation* 2000; **102**: 858–64, reproduced with permission of the American Heart Association.

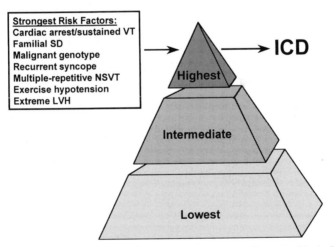

Fig. 1.20 Assessment of risk for sudden cardiac death in the overall hypertrophic cardiomyopathy population. Treatment for prevention of sudden death is limited to that small subset perceived to be at highest risk compared with all other patients with hypertrophic cardiomyopathy on the basis of risk factor analysis. Asymptomatic individuals with mild left ventricular hypertrophy and without ventricular tachycardia on ambulatory Holter ECG, hypotensive blood pressure response to exercise, or a family history of premature hypertrophic cardiomyopathy-related death. ICD = implantable cardioverter–defibrillator; LVH = left ventricular hypertrophy; NSVT = nonsustained ventricular tachycardia; SD = sudden death; VT = ventricular tachycardia. From Maron. Hypertrophic cardiomyopathy. *Lancet* 1997; **350**: 127–33, reproduced with permission of Lancet Ltd.

functional disability often associated with chest pain (and usually in the presence of preserved LV systolic function);[2,3,7,112–115] (3) evolution to the end-stage phase with LV remodeling and systolic dysfunction;[2,66,89] and (4) consequences of atrial fibrillation (AF), including embolic stroke.[31,99,127]

Sudden death

Sudden and unexpected death is the most common mode of demise and the most devastating and unpredictable complication of HCM.[2,3,6,10,23,27,32,35,51–60,103,122–126,128–131] Therefore, within the broad HCM disease spectrum (for which the overall annual mortality rate is about 1%) there are high-risk subsets at much higher risk (perhaps 5% per year or greater),[23] but which constitute only a minority of all HCM patients. Historically, an important but complex objective has been the identification of such individuals among the vast HCM spectrum. For example, sudden death can be the initial manifestation of HCM, and patients in whom sudden death occurs usually have no or only mild prior symptoms.[52–54] While these catastrophes occur most commonly in children and young adults ≤30 years old, risk nevertheless extends across a wide age range through mid-life and beyond.[27] Therefore, achieving a particular age does not itself confer immunity to sudden catastrophe (Fig. 1.19).

Sudden death occurs most commonly during mild exertion or sedentary activities, but is not infrequently related to vigorous physical exertion.[51,54,56–58,120] Indeed, HCM is the most common cause of cardiovascular sudden death in young people, including trained competitive athletes. Furthermore, HCM represents a common cause of sudden death in previously undiagnosed young African–American male athletes, in sharp contrast with the seven-fold less frequent clinical identification of HCM in a hospital-based population.[120] This discrepancy suggests that many HCM cases go unrecognized in the African–American community, underscoring the need for enhanced clinical recognition of HCM in order to create the opportunity for preventive measures to be employed in high-risk patients.

Most HCM patients (55%) do not demonstrate any of the acknowledged risk factors for this disease, and it is exceedingly uncommon for such patients to die suddenly; fewer than 5% of HCM-related sudden deaths occur in the absence of any risk factors.[55] On the other hand, the subset of patients at sufficiently high risk to deserve consideration for an implantable defibrillator may constitute about 10–20% of the overall HCM cohort.[47]

The highest risk for sudden death in HCM has been associated with any of the following noninvasive clinical markers (Fig. 1.20):[2,3] (1) prior cardiac arrest or spontaneous sustained VT; (2) a family history of premature HCM-related death, particularly if sudden, in close relatives, or multiple; (3) syncope (and some cases of near-syncope), particularly when exertional or recurrent, or in young patients and when documented to be arrhythmia-based or clearly unrelated to neurocardiogenic mechanisms; (4) multiple and repetitive, or prolonged bursts of nonsustained VT on serial ambulatory (Holter) ECG; (5) hypotensive blood pressure response to exercise, particularly in patients under

50 years old; and (6) extreme LV hypertrophy with maximum wall thickness ≥30 mm, particularly in adolescents and young adults (such individuals will constitute about 10% of a HCM cohort). The latter risk factor emanates from a continuous, direct relationship between maximum LV wall thickness and sudden death which supports the magnitude of LV hypertrophy as a determinant of prognosis in HCM.[52] Reported exceptions to this association are a few highly selected HCM families with multiple sudden deaths and mild LV hypertrophy due to troponin T mutations.[49,103]

Description of the total HCM risk profile is probably incomplete at present and no single parameter or test is capable of stratifying risk in all patients with this disease. LV outflow gradients (≥30 mm Hg at rest) can only be regarded as a minor risk factor for sudden death in HCM.[7] The impact of the gradient on the risk of sudden death is not sufficiently strong (positive predictive value of only 7%) for LV outflow obstruction to merit a role as the sole (or predominant) deciding clinical parameter and primary basis for a decision to intervene prophylactically with an implantable defibrillator.[7,47] One report suggests that short, tunneled (bridged) segments of left anterior descending coronary artery independently convey an increased risk for cardiac arrest in children with HCM (probably mediated by myocardial ischemia).[32]

Based on genotype–phenotype correlations, it has been proposed that the genetic defects responsible for HCM could represent the primary determinant and stratifying marker for sudden death risk, with specific mutations conferring a favorable or adverse prognosis.[59] For example, some β-myosin heavy-chain mutations (e.g. Arg403Gln, Arg719Gln) and some troponin-T mutations may be associated with higher frequency of premature death compared with certain other mutations, such as those of myosin-binding protein C (InsG791) or α-tropomyosin (Asp175Asn).[3,7,9,11–13,23,24,26,27] However, caution is warranted before strong conclusions are drawn regarding prognosis based solely on the available epidemiologic genetic data, which are still relatively limited and skewed by virtue of patient selection bias toward high-risk families.[2,3,9,45,46] Access to the molecular biology of HCM does not yet represent a clinically relevant strategy that can routinely influence disease management. Prognosis attached to adult gene carriers without LV hypertrophy appears at present to be largely benign.[13,25,53,54] At present, there is no evidence to justify routinely excluding genotype positive–phenotype negative individuals of any age from most employment opportunities or life activities.[3]

The roles of invasive strategies, such as electrophysiologic testing with programmed ventricular stimulation, and the significance of induced arrhythmias in detecting the substrate for VF in individual HCM patients are unresolved.[2,3,37] Limitations include the infrequency with which monomorphic VF is provoked and the nonspecificity of rapid polymorphic VT and VF in HCM.

While the focus in HCM has understandably been on the high-risk patient, the absence of risk factors and certain clinical features can be used to develop a profile of HCM patients who are unlikely to experience sudden death as a result of life-threatening rhythm disturbances, as well as other adverse events.[37]

The adult patients who are most likely at lowest risk are those with no or only very mild heart failure symptoms in the absence of each of the following: (1) a family history of premature death due to HCM; (2) syncope judged unlikely to be neurocardiogenic in origin; (3) nonsustained VT during ambulatory Holter ECG; (4) LV outflow gradient ≥30 mm Hg; (5) substantial LV hypertrophy (wall thickness ≥20 mm); (6) left atrial enlargement (>45 mm); and (7) a hypotensive blood pressure response to exercise. Such patients with a favorable prognosis constitute an important proportion of the overall HCM population, and generally deserve a measure of reassurance regarding their disease. Most HCM patients should undergo a risk stratification assessment (probably with the exception of patients aged more than 60 years) which requires, in addition to careful history and physical examination, noninvasive testing with two-dimensional echocardiography, 24- or 48-hour ambulatory (Holter) ECG, and treadmill (or bicycle) exercise testing. Such evaluation and follow-up should be carried out by (or involve) qualified specialists in cardiovascular medicine.

Intense physical exertion constitutes a sudden death trigger in certain susceptible individuals.[51,54,130] Therefore, disqualification of athletes with unequivocal evidence of HCM from most competitive sports to reduce the level of risk is prudently recommended by a national consensus panel.[132] Strategies for primary and secondary prevention of sudden death with the implantable defibrillator are discussed in Chapter 23.

Atrial fibrillation

AF is the most common sustained arrhythmia in HCM, accounting for unexpected hospital admissions and unscheduled work loss, and it usually justifies aggressive therapeutic strategies[2,3,8,25,31,34,37,99,127] (Fig. 1.18). Paroxysmal episodes or chronic AF ultimately occur in 20–25% of HCM patients and are strongly associated with left atrial enlargement and increasing age.[99] AF may be reasonably well tolerated in about one-third of patients and is not an independent determinant of sudden death.[99] On the other hand, AF is not uncommonly associated with embolic stroke (incidence, 1% per year; prevalence, 6%), leading to death and disability most frequently in the elderly,[31,99] as well as to progressive heart failure, particularly when arrhythmia onset is before 50 years of age and basal outflow obstruction is present.[31]

Paroxysmal AF may occasionally be responsible for acute clinical decompensation and require prompt electrical or pharmacologic cardioversion.[36,37,129] Although data specifically in HCM are limited, amiodarone is regarded as an effective drug for reducing AF recurrences (based on inferences from patients with coronary artery disease). Due to the potential for clot formation and embolization, anticoagulant therapy (with warfarin) is routinely used in patients with either recurrent or chronic AF. Because even one or two paroxysms of AF have been associated with the risk for systemic thromboembolism in HCM, the threshold for initiation of anticoagulant therapy should be low.[31]

Heart failure

Symptoms such as exertional dyspnea, orthopnea, paroxysmal nocturnal dyspnea, and fatigue commonly and characteristically occur in the presence of normal (or supranormal) LV contractility, independent of whether outflow obstruction is present (Fig. 1.18).[2,3,5–8,36,37,109,110,112–115] Such symptoms of HCM-related heart failure, representing an important prognostic pathway in HCM, are usually deferred until adulthood, but may occur at virtually any age and characteristically show substantial day-to-day variability. Marked symptom progression is relatively infrequent, and exertional disability may evolve at varying rates; deterioration is often gradual and punctuated by long periods of stability.

Heart failure symptoms that produce exertional limitation in HCM appear to be largely the consequence of diastolic dysfunction. This results from impaired LV relaxation and increased chamber stiffness and from compromised left atrial systolic performance, leading to elevated left atrial and LV end-diastolic pressures (with reduced stroke volume and cardiac output), and consequently pulmonary congestion with diminished exercise performance[2,3,112–115] (evident by reduced peak oxygen consumption).[96] However, heart failure related to diastolic dysfunction is undoubtedly intertwined with other pathophysiologic mechanisms when present, such as myocardial ischemia, outflow obstruction, and AF.

Chest pain (in the absence of atherosclerotic coronary artery disease) may be atypical or typical of angina pectoris, and suggestive of myocardial ischemia, and is commonly associated with exertional dyspnea.[2,3,10,25,36,37] Myocardial perfusion defects, net lactate release during atrial pacing and blunted coronary flow reserve are evidence of ischemia that is due to the abnormal microvasculature, in which intramural coronary arteries have thickened walls and narrowed lumen.[104,105,107–111,124] Defining the role of myocardial ischemia in risk stratification and disease progression has been difficult, largely because its clinical assessment has been limited by the inability to noninvasively measure these abnormalities with precision. However, long-term follow-up studies after positron emission tomography imaging have provided prognostic evidence that in HCM the degree of coronary microvascular dysfunction (blunted increase in myocardial blood flow in response to dipyridamole infusion) is a strong independent predictor of clinical deterioration with progressive heart failure, and of cardiovascular mortality.[124] Furthermore, severe microvascular dysfunction is often present in patients with mild or no symptoms and precedes clinical deterioration by many years.[124]

Drug treatment strategies (Fig. 1.21) for symptoms in HCM are described in detail in Chapter 14. However, when heart failure symptoms cannot be controlled with maximum medical management, major therapeutic interventions

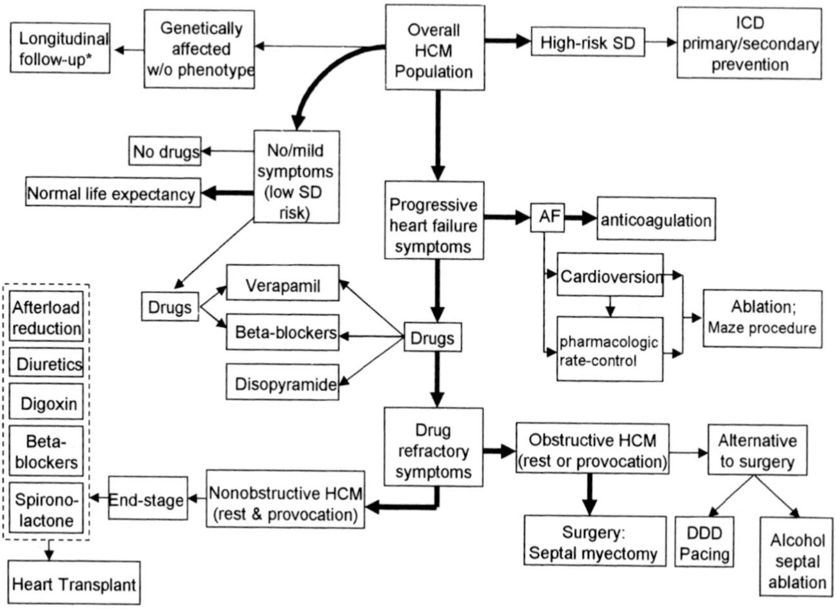

Fig. 1.21 Clinical presentations and treatment strategies for patient subgroups within hypertrophic cardiomyopathy disease. *No specific treatment or intervention indicated, except under exceptional circumstances. AF = atrial fibrillation; ICD = implantable cardioverter–defibrillator; SD = sudden death. From Maron *et al.* American College of Cardiology/European Society of Cardiology Clinical Expert Consensus Document on Hypertrophic Cardiomyopathy. A Report of the American College of Cardiology Task Force on Clinical Expert Consensus Documents and the European Society of Cardiology Committee for Practice Guidelines and Policy Conferences. *J Am Coll Cardiol* 2003; **42** (in press), reproduced with permission of the American College of Cardiology.

are indicated. In such severely symptomatic patients (NYHA classes III/IV) with outflow obstruction the gold standard treatment is the septal myectomy operation, with alcohol septal ablation (and dual-chamber pacing) alternatives for selected patients (Fig. 1.21); these treatment modalities are described in detail in Chapters 15–20.

References

1 Teare D. Asymmetrical hypertrophy of the heart in young adults. *Br Heart J* 1958; **20**: 1–18.

2 Maron BJ. Hypertrophic cardiomyopathy: A systematic review. *JAMA* 2002; **287**: 1308–20.

3 Maron BJ, McKenna WJ, Danielson GK *et al.* American College of Cardiology/European Society of Cardiology Clinical Expert Consensus Document on Hypertrophic Cardiomyopathy. A Report of the American College of Cardiology Task Force on Clinical

Expert Consensus Documents and the European Society of Cardiology Committee for Practice Guidelines and Policy Conferences. *J Am Coll Cardiol* 2003; **42**: 1587–713.

4 Braunwald E, Lambrew CT, Rockoff D *et al*. Idiopathic hypertrophic subaortic stenosis: I. A description of the disease based upon an analysis of 64 patients. *Circulation* 1964; **30** (Suppl. IV): 3–217.

5 Frank S, Braunwald E. Idiopathic hypertrophic subaortic stenosis: Clinical analysis of 126 patients with emphasis on the natural history. *Circulation* 1968; **37**: 759–88.

6 Wigle ED, Sasson Z, Henderson MA *et al*. Hypertrophic cardiomyopathy: The importance of the site and extent of hypertrophy. A review. Prog Cardiovasc Dis 1985; **28**: 1–83.

7 Maron MS, Olivotto I, Betocchi S *et al*. Effect of left ventricular outflow tract obstruction on clinical outcome in hypertrophic cardiomyopathy. *N Engl J Med* 2003; **348**: 295–303.

8 Wigle ED, Rakowski H, Kimball BP *et al*. Hypertrophic cardiomyopathy: Clinical spectrum and treatment. *Circulation* 1995; **92**: 1680–1692.

9 Maron BJ, Moller JH, Seidman CE *et al*. Impact of laboratory molecular diagnosis on contemporary diagnostic criteria for genetically transmitted cardiovascular diseases: Hypertrophic cardiomyopathy, long-QT syndrome, and Marfan syndrome. *Circulation* 1998; **98**: 1460–71.

10 Louie EK, Edwards LC. Hypertrophic cardiomyopathy. *Prog Cardiovasc Dis* 1994; **36**: 275–308.

11 Niimura H, Bachinski LL, Sangwatanaroj S *et al*. Mutations in the gene for human cardiac myosin-binding protein C and late-onset familial hypertrophic cardiomyopathy. *N Engl J Med* 1998; **338**: 1248–57.

12 Maron BJ, Gottdiener JS, Epstein SE. Patterns and significance of distribution of left ventricular hypertrophy in hypertrophic cardiomyopathy: A wide-angle, two-dimensional echocardiographic study of 125 patients. *Am J Cardiol* 1981; **48**: 418–28.

13 Klues HG, Roberts WC, Maron BJ. Anomalous insertion of papillary muscle directly into anterior mitral leaflet in hypertrophic cardiomyopathy: Significance in producing left ventricular outflow obstruction. *Circulation* 1991; **84**: 1188–97.

14 Klues HG, Maron BJ, Dollar AL *et al*. Diversity of structural mitral valve alterations in hypertrophic cardiomyopathy. *Circulation* 1992; **85**: 1651–60.

15 Klues HG, Schiffers A, Maron BJ. Phenotypic spectrum and patterns of left ventricular hypertrophy in hypertrophic cardiomyopathy: Morphologic observations and significance as assessed by two-dimensional echocardiography in 600 patients. *J Am Coll Cardiol* 1995; **26**: 1699–708.

16 Cecchi F, Olivotto I, Gistri R, Lorenzoni R, Chiriatti G, Camici PG. Coronary microvascular dysfunction and prognosis in hypertrophic cardiomyopathy. *N Engl J Med* 2003; **349**: 1027–35.

17 Webb JG, Sasson Z, Rakowski H *et al*. Apical hypertrophic cardiomyopathy: Clinical follow-up and diagnostic correlates. *J Am Coll Cardiol* 1990; **15**: 83–90.

18 Louie EK, Maron BJ. Apical hypertrophic cardiomyopathy: Clinical and two-dimensional echocardiographic assessment. *Ann Intern Med* 1987; **106**: 663–70.

19 Louie EK, Maron BJ. Hypertrophic cardiomyopathy with extreme increase in left ventricular wall thickness: Functional and morphologic features and clinical significance. *J Am Coll Cardiol* 1986; **8**: 57–65.

20 Maron BJ, Mathenge R, Casey SA *et al*. Clinical profile of hypertrophic cardiomyopathy identified de novo in rural communities. *J Am Coll Cardiol* 1999; **33**: 1590–5.

21 Maron BJ, Spirito P, Wesley Y *et al*. Development and progression of left ventricular hypertrophy in children with hypertrophic cardiomyopathy. *N Engl J Med* 1986; **315**: 610–14.

22 Shirani J, Pick R, Roberts WC, Maron BJ. Morphology and significance of the left ventricular collagen network in young patients with hypertrophic cardiomyopathy and sudden cardiac death. *J Am Coll Cardiol* 2000; **35**: 36–44.

23 Maron BJ, Shen W-K, Link MS *et al*. Efficacy of implantable cardioverter-defibrillators for the prevention of sudden death in patients with hypertrophic cardiomyopathy. *N Engl J Med* 2000; **342**: 365–73.

24 Lewis JF, Maron BJ. Elderly patients with hypertrophic cardiomyopathy: A subset with distinctive left ventricular morphology and progressive clinical course late in life. *J Am Coll Cardiol* 1989; **13**: 36–45.

25 Maron BJ, Casey SA, Poliac LC *et al*. Clinical course of hypertrophic cardiomyopathy in a regional United States cohort. *JAMA* 1999; **281**: 650–5.

26 Kofflard MJ, ten Cate FJ, van der Lee C, van Domburg RT. Hypertrophic cardiomyopathy in a large community-based population: Clinical outcome and identification of risk factors for sudden cardiac death and clinical deterioration. *J Am Coll Cardiol* 2003; **41**: 987–93.

27 Maron BJ, Olivotto I, Spirito P *et al*. Epidemiology of hypertrophic cardiomyopathy-related death: Revisited in a large non-referral-based patient population. *Circulation* 2000; **102**: 858–64.

28 Shah PM, Adelman AG, Wigle ED *et al*. The natural (and unnatural) history of hypertrophic obstructive cardiomyopathy. *Circ Res* 1973; **34, 35** (Suppl. II): II-179–II-195.

29 Cecchi F, Olivotto I, Montereggi A *et al*. Hypertrophic cardiomyopathy in Tuscany: Clinical course and outcome in an unselected regional population. *J Am Coll Cardiol* 1995; **26**: 1529–36.

30 Spirito P, Chiarella F, Carratino L *et al*. Clinical course and prognosis of hypertrophic cardiomyopathy in an outpatient population. *N Engl J Med* 1989; **320**: 749–55.

31 Maron BJ, Olivotto I, Bellone P *et al*. Clinical profile of stroke in 900 patients with hypertrophic cardiomyopathy. *J Am Coll Cardiol* 2002; **39**: 301–7.

32 Yetman AT, McCrindle BW, MacDonald LC *et al*. Myocardial bridging in children with hypertrophic cardiomyopathy – a risk factor for sudden death. *N Engl J Med* 1998; **339**: 1201–9.

33 Petrone RK, Klues HG, Panza JA *et al*. Significance of the occurrence of mitral valve prolapse in patients with hypertrophic cardiomyopathy. *J Am Coll Cardiol* 1992; **20**: 55–61.

34 Maron BJ. Hypertrophic cardiomyopathy. *Lancet* 1997; **350**: 127–33.

35 Seidman JG, Seidman CE. The genetic basis for cardiomyopathy. From mutation identification to mechanistic paradigms. *Cell* 2001; **104**: 557–67.

36 Maron BJ, Bonow RO, Cannon RO *et al*. Hypertrophic cardiomyopathy: Interrelation of clinical manifestations, pathophysiology, and therapy. *N Engl J Med* 1987; **316**: 780–9 and 844–52.

37 Spirito P, Seidman CE, McKenna WJ, Maron BJ. Management of hypertrophic cardiomyopathy. *N Engl J Med* 1997; **30**: 775–85.

38 Takagi E, Yamakado T, Nakano T. Prognosis of completely asymptomatic adult patients with hypertrophic cardiomyopathy. *J Am Coll Cardiol* 1999; **33**: 206–11.

39 Zou Y, Song L, Wang Z *et al*. Prevalence of idiopathic hypertrophic cardiomyopathy in Chinese – a cross-sectional population-based echocardiographic analysis of 8080 adults. *Am J Med* 2004; **116**: 14–18.

40 Ho H-H, Lee KLF, Lau C-P, Tso H-F. Clinical characteristics and outcome in Chinese patients with hypertrophic cardiomyopathy. *Am J Med* 2004; **116**: 19–23.

41 Kyriakidis M, Triposkiadis F, Anastasakis A *et al.* Hypertrophic cardiomyopathy in Greece. Clinical course and outcome. *Chest* 1998; **114**: 1091–6.

42 Maron BJ, Casey SA, Hauser RG, Aeppli DM. Clinical course of hypertrophic cardiomyopathy with survival to advanced age. *J Am Coll Cardiol* 2003; **42**: 882–8.

43 Maron BJ, Niimura H, Casey SA *et al.* Development of left ventricular hypertrophy in adults with hypertrophic cardiomyopathy caused by cardiac myosin-binding protein C mutations. *J Am Coll Cardiol* 2001; **38**: 315–21.

44 Richard P, Charron P, Carrier L *et al.* Hypertrophic cardiomyopathy: distribution of disease genes, spectrum of mutations, and implications for a molecular diagnosis strategy. *Circulation* 2003; **107**: 2227–32.

45 Ackerman MJ, Van Driest SL, Ommen SR *et al.* Prevalence and age-dependence of malignant mutations in the beta-myosin heavy chain and troponin T genes in hypertrophic cardiomyopathy. A comprehensive outpatient perspective. *J Am Coll Cardiol* 2002; **39**: 2042–8.

46 Van Driest SL, Ackerman MJ, Ommen SR *et al.* Prevalence and severity of 'benign' mutations in the beta-myosin heavy chain, cardiac troponin T, and alpha-tropomyosin genes in hypertrophic cardiomyopathy. *Circulation* 2002; **106**: 3085–90.

47 Maron BJ, Estes NAM III, Maron MS, Almquist AK, Link MS, Udelson JE. Primary prevention of sudden death as a novel treatment strategy in hypertrophic cardiomyopathy. *Circulation* 2003; **107**: 2872–5.

48 Watkins H, McKenna WJ, Thierfelder L *et al.* The role of cardiac troponin T and -tropomyosin mutations in hypertrophic cardiomyopathy. *N Engl J Med* 1995; **332**: 1058–64.

49 Moolman JC, Corfield VA, Posen B *et al.* Sudden death due to troponin T mutations. *J Am Coll Cardiol* 1997; **29**: 549–55.

50 Niimura H, Patton KK, McKenna WJ *et al.* Sarcomere protein gene mutations in hypertrophic cardiomyopathy of the elderly. *Circulation* 2002; **105**: 446–51.

51 Maron BJ. Sudden death in young athletes. *N Engl J Med* 2003; **3349**: 1064–75.

52 Spirito P, Bellone P, Harris KM, Bernabo P, Bruzzi P, Maron BJ. Magnitude of left ventricular hypertrophy predicts the risk of sudden death in hypertrophic cardiomyopathy. *N Engl J Med* 2000; **342**: 1778–85.

53 Elliott PM, Gimeno JR, Mahon NG, Poloniecki JD, McKenna WJ. Relation between severity of left-ventricular hypertrophy and prognosis in patients with hypertrophic cardiomyopathy. *Lancet* 2001; **357**: 420–4.

54 Maron BJ, Shirani J, Poliac LC *et al.* Sudden death in young competitive athletes: Clinical, demographic and pathological profiles. *JAMA* 1996; **276**: 199–204.

55 Elliott PM, Poloniecki J, Dickie S *et al.* Sudden death in hypertrophic cardiomyopathy: Identification of high risk patients. *J Am Coll Cardiol* 2000; **36**: 2212–18.

56 Maron BJ, Roberts WC, Epstein SE. Sudden death in hypertrophic cardiomyopathy: A profile of 78 patients. *Circulation* 1982; **67**: 1388–94.

57 Maki S. Ikeda H, Muro A *et al.* Predictors of sudden cardiac death in hypertrophic cardiomyopathy. *Am J Cardiol* 1998; **82**: 774–8.

58 Cecchi F, Maron BJ, Epstein SE. Long-term outcome of patients with hypertrophic cardiomyopathy successfully resuscitated after cardiac arrest. *J Am Coll Cardiol* 1989; **13**: 1283–8.

59 Watkins H. Sudden death in hypertrophic cardiomyopathy [editorial]. *N Engl J Med* 2000; **372**: 422–3.

60 Hecht GM, Klues HG, Roberts WC, Maron BJ. Coexistence of sudden cardiac death and end-stage heart failure in familial hypertrophic cardiomyopathy. *J Am Coll Cardiol* 1993; **22**: 489–97.

61 Maron BJ, Harding AM, Spirito P *et al.* Systolic anterior motion of the posterior mitral leaflet: A previously unrecognized cause of dynamic subaortic obstruction in hypertrophic cardiomyopathy. *Circulation* 1983; **68**: 282–93.

62 Maron BJ, Roberts WC. Quantitative analysis of cardiac muscle cell disorganization in the ventricular septum of patients with hypertrophic cardiomyopathy. *Circulation* 1979; **59**: 689–706.

63 Varnava AM, Elliott PM, Mahon N, Davies MJ, McKenna WJ. Relation between myocyte disarray and outcome in hypertrophic cardiomyopathy. *Am J Cardiol* 2001; **88**: 275–9.

64 Lever HM, Kuram RF, Currie PH *et al.* Hypertrophic cardiomyopathy in the elderly: Distinctions from the young based on cardiac shape. *Circulation* 1989; **79**: 580–9.

65 Kitaoka H, Doi Y, Casey SA, Hitomi N, Furuno T, Maron BJ. Comparison of prevalence of apical hypertrophic cardiomyopathy in Japan and USA. *Am J Cardiol* 2003; **92**: 1183–6.

66 Spirito P, Maron BJ, Bonow RO, Epstein SE. Occurrence and significance of progressive left ventricular wall thinning and relative cavity dilatation in hypertrophic cardiomyopathy. *Am J Cardiol* 1987; **60**: 123–9.

67 Maron BJ, Gardin JM, Flack JM *et al.* Prevalence of hypertrophic cardiomyopathy in a general population of young adults: Echocardiographic analysis of 4111 subjects in the CARDIA study. *Circulation* 1995; **92**: 785–9.

68 Maron BJ, Spirito P, Roman MJ *et al.* Evidence that hypertrophic cardiomyopathy is a common genetic cardiovascular disease: Prevalence in a community-based population of middle-aged and elderly American Indians [abstract]. *Circulation* 2003; **108**: IV–664.

69 Hada Y, Sakamoto T, Amano K *et al.* Prevalence of hypertrophic cardiomyopathy in a population of adult Japanese workers as detected by echocardiographic screening. *Am J Cardiol* 1987; **59**: 183–4.

70 Maron BJ, Peterson EE, Maron MS *et al.* Prevalence of hypertrophic cardiomyopathy in an outpatient population referred for echocardiographic study. *Am J Cardiol* 1994; **73**: 577–80.

71 Maron BJ, Epstein SE. Hypertrophic cardiomyopathy: A discussion of nomenclature. *Am J Cardiol* 1979; **43**: 1242–4.

72 Maron BJ, Seidman JS, Seidman CE. Proposal for contemporary screening strategies in hypertrophic cardiomyopathy. *J Am Coll Cardiol.* (In press.)

73 Arad M, Benson DW, Perez-Atayde AR *et al.* Constitutively active AMP kinase mutations cause glycogen storage disease mimicking hypertrophic cardiomyopathy. *J Clin Invest* 2002; **109**: 357–62.

74 Crilley JG, Boehm EA, Blair E *et al.* Hypertrophic cardiomyopathy due to sarcomeric gene mutations is characterized by impaired energy metabolism irrespective of the degree of hypertrophy. *J Am Coll Cardiol* 2003; **41**: 1776–82.

75 Hagège AA, Dubourg O, Desnos M *et al.* Familial hypertrophic cardiomyopathy: Cardiac ultrasonic abnormalities in genetically affected subjects without echocardiographic evidence of left ventricular hypertrophy. *Eur Heart J* 1998; **19**: 489–98.

76 Charron P, Dubourg O, Desnos M *et al.* Diagnostic value of electrocardiography and echocardiography for familial hypertrophic cardiomyopathy in a genotyped adult population. *Circulation* 1997; **96**: 214–19.

77 Charron P, Dubourg O, Desnos M *et al.* Clinical features and prognostic implications of familial hypertrophic cardiomyopathy related to the cardiac myosin-binding protein C gene. *Circulation* 1998; **97**: 2230–6.

78 Ho CY, Sweitzer NK, McDonough B *et al.* Assessment of diastolic function with Doppler tissue imaging to predict genotype in preclinical hypertrophic cardiomyopathy. *Circulation* 2002; **105**: 2992–7.

79 Maron BJ, Thompson PD, Puffer JC *et al.* Cardiovascular preparticipation screening of competitive athletes: Addendum. *Circulation* 1998; **97**: 2294.

80 Maron BJ, Gross BW, Stark SI. Extreme left ventricular hypertrophy. *Circulation* 1995; **92**: 2748.

81 Pelliccia A, Maron BJ, Spataro A *et al.* The upper limit of physiologic cardiac hypertrophy in highly trained elite athletes. *N Engl J Med* 1991; **324**: 295–301.

82 Maron BJ, Pelliccia A, Spirito P. Cardiac disease in young trained athletes: Insights into methods for distinguishing athlete's heart from structural heart disease with particular emphasis on hypertrophic cardiomyopathy. *Circulation* 1995; **91**: 1596–601.

83 Moon JC, McKenna WJ, McCrohon JA, Elliott PM, Smith GC, Pennell DJ. Toward clinical risk assessment in hypertrophic cardiomyopathy with gadolinium cardiovascular magnetic resonance. *J Am Coll Cardiol* 2003; **41**: 1561–7.

84 Panza JA, Maron BJ. Relation of electrocardiographic abnormalities to evolving left ventricular hypertrophy in hypertrophic cardiomyopathy. *Am J Cardiol* 1989; **63**: 1258–65.

85 Maron BJ. The electrocardiogram as a diagnostic tool for hypertrophic cardiomyopathy: Revisited [editorial]. *Ann Noninvas Electrocardiol* 2001; **6**: 277–9.

86 Montgomery JV, Gohman TE, Harris KM, Casey SA, Maron BJ. Electrocardiogram in hypertrophic cardiomyopathy revisited: Does ECG pattern predict phenotypic expression and left ventricular hypertrophy or sudden death? [abstract]. *J Am Coll Cardiol* 2002; **39** (Suppl. A): 161A.

87 Corrado D, Basso C, Schiavon M *et al.* Screening for hypertrophic cardiomyopathy in young athletes. *N Engl J Med* 1998; **339**: 364–9.

88 Obaid AI, Maron BJ. Apical hypertrophic cardiomyopathy developing at a relatively advanced age. *Circulation* 2001; **203**: 1605.

89 Maron BJ, Spirito P. Implications of left ventricular remodeling in hypertrophic cardiomyopathy. *Am J Cardiol* 1998; **81**: 1339–44.

90 Harris KM, Zenovich AG, Casey SA, Wilson J, Maron BJ. Significance and clinical profile of the end-stage phase in a large hypertrophic cardiomyopathy cohort [abstract]. *Circulation* 2003; **108**: IV–626.

91 Maron BJ, Casey SA, Hurrell DG, Aeppli DM. Relation of left ventricular thickness to age and gender in hypertrophic cardiomyopathy. *Am J Cardiol* 2003; **91**: 626–8.

92 Sherrid MV, Chu CK, Delia E *et al.* An echocardiographic study of the fluid mechanics of obstruction in hypertrophic cardiomyopathy. *J Am Coll Cardiol* 1993; **22**: 816–25.

93 Pollick C, Rakowski H, Wigle ED. Muscular subaortic stenosis: The quantitative relationship between systolic anterior motion and pressure gradient. *Circulation* 1984; **69**: 43–9.

94 Shah PM, Taylor RD, Wong M. Abnormal mitral valve coaptation in hypertrophic obstructive cardiomyopathy: Proposed role in systolic anterior motion of mitral valve. *Am J Cardiol* 1981; **48**: 258–62.

95 Panza JA, Maris TJ, Maron BJ. Development and determinants of dynamic obstruction to left ventricular outflow in young patients with hypertrophic cardiomyopathy. *Circulation* 1992; **85**: 1398–405.

96 Sharma S, Elliott PM, Whyte G *et al.* Utility of cardiopulmonary exercise in the assessment of clinical determinants of functional capacity in hypertrophic cardiomyopathy. *Am J Cardiol* 2000; **86**: 162–8.

97 Yu EHC, Omran AS, Wigle ED, Williams WG, Siu SC, Rakowski H. Mitral regurgitation in hypertrophic obstructive cardiomyopathy: Relationship to obstruction and relief with myectomy. *J Am Coll Cardiol* 2000; **36**: 2219–25.

98 Klues HG, Leuner C, Kuhn H. Hypertrophic obstructive cardiomyopathy: No increase of the gradient during exercise. *J Am Coll Cardiol* 1991; **19**: 527–33.

99 Olivotto I, Cecchi F, Casey SA, Dolara A, Traverse JH, Maron BJ. Impact of atrial fibrillation on the clinical course of hypertrophic cardiomyopathy. *Circulation* 2001; **104**; 2517–24.

100 Yamaguchi H, Ishimura T, Nishiyama S *et al.* Hypertrophic nonobstructive cardiomyopathy with giant negative T waves (apical hypertrophy): Ventriculographic and echocardiographic features in 30 patients. *Am J Cardiol* 1979; **44**: 401–12.

101 Maron BJ, Hauser RG, Roberts WC. Hypertrophic cardiomyopathy with left ventricular apical diverticulum. *Am J Cardiol* 1996; **77**: 1263–65.

102 Maron BJ, Verter J, Kapur S. Disproportionate ventricular septal thickening in the developing normal human heart. *Circulation* 1978; **57**: 520–6.

103 Varnava AM, Elliott PM, Baboonian C *et al.* Hypertrophic cardiomyopathy: Histopathological features of sudden death in cardiac troponin T disease. *Circulation* 2001; **104**: 1380–4.

104 Basso C, Thiene G, Corrado D, Buja G, Melacini P, Nava A. Hypertrophic cardiomyopathy and sudden death in the young: Pathologic evidence of myocardial ischemia. *Hum Pathol* 2000; **31**: 988–98.

105 Tanaka M, Fujiwara H, Onodera T *et al.* Quantitative analysis of myocardial fibrosis in normal, hypertensive hearts, and hypertrophic cardiomyopathy. *Br Heart J* 1986; **55**: 575–81.

106 Maron BJ, Wolfson JK, Roberts WC. Relation between extent of cardiac muscle cell disorganization and left ventricular wall thickness in hypertrophic cardiomyopathy. *Am J Cardiol* 1992; **70**: 785–90.

107 Maron BJ, Wolfson JK, Epstein SE *et al.* Intramural ('small vessel') coronary artery disease in hypertrophic cardiomyopathy. *J Am Coll Cardiol* 1986; **8**: 545–57.

108 Tanaka M, Fujiwara H, Onodera T *et al.* Quantitative analysis of narrowings of intramyocardial small arteries in normal hearts, hypertensive hearts, and hearts with hypertrophic cardiomyopathy. *Circulation* 1987; **75**: 1130–9.

109 Cannon RO, Rosing DR, Maron BJ *et al.* Myocardial ischemia in hypertrophic cardiomyopathy: Contribution of inadequate vasodilator reserve and elevated left ventricular filling pressures. *Circulation* 1985; **71**: 234–43.

110 Krams R, Kofflard MJM, Duncker DJ *et al.* Decreased coronary flow reserve in hypertrophic cardiomyopathy is related to remodeling of the coronary microcirculation. *Circulation* 1998; **97**: 230–3.

111 O'Gara PT, Bonow RO, Maron BJ *et al.* Myocardial perfusion abnormalities in patients with hypertrophic cardiomyopathy: Assessment with thallium-201 emission computed tomography. *Circulation* 1987; **76**: 1214–23.

112 Frenneaux MP, Porter A, Caforio ALP *et al.* Determinants of exercise capacity in hypertrophic cardiomyopathy. *J Am Coll Cardiol* 1992; **19**: 1521–6.

113 Bonow RO, Rosing DR, Bacharach SL *et al.* Effects of verapamil on left ventricular systolic function and diastolic filling in patients with hypertrophic cardiomyopathy. *Circulation* 1981; **64**: 787–95.

114 Maron BJ, Spirito P, Green KJ *et al.* Noninvasive assessment of left ventricular diastolic function by pulsed Doppler echocardiography in patients with hypertrophic cardiomyopathy. *J Am Coll Cardiol* 1987; **10**: 733–42.

115 Briguori C, Betocchi S, Romano M *et al.* Exercise capacity in hypertrophic cardiomyopathy depends on left ventricular diastolic function. *Am J Cardiol* 1999; **84**: 309–15.

116 Minakata K, Dearani JA, Nishimura RA, Maron BJ, Danielson GK. Extended septal myectomy for hypertrophic obstructive cardiomyopathy with anomalous mitral papillary muscles or chordae. *J Thorac CV Surg.* (In press.)

117 Klues HG, Roberts WC, Maron BJ. Morphologic determinants of echocardiographic patterns of mitral valve systolic anterior motion in obstructive hypertrophic cardiomyopathy. *Circulation* 1993; **87**: 1570–9.

118 Fay WP, Taliercio CP, Ilstrup DM *et al.* Natural history of hypertrophic cardiomyopathy in the elderly. *J Am Coll Cardiol* 1990; **16**: 821–6.

119 Maron BJ, Spirito P. Impact of patient selection biases on the perception of hypertrophic cardiomyopathy. *J Am Coll Cardiol* 2003; **41**: 974–80.

120 Maron BJ, Carney KP, Lever HM *et al.* Relationship of race to sudden cardiac death in competitive athletes with hypertrophic cardiomyopathy and its natural history. *Am J Cardiol* 1993; **72**: 970–2.

121 Maron BJ, Casey SA, Gohman TE, Aeppli DM. Impact of gender on the clinical and morphologic expression of hypertrophic cardiomyopathy [abstract]. *Circulation* 1999; **100**: I-212.

122 Maron BJ, Savage DD, Wolfson JK, Epstein SE. The prognostic significance of 24 hour ambulatory electrocardiographic monitoring in patients with hypertrophic cardiomyopathy. *Am J Cardiol* 1981; **48**: 252–7.

123 Spirito P, Rapezzi C, Autore C *et al.* Prognosis in asymptomatic patients with hypertrophic cardiomyopathy and nonsustained ventricular tachycardia. *Circulation* 1994; **90**: 2743–7.

124 Cecchi F, Olivotto I, Montereggi A, Squillatini G, Dolara A, Maron BJ. Prognostic value of non-sustained ventricular tachycardia and the potential role of amiodarone treatment in hypertrophic cardiomyopathy: Assessment in an unselected non-referral based patient population. *Heart* 1998; **79**: 331–6.

125 Adabag AS, Casey SA, Maron BJ. Sudden death in hypertrophic cardiomyopathy. Patterns and prognostic significance of tachyarrhythmias on ambulatory Holter ECG [abstract]. *Circulation* 2002; **106**: II-710.

126 Monserrat L, Elliott PM, Sharma S, Virdee M, Penas-Lado M, McKenna WJ. Non-sustained ventricular tachycardia in hypertrophic cardiomyopathy: A marker of sudden death risk in young patients. *J Am Coll Cardiol* 2003; **42**: 873–9.

127 Spirito P, Lakatos E, Maron BJ. Degree of left ventricular hypertrophy in patients with hypertrophic cardiomyopathy and chronic atrial fibrillation. *Am J Cardiol* 1992; **69**: 1217–22.

128 Nicod P, Polikar R, Peterson KL. Hypertrophic cardiomyopathy and sudden death. *N Engl J Med* 1988; **318**: 1255–7.

129 Stafford WJ, Trohman RG, Bilsker M *et al.* Cardiac arrest in an adolescent with atrial fibrillation and hypertrophic cardiomyopathy. *J Am Coll Cardiol* 1985; **7**: 701–4.

130 Corrado D, Basso C, Rizzoli G, Schiavon M, Thiene G. Does sports activity enhance the risk of sudden death in adolescents and young adults? *J Am Coll Cardiol* 2003; **42**: 1959–63.

131 Olivotto I, Maron BJ, Montereggi A *et al.* Prognostic value of systemic blood pressure response during exercise in a community-based patient population with hypertrophic cardiomyopathy. *J Am Coll Cardiol* 1999; **33**: 2044–51.

132 Maron BJ, Isner JM, McKenna WJ. Hypertrophic cardiomyopathy, myocarditis and other myopericardial disease, and mitral valve prolapse. Task Force 3. In: 26th Bethesda Conference. Recommendations for determining eligibility for competition in athletes with cardiovascular abnormalities. *J Am Coll Cardiol* 1994; **24**: 880–5.

CHAPTER 2

Genetic Mutations that Remodel the Heart in Hypertrophic Cardiomyopathy

Carolyn Y. Ho, MD and Christine E. Seidman, MD

Introduction

The observation that hypertrophic cardiomyopathy (HCM) occurs in families led to its recognition as a genetic cardiovascular disorder.[1] Subsequent linkage analysis demonstrated that HCM is caused by mutations in genes that encode components of the sarcomere.[2] Positional cloning techniques and candidate gene screening approaches have enabled an increasingly precise definition of the genetic basis of HCM. More than 200 individual mutations have been identified in all components of the contractile apparatus. However, the precise pathways by which these mutations trigger a hypertrophic response in the myocardium are not clearly defined.

The heart has a limited repertoire of responses to injury. Cardiac hypertrophy is one final common pathway of a variety of stressors on the myocyte. In addition to alterations in sarcomere proteins, recent discoveries have implicated dysregulation of intracellular calcium handling in hypertrophic remodeling of the heart.[3] Furthermore, genetic analyses of families with cardiac hypertrophy and electrophysiologic abnormalities have demonstrated a distinct molecular pathway involving not force generation and transmission but rather glucose metabolism.[4] This defines a new paradigm for approaching genetic mutations that remodel the heart. The fundamental connection between these inherited gene defects and disease phenotype provides a unique opportunity for the translation of molecular discoveries to the clinical management of disease.

Genetics of HCM

Patterns of inheritance

Monogenic (single-gene) disorders typically follow Mendelian patterns of inheritance. Each individual inherits two copies (alleles) of each gene, one from each parent. The particular allele transmitted to each offspring is randomly determined and established at the time of fertilization. Autosomal dominant

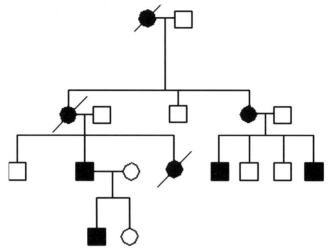

Fig. 2.1 Pedigree of a family with HCM caused by a β-cardiac myosin heavy chain mutation. Circles represent females; squares represent males; solid symbols indicate individuals affected with HCM; slashes indicate deceased individuals. Autosomal dominant transmission is illustrated by approximately 50% of the family inheriting the disorder and equal representation of affected males and females.

disorders require inheritance of only one mutant allele and disease expression occurs despite the presence of the normal or wild-type allele. Autosomal recessive disorders require inheritance of both mutant alleles, so that no normal protein is expressed. Detailed evaluation of kindreds with HCM has defined the presence of *autosomal dominant* transmission of disease (Fig. 2.1): (1) affected males and females are equally represented; (2) 50% of the offspring of affected family members inherit the disorder; (3) father-to-son transmission is present. Clinically affected individuals are heterozygous for the disease-causing mutation present in the family. Genetically unaffected family members and their offspring have no risk of developing or transmitting disease. This dichotomy underlies the power of genetic screening to assign unambiguous disease status to individuals in HCM kindreds who are at risk for developing disease.

In addition to familial disease, sarcomere protein mutations can cause sporadic cases of HCM.[5] In these affected individuals, sarcomere mutations have been identified, but there is no discernible family history of HCM and their parents are clinically and genetically unaffected. Sporadic disease typically occurs as a consequence of *de novo* mutations in the germ line, and consequently carries the same 50% risk of transmission to the offspring.

Identification of gene mutations

Initial studies employed genetic linkage analysis of families with HCM to define disease loci within the human genome. This approach involves determining whether genetic markers of known chromosomal location co-segregate with disease status, meaning that a certain pattern of alleles is inherited by all of the affected but none of the unaffected family members. The likelihood that a particular pattern of inheritance can be ascribed to random chance is quantified by calculating a logarithm of the odds (LOD) score. LOD scores ≥3 indicate less than 1:1000 odds that the observed segregation pattern is due to random chance, and are considered statistically significant evidence for genetic linkage to the locus in question. Performing genome-wide linkage studies on families with HCM led to the identification of four distinct disease loci on chromosomes 14q1, 11q11, 15q2, and 1q3.[6–9]

Candidate genes were then identified at these loci and a common theme was identified: these genes encoded different components of the contractile apparatus, including β-cardiac myosin heavy chain (β-MHC), cardiac troponin T (cTnT), α-tropomyosin (α-TM), and cardiac myosin binding protein C (cMyB-PC). The DNA sequence of each gene was determined and sequence variants identified in affected family members.[2,10–12] Evidence that these sequence variants represented causal mutations for HCM rather than nonfunctional polymorphisms included their absence in unaffected family members as well as normal control chromosomes, and the fact that they resulted in amino acid substitutions in residues that are highly conserved throughout evolution, and are therefore likely to be critical to the structure and function of the protein. Hypothesizing that gene defects in other contractile proteins could also cause HCM, the genes encoding cardiac troponin I,[13] cardiac actin, [14] regulatory myosin light chain, and essential myosin light chain[15] were screened and mutations were identified in HCM kindreds. Thus, the paradigm of HCM as a disease of the sarcomere was established.

To date, more than 200 different mutations in 10 different genes have been reported in individuals and families with HCM (Table 2.1). In addition to the sarcomere proteins listed above, mutations have also been identified in the giant molecule titin, which provides flexibility to the sarcomere and participates in force generation and transmission to the cytoskeleton.[16] As sarcomere proteins are present in all muscle types, the cardiac specificity of most HCM-causing mutations is due to genetic defects in the cardiac-specific isoforms, which are encoded by genes distinct from skeletal and smooth muscle forms. α-TM and titin are expressed in all muscle cells. It is unclear why titin mutations cause only cardiac disease, particularly because so few of these mutations have been identified. Mutations in α-TM may be cardioselective by altering residues that interact with the cardiac isoforms of other proteins. This observation may imply that some domains of α-TM are particularly important for cardiac function.

Many different types of mutations have been identified. Missense mutations (single base-pair changes leading to the substitution of one amino acid for another at the affected codon) occur most commonly, but deletions, insertions, nonsense (substitution of a stop codon), and splice site mutations have been described which may result in the production of a truncated protein. As the normal allele inherited from the genetically unaffected parent is translated into wild-type protein, the mechanisms by which the disease phenotype aris-

Table 2.1 Gene mutations that cause hypertrophic remodeling of the heart. Data are from references 44, 45 and 66, and from http://cardiogenomics.med.harvard.edu/project-detail?project_id=230. CMP = cardiomyopathy

	Gene	Designation	Chromosome	Frequency	No. of mutations	Notes
HCM sarcomere proteins	β-Myosin heavy chain	β-MHC	14q1	~30–40%	>80	Predominantly missense mutations; dilated CMP
	Cardiac myosin binding protein C	cMYBPC	11q1	~30%	>50	Missense, deletions, splice site mutations; elderly-onset HCM
	Cardiac troponin T	cTnT	1q3	~10–15%	>20	Missense, deletions, splice site mutations; dilated CMP
	Cardiac troponin I	cTnI	19p1	<5%	>10	Missense and deletions
	α-Tropomyosin	α-TM	15q2	<5%	8	Missense mutations
	Myosin essential light chain	MLC-1	3p	Rare	2	Missense mutations; skeletal myopathy
	Myosin regulatory light chain	MLC-2	12q	Rare	8	Missense and truncations; skeletal myopathy
	Actin		11q	Rare	5	Missense mutations; dilated CMP
	Titin		2q3	Rare	1	Missense mutation
HCM nonsarcomere proteins	Ryanodine receptor type 2	RyR2	1q4	~5%	4	Intracellular calcium handling
Hypertrophic heart disease	γ-Subunit AMP kinase	PRKAG2	7q3	?	3	Glucose metabolism; pre-excitation catecholaminergic polymorphic ventricular tachycardia

es in dominant disorders are most likely related to either dominant-negative or dominant-activating effects or through haploinsufficiency. Dominant-negative or dominant-activating effects imply that the mutant protein is incorporated into the sarcomere and diminishes or enhances contractile function despite the expression of the remaining wild-type allele. Haploinsufficiency is due to dominant mutations that inactivate an allele leading to a decreased amount of functional protein. Most of the identified mutations in HCM are missense or minor truncations, which are unlikely to result in haploinsufficiency or significant peptide instability; dominant-negative/activating effects are therefore likely to be the predominant mechanism of disease expression.[17]

Current estimates suggest that the incidence of unexplained cardiac hypertrophy in healthy populations is 1/500;[18] however, the proportion attributed to inherited mutations in genes that encode sarcomere proteins remains unknown. Approaches aimed at defining gene mutations from subjects clinically diagnosed with HCM indicate a sarcomere gene mutation in approximately 50–60% (http://cardiogenomics.med.harvard.edu/project-detail?project_id=230). In addition to prototypical HCM caused by sarcomere protein mutations, recent genetic analyses suggest that alterations in proteins involved in myocyte glucose metabolism also result in cardiac hypertrophy. Unlike sarcomere gene mutations, these defects are usually associated with electrophysiologic abnormalities, such as pre-excitation and progressive conduction system disease. Of further intrigue, mutations in sarcomere proteins actin,[19] cardiac β-MHC, and cardiac troponin T[20] have also been associated with familial dilated cardiomyopathy (DCM). The mechanisms by which mutations within the same sarcomere protein culminate in a dilated rather than a hypertrophic phenotype are unclear and may be related to alterations in force transmission in DCM as opposed to force generation in HCM,[14] or to perturbation of signaling molecules, such as calcium. Identification of the full compendium of mutations and pathways that result in the remodeling of the heart is in progress (http://cardiogenomics.med.harvard.edu).

Mutations in sarcomere proteins define HCM

Contractile function: the sarcomere and intracellular calcium

The sarcomere is the functional unit of contraction in muscle cells. Sarcomere proteins are organized as a lattice of interdigitating thick (myosin heavy and light chains) and thin (actin, α-TM and the troponin complex) filaments that cyclically detach and attach during muscle contraction and relaxation, participating in force generation and force transmission.[21,22] Both systole and diastole are active processes powered by the hydrolysis of adenosine triphosphate (ATP) (Fig. 2.2). The complex cascade of molecular events is synchronized by alterations in intracellular calcium levels[23] (Fig. 2.3). Membrane depolarization by the action potential elicits calcium influx through cell membrane L-type calcium channels. Ryanodine receptors on the sarcoplasmic reticulum (SR) are then activated to trigger calcium-induced calcium release. The resulting rise

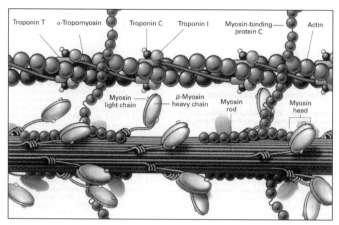

Fig. 2.2 The sarcomere is the basic unit of contraction in the cardiac myocyte. Mutations that cause hypertrophic cardiomyopathy have been identified in cardiac sarcomere proteins. Thin filament elements include actin, α-tropomyosin, and the troponin complex (T, C, and I). The thick filament is composed of myosin heavy and light chains. Actin and myosin crossbridge formation and separation are fueled by the hydrolysis of high-energy phosphates (ATP) and regulated by calcium binding to the troponin complex. Adapted from Spirito *et al.* The management of hypertrophic cardiomyopathy. *N Engl J Med* 1997; **336**: 775–85, ©1997 Massachusetts Medical Society. All rights reserved.

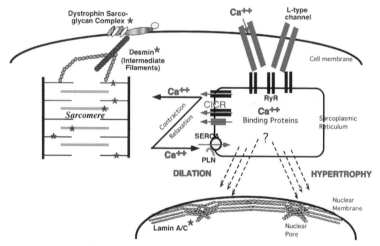

Fig. 2.3 Intracellular calcium trafficking plays a critical role in coordinating excitation–contraction coupling of the cardiac myocyte. Membrane depolarization by the action potential allows entry of calcium via L-type calcium channels. This influx of calcium ions triggers a greater rise in cytoplasmic calcium by calcium-induced calcium release from the SR via ryanodine receptors. Calcium binding to the troponin complex releases inhibition and allows the interaction of the thick and thin filaments, and myocyte contraction occurs. Calcium is then returned to the SR via the sarcoplasmic/endoplasmic calcium ATPase (SERCA) pump, regulated by phospholamban, and relaxation ensues. Adapted from Seidman and Seidman. The genetic basis for cardiomyopathy: from mutation identification to mechanistic paradigms. *Cell* 2001; **104**: 557–67. © 2001, with permission from Elsevier.

in intracellular Ca^{2+} concentration leads to calcium binding of troponin C and causes conformational changes in the troponin complex, releasing troponin I inhibition of actin and allowing actin–myosin crossbridge formation. Myosin then hydrolyzes ATP and undergoes conformational changes that allow the myosin head to be propelled against the thin filament. Activation of the sarcoplasmic/endoplasmic Ca^{2+} ATPase membrane pump, SERCA, causes sequestration of cytosolic Ca^{2+} back into the sarcoplasmic reticulum. The myosin head detaches from actin, troponin I inhibition of actomyosin interaction is re-established, and myocyte relaxation ensues.

Mutations of the thin filament
α-Cardiac actin

α-Cardiac actin is a 375 amino acid protein (41 kilodaltons; kDa) encoded by the cardiac actin gene (ACTC) which is organized into six exons on chromosome 15 (Fig. 2.4).[24] Mutations in actin are typically located in proximity to the putative myosin binding site and are rare causes of HCM.[14,25] The expression of these mutations is relatively mild with respect to both the degree of hypertrophy and the incidence of sudden death. Of note, actin mutations are also a rare cause of familial dilated cardiomyopathy.[19]

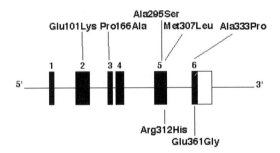

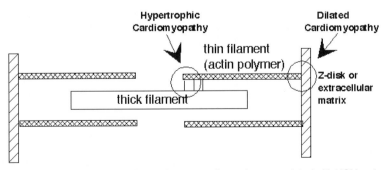

Fig. 2.4 Organization of the α-cardiac actin gene and mutations associated with HCM and dilated cardiomyopathy.

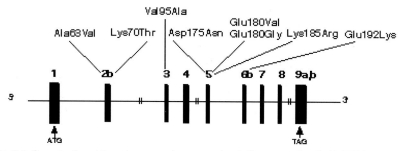

Fig. 2.5 Organization of the α-tropomyosin gene and mutations associated with HCM.

α-Tropomyosin

The α-TM gene (*TPM1*) is organized into 15 exons on chromosome 15 (Fig. 2.5)[26] and encodes a 284 amino acid protein expressed in fast skeletal and cardiac muscle.[27] α-TM forms a complex with troponin T and regulates actin–myosin interaction in response to intracellular Ca^{2+} concentration. Calcium binding to troponin C leads to conformational changes in troponins I and T that release tropomyosin inhibition of actin–myosin crossbridge formation. Mutations in *TPM1* are thought to account for a small proportion (<5%) of familial and sporadic HCM, including a potential founder effect in the Finnish population.[2,9,11,28–31] The clinical phenotype of HCM caused by *TPM1* mutations is difficult to accurately characterize because of the small number of identified families, but has been associated with variable degrees of left ventricular hypertrophy (LVH) and relatively good survival.[11,30]

Although α-TM is expressed in both cardiac and skeletal muscle, the clinical expression of *TPM1* mutations is dominated by HCM rather than skeletal myopathy. The cardiac specificity of phenotype may be due to the fact that the identified mutations alter the portions of the α-TM molecule that interact with the cardiac-specific isoform of troponin T. Alterations in calcium sensitivity may also play a role in the tissue-specificity of *TPM1* mutations.[32]

Cardiac troponin T

Troponin T links the troponin complex to α-TM and therefore plays a central role in the regulation of contraction. The cTnT gene (*TNNT2*) encompasses 17 kilobases (kb) of DNA on chromosome 1 and encodes a 288 amino acid peptide (36–39 kDa) over 16 exons (Fig. 2.6). Several distinct isoforms are expressed in cardiac tissue via alternative splicing.[33] Approximately 10–15% of HCM is thought to be attributable to mutations in cTnT,[11] which have predominantly been of the missense variety, although splice signal mutations, insertions, and deletions have been reported (Fig. 2.6).[2,11,34–36] Historically, the clinical phenotype resulting from cTnT mutations has been characterized by modest or clinically inapparent amounts of LVH, but increased risk of sudden death. However, this classic description is based on information from a highly selected, referral-based population, and benign cTnT mutations have been reported.[37,38]

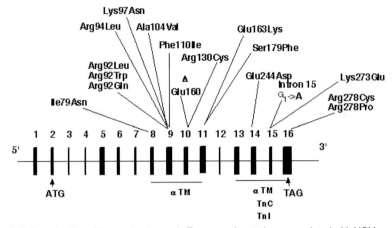

Fig. 2.6 Organization of the cardiac troponin T gene and mutations associated with HCM.

Cardiac troponin I

Troponin I is the inhibitory subunit of the troponin complex. In conditions of low intracellular Ca^{2+}, troponin I (TnI) inhibits actin–myosin interaction. When calcium ions bind to troponin C, conformational changes occur in TnI which release the inhibition of TnT and α-TM, thereby allowing actomyosin crossbridge formation. The gene for the cardiac-specific isoform of troponin I (*TNNI3*) spans eight exons on chromosome 19 and encodes a 210 amino acid (27–31 kDa) protein (Fig. 2.7).[39] Direct DNA sequence analysis of carciac TnI (cTnI) in patients with HCM suggests that mutations in this gene account for approximately 5% of disease (http://cardiogenomics.med.harvard.edu), but this gene has only recently had comprehensive analyses. A more precise assessment of the contribution of cTnI to HCM is still uncertain. Although early reports suggested that apical hypertrophy and ventricular pre-excitation were

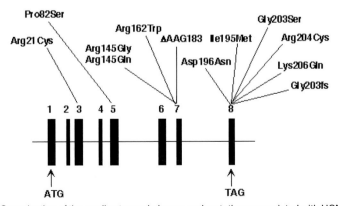

Fig. 2.7 Organization of the cardiac troponin I gene and mutations associated with HCM.

associated with HCM caused by cTnI mutations,[13] more recent clinical studies of patients with these defects have not confirmed them as specific features of cTnI defects. Detailed survival analyses have not been performed.

Mutations of the thick filament
β-Cardiac myosin heavy chain

Myosin heavy chains account for approximately 1% of total myocyte protein. They are large molecules (>200 000 kDa) organized into two functional domains: an amino-terminal globular head that interacts with actin and a carboxyl terminal rod.[21,40] Force is transduced via a hinge region between these two domains. There are two cardiac-specific myosin heavy-chain isoform genes: α-cardiac MHC (*MYH6*) and β-cardiac MHC (*MYH7*). Both genes are encoded in tandem on chromosome 14. The α-isoform predominates in fetal life and in the adult atria; the β-isoform predominates in the adult ventricles, accounting for more than 70% of total ventricular myosin.[41]

The genetic basis of HCM was first described by linkage analysis and the subsequent identification of a missense mutation, Arg403Gln (a single base-pair change resulting in the substitution of glutamine for arginine at residue 403), in the β-MHC gene.[6,10] Consequently, β-MHC mutations serve as a prototype for HCM and are thought to account for approximately 35% of cases of the disease. To date, more than 80 unique mutations have been identified in familial and sporadic disease.[5,10,42–45] The majority of mutations are missense and clustered within the globular head domain (Fig. 2.8).

The phenotype associated with β-MHC mutations is generally quite striking. Significant LVH is apparent in nearly all genetically affected individuals by late adolescence.[46] Moreover, the clinical course of selected myosin mutations has been severe, with markedly attenuated survival due to the development of end-stage heart failure and sudden death (Fig. 2.9).[42,47] The precise determinants driving prognosis from heritable gene mutations are likely to be manifold and incompletely understood. At the molecular level, mutations that result in a change in the charge of the substituted amino acid may give rise to a more severe disease, ostensibly because charge-changing substitutions result in more profound perturbations of protein structure and function. Nonconservative β-MHC mutations (including Arg403Gln and Arg719Trp) have been associated with more severe phenotypic effects, compared to conservative mutations (e.g. Val606Met) that appear to have minimal impact on overall survival.

Cardiac myosin binding protein C

The cardiac myosin binding protein C gene (*MYBPC3*) contains 37 exons spanning 24 kb of chromosome 11 and encoding a 1274 amino acid (137 kDa) protein (Fig. 2.10). cMyBPC is transversely arrayed in strips that provide structural support to the sarcomere by binding MHC and titin.[48,49] Functionally, MyBPC may provide structural integrity to the sarcomere in addition to

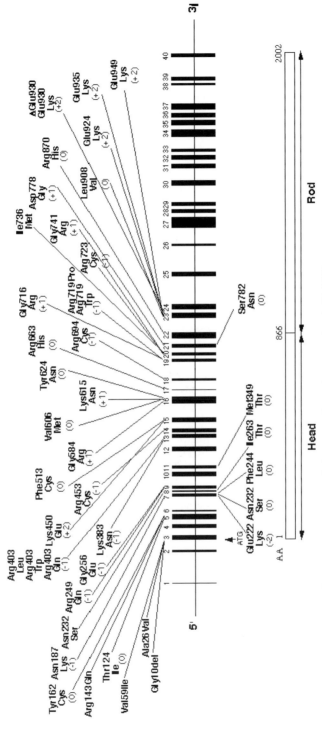

Fig. 2.8 Organization of the β-cardiac myosin heavy chain gene and mutations associated with HCM.

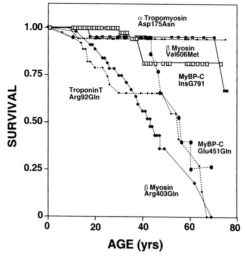

Fig. 2.9 Survival with HCM is influenced by genetic etiology. Kaplan–Meier curves demonstrate differences in life expectancy in HCM caused by α-TM, cMYBPC and β-MHC mutations. Survival related to mutations in α-TM and cMYBPC is generally better than that related to β-MHC mutations. However, some mutations in β-MHC are associated with a more benign prognosis, possibly related to conservation of charge with Val606Met compared with Arg403Gln. Adapted from Seidman and Seidman. Hypertrophic cardiomyopathy. In: Scriver *et al.*, eds. *The Metabolic and Molecular Bases of Inherited Disease*: McGraw-Hill, 2000: 5433–52, with permission from the McGraw-Hill Companies.

modulating myosin ATPase activity and cardiac contractility in response to adrenergic stimulation.[48]

Missense, splice site, and deletion/insertion mutations in *MYBPC3* have been described and appear to be a prevalent cause of HCM, accounting for 20–30% of cases of the disease.[12,46,50,51] As with HCM caused by mutations in other elements of the contractile apparatus, the phenotype of cMyBPC-related disease is heterogeneous, but recurring themes emerge. Most strikingly, the age at onset of clinically apparent hypertrophy is delayed by several decades compared with HCM caused by mutations in cTnT and β-MHC. Approximately half of adults under the age of 50 years with cMyBPC mutations have detectable LVH (maximal wall thickness >13 mm), compared with nearly all patients with mutations in other genes.[46,52] The disease course has typically been relatively mild and not associated with decreased life expectancy, but there are reports of sudden death related to mutations in this gene.[46]

α-Cardiac myosin heavy chain

Although β-MHC is the predominant isoform expressed by the adult human ventricular myocardium, the α-isoform is also present and may account for up to 30% of adult ventricular myosin heavy chain.[53] The α-MHC gene is encoded on chromosome 14q12 in tandem with the β-isoform. Expression is developmentally regulated such that the α-isoform is abundant in the atria

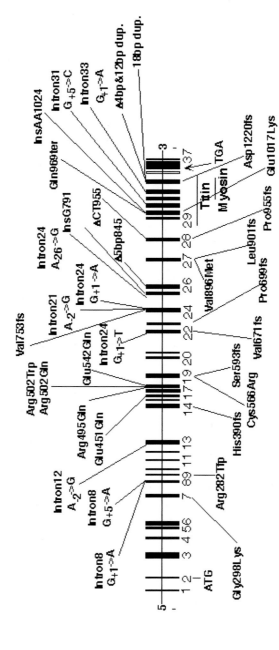

Fig. 2.10 Organization of the cardiac myosin binding protein C gene and mutations associated with HCM.

and ventricles during fetal development. After birth, the ventricles express predominantly the β-isoform.[54,55] Mutations in α-MHC have been associated with sporadic cases of elderly-onset HCM.[52] There is speculation that the lower amounts of this isoform expressed in the adult ventricle may account for the delayed onset of hypertrophy.

Myosin light chains

The regulatory (*MYL2*, chromosome 12) and essential (*MYL3*, chromosome 19) myosin light chains belong to the EF-hand superfamily of proteins with a helix–loop–helix motif.[56] They are thought to play a role in determining the speed and force of actomyosin sliding by interacting with the head–rod junction of the myosin heavy chain.[57,58] Mutations in myosin light chains are rarely reported genetic etiologies of HCM, accounting for less than 5% of the entire HCM population.[15] These defects may particularly predispose to cardiac remodeling with midcavitary obliteration (hour-glass morphology).

Experimental models of HCM

Mutations in contractile proteins may affect actin–myosin crossbridge formation, calcium cycling in the sarcomere, the energetics of force generation, or force transmission.[59–61] The heterogeneity of HCM in the human population indicates significant intra- and intergenic variability in the response to inherited gene mutations. To evaluate the consequences of specific sarcomere mutations in a more precise and controlled manner, a variety of experimental models of HCM have been developed, ranging from isolated myofibrils to genetically modified animals.[44,45] Information gained from interrogating these models provides a great opportunity to identify factors that may exacerbate or ameliorate disease and may thereby provide new insights into understanding and treating HCM.

In vitro studies

β-MHC and cTnT proteins genetically engineered to contain point mutations represented in human HCM have been most extensively studied *in vitro*. Limitations of these models include the diversity of systems employed (skinned muscle strips, cardiomyocytes, and myotubes) and that myocyte function is tested in the absence of mechanical load. Therefore, the direct applicability of findings to the disease state in intact organisms is unclear. These mutated proteins appear to be incorporated into sarcomeres without major disruption of sarcomeric or myofibrillar structure.[17,62] Their expression in primary cultures of ventricular myocytes or quail myotubes has been shown to exert complicated effects on ATPase activity, calcium sensitivity, and motility.[44,61,63–66] The perturbation of actin–myosin motility has been particularly difficult to interpret. *In vitro* sliding filament assays assess the force and velocity of actin translocation along myosin. Altered crossbridge kinetics have been observed[67] along with both impaired and enhanced force generation and sliding velocities.[61,64,68–70] Whether the gain or loss of function relates to the specific biophysical consequences of each distinct mutation or some other mechanism remains unclear.

Animal models of HCM

Genetically modified animals bearing mutations identified in human HCM are invaluable models for studying the consequences of gene mutations at the level of the heart and the intact organism. In addition to enabling basic structure–function information to be obtained, animal models allow the unique opportunity to study the influence of genetic background, environment, and pharmacologic therapy on these inherited monogenic defects.

The oldest and best-characterized animal model of HCM is the α-MHC[403/+] knock-in mouse, in which the human β-MHC mutation Arg403Gln is introduced into one allele of the mouse α-MHC gene via techniques of homologous recombination.[71] This mutation is associated with a severe form of HCM in humans, with a 50% mortality rate by the age of 45 years.[42] The resulting genetically modified mice express a phenotype that closely recapitulates the human disorder, developing myocardial disarray, hypertrophy and fibrosis in an age-dependent manner. Although general life expectancy is not significantly altered, heterozygous mice manifest increased arrhythmogenicity and risk for exercise-induced sudden death compared with their wild-type littermates.[72] Enhanced systolic contractile performance (the dominant-activating effect) was identified by examining isolated myocytes and intact heart preparations.[61,70,73] Interestingly, diastolic function was significantly impaired even before the development of hypertrophy.[71,73]

The α-MHC[403/+] mouse has been used to investigate the effects of medication administration on phenotype. Such studies have highlighted the importance of intracellular calcium in mediating signal transduction, linking alterations of muscle contraction to myocyte growth. Calcineurin A is a calcium-dependent phosphatase that may be critically involved in the molecular pathways of hypertrophic remodeling.[23,74] Non-HCM transgenic mice engineered to overexpress calcineurin develop LVH, possibly due to dephosphorylation and nuclear translocation of the transcription factor NF-AT3 (nuclear factor of activated T cells) and the subsequent activation of growth-promoting pathways.[74] The development of hypertrophy in this model could be abrogated by inhibition of calcineurin by administering cyclosporin A.

This finding sparked interest in the use of cyclosporin A as a potential treatment for HCM. However, administration of this agent to α-MHC[403/+] HCM mice was, paradoxically, associated with marked worsening of the clinical expression of this sarcomere protein mutation, including more rapid and severe development of LVH, more extensive histopathologic changes, and increased risk for premature death.[75] The underlying mechanism is unclear but may be related to failure of the normal increase in the resting intracellular Ca^{2+} concentration in α-MHC[403/+] mice. This exaggerated phenotypic response was attenuated by co-administration of the L-type calcium channel blocker diltiazem.[75] Furthermore, short-term administration of diltiazem alone to young α-MHC[403/+] mice prior to the development of histologic or morphologic abnormalities (prehypertrophic phase, 6–8 weeks of age) attenuates the development of hypertrophy and other morphologic changes.[3] One consequence of the Arg403Gln mutation appears to be abnormal sequestration of calcium by the mutant sarcomere, possibly related to diminished levels of calcium transport proteins such as calsequestrin and ryanodine receptors, with ultimate depletion of sarcoplasmic reticulum calcium levels.[3] Diltiazem may serve to blunt this effect by restoring normal calcium cycling between the sarcoplasmic reticulum and the cytoplasm, thereby interrupting the signals leading to hypertrophic remodeling. Fundamental dysregulation of calcium handling caused by myosin mutations may, in part, mediate the hypertrophic response of the myocyte.

In addition to the α-MHC[403/+] mouse model, a variety of other genetically modified mice, rats, and rabbits have been developed, incorporating mutations in β-MHC, cMyBPC, α-TM, and cTnT (Table 2.2).[76–82] These models typically show myocyte disarray, variable degrees of hypertrophy, and systolic and diastolic dysfunction with functional and biochemical abnormalities generally preceding the development of structural abnormalities. The β-MHC[403/+] transgenic rabbit model[77] may be a particularly attractive model, as the β-isoform of MHC is predominant in rabbit and human hearts, whereas the α-isoform predominates in mice and rats. These rabbits show significant hypertrophy, fibrosis, diastolic dysfunction and an increased risk of sudden death.[77] Impaired myocardial relaxation develops in advance of hypertrophy,[83] a finding recently replicated in patients with HCM.[84,85]

The specificity and precision with which disease processes can be studied in these animal models will allow continued refinement of our understanding of the nature of the true phenotype of HCM and further investigation into basic questions about this complex disease: (1) the question of whether LVH in HCM is a primary or secondary response to either impaired or enhanced contractility; (2) the influence of genetic background, modifier genes, environmental factors, and pharmacologic intervention on disease expression; and (3) the elucidation of early molecular events that precede the development of overt hypertrophy and the pathways leading from sarcomere dysfunction to myocyte hypertrophy.

Genotype–phenotype correlations

When the genetic basis of HCM was initially revealed, there was optimism that a discrete number of mutations would exist, each with a characteristic phenotype that would allow prediction of the clinical course by identification of the causal gene defect. The reality is far more complex. Over 200 individual mutations have been reported and the compilation is far from complete. Moreover, the vast majority of these mutations are private, meaning that they are unique to a given family and, except in rare circumstances, without significant founder effect.[30,31]

Table 2.2 Animal models of hypertrophic cardiomyopathy. LVH = left ventricular hypertrophy; CMP = cardiomyopathy. Adapted from Marian and Roberts. The molecular genetic basis for hypertrophic cardiomyopathy with permission. *J Mol Cell Cardiol* 2001; **33**: 655–70, with permission from Elsevier

Gene	Mutation	Phenotype
α-Myosin heavy chain	Arg403Gln (knock-in)[71,73]	Myocyte disarray/fibrosis; systolic and diastolic dysfunction; left ventricular hypertrophy and left atrial enlargement; altered force generation (intact animal and single molecule); abnormal conduction. Homozygous neonates have lethal dilated CMP
	Deletion actin binding domain[88]	Myocyte disarray/fibrosis; LVH in females; dilatation in males
	Knock-out[109]	Homozygotes: embryonic lethality. Heterozygotes: fibrosis, disarray, impaired contractility and relaxation
Cardiac troponin T	Deletion C-terminal[110]	Myocyte disarray/fibrosis; diastolic dysfunction; myocyte atrophy
	Arg92Gln[76,81]	Myocyte disarray/fibrosis; hypercontractility; diastolic dysfunction
	Deletion exon 16 (rat model)[82]	Systolic and diastolic dysfunction; exercise-induced hypertrophy, disarray and sudden death
Cardiac myosin binding protein C	Deletion C-terminal[78]	Myocyte disarray and fibrosis without hypertrophy; contractile dysfunction
	Truncation[111]	Neonatal dilated cardiomyopathy in homozygous mice; hypertrophic cardiomyopathy in heterozygous mice
α-Tropomyosin	Asp175Asn[79]	Myocyte disarray/hypertrophy; impaired contractility and relaxation; increased Ca^{2+} sensitivity
	Knock-out[112]	Homozygotes: embryonic lethality. Heterozygotes: no phenotype
β-Myosin heavy chain	Arg403Gln (rabbit model)[77]	Hypertrophy/disarray/fibrosis; diastolic > systolic dysfunction; increased risk of premature death

Clinical studies of families and individuals with HCM are remarkable not only for the genetic diversity found, but also for the phenotypic heterogeneity. There is marked variation in disease penetrance and expressivity, both between mutations and within families with the same mutation.[42,86] In the two decades since the initial identification of the genetic basis of HCM, answers to fundamental questions, such as why some sarcomere protein mutations cause more severe disease than others and why individuals with the same mutation have a wide range of clinical features, remain unanswered. Clinical manifestations of specific genetic mutations indicate that the age at disease onset, the degree of hypertrophy, and the prognosis are all shaped by genotype, but numerous confounding factors limit the ability to generalize genotype–phenotype correlations described for specific mutations. Using family studies, attempts have been made to establish broad genotype–phenotype correlations in the three most thoroughly studied genes: β-myosin heavy chain, cardiac myosin binding protein C, and cardiac troponin T. These general observations are summarized in Table 2.3. Identification of wider genetic and environmental influences that affect disease expression is an active area of investigation.

Penetrance

Most gene mutations that cause HCM are highly penetrant, meaning that nearly all individuals who inherit a sarcomere mutation will ultimately develop clinical disease. However, penetrance is clearly age-dependent.[46,51,52,87] Although the causal gene mutation is present at the time of fertilization, characteristic clinical manifestations of HCM are rarely seen in genetically affected children. Signs and symptoms of disease generally become apparent during adolescence; hence, the pubertal growth spurt and accompanying changes in the hormonal milieu may influence pathways that lead to hypertrophic remodeling of the heart. In addition, gender may play a role in altering phenotypic expression of HCM with evidence suggesting greater degrees of penetrance in males than females.[88–90]

The underlying gene mutation also appears to play an important role in the age at disease onset. Mutations in β-MHC are generally fully penetrant by the

Table 2.3 Established genotype–phenotype correlations in hypertrophic cardiomyopathy. LVH = left ventricular hypertrophy

Gene	Phenotypic characteristics
β-Myosin heavy chain	Early-onset disease; more extensive hypertrophy Higher incidence of sudden death Phenotypic heterogeneity
Myosin binding protein C	Mild hypertrophy (60% have LVH by standard criteria) Later onset of LVH and clinical manifestations Lower incidence of sudden death Malignant mutations have been identified
Cardiac troponin T	Mild LVH Higher incidence of sudden death

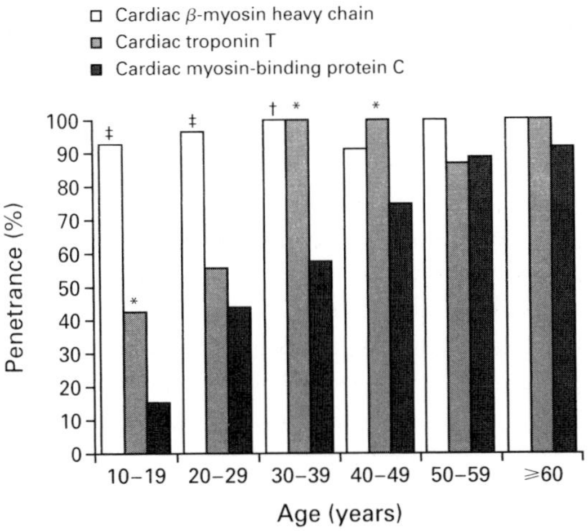

Cardiac β-myosin heavy chain
Cardiac troponin T
Cardiac myosin-binding protein C

Fig. 2.11 Penetrance of left ventricular hypertrophy in HCM caused by sarcomere protein mutations is dependent on age. Disease caused by β-MHC mutations (solid black bars) is typically evident by the second decade of life, whereas disease caused by cMyBPC mutations (dark grey bars) is generally not expressed until middle age or older. ($^{†}P < 0.05$; $^{§}P < 0.005$; $^{¶}P < 0.0005$). From Niimura *et al.* Mutations in the gene for cardiac myosin-binding protein C and late-onset familial hypertrophic cardiomyopathy. *N Engl J Med* 1998; **338**: 1248–57. © 1998 Massachusetts Medical Society. All rights reserved. Adapted with permission.

second decade of life. In contrast, the expression of cMyBPC mutations may be delayed until middle or elderly age (Fig. 2.11).[46] In a study of elderly patients with sporadic, late-onset HCM, sarcomere mutations were identified in ~20% (7/31), a proportion similar to typical HCM. The majority of mutations (5/7) were in cMyBPC; 2 novel mutations were found in cTnI, and 1 mutation was identified in the α-isoform of MHC.[52] Despite their prevalence in earlier-onset disease, no mutations were identified in the genes encoding β-MHC, cTnT, or α-TM. The recognition that primary hypertrophic heart disease which develops in late adult life may be caused by a genetically programmed event has important implications for elucidating factors that modify the expression of gene defects (e.g. environment, effects of aging and coexistent disease) as well as the fundamental molecular mechanisms of hypertrophy. Important also are implications for the patient's family as the mutation likely arose as a germ-line event and as such offspring are at risk for inheriting the disorder.

Degree of hypertrophy

The degree of LVH is probably influenced by the underlying genetic cause of HCM. In general, HCM caused by β-MHC mutations seems to be associated with greater degrees of LVH than disease caused by mutations in cTnT. In studies examining small numbers of families with different mutations in these two genes, the mean maximal left ventricular wall thickness for myosin mutations was 23.7 ± 7.7 mm, compared with 16.7 ± 5.5 mm for cTnT mutations.[11,19] Gene dosage appears to be directly correlated with clinical expression of disease.

Individuals homozygous for sarcomere protein mutations have been rarely reported in HCM; this is probably related to the lethality of this state. In two reported instances of homozygosity involving β-MHC and cTnT mutations, the clinical expression was dramatic and far more severe than the corresponding heterozygous state with respect to both degree of LVH and survival.[38,92]

In addition to specific genetic mutations, modifier genes and the background genetic milieu also affect the phenotype. The role of the genetic background has been evaluated in the α-MHC[403/+] mouse model of HCM by introducing the same mutation into different strains of mice. The degree of LVH and exercise capacity were significantly worse in inbred compared with outbred strains of mice, suggesting that modifying genes play a role in shaping the phenotypic response to this genetic stimulus to remodeling.[93] Data from human HCM are harder to interpret. There is a suggestion that polymorphisms in the renin–angiotensin–aldosterone system may modify the expression of sarcomere mutations.[94–97] The D allele of the insertion/deletion polymorphism in the angiotensin I converting enzyme gene has been associated with greater degrees of hypertrophy and sudden death risk in myosin heavy chain disease.[95,98] Full elucidation of the myriad of genetic modifiers influencing expression of sarcomere protein mutations is in progress.

Survival and risk for sudden cardiac death

Premature and sudden cardiac death are the most dramatic and feared sequelae of HCM, and there has therefore been great interest in improving capabilities for accurate risk stratification. There have been attempts to make general observations between genotype and survival in HCM: (1) mutations in cTnT may be associated with higher degrees of sudden death and decreased survival; (2) life expectancy may not be significantly altered in disease caused by α-TM or cardiac myosin binding protein C compared with certain severe β-MHC mutations.[11,35,44,46,65,99] However, these observations have typically been based on a small number of mutations identified in relatively small, highly selected families.

Contradictory phenotypes have been identified in all classes of mutations; for example, β-MHC and cTnT mutations associated with a benign clinical course and cMyBPC mutations associated with a more severe form of disease.[37,100,101] More typically, the correlation between genetic etiology and survival may be mutation-specific, potentially related to whether the resulting amino acid substitution results in a change in charge of the residue and hence has a more significant impact on protein structure (Fig. 2.9).[11,37,42] Despite the complexity of acquiring more data on the relevance of genotype to the propensity of sudden death, there is considerable evidence that the family history provides an important parameter for predicting risk. Because affected individuals from the same family always share the same genetic cause for HCM (despite vast differences in other genes and lifestyles), these data strongly indicate an important contributory role for the underlying gene defect in modulating the risk of sudden death in HCM.

New paradigms of inherited cardiac hypertrophy: glucose metabolism

PRKAG2 mutations and cardiac hypertrophy

Approximately 5–10% of patients with HCM have associated ventricular pre-excitation or Wolff–Parkinson–White syndrome.[102] Recent genetic studies of families and sporadic cases of hypertrophic heart disease with conduction abnormalities have identified a novel disease entity distinct from HCM caused by sarcomere protein mutations. Affected individuals inherit an autosomal dominant mutation in the γ2 regulatory subunit (PRKAG2) of adenosine monophosphate (AMP)-activated protein kinase, an enzyme involved in glucose uptake and glycolysis.[4,103,104] Affected individuals manifest cardiac hypertrophy and a spectrum of disordered intracardiac conduction, particularly ventricular pre-excitation, atrial fibrillation, and progressive atrioventricular block. Pre-excitation typically occurred early in life, often associated with supraventricular tachyarrhythmias and occasionally with syncope. The presence of an accessory pathway was verified on electrophysiologic studies in ten individuals.[4] Progressive conduction system disease occurred with increasing age, including sinus bradycardia and atrioventricular block, such that permanent pacemaker implantation was necessary in over 30% of affected individuals.[4] This high prevalence of heart block or pacemaker use serves as a discriminating feature from sarcomeric HCM. Severe clinical outcomes were also noted as a consequence of *PRKAG2* mutations, including progression to end-stage heart failure in 5/95 and cardiac transplantation in one patient; sudden cardiac death was reported in 4/95 affected individuals.[4]

Histopathologic and biochemical analyses on these patients have demonstrated that this disease is not a variant of HCM, but rather a novel glycogen storage disease of the myocardium, more similar to Pompe or Danon disease.[105] The pathologic hallmark of HCM is myocyte hypertrophy with disarray and fibrosis. In contrast, myocardial specimens from individuals with *PRKAG2* mutations show myocyte enlargement without disarray or fibrosis. Prominent vacuoles filled with glycogen-associated granules are also a key feature (Fig. 2.12). Mutations in *PRKAG2* may lead to constitutive activation of AMP kinase and subsequent increase in glucose uptake and glycogen accumulation in myocytes (causing hypertrophy) and in the conduction system (causing sinus and AVN dysfunction).[106,107]

Hypertrophic heart disease caused by *PRKAG2* mutations represents a distinct disease entity from HCM resulting from mutations in sarcomere proteins (Table 2.4). Different signaling pathways are involved in each of these conditions and thus the clinical approach for individuals with *PRKAG2* mutations should not necessarily be based on tenets derived from the management of HCM.

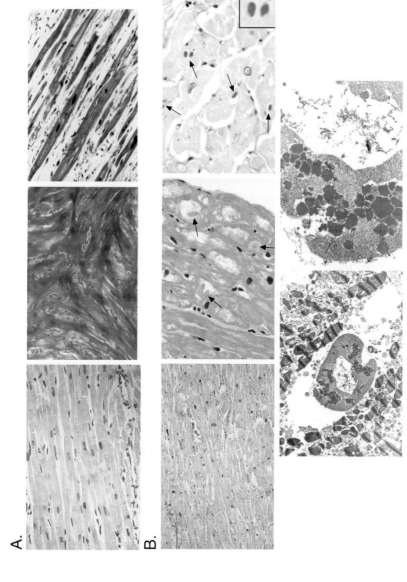

Fig. 2.12 The histopathologic features of HCM (**A**) and hypertrophic heart disease caused by *PRKAG2* mutations (**B**) are distinct. In contrast to the characteristic findings of myocyte disarray and fibrosis in HCM (**A**), *PRKAG2* mutations cause myocyte enlargement with prominent vacuoles filled with glycogen-associated granules. Disarray and fibrosis are not typical.

Table 2.4 Clinical features of cardiac hypertrophy caused by inherited gene mutations. Adapted from SeidmanC. Genetic causes of inherited cardiac hypertrophy: Robert L. Frye lecture. *Mayo Clinic Proceedings* 2002; **77**: 1315–19, with permission from *Mayo Clinic Proceedings*

Clinical findings	Sarcomere mutation	PRKAG2 mutation
Mode of inheritance	Autosomal dominant	Autosomal dominant
Left ventricular hypertrophy	Variable severity, generally asymmetric	Variable severity, generally concentric
Histopathology	Myocyte hypertrophy, disarray and interstitial fibrosis	Myocyte hypertrophy with vacuoles filled with glycogen-associated granules
Bradycardia	Uncommon	Common
Ventricular pre-excitation	Infrequent (~5–10%)	Common
Atrial fibrillation	Late onset	Early onset
Atrioventricular block	Rare	Frequent and progressive
Pacemaker requirement	Rare	Common

Conclusions and future directions

Given the heterogeneous clinical features of HCM and age-dependent penetrance, genotype analysis is uniquely positioned to allow the early and unequivocal diagnosis of disease status. In addition to implications for genetic counseling, such information may ultimately have a direct effect on clinical management to guide decisions regarding pharmacologic and device-based therapy as well as the potential for preclinical interventions designed to interrupt the natural history of disease. Causal mutations for HCM can be identified by direct DNA sequence analysis of sarcomere protein genes. This approach is reliable and sensitive but remains laborious and time-consuming, and is therefore not yet practical for population-based genetic screening efforts. A complete inventory of the spectrum of mutations and their attendant clinical outcomes is necessary for a fuller understanding of genotype–phenotype correlations.

Our comprehension of the phenotypic effect of sarcomere mutations has been predicated by the tools available to assess disease manifestations clinically. Historically, the diagnosis and definition of HCM have been dominated by describing outflow tract gradients and unexplained LVH. In fact, abnormalities of diastolic function and more subtle alterations of biochemical pathways, including intracellular calcium handling,[3] may be more fundamental manifestations of sarcomere protein mutations. Recent echocardiographic studies on families with HCM have demonstrated that diastolic dysfunction develops in advance of LVH and may be an earlier manifestation of the underlying genetic defect.[84,85] Our understanding and definition of the true phenotype of HCM thus continue to evolve.

Unraveling the molecular mechanisms that shape the clinical expression of inherited gene defects has consequences for secondary cardiac hypertrophy. The critical pathways that participate in primary cardiac remodeling may be the same as those that are activated in much more prevalent forms of acquired cardiovascular disease. Thus, gaining information about the fundamental events and genes involved in remodeling the heart may promote understanding of the development of heart failure in general.

Advances in defining the molecular and genetic processes underlying HCM provide insights germane to both clinical cardiology and basic cardiac myocyte biology. In the clinical realm, identifying the causal role of sarcomere gene mutations allows the unequivocal and early diagnosis of affected individuals. Early, genetic-based diagnosis may allow the identification of individuals at risk for developing the most severe consequences of this disorder, and ultimately may also allow early intervention. From the basic science perspective, elucidation of pathways of hypertrophic remodeling will foster understanding of the basic processes that govern myocyte growth and death and inspire treatments to abrogate the natural history of HCM.

References

1 Hollman A, Goodwin JF, Teare D, Renwick JW. A family with obstructive cardiomyopathy (asymmetrical hypertrophy). *Br Heart J* 1960; **22**: 449–56.
2 Thierfelder L, Watkins H, MacRae C *et al.* Alpha-tropomyosin and cardiac troponin T mutations cause familial hypertrophic cardiomyopathy: A disease of the sarcomere. *Cell* 1994; **77**: 701–12.
3 Semsarian C, Ahmad I, Giewat M *et al.* The L-type calcium channel inhibitor diltiazem prevents cardiomyopathy in a mouse model. *J Clin Invest* 2002; **109**: 1013–20.
4 Arad M, Benson DW, Perez-Atayde AR *et al.* Constitutively active AMP kinase mutations cause glycogen storage disease mimicking hypertrophic cardiomyopathy. *J Clin Invest* 2002; **109**: 357–62.
5 Watkins H, Thierfelder L, Hwang DS *et al.* Sporadic hypertrophic cardiomyopathy due to de novo myosin mutations. *J Clin Invest* 1992; **90**: 1666–71.
6 Jarcho JA, McKenna W, Pare JA *et al.* Mapping a gene for familial hypertrophic cardiomyopathy to chromosome 14q1. *N Engl J Med* 1989; **321**: 1372–8.
7 Carrier L, Hengstenberg C, Beckmann JS *et al.* Mapping of a novel gene for familial hypertrophic cardiomyopathy to chromosome 11. *Nat Genet* 1993; **4**: 311–13.
8 Thierfelder L, MacRae C, Watkins H *et al.* A familial hypertrophic cardiomyopathy locus maps to chromosome 15q2. *Proc Natl Acad Sci USA* 1993; **90**: 6270–4.
9 Watkins H, MacRae C, Thierfelder L *et al.* A disease locus for familial hypertrophic cardiomyopathy maps to chromosome 1q3. *Nat Genet* 1993; **3**: 333–7.
10 Geisterfer-Lowrance AA, Kass S, Tanigawa G *et al.* A molecular basis for familial hypertrophic cardiomyopathy: A beta cardiac myosin heavy chain gene missense mutation. *Cell* 1990; **62**: 999–1006.

11 Watkins H, McKenna WJ, Thierfelder L *et al.* Mutations in the genes for cardiac tropo-nin T and alpha-tropomyosin in hypertrophic cardiomyopathy. *N Engl J Med* 1995; **332**: 1058–64.

12 Watkins H, Conner D, Thierfelder L *et al.* Mutations in the cardiac myosin binding pro-tein-C gene on chromosome 11 cause familial hypertrophic cardiomyopathy. *Nat Genet* 1995; **11**: 434–7.

13 Kimura A, Harada H, Park J-E *et al.* Mutations in the cardiac troponin I gene associated with hypertrophic cardiomyopathy. *Nat Genet* 1997; **16**: 379–82.

14 Mogensen J, Klausen IC, Pedersen AK *et al.* Alpha-cardiac actin is a novel disease gene in familial hypertrophic cardiomyopathy. *J Clin Invest* 1999; **103**: R39–R43.

15 Poetter K, Jiang H, Hassanzadeh S *et al.* Mutations in either the essential or regulatory light chains of myosin are associated with a rare myopathy in human heart and skeletal muscle. *Nat Genet* 1996; **13**: 63–9.

16 Satoh M, Takahashi M, Sakamoto T *et al.* Structural analysis of the titin gene in hyper-trophic cardiomyopathy: Identification of a novel disease gene. *Biochem Biophys Res Commun* 1999; **262**: 411–17.

17 Watkins H, Seidman CE, Seidman JG *et al.* Expression and functional assessment of a truncated cardiac troponin T that causes hypertrophic cardiomyopathy. Evidence for a dominant negative action. *J Clin Invest* 1996; **98**: 2456–61.

18 Maron BJ, Gardin JM, Flack JM *et al.* Prevalence of hypertrophic cardiomyopathy in a general population of young adults—echocardiographic analysis of 4111 subjects in the CARDIA study. *Circulation* 1995; **92**: 785–9.

19 Olson TM, Michels VV, Thibodeau SN *et al.* Actin mutations in dilated cardiomyopathy, a heritable form of heart failure. *Science* 1998; **280**: 750–2.

20 Kamisago M, Sharma SD, DePalma SR *et al.* Mutations in sarcomere protein genes as a cause of dilated cardiomyopathy. *N Engl J Med* 2000; **343**: 1688–96.

21 Rayment I, Holden HM, Whittaker M *et al.* Structure of the actin–myosin complex and its implications for muscle contraction. *Science* 1993; **261**: 58–65.

22 Filatov VL, Katrukha AG, Bulargina TV, Gusev NB. Troponin: Structure, properties, and mechanism of functioning. *Biochemistry (Mosc.)* 1999; **64**: 969–85.

23 MacKrill JJ. Protein-protein interactions in intracellular Ca2+-release channel function. *Biochem J* 1999; **337**: 345–61.

24 Hamada H, Petrino MG, Kakunaga T. Molecular structure and evolutionary origin of human cardiac muscle actin gene. *Proc Natl Acad Sci USA* 1982; **79**: 5901–5.

25 Olson TM, Doan TP, Kishimoto NY, Whitby FG, Ackerman MJ, Fananapazir L. Inherited and de novo mutations in the cardiac actin gene cause hypertrophic cardiomyopathy. *J Mol Cell Cardiol* 2000; **32**: 1687–94.

26 Mogensen J, Kruse TA, Borglum AD. Refined localization of the human alpha-tropo-myosin gene (TPM1) by genetic mapping. *Cytogenet Cell Genet* 1999; **84**: 35–6.

27 Schultheiss T, Lin ZX, Lu MH *et al.* Differential distribution of subsets of myofibrillar proteins in cardiac nonstriated and striated myofibrils. *J Cell Biol* 1990; **110**: 1159–72.

28 Watkins H, Anan R, Coviello DA, Spirito P, Seidman JG, Seidman CE. A de novo muta-tion in alpha-tropomyosin that causes hypertrophic cardiomyopathy. *Circulation* 1995; **91**: 2302–5.

29 Yamauchi-Takihara K, Nakajima-Taniguchi C, Matsui H *et al.* Clinical implications of hypertrophic cardiomyopathy associated with mutations in the alpha-tropomyosin gene. *Heart* 1996; **76**: 63–5.

30 Coviello DA, Maron BJ, Spirito P *et al*. Clinical features of hypertrophic cardiomyopathy caused by mutation of a 'hot spot' in the alpha-tropomyosin gene. *J Am Coll Cardiol* 1997; **29**: 635–40.

31 Jaaskelainen P, Soranta M, Miettinen R *et al*. The cardiac beta-myosin heavy chain gene is not the predominant gene for hypertrophic cardiomyopathy in the Finnish population. *J Am Coll Cardiol* 1998; **32**: 1709–16.

32 Bottinelli R, Coviello DA, Redwood CS *et al*. A mutant tropomyosin that causes hypertrophic cardiomyopathy is expressed in vivo and associated with an increased calcium sensitivity. *Circ Res* 1998; **82**: 106–15.

33 Anderson PA, Greig A, Mark TM *et al*. Molecular basis of human cardiac troponin T isoforms expressed in the developing, adult, and failing heart. *Circ Res* 1995; **76**: 681–6.

34 Forissier JF, Carrier L, Farza H *et al*. Codon 102 of the cardiac troponin T gene is a putative hot spot for mutations in familial hypertrophic cardiomyopathy. *Circulation* 1996; **94**: 3069–73.

35 Moolman JC, Corfield VA, Posen B *et al*. Sudden death due to troponin T mutations. *J Am Coll Cardiol* 1997; **29**: 549–55.

36 Nakajima-Taniguchi C, Matsui H, Fujio Y, Nagata S, Kishimoto T, Yamauchi-Takihara K. Novel missense mutation in cardiac troponin T gene found in Japanese patient with hypertrophic cardiomyopathy. *J Mol Cell Cardiol* 1997; **29**: 839–43.

37 Anan R, Greve G, Thierfelder L *et al*. Prognostic implications of novel beta cardiac myosin heavy chain gene mutations that cause familial hypertrophic cardiomyopathy. *J Clin Invest* 1994; **93**: 280–5.

38 Ho CY, Lever HM, DeSanctis R, Farver CF, Seidman JG, Seidman CE. Homozygous mutation in cardiac troponin T: Implications for hypertrophic cardiomyopathy. *Circulation* 2000; **102**: 1950–5.

39 Mogensen J, Kruse TA, Borglum AD. Assignment of the human cardiac troponin I gene (TNNI3) to chromosome 19q13.4 by radiation hybrid mapping. *Cytogenet Cell Genet* 1997; **79**: 272–3.

40 Sata M, Stafford WF 3rd, Mabuchi K, Ikebe M. The motor domain and the regulatory domain of myosin solely dictate enzymatic activity and phosphorylation-dependent regulation, respectively. *Proc Natl Acad Sci USA* 1997; **94**: 91–6.

41 Saez LJ, Gianola KM, McNally EM *et al*. Human cardiac myosin heavy chain genes and their linkage in the genome. *Nucleic Acids Res* 1987; **15**: 5443–59.

42 Watkins H, Rosenzweig A, Hwang DS *et al*. Characteristics and prognostic implications of myosin missense mutations in familial hypertrophic cardiomyopathy. *N Engl J Med* 1992; **326**: 1108–14.

43 Fananapazir L, Dalakas MC, Cyran F, Cohn G, Epstein ND. Missense mutations in the beta-myosin heavy-chain gene cause central core disease in hypertrophic cardiomyopathy. *Proc Natl Acad Sci USA* 1993; **90**: 3993–7.

44 Marian AJ, Roberts R. The molecular genetic basis for hypertrophic cardiomyopathy. *J Mol Cell Cardiol* 2001; **33**: 655–70.

45 Seidman JG, Seidman C. The genetic basis for cardiomyopathy: From mutation identification to mechanistic paradigms. *Cell* 2001; **104**: 557–67.

46 Niimura H, Bachinski LL, Sangwatanaroj S *et al*. Mutations in the gene for cardiac myosin-binding protein C and late-onset familial hypertrophic cardiomyopathy. *N Engl J Med* 1998; **338**: 1248–57.

47 Epstein ND, Cohn GM, Cyran F, Fananapazir L. Differences in clinical expression of hypertrophic cardiomyopathy associated with two distinct mutations in the beta-myosin

heavy chain gene. A 908Leu–Val mutation and a 403Arg–Gln mutation. *Circulation* 1992; **86**: 345–52.

48 Freiburg A, Gautel M. A molecular map of the interactions between titin and myosin-binding protein C. Implications for sarcomeric assembly in familial hypertrophic cardiomyopathy. *Eur J Biochem* 1996; **235**: 317–23.

49 Carrier L, Bonne G, Bahrend E, Yu B *et al.* Organization and sequence of human cardiac myosin binding protein C gene (MYBPC3) and identification of mutations predicted to produce truncated proteins in familial hypertrophic cardiomyopathy. *Circ Res* 1997; **80**: 427–34.

50 Bonne G, Carrier L, Bercovici J *et al.* Cardiac myosin binding protein-C gene splice acceptor site mutation is associated with familial hypertrophic cardiomyopathy. *Nat Genet* 1995; **11**: 438–40.

51 Charron P, Dubourg O, Desnos M *et al.* Clinical features and prognostic implications of familial hypertrophic cardiomyopathy related to the cardiac myosin-binding protein C gene. *Circulation* 1998; **97**: 2230–6.

52 Niimura H, Patton KK, McKenna WJ *et al.* Sarcomere protein gene mutations in hypertrophic cardiomyopathy of the elderly. *Circulation* 2002; **105**: 446–51.

53 Nakao K, Minobe W, Roden R, Bristow MR, Leinwand LA. Myosin heavy chain gene expression in human heart failure. *J Clin Invest* 1997; **100**: 2362–70.

54 Schiaffino S, Reggiani C. Molecular diversity of myofibrillar proteins: Gene regulation and functional significance. *Physiol Rev* 1996; **76**: 371–423.

55 Nadal-Ginard B, Mahdavi V. Molecular basis of cardiac performance. Plasticity of the myocardium generated through protein isoform switches. *J Clin Invest* 1989; **84**: 1693–700.

56 Kretsinger RH. Structure and evolution of calcium-modulated proteins. *CRC Crit Rev Biochem* 1980; **8**: 119–74.

57 Lowey S, Waller GS, Trybus KM. Skeletal muscle myosin light chains are essential for physiological speeds of shortening. *Nature* 1993; **365**: 454–6.

58 VanBuren P, Waller GS, Harris DE, Trybus KM, Warshaw DM, Lowey S. The essential light chain is required for full force production by skeletal muscle myosin. *Proc Natl Acad Sci USA* 1994; **91**: 12403–7.

59 Sweeney HL, Feng HS, Yang Z, Watkins H. Functional analyses of troponin T mutations that cause hypertrophic cardiomyopathy: Insights into disease pathogenesis and troponin function. *Proc Natl Acad Sci USA* 1998; **95**: 14406–10.

60 Redwood CS, Moolman-Smook JC, Watkins H. Properties of mutant contractile proteins that cause hypertrophic cardiomyopathy. *Cardiovasc Res* 1999; **44**: 20–36.

61 Tyska MJ, Hayes E, Giewat M, Seidman CE, Seidman JG, Warshaw DM. Single-molecule mechanics of R403Q cardiac myosin isolated from the mouse model of familial hypertrophic cardiomyopathy. *Circ Res* 2000; **86**: 737–44.

62 Becker KD, Gottshall KR, Hickey R, Perriard JC, Chien KR. Point mutations in human beta cardiac myosin heavy chain have differential effects on sarcomeric structure and assembly: An ATP binding site change disrupts both thick and thin filaments, whereas hypertrophic cardiomyopathy mutations display normal assembly. *J Cell Biol* 1997; **137**: 131–40.

63 Sweeney HL, Straceski AJ, Leinwand LA, Tikunov BA, Faust L. Heterologous expression of a cardiomyopathic myosin that is defective in its actin interaction. *J Biol Chem* 1994; **269**: 1603–5.

64 Fujita H, Sugiura S, Momomura S, Omata M, Sugi H, Sutoh K. Characterization of mutant myosins of Dictyostelium discoideum equivalent to human familial hypertrophic

cardiomyopathy mutants. Molecular force level of mutant myosins may have a prognostic implication. *J Clin Invest* 1997; **99**: 1010–15.

65 Bonne G, Carrier L, Richard P, Hainque B, Schwartz K. Familial hypertrophic cardiomyopathy: From mutations to functional defects. *Circ Res* 1998; **83**: 580–93.

66 Roberts R, Sigwart U. New concepts in hypertrophic cardiomyopathies, Part I. *Circulation* 2001; **104**: 2113–16.

67 Blanchard E, Seidman C, Seidman JG, LeWinter M, Maughan D. Altered crossbridge kinetics in the alphaMHC403/+ mouse model of familial hypertrophic cardiomyopathy. *Circ Res* 1999; **84**: 475–83.

68 Cuda G, Fananapazir L, Epstein ND, Sellers JR. The in vitro motility activity of beta-cardiac myosin depends on the nature of the beta-myosin heavy chain gene mutation in hypertrophic cardiomyopathy. *J Muscle Res Cell Motil* 1997; **18**: 275–83.

69 Sata M, Ikebe M. Functional analysis of the mutations in the human cardiac beta-myosin that are responsible for familial hypertrophic cardiomyopathy. Implication for the clinical outcome. *J Clin Invest* 1996; **98**: 2866–73.

70 Palmiter KA, Tyska MJ, Haeberle JR, Alpert NR, Fananapazir L, Warshaw DM. R403Q and L908V mutant beta-cardiac myosin from patients with familial hypertrophic cardiomyopathy exhibit enhanced mechanical performance at the single molecule level. *J Muscle Res Cell Motil* 2000; **21**: 609–20.

71 Geisterfer-Lowrance AA, Christe M, Conner DA *et al.* A mouse model of familial hypertrophic cardiomyopathy. *Science* 1996; **272**: 731–4.

72 Berul CI, Christe ME, Aronovitz MJ, Seidman CE, Seidman JG, Mendelsohn ME. Electrophysiological abnormalities and arrhythmias in alpha MHC mutant familial hypertrophic cardiomyopathy mice. *J Clin Invest* 1997; **99**: 570–6.

73 Spindler M, Saupe KW, Christe ME *et al.* Diastolic dysfunction and altered energetics in the alphaMHC403/+ mouse model of familial hypertrophic cardiomyopathy. *J Clin Invest* 1998; **101**: 1775–83.

74 Molkentin JD, Lu JR, Antos CL *et al.* A calcineurin-dependent transcriptional pathway for cardiac hypertrophy. *Cell* 1998; **93**: 215–28.

75 Fatkin D, McConnell BK, Mudd JO *et al.* An abnormal Ca(2+) response in mutant sarcomere protein-mediated familial hypertrophic cardiomyopathy. *J Clin Invest* 2000; **106**: 1351–9.

76 Oberst L, Zhao G, Park JT *et al.* Dominant-negative effect of a mutant cardiac troponin T on cardiac structure and function in transgenic mice. *J Clin Invest* 1998; **102**: 1498–505.

77 Marian AJ, Wu Y, Lim DS *et al.* A transgenic rabbit model for human hypertrophic cardiomyopathy. *J Clin Invest* 1999; **104**: 1683–92.

78 Yang Q, Sanbe A, Osinska H, Hewett TE, Klevitsky R, Robbins J. In vivo modeling of myosin binding protein C familial hypertrophic cardiomyopathy. *Circ Res* 1999; **85**: 841–7.

79 Muthuchamy M, Pieples K, Rethinasamy P *et al.* Mouse model of a familial hypertrophic cardiomyopathy mutation in alpha-tropomyosin manifests cardiac dysfunction. *Circ Res* 1999; **85**: 47–56.

80 Georgakopoulos D, Christe ME, Giewat M, Seidman CM, Seidman JG, Kass DA. The pathogenesis of familial hypertrophic cardiomyopathy: Early and evolving effects from an alpha-cardiac myosin heavy chain missense mutation. *Nat Med* 1999; **5**: 327–30.

81 Tardiff JC, Hewett TE, Palmer BM *et al.* Cardiac troponin T mutations result in allele-specific phenotypes in a mouse model for hypertrophic cardiomyopathy. *J Clin Invest* 1999; **104**: 469–81.

82 Frey N, Franz WM, Gloeckner K *et al.* Transgenic rat hearts expressing a human cardiac troponin T deletion reveal diastolic dysfunction and ventricular arrhythmias. *Cardiovasc Res* 2000; **47**: 254–64.

83 Nagueh SF, Kopelen HA, Lim DS *et al.* Tissue Doppler imaging consistently detects myocardial contraction and relaxation abnormalities, irrespective of cardiac hypertrophy, in a transgenic rabbit model of human hypertrophic cardiomyopathy. *Circulation* 2000; **102**: 1346–50.

84 Nagueh SF, Bachinski LL, Meyer D *et al.* Tissue Doppler imaging consistently detects myocardial abnormalities in patients with hypertrophic cardiomyopathy and provides a novel means for an early diagnosis before and independently of hypertrophy. *Circulation* 2001; **104**: 128–30.

85 Ho CY, Sweitzer NK, McDonough B *et al.* Assessment of diastolic function with Doppler tissue imaging to predict genotype in preclinical hypertrophic cardiomyopathy. *Circulation* 2002; **105**: 2992–7.

86 Spirito P, Seidman CE, McKenna WJ, Maron BJ. The management of hypertrophic cardiomyopathy. *N Engl J Med* 1997; **336**: 775–85.

87 Rosenzweig A, Watkins H, Hwang DS *et al.* Preclinical diagnosis of familial hypertrophic cardiomyopathy by genetic analysis of blood lymphocytes. *N Engl J Med* 1991; **325**: 1753–60.

88 Vikstrom KL, Factor SM, Leinwand LA. Mice expressing mutant myosin heavy chains are a model for familial hypertrophic cardiomyopathy. *Mol Med* 1996; **2**: 556–67.

89 Charron P, Carrier L, Dubourg O *et al.* Penetrance of familial hypertrophic cardiomyopathy. *Genet Couns* 1997; **8**: 107–14.

90 Maron BJ, Casey SA, Gohman TE, Aeppli DM. Impact of gender on the clinical and morphologic expression of hypertrophic cardiomyopathy [abstract]. *Circulation* 1999; **100** (Suppl. 1): Abstract 1098.

91 Solomon SD, Wolff S, Watkins H *et al.* Left ventricular hypertrophy and morphology in familial hypertrophic cardiomyopathy associated with mutations of the beta-myosin heavy chain gene. *J Am Coll Cardiol* 1993; **22**: 498–505.

92 Nishi H, Kimura A, Harada H *et al.* Possible gene dose effect of a mutant cardiac beta-myosin heavy chain gene on the clinical expression of familial hypertrophic cardiomyopathy. *Biochem Biophys Res Commun* 1994; **200**: 549–56.

93 Semsarian C, Healey MJ, Fatkin D *et al.* A polymorphic modifier gene alters the hypertrophic response in a murine model of familial hypertrophic cardiomyopathy. *J Mol Cell Cardiol* 2001; **33**: 2055–60.

94 Marian AJ, Yu QT, Workman R, Greve G, Roberts R. Angiotensin-converting enzyme polymorphism in hypertrophic cardiomyopathy and sudden cardiac death. *Lancet* 1993; **342**: 1085–6.

95 Tesson F, Dufour C, Moolman JC *et al.* The influence of the angiotensin I converting enzyme genotype in familial hypertrophic cardiomyopathy varies with the disease gene mutation. *J Mol Cell Cardiol* 1997; **29**: 831–8.

96 Marian AJ. Modifier genes for hypertrophic cardiomyopathy. *Curr Opin Cardiol* 2002; **17**: 242–52.

97 Ortlepp JR, Vosberg HP, Reith S *et al.* Genetic polymorphisms in the renin–angiotensin–aldosterone system associated with expression of left ventricular hypertrophy in hypertrophic cardiomyopathy: A study of five polymorphic genes in a family with a disease causing mutation in the myosin binding protein C gene. *Heart* 2002; **87**: 270–5.

98 Brugada R, Kelsey W, Lechin M et al. Role of candidate modifier genes on the phenotypic expression of hypertrophy in patients with hypertrophic cardiomyopathy. *J Investig Med* 1997; **45**: 542–51.

99 Seidman C. Genetic causes of inherited cardiac hypertrophy: Robert L. Frye Lecture. *Mayo Clin Proc* 2002; **77**: 1315–19.

100 Anan R, Shono H, Kisanuki A, Arima S, Nakao S, Tanaka H. Patients with familial hypertrophic cardiomyopathy caused by a Phe110Ile missense mutation in the cardiac troponin T gene have variable cardiac morphologies and a favorable prognosis. *Circulation* 1998; **98**: 391–7.

101 Van Driest SL, Ackerman MJ, Ommen SR et al. Prevalence and severity of 'benign' mutations in the beta-myosin heavy chain, cardiac troponin T, and alpha-tropomyosin genes in hypertrophic cardiomyopathy. *Circulation* 2002; **106**: 3085–90.

102 Fananapazir L, Tracy CM, Leon MB et al. Electrophysiologic abnormalities in patients with hypertrophic cardiomyopathy. A consecutive analysis in 155 patients. *Circulation* 1989; **80**: 1259–68.

103 Blair E, Redwood C, Ashrafian H et al. Mutations in the gamma(2) subunit of AMP-activated protein kinase cause familial hypertrophic cardiomyopathy: Evidence for the central role of energy compromise in disease pathogenesis. *Hum Mol Genet* 2001; **10**: 1215–20.

104 Gollob MH, Green MS, Tang AS et al. Identification of a gene responsible for familial Wolff-Parkinson-White syndrome. *N Engl J Med* 2001; **344**: 1823–31.

105 Francesconi M, Auff E. Cardiac arrhythmias and the adult form of type II glycogenosis. *N Engl J Med* 1982; **306**: 937–8.

106 Holmes BF, Kurth-Kraczek EJ, Winder WW. Chronic activation of 5'-AMP-activated protein kinase increases GLUT-4, hexokinase, and glycogen in muscle. *J Appl Physiol* 1999; **87**: 1990–5.

107 Bergeron R, Russell RR 3rd, Young LH et al. Effect of AMPK activation on muscle glucose metabolism in conscious rats. *Am J Physiol* 1999; **276**: E938–44.

108 Seidman CE, Seidman JG. Hypertrophic cardiomyopathy. In: Scriver CR, Beaudet AL, Valle D et al., eds. *The Metabolic and Molecular Bases of Inherited Disease*. New York: McGraw-Hill, 2000: 5433–52.

109 Jones WK, Grupp IL, Doetschman T et al. Ablation of the murine alpha myosin heavy chain gene leads to dosage effects and functional deficits in the heart. *J Clin Invest* 1996; **98**: 1906–17.

110 Tardiff JC, Factor SM, Tompkins BD et al. A truncated cardiac troponin T molecule in transgenic mice suggests multiple cellular mechanisms for familial hypertrophic cardiomyopathy. *J Clin Invest* 1998; **101**: 2800–11.

111 McConnell BK, Jones KA, Fatkin D et al. Dilated cardiomyopathy in homozygous myosin-binding protein-C mutant mice. *J Clin Invest* 1999; **104**: 1235–44.

112 Rethinasamy P, Muthuchamy M, Hewett TE et al. Molecular and physiological effects of alpha-tropomyosin ablation in the mouse. *Circ Res* 1998; **82**: 116–23.

CHAPTER 3

Genetic Basis and Genotype–Phenotype Relationships in Familial Hypertrophic Cardiomyopathy

Albert A. Hagège, MD, PhD, Ketty Schwartz, PhD, Michel Desnos, MD, and Lucie Carrier, PhD

Knowledge about hypertrophic cardiomyopathy (HCM) has been established through three consecutive historical phases: the clinical description of the disease (1898–1958), the genetic approach with the individualization of familial HCM (FHCM) (since 1989),[1] and the studies of the relationships between genotype and phenotype in FHCM (since 1992). A familial history is found in approximately two-thirds of patients. In others, HCM is sporadic, which is due also in part to mutations that arise *de novo*. Therefore, sporadic cases are genetic and transmit the mutation and the disease to their offspring. The transmission is mainly autosomal dominant with incomplete and age-dependent penetrance. The study of the consequences for the phenotype of different morbid mutations marks the transition from science to medicine. This is a recent challenge and could have important clinical consequences.

Genetic basis

Morbid genes and mutations

None of the previous pathogenic hypotheses have predicted that defects in genes encoding contractile proteins could be the cause of the disease. Linkage analysis provided the first evidence for genetic heterogeneity, with sequential discovery of disease loci on chromosome 14q11,[1] 1q32,[2] 15q22[3] and 11p11-q13.[4] The first demonstration that human mutations in the genes for β-myosin heavy chain (β-MyHC),[5] cardiac troponin T (cTnT),[6] α-tropomyosin (α-TM)[6] and cardiac myosin-binding protein C (cMyBP-C)[7,8] occurred at these chromosomal loci led to the conclusion that FHCM is a disease of the sarcomere.[9,10] Thereafter, mutations in the essential (MLC-1) and regulatory (MLC-2) myosin light chains,[11,12] cardiac α-actin,[13] cardiac troponin I (cTnI),[14] titin,[15] and probably cardiac troponin C (cTnC; only one case reported)[16] were found as rare causes of FHCM. These genes (Table 3.1) certainly do not represent the whole spectrum of FHCM disease genes, and one might reasonably hypothesize that disease genes yet to be identified include additional components of the sarcomere. Indeed, one FHCM patient was recently reported as presenting a muta-

Table 3.1 Disease genes and proteins involved in familial hypertrophic cardiomyopathy (FHCM)

Protein	Gene	Locus	Reference
Pure form of FHCM			
β-Myosin heavy chain (β-MyHC)	MYH7	*CMH1* 14q11-q12	Geisterfer-Lowrance *et al.* (1990)[5]
α-Myosin heavy chain (α-MyHC)	MYH6	*CMH10* 14q11-q12	Patton *et al.* (2000)[17]
Ventricular essential myosin light chain (MLC-1s/v)	MYL3	*CMH5* 3p	Poetter *et al.* (1996)[11]
Ventricular regulatory myosin light chain (MLC-2s/v)	MYL2	*CMH6* 12q23-q24.3	Poetter *et al.* (1996)[11] Flavigny *et al.* (1998)[12]
α-Cardiac actin (α-cAct)	ACTC	*CMH8* 15q14	Mogensen *et al.* (1999)[13]
Cardiac troponin T (cTnT)	TNNT2	*CMH2* 1q32	Thierfelder *et al.* (1994)[6]
Cardiac troponin I (cTnI)	TNNI3	*CMH7* 19p13.4	Kimura *et al.* (1997)[14]
Cardiac troponin C (cTnC)	TNNC1	*CMH11*	Hoffmann *et al.* (2001)[16]
α-Tropomyosin (α-TM)	TPM1	*CMH3* 15q22.1	Thierfelder *et al.* (1994)[6]
Cardiac myosin-binding protein C (cMyBP-C)	MYBPC3	*CMH4* 11p11.2	Bonne *et al.* (1995)[7] Watkins *et al.* (1995)[8]
Titin	TTN	*CMH9* 2q24.3	Satoh *et al.* (1999)[15]
FHCM associated with Wolff–Parkinson– White syndrome			
γ$_2$ subunit of AMP-activated protein kinase	PRKAG2	*CMH11* 7q36	Blair *et al.* (2001);[18] Gollob *et al.* (2001)[19]

tion in the α-myosin heavy chain gene, which is located in tandem with the β-MyHC gene on chromosome 14.[17] In addition to these 'pure' forms of FHCM, mutations in the γ$_2$-subunit of the AMP-activated protein kinase have been shown to be involved in families with FHCM plus the Wolff–Parkinson–White syndrome.[18,19] Besides the large locus heterogeneity, there is wide allelic heterogeneity, because at least 143 mutations have been found in the different genes and entered in the FHCM database (Table 3.2).[20] The two major genes appear to be the β-MyHC (around 35% of patients) and cMyBP-C (at least 20% of patients) genes. Mutations of the β-MyHC, cMyBP-C and cTnT genes account for about two-thirds of all cases of FHCM, but it should be noted that in previous reports not necessarily all the genes were screened. Most of the FHCM mutations are missense mutations or small deletions that do not disrupt the reading frame, with the exception of the cMyBP-C gene, in which most are frame-shift mutations, i.e., splice-site mutations, insertions, or deletions. Genetic studies have allowed the identification of patients with double mutations who develop a more severe form of the disease – patients who are compound heterozygous for β-MyHC mutations,[21,22] double heterozygous for β-MyHC and cMyBP-C

Table 3.2 Distribution of the familial hypertrophic cardiomyopathy database mutations. From the DNA Mutation Database web site (http://morgan.angis.su.oz.au/Databases/Heart/heartbreak.html)

Gene locus	Number of mutations	Number of missense mutations or deletions in frame	Number of frameshift or nonsense mutations
MYH7	70	67	3
MYBPC3	30	8	22
TNNT2	14	13	1
MYL2	8	7	1
TNNI3	8	8	–
ACTC	5	5	–
TPM1	5	5	–
MYL3	2	2	–
TTN	1	1	–

mutations,[23] or homozygous for mutations of β-MyHC[24] or cTnT.[25] In addition, a detailed analysis of a *de novo* mutation in a French family led to the first description of germ-line mosaicism in FHCM.[26] This mosaicism had been inherited by the mother but did not affect her somatic cells.

Functional consequences

FHCM is caused by a structural and/or functional impairment of the sarcomere, which is the contractile unit of striated muscle (Fig. 3.1, Table 3.2). The sarcomeric proteins are organized into thick and thin filaments, which account for the microscopic appearance of cross-striations in striated muscle cells. Contraction occurs by sliding of the thick and thin filaments. The sar-

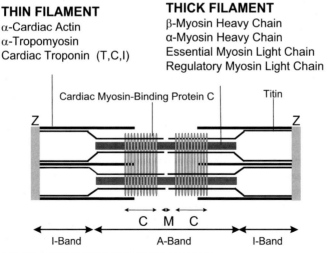

THIN FILAMENT
α-Cardiac Actin
α-Tropomyosin
Cardiac Troponin (T,C,I)

THICK FILAMENT
β-Myosin Heavy Chain
α-Myosin Heavy Chain
Essential Myosin Light Chain
Regulatory Myosin Light Chain

Cardiac Myosin-Binding Protein C   Titin

Z   Z

C   M   C

I-Band   A-Band   I-Band

Fig. 3.1 Localization of the FHCM proteins in the sarcomere.

comeric gene mutations may also be associated with either the transition between HCM and dilated cardiomyopathy[27] or with primary dilated cardiomyopathy.[28,29] This finding suggests that the position of the mutated amino acid triggers the development of either HCM (by impaired force generation) or dilated cardiomyopathy (by impaired force transmission).

The molecular mechanism by which the mutations lead to FHCM has not been completely elucidated. It is generally accepted that FHCM can be explained by either the production of a poison polypeptide that interferes with normal protein function (a dominant negative mechanism) or the inactivation of an allele resulting in a reduced amount of functional protein (haploinsufficiency). One of the major problems in our understanding of the molecular mechanisms of FHCM has been the difficulty in obtaining cardiac endomyocardial tissue from affected patients. Nevertheless, the incorporation of the mutant protein *in vivo* has been demonstrated for two missense mutations, the Arg[403]Gln β-MyHC and the Asp[175]Asn α-TM mutations. The first could be distinguished in extracts from skeletal muscle because it induces the loss of an arginine-specific endoproteinase digest site,[30] and the second as it exhibits a specific electrophoretic band.[31] This 'poison polypeptide' hypothesis has been also demonstrated by several *in vitro*, *ex vivo* and *in vivo* analyses in which missense mutations produce stable polypeptides that are incorporated into the sarcomere and produce functional impairment and/or sarcomere disassembly.[9,10] The mechanisms by which the frameshift mutations lead to FHCM are not understood well because neither the truncated protein nor a decrease in the wild-type protein was detected in the myocardial tissue of two patients with cMyBP-C mutations.[32,33] However, several *ex vivo* analyses and mouse transgenic models have shown that truncated proteins are present in the sarcomere and may act as poison polypeptides in a dominant negative manner, at least on the structure of the sarcomere.[34,38]

Genotype–phenotype correlations

Aims
There is a complex relationship between a genotype and a particular phenotype in families with HCM sharing the same mutation or different mutations of the same morbid gene. Studies have essentially tried to differentiate families with benign or malignant mutations [short or near-normal life expectancy, occurrence of sustained ventricular tachycardia, sudden cardiac death (SCD), congestive heart failure, the need for transplantation or implantation of a cardiac defibrillator]. Moreover, they assessed the mutation-specific clinical features [distribution and degree of left ventricular hypertrophy (LVH), atrial fibrillation] and penetrance of the disease (Table 3.3).

Techniques
Correlations are based on studies of the genotyped families and the establishment of a clinical diagnosis (examination, ECG, echocardiography) and a fol-

Table 3.3 Summary of the genotype–phenotype relations in familial hypertrophic cardiomyopathy. DCM = dilated cardiomyopathy; LV = left ventricle; SCD = sudden cardiac death; VT = ventricular tachycardia; WPW, Wolff–Parkinson–White syndrome

Gene	Penetrance	LVH	SCD
β-MyHC	Variable	Moderate/severe	Variable
MyBP-C	Low penetrance, late onset	Usually mild	Usually low
cTnT	Lethal (young male)	Mild/absent	Frequent
α-TM	Low penetrance DCM-like pattern	Mild or absent	Often frequent (VT)
cTnI	DCM-like pattern High penetrance	Moderate Apical or typical	Variable
MYL3/MYL2	Skeletal myopathy	Mid-LVH + obstruction	?
α-Actin	High penetrance	Apical LVH + obstruction	?

low-up study for each of the relatives. Genetic status is beginning to be used as the criterion of reference to reassess diagnostic criteria and penetrance. The diagnosis of FHCM is usually based on ECG and echocardiography, and it is generally accepted that echocardiography is a more accurate technique than ECG for diagnosis in adults. However, analysis of a large genotyped population showed that, in adults, ECG and echocardiography have similar diagnostic values for FHCM, with excellent specificity but lower sensitivity.[39] Proposed diagnosis criteria for the disease in family relatives of a propositus with HCM are defined by consensus, using echocardiography [major criterion: maximal wall thickness (LVWT) of at least one left ventricular segment >13 mm on two-dimensional echographic views; minor criterion: LVWT = 13 mm] and ECG [major criteria: pathologic Q waves, LVH, major ST-T changes; minor criteria: left atrial hypertrophy, small q waves, short PR interval, microvoltage, bundle block branch].[39] The prognosis linked to morbid mutations on the more frequent causal genes has been extensively studied.

β-MyHC gene mutations
Some mutations are classified as malignant ($Arg^{403}Gln$, $Arg^{453}Cys$, $Arg^{719}Trp$), and are characterized by high penetrance, early onset of symptoms, severe LVH and a high incidence of SCD at a young age (mean 40 years) or heart failure ($Arg^{719}Gln$). Others are classified as benign ($Gly^{256}Glu$, $Val^{606}Met$, $Leu^{908}Val$), with low penetrance, late onset of symptoms, mild LVH, near-normal life expectancy and a low incidence of SCD (<2% at 50 years).[40,41] Initially, studies showed a correlation between the prognosis and the degree of LVH.[42]

However, the Arg[723]Cys mutation in the β-MyHC gene, for example, causes marked LVH [mean maximal wall thickness (LVWT) 20 mm] without decreasing life expectancy, while the Arg[719]Trp mutation causes moderate LVH (LVWT 15 mm) and has 75% survival at 40 years (and a mean age of death of 36 years).[43] Similarly, the Arg[403]Leu mutation causes only mild LVH, with 42% survival at 50 years (mean age of death 38 years), while the Arg[403]Trp mutation causes more severe LVH, but 100% survival at 50 years.[44] Finally, the Arg[869]Gly mutation causes mild LVH while the Arg[663]His mutation causes marked LVH, both with nearly normal life expectancy and frequent atrial fibrillation.[24,45] The complexity of the relationships between genotype and prognosis is underlined by numerous publications. (1) The Arg[403]Gln and Leu[908]Val mutations, which were reported in US families, carry identical morphologic appearances but highly different penetrances (100 vs 61% respectively in adults by echography and ECG) and incidences of SCD (40 vs 4% respectively).[46] (2) Even if the Arg[403]Gln mutation is in general malignant, it has been reported as benign in a Korean family with neither SCD nor syncope, underlining the influence of the genetic background on the phenotypic expression of a mutation.[41] (3) Moreover, although the Val[606]Met mutation is benign in most families with low penetrance and low incidence of SCD[47,48], it has been considered as malignant in others, with full penetrance and a 50% incidence of SCD before 30 years.[41,49,50]

MyBP-C gene mutations

Two large observational studies involve mutations on the MyBP-C gene. The first includes nine families with seven mutations.[14] When compared with families with β-MHC mutations, the phenotype appears similar but there is milder LVH (12 vs 16 mm), a better prognosis, with no deaths before 40 years, delayed onset (41 vs 35 years) and lower penetrance in adults before 30 years (41 vs 62%).[51] However, some mutations (SASint20A or SASint7) carry a higher mortality rate (survival >50% at 60 years).[51] A second study includes 15 families with 13 mutations.[52] It underlines the broad spectrum of phenotypes, the low incidence of SCD (although it was present in 4/15 families) and the fact that protein truncation mutations show earlier manifestations (33 vs 49 years), more frequent invasive procedures (septal ablation or implantation of a cardiac defibrillator), delayed onset and low penetrance when compared with missense mutations or in-frame deletions.[52]

cTnT gene mutations

Mutations of the cTnT gene may or may not cause LVH, which is variable in degree but is usually mild, with a high incidence of SCD (64% at 28 years in males for the Arg[92]Trp mutation[53] and 80% before 45 years for the Arg[94]Leu mutation).[54] For five mutations (Arg[92]Gln, Ile[79]Asn, Ala[104]Val, Glu[160]del, Intron15G1-A), average life expectancy is only 35 years, with a 35% incidence in SCD.[55] Penetrance is variable by ECG (66–100%) and low by echography (0–40%).[53,54] However, the Phe[110]Ile mutation carries a lower risk of SCD (about 10%) and higher penetrance (>80%),[55] and the prognosis is also good for the Ser[179]Phe mutation.

cTnI gene mutations

The Lys[183]deletion has been studied extensively. Penetrance is high in adults (around 90% by echography or ECG)[56] with moderate LVH (14 mm), there is great variability in distribution between and within families (apical LVH or typical forms may occur in the same family) and SCD could occur at any age between 10 and 70 years in 4/7 families.[15] Moreover, left ventricular dysfunction with wall thinning is frequent, occurring in almost half of patients after 40 years (dilated cardiomyopathy-like forms in one-fifth of cases).[56]

α-TM gene mutations

Five mutations were described, all carrying mild LVH, low penetrance (about 50% for the V95A mutation),[57] an overall poor prognosis with sustained ventricular tachycardia and SCD,[3,27,57,58] and frequent progression towards the dilated form with wall thinning.[58] However, one benign mutation has also been described.[59]

Other morbid genes

Alpha-cardiac actin mutations carry a high penetrance, with apical LVH and/or subaortic obstruction.[14,60] *MYL3* (ventricular essential myosin light chain) gene mutations have various degrees of penetrance and a classical morphologic form.[61] *MYL2* (ventricular regulatory myosin light chain) gene mutations cause obstruction, with mid-ventricular[12] or classical forms[13] of LVH. Skeletal myopathy has been associated with these mutations. Moreover, it has been recently suggested that mutations in the CRP3 gene, encoding for the muscle LIM protein (MLP), which is an essential nuclear regulator of myogenic differentiation, can also cause HCM.[76]

Penetrance

Genetic studies have revealed the presence of clinically healthy individuals carrying a mutant allele (healthy carriers) that is associated in first-degree relatives with a typical phenotype of the disease. This situation is well known for children, in whom LVH may appear as they grow up, but was thought to be uncommon in adults. In adult healthy carriers, clinical and echocardiographic (and less frequently ECG) examinations are normal and the prognosis is usually benign (no SCD), except for cTnT mutations.[55] Recent studies have shown that these subjects represent 20–50% of the adult relatives with the mutation, depending on the morbid mutation.[62,63] The high incidence of healthy carriers has been particularly underlined for the MyBP-C mutations.[51,52,62,63] Penetrance in these subjects decreases with age and is incomplete until 60 years.[63] The frequency of a normal echocardiogram has been reported to be high (between 25%[64] and 42%[63]) particularly in adults (47% after 18 years,[62] 40% between 18 and 29 years,[51] 35% at 20–39 years).[64] These subjects may sometimes develop LVH as adults, as shown in three out of five patients (age >25 years) with a normal echocardiographic examination at inclusion and who exhibited development of LVH in mid-life without obstruction or symptoms and preceded by ECG abnormalities.[64] In cases of β-MyHC mutations, penetrance is usually higher in adults: as high as 90%.[44,63] In cases of cTnT mutations, penetrance is usually low (about 50%) between 20 and 30 years but increases with age.[63] Finally, it is a striking fact that penetrance varies not only with the morbid gene but also for different mutations within the same gene.[51]

Molecular basis

The initial hypothesis—that non-conservative mutations (which, after substitution of an amino acid, change the net electrical charge of the sarcomeric protein) are malignant and that conservative mutations are benign—is not supported by observation studies. For example, the Arg[453]Cys mutation in the β-MyHC gene is malignant whereas the Arg[403]Gln mutation is benign, but neither of them changes the net electrical charge of the mutant protein. A gene dose effect (the influence of the relative quantities of mutant and wild proteins) is supported by the fact that homozygous mutations lead to more severe disease: the Arg[869]Gly mutation of the β-MyHC gene causes severe disease in the young, frequent atrial fibrillation and dilated cardiomyopathy-like forms,[24] and the Ser[179]Phe and the Phe[110]Ile mutations on the cTnT gene occur in the young, causing severe LVH and right ventricular hypertrophy with a high frequency of SCD.[25,65] Similarly, the coexistence of double heterozygosity (morbid mutations of β-MyHC and MyBP-C) causes marked LVH.[23]

Limitations

The causes of the complexity of the correlations between genotype and phenotype are multiple: genetic and clinical heterogeneity of the disease; unpublished and unknown, spontaneous mutations; the low frequency of known mutations (often less than 5%, or a 'private' mutation is limited to one single family); the small size of genotyped families, who come from different countries (influence of the genetic background on the phenotype); limited and retrospective follow-up; interference by therapeutic interventions (myectomy and dilated forms, amiodarone and SCD); and the influence of environmental factors (competitive sports, blood pressure or alcoholic ingestion) and of other genetic factors. It is now well established that genetic factors, named as modifier genes, may modulate the phenotypic expression of FHCM induced by the causal major gene mutations. For example, for the same mutation, the extent of LVH varies not only among members of different families but also among members of each family. The major significant results obtained so far concern the influence of the angiotensin I converting enzyme insertion/deletion (I/D) polymorphism. Association studies showed that, compared with a control population, the D allele is more common in patients with HCM and in patients with a high incidence of sudden cardiac death.[66–68] It was also shown that the association between the D allele and the severity of LVH is observed in patients with a *MYH7* R403 codon mutation, but not in *MYBPC3* mutation carriers,[69] raising the concept of multiple genetic modifiers in FHCM. Variants of endothelin-1 and tumor necrosis factor-α were also found to be modulators of cardiac hypertrophy.[70,71] However, these variants account in general for less than 5% of the variability of LVH.[66,70] Gender also influences the phenotype. In a large French genotyped population, penetrance is incomplete, age-related and greater in males than in females.[72] This has very important implications for genetic counseling, especially for women under the age of 50. One of the transgenic mouse models of FHCM also shows a gender difference[73] and now provides a good genetic model with which to look for a direct role of sexual hormones in the myocardium and to study the role of putative modifier genes on the sex chromosomes.

Potential interests

The potential clinical interests of the phenotype–genotype correlation studies are the following: diagnosis (familial screening, preclinical diagnosis) and clinical description (penetrance, ECG/echo patterns); prognosis (functional status, life expectancy); genetic counseling (pregnancy); and clinical counseling (physical activities, adequate therapy with amiodarone, implantation of a cardiac defibrillator). However, in current clinical practice the interest of genotype–phenotype relationships in FHCM remains limited. Such information could perhaps aid in the management of patients by facilitating the determination of a morbid mutation in a non-genotyped family, although there is no gene-specific phenotype. It would also be useful for risk stratification despite the fact that clinical genotyping is generally unavailable at present. However, only 1% of a cohort of unrelated HCM patients seen at a tertiary referral center possessed one of the five malignant mutations that were routinely tested on the β-MyHC or cTnT gene,[74] while the prevalence of eight 'benign' mutations in the β-MyHC, cTNT and α-TM genes was found to be only 1.7% (5 out of 293 patients, all of whom had a severe form of the disease).[75] These findings hinder the future widespread application of genetic testing in HCM.

Summary

FHCM is an extremely heterogeneous disease that is associated in its pure form with mutations in genes encoding proteins of the contractile apparatus. Morbid mutations affect the phenotypic expression of hypertrophic cardiomyopathy, although there is no phenotype locus-specific for the disease. Some mutations confer a high risk and others do not, but the prognosis may differ between families with similar mutations. Moreover, there is great variability in expression (symptoms, ECG, degree/distribution of LVH) for a given mutation between and within families. In the near future, the objective should be to identify new (major or modifier) genes involved in FHCM and to reach a better understanding of the molecular mechanisms by which mutations lead to the disease. The analyses of human endomyocardial tissue, *ex vivo* and *in vitro* studies, and the development of animal models by the use of a homologous recombination strategy will help in investigations of the pathogenesis of human FHCM mutations.

References

1 Jarcho JA, McKenna W, Pare JAP *et al.* Mapping a gene for familial hypertrophic cardio-myopathy to chromosome 14ql. *N Engl J Med* 1989; **321**: 1372–8.
2 Watkins H, MacRae C, Thierfelder L *et al.* A disease locus for familial hypertrophic car-diomyopathy maps to chromosome 1q3. *Nat Genet* 1993; **3**: 333–7.
3 Thierfelder L, MacRae C, Watkins H *et al.* A familial hypertrophic cardiomyopathy locus maps to chromosome 15q2. *Proc Natl Acad Sci USA* 1993; **90**: 6270–4.
4 Carrier L, Hengstenberg C, Beckmann JS *et al.* Mapping of a novel gene for familial hy-pertrophic cardiomyopathy to chromosome 11. *Nat Genet* 1993; **4**: 311–13.
5 Geisterfer-Lowrance AAT, Kass S, Tanigawa G *et al.* A molecular basis for familial hyper-trophic cardiomyopathy: A β cardiac myosin heavy chain gene missense mutation. *Cell* 1990; **62**: 999–1006.
6 Thierfelder L, Watkins H, MacRae C *et al.* Alpha-tropomyosin and cardiac troponin T mutations cause familial hypertrophic cardiomyopathy: A disease of the sarcomere. *Cell* 1994; **77**: 701–12.
7 Bonne G, Carrier L, Bercovici J *et al.* Cardiac myosin binding protein-C gene splice ac-ceptor site mutation is associated with familial hypertrophic cardiomyopathy. *Nat Genet* 1995; **11**: 438–40.
8 Watkins H, Conner D, Thierfelder L *et al.* Mutations in the cardiac myosin binding pro-tein-C gene on chromosome 11 cause familial hypertrophic cardiomyopathy. *Nat Genet* 1995; **11**: 434–7.
9 Bonne G, Carrier L, Richard P *et al.* Familial hypertrophic cardiomyopathy: From muta-tions to functional defects. *Circ Res* 1998; **83**: 579–593.
10 Seidman JG, Seidman CE. The genetic basis for cardiomyopathy: From mutation identifi-cation to mechanistic paradigms. *Cell* 2001; **104**: 557–67.
11 Poetter K, Jiang H, Hassanzadeh S *et al.* Mutation in either the essential or regulatory light chains of myosin are associated with a rare myopathy in human heart and skeletal muscle. *Nat Genet* 1996; **13**: 63–9.
12 Flavigny J, Richard P, Isnard R *et al.* Identification of two novel mutations in the ventricu-lar regulatory myosin light chain gene (MYL2) associated with familial and classical forms of hypertrophic cardiomyopathy. *J Mol Med* 1998; **76**: 208–14.
13 Mogensen J, Klausen IC, Pedersen AK *et al.* Alpha-cardiac actin is a novel disease gene in familial hypertrophic cardiomyopathy. *J Clin Invest* 1999; **103**: R39–R43.
14 Kimura A, Harada H, Park JE *et al.* Mutations in the cardiac troponin I gene associated with hypertrophic cardiomyopathy. *Nat Genet* 1997; **16**: 379–82.
15 Satoh M, Takahashi M, Sakamoto T *et al.* Structural analysis of the titin gene in hypertro-phic cardiomyopathy: Identification of a novel disease gene. *Biochem Biophys Res Commun* 1999; **262**: 411–17.
16 Hoffmann B, Schmidt-Traub H, Perrot A *et al.* First mutation in cardiac troponin C, L29Q, in a patient with hypertrophic cardiomyopathy. *Hum Mutat* 2001; **17**: 524.
17 Patton KK, Niimura H, Soults J *et al.* Sarcomere protein gene mutations: A frequent cause of elderly-onset hypertrophic cardiomyopathy. *Circulation* 2000; **102** (Suppl. II): 178.
18 Blair E, Redwood C, Ashrafian H *et al.* Mutations in the γ2-subunit of AMP-activated pro-tein kinase cause familial hypertrophic cardiomyopathy: Evidence for the central role of energy compromise in disease pathogenesis. *Hum Mol Genet* 2001; **10**: 1215–20.
19 Gollob MH, Green MS, Tang ASL *et al.* Identification of a gene responsible for familial Wolff–Parkinson–White syndrome. *N Engl J Med* 2001; **344**: 1823–64.

20 Fung DC, Yu B, Littlejohn T *et al*. An online locus-specific mutation database for familial hypertrophic cardiomyopathy. *Hum Mutat* 1999; **14**: 326–32.

21 Nishi H, Kimura A, Harada H *et al*. Possible gene dose effect of a mutant cardiac β-myosin heavy chain gene on the clinical expression of familial hypertrophic cardiomyopathy. *Biochem Biophys Res Commun* 1994; **200**: 549–56.

22 Jeschke B, Uhl K, Weist B *et al*. A high risk phenotype of hypertrophic cardiomyopathy associated with a compound genotype of two mutated β-myosin heavy chain genes. *Hum Genet* 1998; **102**: 299–304.

23 Richard P, Isnard R, Carrier L *et al*. Double heterozygosity for mutations in the beta myosin heavy chain and in the cardiac myosin binding protein C genes in a family with hypertrophic cardiomyopathy. *J Med Genet* 1999; **36**: 542–5.

24 Richard P, Charron P, Leclercq C *et al*. Homozygotes for a R869G mutation in the beta-myosin heavy chain gene have a severe form of familial hypertrophic cardiomyopathy. *J Mol Cell Cardiol* 2000; **32**: 1575–83.

25 Ho CY, Lever HM, DeSanctis R *et al*. Homozygous mutation in cardiac troponin T. Implications for hypertrophic cardiomyopathy. *Circulation* 2000; **102**: 1950–5.

26 Forissier J-F, Richard P, Briault S *et al*. First description of a germ line mosaicism in familial hypertrophic cardiomyopathy. *J Med Genet* 2000; **37**: 132–4.

27 Regitz-Zagrosek V, Erdmann J, Wellnhofer E *et al*. Novel mutation in the α-tropomyosin gene and transition from hypertrophic to hypocontractile dilated cardiomyopathy. *Circulation* 2000; **102**: e112–6.

28 Olson TM, Michels VV, Thibodeau SN *et al*. Actin mutations in dilated cardiomyopathy, a heritable form of heart failure. *Science* 1998; **280**: 750–2.

29 Kamisago M, Sharma SD, DePalma SR *et al*. Mutations in sarcomere protein genes as a cause of dilated cardiomyopathy. *N Engl J Med* 2000; **343**: 1688–96.

30 Cuda G, Fananapazir L, Zhu WS *et al*. Skeletal muscle expression and abnormal function of β-myosin in hypertrophic cardiomyopathy. *J Clin Invest* 1993; **91**: 2861–5.

31 Bottinelli R, Coviello DA, Redwood CS *et al*. A mutant tropomyosin that causes hypertrophic cardiomyopathy is expressed in vivo and associated with increased calcium sensitivity. *Circ Res* 1998; **82**: 106–15.

32 Rottbauer W, Gautel M, Zehelein J *et al*. Novel splice donor site mutation in the cardiac myosin-binding protein-C gene in familial hypertrophic cardiomyopathy. Characterization of cardiac transcript and protein. *J Clin Invest* 1997; **100**: 475–82.

33 Moolman JA, Reith S, Uhl K *et al*. A newly created splice donor site in exon 25 of the MyBP-C gene is responsible for inherited hypertrophic cardiomyopathy with incomplete disease penetrance. *Circulation* 2000; **101**: 1396–402.

34 Yang Q, Sanbe A, Osinska H *et al*. A mouse model of myosin binding protein C human familial hypertrophic cardiomyopathy. *J Clin Invest* 1998; **102**: 1292–300.

35 Flavigny J, Souchet M, Sébillon P *et al*. COOH-terminal truncated cardiac myosin-binding protein C mutants resulting from familial hypertrophic cardiomyopathy mutations exhibit altered expression and/or incorporation in fetal rat cardiomyocytes. *J Mol Biol* 1999; **294**: 443–56.

36 Yang Q, Sanbe A, Osinska H *et al*. In vivo modeling of myosin binding protein C familial hypertrophic cardiomyopathy. *Circ Res* 1999; **85**: 841–7.

37 McConnell BK, Fatkin D, Semsarian C *et al*. Comparison of two murine models of familial hypertrophic cardiomyopathy. *Circ Res* 2001; **88**: 383–9.

38 Sebillon P, Bonne G, Flavigny J *et al*. COOH-terminal truncated human cardiac MyBP-C alters myosin filament organization. *C R Acad Sci* 2001; **324**: 251–60.

39 Charron P, Dubourg O, Desnos M *et al.* Diagnostic value of electrocardiography and echocardiography for familial hypertrophic cardiomyopathy in a genotyped adult population. *Circulation* 1997; **96** : 214–19.

40 Ko YL, Chen JJ, Tang TK *et al.* Malignant familial hypertrophic cardiomyopathy in a family with a Arg453Cys mutation in the β-myosin heavy chain gene: Coexistence of sudden death and end-stage heart failure. *Hum Gen* 1996; **97**: 585–90.

41 Fananapazir L, Epstein ND. Genotype–phenotype correlations in hypertrophic cardiomyopathy: Insights provided by comparisons of kindreds with distinct and identical β-myosin heavy chain gene mutations. *Circulation* 1994; **89** : 22–32.

42 Abchee A, Marian AJ. Prognostic significance of beta-myosin heavy chain mutations is reflective of their hypertrophic expressivity in patients with hypertrophic cardiomyopathy. *J Invest Med* 1997; 45: 191–6.

43 Tesson F, Richard P, Charron P *et al.* Genotype–phenotype analysis in four families with mutations in beta-myosin heavy chain gene responsible for familial hypertrophic cardiomyopathy. *Hum Mutat* 1998; **12** : 385–92.

44 Charron P, Dubourg O, Desnos M *et al.* Genotype–phenotype correlations in familial hypertrophic cardiomyopathy. A comparison between mutations in the cardiac protein C and the β-myosin heavy chain genes. *Eur Heart J* 1998; **19** : 139–45.

45 Gruver EJ, Fatkin D, Dodds GA *et al.* Familial hypertrophic cardiomyopathy and atrial fibrillation caused by Arg663His β-cardiac myosin heavy chain mutation. *Am J Cardiol* 1999; **83** (12A): 13H–18H.

46 Epstein ND, Cohn GM, Cyran F *et al.* Difference in clinical expression of hypertrophic cardiomyopathy associated with two distinct mutations in the β-myosin heavy chain gene: A Leu908Val mutation and an Arg403Gly mutation. *Circulation* 1992; **86**: 345–52.

47 Watkins H, McKenna WJ, Thierfelder L *et al.* Mutations in the genes for cardiac troponin T and α-tropomyosin in hypertrophic cardiomyopathy. *N Engl J Med* 1995; **332**: 1058–64.

48 Marian AJ, Mares A Jr, Kelly DP *et al.* Sudden cardiac death in familial hypertrophic cardiomyopathy. Variability in phenotypic expression of β-myosin heavy chain mutations. *Eur Heart J* 1995; **16**: 368–76.

49 Havndrup O, Bundgaard H, Andersen PS *et al.* The Val606Met mutation in the cardiac β-myosin heavy chain gene in patients with familial hypertrophic cardiomyopathy is associated with a high risk of sudden death at young age. *Am J Cardiol* 2001; **87**: 1315–17.

50 Semsarian C, Yu B, Ryce C, Lawrence C *et al.* Sudden cardiac death in familial hypertrophic cardiomyopathy: Are 'benign' mutations really benign? *Pathology* 1997; **29** : 305–8.

51 Charron P, Dubourg O, Desnos M *et al.* Clinical features and prognostic implications of familial hypertrophic cardiomyopathy related to the cardiac myosin-binding protein C gene. *Circulation* 1998; **97**: 2230–6.

52 Erdmann J, Raible J, Maki-Abadi J *et al.* Spectrum of clinical phenotypes and gene variants in cardiac myosin-binding protein C mutation carriers with hypertrophic cardiomyopathy. *J Am Coll Cardiol* 2001; **38**: 322–30.

53 Moolman JC, Corfield VA, Posen B *et al.* Sudden death due to troponin T mutations. *J Am Coll Cardiol* 1997; **29** : 549–55.

54 Varnava A, Baboonian C, Davison F *et al.* A new mutation of the cardiac troponin T gene causing familial hypertrophic cardiomyopathy without left ventricular hypertrophy. *Heart* 1999; **82** : 621–4.

55 Anan R, Shono H, Kisanuki A *et al.* Patients with familial hypertrophic cardiomyopathy caused by a Phe[110]Ile missense mutation in the cardiac troponin T gene have variable cardiac morphologies and a favorable prognosis. *Circulation* 1998; **98** : 391–7.

56 Kokado H, Shimizu M, Yoshio H *et al.* Clinical features of hypertrophic cardiomyopathy caused by a Lys183 deletion mutation in the cardiac troponin I gene.*Circulation* 2000; **102**: 663–9.

57 Karibe A, Tobacman LS, Strand J *et al.* Hypertrophic cardiomyopathy caused by a novel α-tropomyosin mutation (V95A) is associated with mild cardiac phenotype, abnormal calcium binding to troponin, abnormal myosin cycling and poor prognosis. *Circulation* 2001; **103**: 65–71.

58 Yamauchi-Takihara K, Nakajima-Taniguchi C, Matsui H *et al.* Clinical implications of hypertrophic cardiomyopathy associated with mutations in the α-tropomyosin gene. *Heart* 1996; **76**: 63–5.

59 Coviello DA, Maron BJ, Spirito P *et al.* Clinical features of hypertrophic cardiomyopathy caused by mutation of a 'hot spot' in the α-tropomyosin gene. *J Am Coll Cardiol* 1997; **29**: 635–40.

60 Mogensen J, Klausen IC, Pedersen AK *et al.* Alpha-cardiac actin is a novel disease gene in familial hypertrophic cardiomyopathy. *J Clin Invest* 1999; **103**: R39–43.

61 Lee W, Hwang TH, Kimura A *et al.* Different expressivity of a ventricular essential myosin light chain gene Ala57Gly mutation in familial hypertrophic cardiomyopathy. *Am Heart J* 2001; **141**: 184–9.

62 Hagège AA, Dubourg O, Desnos M *et al.* Familial hypertrophic cardiomyopathy. Cardiac ultrasonic abnormalities in genetically affected subjects without echocardiographic evidence of left ventricular hypertrophy. *Eur Heart J* 1998; **19**: 490–9.

63 Niimura H, Bachinski LL, Sangwatanaroj S *et al.* Mutations in the gene for human cardiac myosin-binding protein C and late-onset familial hypertrophic cardiomyopathy. *N Engl J Med* 1998; **338**: 1248–57.

64 Maron BJ, Niimura H, Casey SA *et al.* Development of left ventricular hypertrophy in adults with hypertrophic cardiomyopathy caused by cardiac myosin-binding protein C gene mutations. *J Am Coll Cardiol* 2001; **38**: 315–21.

65 Lin T, Ichihara S, Yamada Y *et al.* Phenotypic variation of familial hypertrophic cardiomyopathy caused by the Phe(110)Ile mutation in cardiac troponin T. *Cardiology* 2000; **93**: 155–62.

66 Marian AJ, Yu Q-T, Workman R *et al.* Angiotensin-converting enzyme polymorphism in hypertrophic cardiomyopathy and sudden cardiac death. *Lancet* 1993; **342**: 1085–6.

67 Lechin M, Quinones MA, Omran A *et al.* Angiotensin-I converting enzyme genotypes and left ventricular hypertrophy in patients with hypertrophic cardiomyopathy. *Circulation* 1995; **92**: 1802–12.

68 Yonega K, Okamoto H, Machida M *et al.* Angiotensin-converting enzyme gene polymorphism in Japanese patients with hypertrophic cardiomyopathy. *Am Heart J* 1995; **130**: 1089–93.

69 Tesson F, Dufour C, Moolman JC *et al.* The influence of the angiotensin I converting enzyme genotype in familial hypertrophic cardiomyopathy varies with the disease gene mutation. *J Mol Cell Cardiol* 1997; **29**: 831–8.

70 Brugada R, Kelsey W, Lechin M *et al.* Role of candidate modifier genes on the phenotypic expression of hypertrophy in patients with hypertrophic cardiomyopathy. *J Investig Med* 1997; **45**: 542–51.

71 Patel R, Lim DS, Reddy D *et al.* Variants of trophic factors and expression of cardiac hypertrophy in patients with hypertrophic cardiomyopathy. *J Mol Cell Cardiol* 2000; **32**: 2369–677.

72 Charron P, Carrier L, Dubourg O *et al.* Penetrance of familial hypertrophic cardiomyopathy. *Genet Couns* 1997; **8**: 107–14.

73 Vikstrom KL, Factor SM, Leinwand LA. Mice expressing mutant myosin heavy chains are a model for familial hypertrophic cardiomyopathy. *Mol Med* 1996; **2**: 556–67.

74 Ackerman MJ, VanDriest SL, Ommen SR *et al.* Prevalence and age-dependence of malignant mutations in the beta-myosin heavy chain and troponin T gene in hypertrophic cardiomyopathy: A comprehensive outstanding perspective. *J Am Coll Cardiol* 2002; **39**: 2049–51.

75 Van Driest BA, Ackerman MJ, Ommen SR *et al.* Prevalence and severity of 'benign' mutations in the β-myosin heavy chain, cardiac troponin T and α-tropomyosin genes in hypertrophic cardiomyopathy. *Circulation* 2002; **106**: 3085.

76 Geier C, Perrot A, Özcelik C *et al.* Mutations in the human muscle LIM protein gene in families with hypertrophic cardiomyopathy. *Circulation* 2003; **107**: 1390–5.

CHAPTER 4

Historical Perspective, Mechanism, and Clinical Significance of Left Ventricular Outflow Tract Obstruction in Hypertrophic Cardiomyopathy

Martin S. Maron, MD, Iacopo Olivotto, MD, and Barry J. Maron, MD

Introduction

Since the initial descriptions of hypertrophic cardiomyopathy (HCM) 45 years ago, left ventricular (LV) outflow tract obstruction has been a prominent and quantifiable feature of the disease.[1-23] However, throughout the history of the disease, dynamic outflow obstruction has been an aspect of HCM that has generated much confusion and, at times, heated controversy.[8,15,18-20] Periodically, the very existence of mechanical impedance as the etiology of obstruction has been a source of continued debate.[15,18-20] This is evident in the constellation of names that have described HCM as either an obstructive or nonobstructive disease.[4]

Our understanding of the pathophysiology and mechanism of obstruction has evolved greatly over the years, and we have arrived today at a pivotal junction with respect to our knowledge and treatment of this unique feature of HCM. However, the relationship between outflow obstruction and clinical events, such as progression to heart failure symptoms and sudden death, has until recently remained in part unresolved. Previous studies addressing the clinical significance of outflow tract obstruction in HCM have been relatively small, with sometimes conflicting data.[4,6-11] Recently, however, a large multicenter retrospective study clarified the relationship between obstruction and the clinical course in patients with HCM.[21] These data and their impact on the treatment of patients with obstructive HCM are the subject of the present discussion.

Historical perspectives

The introduction of intracardiac hemodynamic monitoring in the late 1950s led to the initial description of outflow tract gradients in patients with HCM.

In the cardiac catheterization laboratory, through direct puncture of the left ventricle, Dr Russell Brock described a series of patients with a murmur suggestive of aortic stenosis and a pressure gradient between the LV and peripheral artery.[22,23] On autopsy, most of these patients were found to be free of valve disease (as well as the absence of a subaortic band), but nevertheless were noted to have extreme septal hypertrophy. This led Brock, in 1957, to conclude that a 'functional obstruction' of the subaortic area was present but that its etiology was unclear. Brock proposed that the mechanism for this 'functional obstruction' was massive hypertrophy of the LV (secondary to hypertension) causing systolic cavity obliteration.[19,22,23] The idea that ventricular muscular hypertrophy was a cause of pressure gradients inspired the early surgical treatment of obstructive HCM for the relief of outflow obstruction. During the same period, Dr Donald Teare (a British pathologist and coroner of London) published the first autopsy report of the modern era, describing nine patients with asymmetric septal hypertrophy and sudden death.[24] The explanation for this pathologic process of myocardial hypertrophy was thought to be a 'benign tumour' of the heart. Obviously, the possibility of linking the patients of both Brock and Teare under a single disease entity was unlikely at the time, given the absence on autopsy of an obvious anatomical cause of the etiology of outflow obstruction.

Throughout the early 1960s, a substantial number of reports regarding patients with dynamic pressure gradients without an identifiable anatomical cause for subaortic obstruction were noted in the world literature. The idea that a yet to be identified 'muscular contraction ring' was responsible for these pressure gradients led to a nomenclature describing the disease as both obstructive and nonobstructive. In 1964, Braunwald and colleagues published the seminal monograph from the National Institutes of Health describing in detail 64 patients with idiopathic hypertrophic subaortic stenosis.[1] This study, unprecedented in scope and detail, included left heart catheterization with physiologic and pharmacologic challenges, intracardiac hemodynamic recordings, and selective ventriculograms. For the first time, the scope and magnitude of the dynamic nature of the outflow tract gradient was described in relation to a multitude of interventions. This eventually led to our understanding of the classic maneuvers that may alter the pressure gradient. However, during this period, the validity of catheter-derived pressure gradients (and therefore the presence of elevated LV pressures) was challenged. The concept of 'catheter entrapment', whereby catheters in the LV cavity were thought to be embedded in the ventricular wall, thereby reflecting only artificially elevated intramyocardial pressures (and not true intracavitary pressures), was proposed to explain the high LV pressures being recorded.[18–20] However, by documenting elevated pressures and gradients by the placement of catheters also in the submitral area by transeptal approach (an area of LV unaffected by cavity obliteration), this hypothesis was refuted.[16]

In the late 1960s, with the advent of M-mode echocardiography, the muscular contraction ring which had been considered the anatomic cause of subaortic obstruction up to this time was replaced with systolic anterior motion (SAM) of the mitral valve.[25] The 1970s brought further technologic advances in imaging, including the advent of two-dimensional echocardiography, which for the first time allowed a more precise diagnosis of HCM based on asymmetric distribution of LV hypertrophy as well as direct visualization of SAM and its contact with the ventricular septum in real time.[26–31] In addition, Doppler-derived outflow tract velocities were used to estimate in quantitative terms the pressure gradient noninvasively.[14] As a result, echocardiography eventually supplanted cardiac catheterization for the serial hemodynamic evaluation of patients with HCM.

Interestingly, the advent of echocardiography did not eliminate controversy concerning the etiology of pressure gradients in HCM. The concept of systolic 'cavity obliteration' has been proposed to challenge the established notion that dynamic gradients are produced by a true mechanical impedance due to SAM–septal contact. The theory of cavity obliteration is based on the idea that the initial rapid contraction of the ventricle produces such a substantial ejection of blood in early systole that in the later phases of systole there remains little of the stroke volume to be obstructed.[11] Therefore, it was proposed that 'as the LV cavity becomes smaller, the body and outflow tract of the ventricle become progressively isolated from one another, and a pressure difference develops between these two areas. These two regions are not separated by obstruction but by the tightly opposed walls of the essentially empty ventricle below.'[15,19,20] However, it has subsequently been shown that a significant proportion of the forward stroke volume remains in the LV cavity at the time of SAM–septal contact and therefore true mechanical impedance to outflow occurs.

In addition, perhaps the strongest circumstantial evidence that the mechanical impedance created by SAM–septal contact is responsible for clinically significant outflow gradients is 40 years of surgical experience in the treatment of obstructive HCM. Ventricular septal myectomy has been performed at experienced surgical centers with excellent outcomes (as well as low mortality), resulting in the abolition of SAM–septal contact and outflow gradient, normalization of LV systolic pressures and, most importantly, dramatic improvement in clinical symptoms.[31–33]

Mechanism of obstruction

With the advent of echocardiography in the early 1970s, it became evident that LV outflow tract obstruction in HCM was predominantly due to SAM of the mitral leaflets making contact with the ventricular septum[25–31] (Fig. 4.1). In most instances the anterior leaflet of the mitral valve is responsible for septal contact, but SAM, preferentially of the posterior leaflet, occurs in about 5% of obstructive patients.[26,27] The occurrence of SAM–septal contact creates a pressure gradient between the LV and outflow tract that is easily quantifiable noninvasively by continuous-wave Doppler echocardiography.[14] Using the modified Bernoulli equation, Doppler-derived outflow tract velocities can

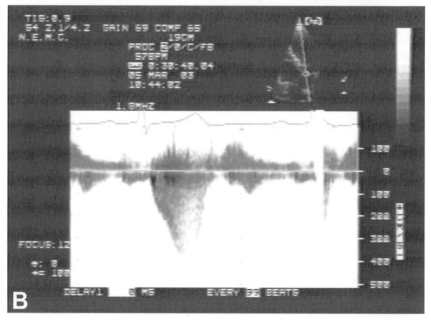

Fig. 4.1 Left ventricular outflow obstruction in hypertrophic cardiomyopathy. (**A**) Parasternal long-axis image obtained in mid-systole showing systolic anterior motion (SAM) of the anterior mitral leaflet making a sharp right-angled bend and contact with the hypertrophied basal ventricular septum (VS). (**B**) Continuous-wave Doppler recording through the left ventricular outflow tract, demonstrating a waveform with typical late-peaking mid-systolic configuration and 4 m/s velocity (estimated gradient, 64 mm Hg).

be converted to estimated pressure gradients. It is important to note that, in contrast to aortic stenosis, which is a fixed anatomic obstruction, SAM–septal contact is a dynamic process. As a result, at any one point in time the magnitude of the pressure gradient is dependent on a variety of loading conditions. Examples include the classic physiologic maneuvers or conditions that accentuate the gradient by decreased filling of the LV (Valsalva strain, hypovolemia), decreased aortic impedance, or increased contractile states (inotropic drugs, postextrasystolic beats). In contrast, interventions and conditions that decrease gradient include increased filling of the LV (leg raising, squatting or volume expansion), increased aortic impedance and decreased contractile states (negative inotropic drugs). In addition, ingestion of heavy meals or even moderate amounts of alcohol have been shown to acutely increase gradients by more than 50% from baseline.[12,13]

The mechanism by which SAM–septal contact occurs is the source of continued controversy. To date, two pathophysiologic explanations have been proposed: the Venturi effect and drag forces.[29,31] We do not know which of these mechanisms is primarily responsible for the generation of outflow tract obstruction in HCM, and most likely both are present to some extent concurrently in individual patients. Regardless, it is important to emphasize that there are a number of morphologic and hemodynamic variables unique to HCM that are necessary for either mechanism to produce obstruction. These include the following potential variables: hypertrophied basal anterior ventricular septum; decreased area of the LV outflow tract; increased ejection velocity; elongated mitral valve leaflets; and altered geometry of the papillary muscle–mitral valve apparatus. A number of these morphologic features can together create a structural milieu in the LV outflow tract that predisposes to the development of subaortic obstruction.[27–31]

The Venturi effect was initially proposed as the mechanism of outflow tract obstruction in HCM.[30] This theory is based on the concept that the hypertrophied basal septum creates a local under-pressure in the outflow tract that acts to suck the mitral valve anteriorly toward the septum. However, the Venturi concept fails to take into account the variety of other structural abnormalities that lead to obstruction, and therefore remains an incomplete explanation for all circumstances under which obstruction occurs. Thus, the Venturi phenomenon has largely been supplanted by the drag effect hypothesis.[31]

Appreciation of how the drag effect explains obstruction requires an understanding of the abnormalities of the papillary muscle–mitral valve apparatus in HCM. In most patients with HCM, the papillary muscles are hypertrophied and fused with the ventricular septum, each other, or the LV free wall. This leads to an abnormal anterior displacement of the mitral valve apparatus, permitting a significant portion of the mitral leaflet surface area to be exposed to blood flow in the LV outflow tract. In addition, the hypertrophied basal septum acts to redirect blood flow posteriorly and laterally, thereby creating an opportunity for this flow to 'catch' the mitral leaflet and 'drag' it toward the septum. As described by Sherrid and colleagues,[31] the initial occurrence of

SAM–mitral septal contact creates a new pressure difference between LV cavity and outflow tract, which in turn acts to further decrease the area of septal contact. This cascade of events creates an amplifying feedback loop that will further increase the gradient the longer there is mitral valve-septal contact; i.e., 'obstruction begets more obstruction.'[31] Pharmacologic therapy with negative inotropic agents (β-blockers, calcium channel blockers, and disopyramide) acts to decrease rapid acceleration of ejection, thereby delaying the onset of mitral–septal contact to later in systole. This lessens the time for the amplifying loop to occur in systole, thereby decreasing the outflow gradient.[34]

In the majority of obstructive HCM patients, the presence of mitral regurgitation is due to mitral leaflet incompetence secondary to SAM of the mitral valve. When mitral regurgitation is due to SAM, the regurgitant jet is usually mild to moderate (it is only occasionally severe) and posteriorly directed into the left atrium. The presence of severe mitral regurgitation with centrally projected jets is highly suggestive of intrinsic (primary) mitral valve disease. Septal myectomy greatly reduces or eliminates the presence of SAM-related mitral regurgitation. It was previously thought that mitral regurgitation due to intrinsic mitral valve disease was suitable only for prosthetic (low profile) mitral valve replacement, but experienced surgical centers have shown that myectomy alone, with or without mitral valve repair, is sufficient to abolish mitral regurgitation.[33]

Clinical data

Prior studies that assessed the relationship between LV outflow tract gradients and prognosis in HCM have been relatively small, have included highly selected patient populations, and have often reached contradictory conclusions.[6–11] These facts, as well as the continued controversy surrounding the clinical importance of outflow obstruction, provided the impetus for a recent multicenter retrospective analysis of the influence of basal LV outflow tract obstruction on clinical outcome in HCM.[21] This analysis consisted of 1101 consecutive HCM patients, initially evaluated by continuous-wave Doppler echocardiography, who were followed for an average of 6 years at three HCM centers in the USA and Italy. In this study, 25% of the study population had resting LV outflow tract obstruction (defined as a gradient ≥30 mm Hg) and 75% were considered nonobstructed (gradient <30 mm Hg). Only gradient measurements obtained under basal conditions were included in this study as it is not standard practice at the participating institutions to routinely and systematically measure provoked gradients. The three primary clinical end-points were: death related to HCM (sudden death or death as a consequence of heart failure or stroke); the combined end-point of death from heart failure or stroke and progression to severe symptoms in New York Heart Association (NYHA) functional classes III/IV; and sudden death alone. Patients with severe and marked obstructive symptoms who underwent invasive therapy (surgical myectomy or alcohol septal ablation) were censored from the analysis at the time of their intervention. Therefore, this study did not assess the effect of such treatment interventions on obstruction and prognosis.

Of note, patients with LV outflow obstruction were twice as likely as patients without obstruction to incur HCM-related death (relative risk, 2.0) (Fig. 4.2). When progression to NYHA classes III/IV and death from heart failure or stroke were analyzed together, patients with obstruction had more than a four-fold greater likelihood of reaching this combined primary end-point compared with patients without obstruction (relative risk, 4.4) (Fig. 4.3). In addition, those patients with obstruction and NYHA class II at study entry were more likely to progress to severe heart failure symptoms or heart failure or stroke death than asymptomatic obstructive patients or those patients without obstruction. Finally, patients with LV outflow obstruction who were 40 years of age or older had a significantly higher probability of progressing to severe heart failure symptoms or heart failure or stroke death than younger patients or those without obstruction (Fig. 4.4).

The probability of sudden cardiac death was greater in obstructive patients than in nonobstructive patients (Fig. 4.5). However, the overall annual sudden death rate in the cohort was low. Also, similar to other clinical markers previously identified to portend high risk for sudden death in HCM (i.e., nonsustained ventricular tachycardia on Holter, extreme LV hypertrophy ≥30 mm thickness, syncope, hypotensive blood pressure response to exercise, and a family history of HCM-related death), obstruction was associated with a

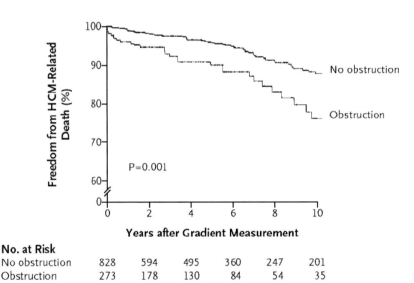

No. at Risk

No obstruction	828	594	495	360	247	201
Obstruction	273	178	130	84	54	35

Fig. 4.2 Probability of hypertrophic cardiomyopathy-related death among 273 patients with a left ventricular outflow gradient ≥30 mm Hg under basal conditions and 828 hypertrophic cardiomyopathy patients without obstruction at study entry. From Maron *et al.* Effect of left ventricular outflow tract obstruction on clinical outcome in hypertrophic cardiomyopathy. *N Engl J Med* 2003; **348**: 295–303, © 2003 Massachusetts Medical Society. All rights reserved.

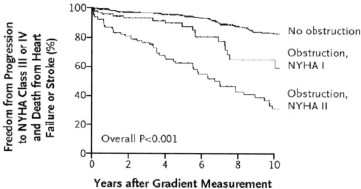

Fig. 4.3 Probability of progression to severe heart failure (NYHA classes III or IV) or death from heart failure or stroke among 224 hypertrophic cardiomyopathy patients with left ventricular outflow tract obstruction and 770 hypertrophic cardiomyopathy patients without obstruction. From Maron *et al.* Effect of left ventricular outflow tract obstruction on clinical outcome in hypertrophic cardiomyopathy. *N Engl J Med* 2003; **348**: 295–303, Copyright © 2003 Massachusetts Medical Society. All rights reserved.

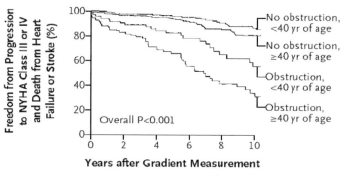

No. at Risk

No obstruction, <40 yr of age	349	251	206	146	103	80
No obstruction, ≥40 yr of age	421	306	258	188	128	108
Obstruction, <40 yr of age	106	70	52	37	21	15
Obstruction, ≥40 yr of age	118	74	51	29	18	10

Fig. 4.4 Effect of age and the presence or absence of left ventricular outflow tract obstruction ≥30 mm Hg on the probability of progression to severe heart failure (NYHA classes III or IV) or death from heart failure or stroke. Patients who were already in NYHA classes III or IV at entry were excluded from this analysis. From Maron *et al.* Effect of left ventricular outflow tract obstruction on clinical outcome in hypertrophic cardiomyopathy. *N Engl J Med* 2003; **348**: 295–303, © 2003 Massachusetts Medical Society. All rights reserved.

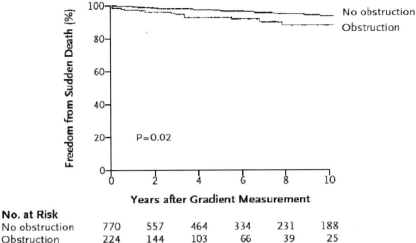

No. at Risk						
No obstruction	770	557	464	334	231	188
Obstruction	224	144	103	66	39	25

Fig. 4.5 Probability of sudden death among 224 hypertrophic cardiomyopathy patients with a left ventricular outflow tract gradient ≥30 mm Hg and 770 hypertrophic cardiomyopathy patients without obstruction. Patients who were already in NYHA classes III or IV at study entry were excluded from this analysis. From Maron *et al.* Effect of left ventricular outflow tract obstruction on clinical outcome in hypertrophic cardiomyopathy. *N Engl J Med* 2003; **348**: 295–303, © 2003 Massachusetts Medical Society. All rights reserved.

particularly low positive predictive value for sudden death (7%), although the negative predictive value was high (95%). Based on both this low annual event rate and low positive predictive value, at present there is insufficient evidence to consider outflow obstruction (gradient, ≥30 mm Hg) a sole, independent marker for future sudden cardiac death in HCM. Therefore, the decision to prophylactically implant an implantable cardioverter defibrillator in this disease should not be based only on the presence of LV outflow obstruction, but rather should still be considered in the framework of the previously defined high-risk clinical markers.

Increasing magnitude of outflow gradient (30–49 mm Hg; 50–69 mm Hg; ≥70 mm Hg) did not add to the likelihood of overall HCM-related death or progression to severe heart failure symptoms (Fig. 4.6). These results most likely reflect the dynamic nature of obstruction in HCM. Small gradients of 30 mm Hg or more at rest will most likely increase significantly to ≥50 mm Hg with physiologic exercise (conditions similar to those that generate symptoms in patients with HCM). Although these data show no difference in outcome with regard to the magnitude of the gradient, it is imperative to underscore that the traditional threshold for invasive interventions in patients with drug-refractory heart failure symptoms remains a gradient of at least 50 mm Hg (at rest or with physiologic provocation). Indeed, for symptomatic patients with minimal basal gradients, it remains the standard practice to document a gradient of ≥50 mm Hg with physiological provocation (i.e. the standard Bruce

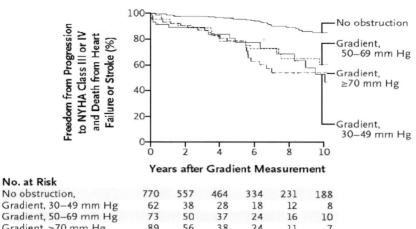

No. at Risk

No obstruction,	770	557	464	334	231	188
Gradient, 30–49 mm Hg	62	38	28	18	12	8
Gradient, 50–69 mm Hg	73	50	37	24	16	10
Gradient, ≥70 mm Hg	89	56	38	24	11	7

Fig. 4.6 Relation of the magnitude of left ventricular outflow tract gradient or the absence of a gradient to the probability of progression to severe heart failure (NYHA classes III or IV) or death from heart failure or stroke. $P < 0.001$ for the comparison of the patient group without obstruction with each patient subgroup with obstruction; $P > 0.30$ for each comparison among the subgroups with obstruction. Patients who were already in NYHA classes III or IV at study entry were excluded from this analysis. From Maron *et al.* Effect of left ventricular outflow tract obstruction on clinical outcome in hypertrophic cardiomyopathy. *N Engl J Med* 2003; **348**: 295–303, © 2003 Massachusetts Medical Society. All rights reserved.

treadmill exercise echocardiogram) prior to recommending septal myectomy or alcohol septal ablation to relieve obstruction.

These multicenter data show for the first time in a large cohort of prospectively enrolled HCM patients that LV outflow tract obstruction is a strong independent marker for progression to heart failure symptoms and mortality related to heart failure and stroke.[21] Since the effect of major treatments on the primary end-points were not assessed in this investigation, the extent to which therapeutic interventions such as septal myectomy alter the natural history of patients with outflow obstruction is not yet definitively resolved. However, a preliminary retrospective, nonrandomized longitudinal analysis of Mayo Clinic patients after surgical septal myectomy shows excellent long-term survival of 98, 96, and 88% at 5, 10, and 15 years, respectively. The survival of the operated patients was similar to the life expectancy of the general population and of nonobstructive patients, but superior to that of nonoperated patients with obstruction.

To what extent do these data affect the current treatment algorithm for symptomatic patients with obstructive HCM? The initial treatment option for all symptomatic patients with obstruction is an aggressive pharmacologic trial. Generally, β-blockers are considered first-line agents as these drugs are capable of blunting exertional gradients. If there is suboptimal symptom benefit with β-blockers, a calcium channel blocker such as verapamil can be substituted. Finally, if the previous two classes of drug therapy fail the third-line agent should be the class Ia anti-arrythmic agent disopyramide.[4,5,35] Traditionally, the subgroup of HCM patients who continue to have progressive, severe heart failure symptoms despite maximal medical management become candidates for surgical myectomy (or alcohol septal ablation) to relieve obstruction and improve symptoms.[35]

We do not, however, believe that the aforementioned obstruction data confer a sweeping alteration of these management strategies. Nonetheless, it may be reasonable to infer from these data that major interventions should be considered earlier and at a lower gradient cut-off than is current standard clinical practice. For example, instead of deferring interventions until particularly severe and disabling symptoms develop, it may be prudent to offer a strategy of somewhat earlier invasive treatment, especially in patients with long-standing gradients and relatively recent symptomatic progression. As always, the decision to offer surgery (or alcohol ablation) to any patient with obstructive HCM should be predicated on the balance between the risks of the procedure and the benefit that can be achieved in terms of quality of life for individual patients.[32,33,35]

The pathophysiology of progressive heart failure symptoms due to obstruction importantly involves the resultant elevation in LV systolic pressures. Such pressures will create increased LV wall stress and microvascular-based myocardial ischemia, which, over long periods of time, probably results in cell death and replacement scarring.[4,36–38] Such cellular changes lead to increased chamber stiffness, worsening of LV compliance, and eventually diastolic dysfunction with elevated LV filling pressures. Outflow obstruction is a disease feature that is usually present early in life. Therefore, if we assume that patient age approximates the duration of an individual's exposure to subaortic obstruction, then the available data showing increased progression to heart failure symptoms in patients aged 40 years or older is consistent with the hypothesis that longer periods of exposure to elevated LV systolic pressures are more deleterious. With regard to the relationship between sudden death and obstruction, it is possible that cellular remodeling that produces fibrosis and scarring also increases the electrical instability of the myocardium and creates a nidus for the generation of ventricular re-entry arrhythmias.[38]

Conclusions

The pathophysiology and clinical significance of LV outflow obstruction in HCM has been a source of controversy for almost 50 years. However, it is only recently that we have come to appreciate more precisely, and in a reasonably definitive fashion, the role obstruction plays within the context of HCM disease progression. The recent multicenter investigation of subaortic obstruction has unequivocally demonstrated for the first time that outflow obstruction is an important pathophysiologic feature of HCM, which, over extended periods of time, is an independent determinant of limiting symptoms and cardiovascular death. These data provide a strong foundation to legitimize the role of invasive treatment (such as septal myectomy), which has been part of the management strategies for obstructive HCM for over 40 years. Furthermore, long-term postoperative follow-up data showing that septal myectomy patients have a life expectancy that is similar to that of the general population (and superior to that of nonoperated obstructive patients) raises the possibility that surgery also has a survival benefit. Finally, as the clinical consequences of the available data pertain only to gradients present under resting conditions, clarification of the prevalence and long-term significance of provocable gradients remains an important future endeavor.

References

1 Braunwald E, Lambrew CT, Rockoff D *et al.* Idiopathic hypertrophic subaortic stenosis: I. A description of the disease based upon an analysis of 64 patients. *Circulation* 1964; **30** (Suppl. IV): 3–217.

2 Wigle ED, Rakowski H, Kimball BP *et al.* Hypertrophic cardiomyopathy: Clinical spectrum and treatment. *Circulation* 1995; **92**: 1680–92.

3 Frank S, Braunwald E. Idiopathic hypertrophic subaortic stenosis: Clinical analysis of 126 patients with emphasis on the natural history. *Circulation* 1968; **37**: 759–88.

4 Maron BJ. Hypertrophic cardiomyopathy: A systematic review. *JAMA* 2002; **287**: 1308–20.

5 Spirito P, Seidman CE, McKenna WJ, Maron BJ. Management of hypertrophic cardiomyopathy. *N Engl J Med* 1997; **30**: 775–85.

6 Murgo J, Alter BR, Dorethy JF, Altobelli SA, McGranahan GM. Dynamics of left ventricular ejection in obstructive and nonobstructive hypertrophic cardiomyopathy. *J Clin Invest* 1980; **66**: 1369–82.

7 Kizilbash AM, Heinle SK, Grayburn PA. Spontaneous variability of left ventricular outflow tract gradient in hypertrophic obstructive cardiomyopathy. *Circulation* 1998; **97**: 461–6.

8 Romeo F, Pelliccia F, Cristofani R, Martuscelli E, Reale A. Hypertrophic cardiomyopathy: Is a left ventricular outflow tract gradient a major prognostic determinant? *Eur Heart J* 1990; **11**: 233–40.

9 Klues HG, Leuner C, Kuhn H. Hypertrophic obstructive cardiomyopathy: No increase of the gradient during exercise. *J Am Coll Cardiol* 1991; **19**: 527–33.

10 Panza JA, Maris TJ, Maron BJ. Development and determinants of dynamic obstruction to left ventricular outflow in young patients with hypertrophic cardiomyopathy. *Circulation* 1992; **85**: 1398–405.

11 Maron BJ, Gottdiener JS, Arce J, Rosing DR, Wesley YE, Epstein SE. Dynamic subaortic obstruction in hypertrophic cardiomyopathy: Analysis by pulsed Doppler echocardiography. *J Am Coll Cardiol* 1985; **6**: 1–15.

12 Gilligan DM, Chan WL, Ang EL, Oakley CM. Effects of a meal on hemodynamic function at rest and during exercise in patients with hypertrophic cardiomyopathy. *J Am Coll Cardiol* 1991; **18**: 429–36.

13 Paz R, Jortner R, Tunick PA *et al.* The effect of the ingestion of ethanol on obstruction of the left ventricular outflow tract in hypertrophic cardiomyopathy. *N Engl J Med* 1996; **335**: 938–41.

14 Panza JA, Petrone RK, Fananapazir L, Maron BJ. Utility of continuous wave Doppler echocardiography in the noninvasive assessment of left ventricular outflow tract pres-

sure gradient in patients with hypertrophic cardiomyopathy. *J Am Coll Cardiol* 1992; **19**: 91–9.

15 Criley JM, Siegel RJ. Has 'obstruction' hindered our understanding of hypertrophic cardiomyopathy? *Circulation* 1985; **72**: 1148–54.

16 Ross J Jr, Braunwald E, Gault JH, Mason DT, Morrow AG. The mechanisms of the intraventricular pressure gradient in idiopathic hypertrophic subaortic stenosis. *Circulation* 1966; **34**: 558–78.

17 Wigle ED, Marquis Y, Auger P. Muscular subaortic stenosis: initial left ventricular inflow tract pressure in the assessment of intra-ventricular pressure differences in man. *Circulation* 1967; **35**: 1100–17.

18 Murgo JP. Does outflow obstruction exist in hypertrophic cardiomyopathy? *N Engl J Med* 1982; **307**: 1008.

19 Criley JM, Siegel RJ. Obstruction is unimportant in the pathophysiology of hypertrophic cardiomyopathy. *Postgrad Med J* 1986; **62**: 515–29.

20 Criley JM. Unobstructed thinking (and terminology) is called for in the understanding and management of hypertrophic cardiomyopathy. *J Am Coll Cardiol* 1997; **29**: 741–3.

21 Maron MS, Olivotto I, Betocchi S *et al.* Effect of left ventricular outflow tract obstruction on clinical outcome in hypertrophic cardiomyopathy. *N Engl J Med* 2003; **348**: 295–303.

22 Brock R. Functional obstruction of the left ventricle (acquired aortic subvalvular stenosis). *Guy's Hosp Rep* 1957; **106**: 221–38.

23 Brock R. Functional obstruction of the left ventricle (acquired aortic subvalvular stenosis). *Guy's Hosp Rep* 1959; **108**: 126–43.

24 Teare D. Asymmetric hypertrophy of the heart in young adults. *Br Heart J* 1958; **20**: 1–8.

25 Shah PM, Gramiak R, Kramer DH. Ultrasound localization of left ventricular outflow obstruction in hypertrophic obstructive cardiomyopathy. *Circulation* 1969; **40**: 3–11.

26 Maron BJ, Harding AM, Spirito P, Roberts WC, Waller BF. Systolic anterior motion of the posterior mitral leaflet: A previously unrecognized cause of dynamic subaortic obstruction. *Circulation* 1983; **68**: 282–93.

27 Klues HG, Roberts WC, Maron BJ. Morphological determinants of echocardiographic patterns of mitral valve systolic anterior motion in obstructive hypertrophic cardiomyopathy. *Circulation* 1993; **87**: 1570–9.

28 Spirito P, Maron BJ. Patterns of systolic anterior motion of the mitral valve in hypertrophic cardiomyopathy: assessment by two-dimensional echocardiography. *Am J Cardiol* 1984; **54**: 1039–46.

29 Sherrid MV, Gunsburg DZ, Moldenhauer S, Pearle G. Systolic anterior motion begins at low left ventricular outflow tract velocity in obstructive hypertrophic cardiomyopathy. *J Am Coll Cardiol* 2000; **36**: 1344–54.

30 Cape EG, Simons D, Jimoh A, Weyman AE, Yoganathan AP, Levine RA. Chordal geometry determines the shape and extent of systolic anterior mitral motion: in vitro studies. *J Am Coll Cardiol* 1989; **13**: 1438–48.

31 Sherrid MV, Chaudhry FA, Swistel DG. Obstructive hypertrophic cardiomyopathy: Echocardiography, pathophysiology, and the continuing evolution of surgery for obstruction. *Ann Thorac Surg* 2003; **75**: 620–32.

32 McCully RB, Nishimura RA, Tajik AJ *et al.* Extent of clinical improvement after surgical treatment of hypertrophic obstructive cardiomyopathy. *Circulation* 1996; **94**: 467–71.

33 Yu EHC, Omran AS, Wigle ED, Williams WG, Siu SC, Rakowski H. Mitral regurgitation in hypertrophic obstructive cardiomyopathy: relationship to obstruction and relief with myectomy. *J Am Coll Cardiol* 2000; **36**: 2219–25.

34 Sherrid MV, Pearle G, Gunsberg DZ. Mechanism of benefit of negative inotropes in obstructive hypertrophic cardiomyopathy. *Circulation* 1998; **97**: 41–7.

35 Maron BJ, McKenna WJ, Danielson GK *et al.* American College of Cardiology/European Society of Cardiology Clinical Expert Consensus Document on Hypertrophic Cardiomyopathy. *J Am Coll Cardiol* 2003; 42: 1687–713.

36 Maron BJ, Wolfson JK, Epstein SE *et al.* Intramural ('small vessel') coronary artery disease in hypertrophic cardiomyopathy. *J Am Coll Cardiol* 1986; **8**: 545–57.

37 Cannon RO, Rosing DR, Maron BJ *et al.* Myocardial ischemia in hypertrophic cardiomyopathy: Contribution of inadequate vasodilator reserve and elevated left ventricular filling pressures. *Circulation* 1985; **71**: 234–43.

38 Shirani J, Pick R, Roberts WC, Maron BJ. Morphology and significance of the left ventricular collagen network in young patients with hypertrophic cardiomyopathy and sudden cardiac death. *J Am Coll Cardiol* 2000; **35**: 36–44.

CHAPTER 5

Hypertrophic Cardiomyopathy with Latent (Provocable) Obstruction: Pathophysiology and Management

E. Douglas Wigle, MD, Maria Eriksson, MD, PhD,
Paul Rakowski, David Focsaneanu, Cairrine Sloggett, RN,
Anna Woo, MD, and Harry Rakowski, MD

Introduction

Hypertrophic cardiomyopathy (HCM) may be hemodynamically classified as being either nonobstructive (NO) or obstructive (Table 5.1).[1,2] Subaortic obstruction in HCM is more than ten times as common as midventricular obstruction, which in 50% of cases is also associated with subaortic obstruction. This chapter deals only with the subaortic obstruction due to mitral leaflet–septal contact, which may be latent (provocable) (LO) (Fig. 5.1), labile (spontaneously variable) or present at rest (RO).[1–3]

Definition of latent obstruction

In the hemodynamic era, we defined latent or provocable obstructive HCM as the circumstance in which there was no pressure gradient at rest between the left ventricle and aorta, but one which could be induced with appropriate provocations[1] (Fig. 5.1). In this age of Doppler calculation of pressure gradients, patients with latent obstruction would have outflow tract velocities of less than 2 m/s at rest and 2.5 m/s or greater on provocation. It is extremely important

Table 5.1 Hemodynamic classification of HCM

Obstructive HCM
Subaortic obstruction
Midventricular obstruction
Nonobstructive HCM
Normal (supranormal) systolic function
Impaired systolic function (end-stage HCM)

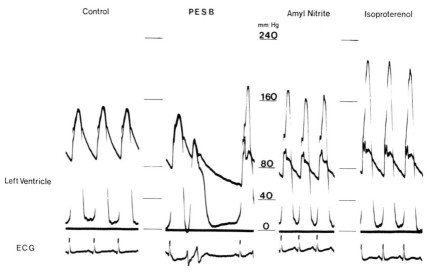

Fig. 5.1 Simultaneous left ventricular and aortic pressure tracings from a typical patient with latent obstruction showing the absence of a pressure gradient under control conditions, but the development of a pressure gradient in the post-extrasystolic beat (PESB), following amyl nitrite inhalation or isoproterenol infusion. Note the normal shape of the aortic pressure pulse under the control condition and the typical spike and dome configuration of the pressure pulse following provocation of the obstruction. Reproduced with permission from Wigle *et al.* Hypertrophic cardiomyopathy. The importance of the site and the extent of hypertrophy. A review. *Progr Cardiovasc Dis* 1985; **28**: 1–83, © 1985.

that provocative maneuvers be carried out when all negative inotropic therapy has been withdrawn, which may itself prevent obstruction.

Pathophysiology of latent obstruction

Site and extent of hypertrophy
In a series of reports dating from 1963 to 1985[1,3–5] we described the features of LO that distinguish these patients from those with RO or NO. Using an echocardiographic point score system to quantitate the extent of hypertrophy in 100 cases of HCM (Table 5.2), we demonstrated that the extent of hypertrophy in LO was significantly less than in NO or RO (Table 5.3). These studies also demonstrated that the left ventricular end-diastolic pressure (LVEDP) correlated with the extent of hypertrophy, i.e. the LVEDP in LO was significantly less than in NO or RO (Table 5.3).

We then analyzed the distribution of septal hypertrophy in these 100 cases of HCM[1] (Table 5.4). In 25 cases, only the basal one-third of the septum was hypertrophied (Fig. 5.2), whereas in 27 cases the hypertrophy involved the basal two-thirds of the septum, and in the remaining 48 cases the septum was hypertrophied from base to apex (Table 5.4). Of note was the fact that anterolateral extension of the hypertrophy was not observed when only basal

Table 5.2 Extent of hypertrophy in hypertrophic cardiomyopathy according to an echocardiographic point score system. Reproduced with permission from Wigle *et al.* Hypertrophic cardiomyopathy. The importance of the site and the extent of hypertrophy. A review. *Progr Cardiovasc Dis* 1985; **28**: 1–83, © 1985

Extent of hypertrophy		Points
Septal thickness (mm)	15–19	1
(basal 1/3 of septum)	20–24	2
	25–29	3
	>30	4
Extension to papillary muscles (basal 2/3 of septum)		2
Extension to apex (total septal involvement)		2
Anterolateral wall extension		2
Total		10

Table 5.3 Hemodynamic subgroups of hypertrophic cardiomyopathy: extent of hypertrophy correlated with left ventricular end-diastolic pressure (LVEDP). Reproduced with permission from Wigle *et al.* Hypertrophic cardiomyopathy. The importance of the site and the extent of hypertrophy. A review. *Progr Cardiovasc Dis* 1985; **28**: 1–83, © 1985

Hemodynamic subgroup	Hypertrophy point score (1–10 ± SD)	LVEDP (± SD) (mm Hg)
Latent obstruction	**2.9 ± 2.1*	**12.4 ± 5.2*
Nonobstructive hypertrophic cardiomyopathy	6.0 ± 2.9*	16.6 ± 7.3*
Resting obstruction	**8.6 ± 2.3	**18.4 ± 7.0*

*$P < 0.05$, **$P < 0.001$.

septal hypertrophy was present and the occurrence of anterolateral extension of hypertrophy increased progressively as the extent of septal hypertrophy increased, being present in 91% of cases with full-length septal hypertrophy (Table 5.4).

The hemodynamic subgroups of HCM were correlated with the extent of septal hypertrophy[1] (Table 5.5). In the presence of basal septal hypertrophy, 72% of cases had LO, whereas 28% had NO or RO. The incidence of LO decreased progressively as the extent of hypertrophy increased; only 8% of cases of full-length septal hypertrophy had LO whereas 58% had RO (Table 5.5).

We then analyzed the extent of hypertrophy in each of the three hemodynamic subgroups[1] (Table 5.6). In 34 cases with LO, 53% had only basal septal hypertrophy and in 35% the hypertrophy involved the basal two-thirds of the

Table 5.4 Extent of hypertrophy in 100 cases of ventricular septal hypertrophy determined by two-dimensional echocardiography. The presence of septal hypertrophy was determined by one-dimensional echocardiographic criteria in all cases (ventricular septum ≥15 mm and septal–posterior wall ratio ≥1.5:1). †In eight cases it was not possible to comment on anterolateral wall extension; thus only 92 of these cases were analyzed in this respect. Reproduced with permission from Wigle *et al.* Hypertrophic cardiomyopathy. The importance of the site and the extent of hypertrophy. A review. *Progr Cardiovasc Dis* 1985; **28**: 1–83, © 1985

Extent of hypertrophy	Number of cases	Anterolateral wall extension†
Basal 1/3 of septum (subaortic area)	25	0/23 (0%)
Basal 2/3 of septum (down to papillary muscles)	27	8/23 (35%)
Whole septum (from base to apex)	48	42/46 (91%)
Total	100	50/92 (54%)

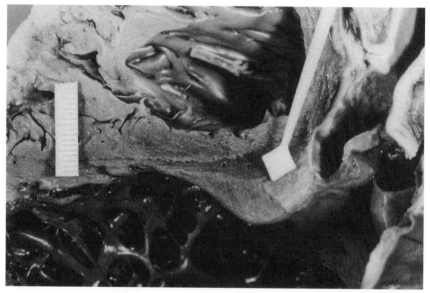

Fig. 5.2 Pathologic appearance of basal septal hypertrophy (involving the basal one-third of the septum) (arrow) as would be seen in the parasternal long-axis echocardiographic view. The aortic valve is immediately to the right of the arrow and the apex of the LV to the left. During life the patient had latent (provocable) obstruction and died of disseminated malignancy. Reproduced with permission from Wigle *et al.* Hypertrophic cardiomyopathy. The importance of the site and the extent of hypertrophy. A review. *Progr Cardiovasc Dis* 1985; **28**: 1–83, © 1985.

Table 5.5 Hemodynamic subgroups related to the extent of ventricular septal hypertrophy in hypertrophic cardiomyopathy. Table 4 indicates that localized subaortic septal hypertrophy is not associated with anterolateral wall extension, whereas full septal hypertrophy has anterolateral wall extension in 91% of cases. LO = latent obstruction; NO = nonobstructive hypertrophic cardiomyopathy; RO = resting obstruction. Reproduced with permission from Wigle *et al.* Hypertrophic cardiomyopathy. The importance of the site and the extent of hypertrophy. A review. *Progr Cardiovasc Dis* 1985; **28**: 1–83, © 1985

Extent of hypertrophy	Number of cases	Hemodynamic subgroups		
Basal 1/3 of septum	25	LO	18	72%
(localized subaortic hypertrophy)		NO	4	16%
		RO	3	12%
Basal 2/3 of septum	27	LO	12	44%
(down to papillary muscles)		NO	7	26%
		RO	8	30%
Base-to-apex hypertrophy	48	LO	4	8%
		NO	16	34%
		RO	28	58%

Table 5.6 Extent of ventricular septal hypertrophy related to the hemodynamic subgroups in hypertrophic cardiomyopathy. Reproduced with permission from Wigle *et al.* Hypertrophic cardiomyopathy. The importance of the site and the extent of hypertrophy. A review. *Progr Cardiovasc Dis* 1985; **28**: 1–83, © 1985

Hemodynamic subgroup	Number of cases	Extent of septal hypertrophy		
Latent obstruction	34	Basal 1/3	18	53%
		Basal 2/3	12	35%
		Whole septum	4	12%
Nonobstructive	27	Basal 1/3	4	14%
hypertrophic		Basal 2/3	7	26%
cardiomyopathy		Whole septum	16	60%
Resting obstruction	39	Basal 1/3	3	8%
		Basal 2/3	8	20%
		Whole septum	28	72%

septum. Thus, 88% of cases with LO had a limited extent of septal hypertrophy and only 12% had full-length septal hypertrophy (Table 5.6). In contrast, 60% of NO and 72% of RO cases had full-length septal hypertrophy whereas only 8–14% of NO or RO cases had only basal septal hypertrophy. It is evident from these studies that LO was associated with less extensive hypertrophy and that hypertrophy predominantly involved the base of the septum.[1] These observations have subsequently been confirmed by others.[6]

Other features of latent obstruction

Subsequently, we carried out echocardiographic studies on 80 patients who had previously been hemodynamically classified as to whether they had LO, NO, or RO.[4] In these studies, we quantitated basal septal thickness, LV outflow tract diameter at the onset of systole, anterior displacement of the anterior mitral leaflet in the LV, and compared these values with those of normal controls. In addition, we quantitated the degree of mitral leaflet systolic anterior motion (SAM), the occurrence of aortic valve notching and left atrial diameter in the three hemodynamic subgroups.[4] These studies revealed a statistically significant and progressive increase in basal septal thickness and a decrease in LV outflow tract diameter in patients with NO, LO and RO.[4] Thus, although cases with LO had less extensive hypertrophy than in NO or RO, the basal septal hypertrophy in LO was greater than in NO but less than in RO: LV outflow tract diameter in LO was less than in NO but greater than in RO. There was anterior displacement of the anterior mitral leaflet in all groups of HCM compared with controls.[4]

We next classified the degree of mitral leaflet SAM in the three hemodynamic subgroups as being absent, mild (more than 10 mm from the septum), moderate (within 10 mm of the septum or established brief, leaflet–septal contact less than 30% of echocardiographic systole), or severe with prolonged mitral leaflet–septal contact greater than 30% of echocardiographic systole.[4] Table 5.7 shows the degree of mitral leaflet SAM in NO, LO, and RO. Patients with NO had no or only mild SAM, whereas patients with RO always had severe SAM. In 90% of patients with LO, the degree of SAM was mild (30%) or moderate (60%), and became more severe with provocation. We subsequently demonstrated that the onset of the obstructive pressure gradient in RO is virtually simultaneous with the onset of mitral leaflet–septal contact, and that the magnitude of the pressure gradient correlated with the time of onset and duration of mitral leaflet septal–contact.[1,7] If mitral leaflet–septal contact occurred after 55% of echocardiographic systole, no pressure gradient developed, which correlated with the fact that moderate SAM does not cause an obstructive pressure gradient.[4]

Table 5.7 Degree of systolic anterior motion in the hemodynamic subgroups of hypertrophic cardiomyopathy. See text for definitions of mild, moderate and severe systolic anterior motion. Reproduced with permission from Wigle *et al.* Hypertrophic cardiomyopathy. The importance of the site and the extent of hypertrophy. A review. *Progr Cardiovasc Dis* 1985; **28**: 1–83, © 1985

Subgroups	Cases (n)	Absent	Mild	Moderate	Severe
Nonobstructive hypertrophic cardiomyopathy	15	13	2	–	–
Latent obstruction	28	2	9	17	–
Resting obstruction	27	–	–	–	27

Aortic valve notching occurred in all patients with RO, in only three of 17 patients with LO and in no patient with NO. Left atrial enlargement was present in 94% of patients with RO (presumably because of the concomitant mitral regurgitation)[8-10] but in only 13–14% of patients with LO or NO.[4]

Provocation of latent obstruction

In LO the outflow tract obstruction may be provoked by amyl nitrite inhalation,[5,6,11] isoproterenol[12,13] or dobutamine infusion, in a post-extrasystolic beat[14] during the Valsalva maneuver or exercise, and by standing from the squatting position. These provocative maneuvers, which should be performed off medication, may be carried out during the clinical examination or during echo/Doppler or hemodynamic investigation. We believe strongly that all patients with no evidence of obstruction at rest should be provoked in order to determine whether LO is present and to distinguish LO from NO. Indeed, in one series of 47 patients with no obstruction at rest, an obstruction was stimulated by amyl nitrite inhalation in 25 (53%).[11]

During the clinical examination, patients with no obstruction at rest should be examined supine and when standing in full expiration[15] following squatting, during the Valsalva maneuver or preferably following amyl nitrite inhalation. Patients with NO have either no or at most a grade 1/6 apical murmur that does not intensify with provocation. Patients with LO usually have a grade 1–2/6 apical murmur at rest that becomes grade 3/6 with provocation, signifying obstruction. During echo/Doppler examination, we favor provocation with amyl nitrite, and during hemodynamic investigation we favor amyl nitrite inhalation and determination of the gradient in a post-extrasystolic beat.

Clinical features of latent obstruction

We currently have approximately 1500 patients registered in our HCM clinic, of whom 127 have LO, an incidence of 8.5%, which is approximately the same incidence as apical HCM[16] in our clinic population. In our earlier report[1] of 34 patients with LO, 62% were male, the average age was 49.7 ± 13.9 years and 88% of patients had either basal septal hypertrophy (53%) or hypertrophy limited to the basal two-thirds of the septum (35%). In the follow-up of the 127 patients with LO, 73% were male, the average age was 45.1 ± 15.8 years and 87% of patients had either basal septal hypertrophy (58%) or hypertrophy limited to the basal two-thirds of the septum (29%). Thus, the limited extent of hypertrophy in LO has remained remarkably consistent over the years, as has the male predominance and age range.

Patients with LO usually present with dyspnea, angina, and presyncope/syncope on exertion, but their symptoms are usually less severe than those of patients with RO or NO, in whom the degree of hypertrophy is more severe.[1-3] On clinical examination, the apical murmur is usually grade 1–2/6 in intensity but becomes grade 3/6 in intensity with provocation. The ECG may be normal or demonstrate only mild changes in keeping with the less severe degree of hypertrophy in LO, compared with RO or NO, in which the ECG typically reveals evidence of LVH, reflecting the greater extent of hypertrophy in these cases. As indicated, echo/Doppler examination usually reveals basal septal hypertrophy or hypertrophy involving the basal two-thirds of the septum, a mild or moderate degree of mitral leaflet SAM that becomes more severe on provocation, an outflow tract obstruction only on provocation with amyl nitrite, lack of aortic valve notching, and normal left atrial size. Presently, hemodynamic or angiographic investigation of LO is rarely required unless other cardiac conditions are suspected.

Management of latent obstruction

β-Adrenergic blocking agents have been demonstrated to prevent the provocation of the obstructive pressure gradient in LO and thus are the preferred form of medical therapy[1–3] (Fig. 5.3). These agents are administered in a dose sufficient to give a resting heart rate of 60 beats/min but no slower. We have previously demonstrated the efficacy of such therapy in patients with LO, whereas the benefits of such therapy are usually unimpressive in patients with RO and significant symptoms.[3] β-Adrenergic blocking agents are not tolerated or are less effective in a small percentage of patients with LO. In such patients we would add the type 1-A anti-arrhythmic agent disopyramide, not for its anti-arrhythmic properties but rather for its negative inotropic properties.[1,2]

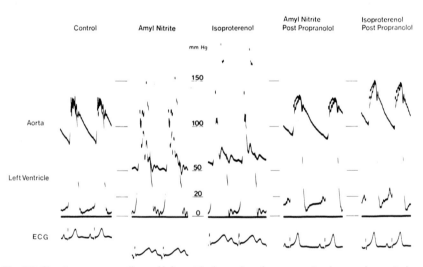

Fig. 5.3 Simultaneous recordings of left ventricular and aortic pressure tracings under control conditions and following amyl nitrite inhalation and isoproterenol infusion, before and after intravenous infusion of the β-adrenergic blocking agent propranolol. Propranolol blocked the provocation of the obstruction.

We advise against the use of all calcium antagonists in LO because of the uncertainty regarding whether the negative inotropic properties of these agents would prevent provocation of the obstruction, versus their afterload reducing properties, leading to provocation of the obstruction.[2] Indeed, we are aware of cases of LO in which verapamil administration provoked an obstructive pressure gradient of 100 mm Hg.

Rarely, patients with LO progress to RO and/or are intolerant of drug therapy, or fail to respond satisfactorily to medical therapy, and an intervention with myectomy surgery or septal ethanol ablation is required. We have carried out myectomy surgery in 11 such cases and septal ethanol ablation in three, an intervention rate of 11% in 127 patients with LO.

Prognosis

The average follow-up of the 127 patients with LO was 12.8 ± 8.3 years. There were eight deaths due to cardiovascular causes: four sudden deaths (in three of which there was extensive hypertrophy), three deaths due to congestive heart failure and one death due to stroke. Cardiovascular mortality was 6% and annual cardiovascular mortality was 0.4% per annum, which is similar to our experience with apical HCM (0.1% per annum).[16] Thus, the prognosis in LO is very favorable in the absence of severe hypertrophy, which is an established risk factor for sudden death.[1,17]

Although mortality is low in LO, there is very significant morbidity, morbid events occurring in 59 of 127 patients (46%).[20] The commonest of these were atrial fibrillation (36/127; 28%) and cerebrovascular accidents (15/127; 12%). The predictors of cardiovascular morbidity were left atrial enlargement and older age.

Summary

Of the approximately 1500 patients currently registered in our HCM clinic, 127 (8%) have been documented to have LO, which is the same incidence as that of apical HCM in the clinic population. LO is defined as the absence of outflow tract obstruction at rest and its presence on provocation. LO characteristically has significantly less extensive hypertrophy than other HCM hemodynamic subgroups, but the hypertrophy involves the basal septum, resulting in a narrowed LV outflow tract and the presence of provocable obstruction. These patients are often significantly symptomatic on exertion and usually respond to β-adrenergic blocking therapy which prevents the provocation of the obstruction. Rarely are other therapeutic interventions required in the management, and the prognosis is generally favorable.

References

1 Wigle ED, Sasson Z, Henderson MA *et al*. Hypertrophic cardiomyopathy. The importance of the site and the extent of hypertrophy. A review. *Prog Cardiovasc Dis* 1985; **28**: 1–83.
2 Wigle ED, Rakowski H, Kimball BP, Williams WG. Hypertrophic cardiomyopathy. Clinical spectrum and treatment. *Circulation* 1995; **92**: 1680–92.
3 Wigle ED, Adelman AG, Felderhof CH. Medical and surgical treatment of the cardiomyopathies. *Circ Res* 1974; **34, 35**: (Suppl. II): 196–207.
4 Gilbert BW, Pollick C, Adelman AG, Wigle ED. Hypertrophic cardiomyopathy: Subclassification by M-mode echocardiography. *Am J Cardiol* 1980: **45**: 861–71.
5 Wigle ED, Lenkei S, Chrysohou A, Wilson DR. Muscular subaortic stenosis: The effect of peripheral vasodilatation. *Can Med Assoc J* 1963; **80**: 896–9.
6 Nakatani S, Marwick TH, Lever HM, Thomas JD. Resting echocardiographic features of latent left ventricular outflow obstruction in hypertrophic cardiomyopathy. *Am J Cardiol* 1996; **78**: 662–7.
7 Pollick C, Rakowski H, Wigle ED. Muscular subaortic stenosis: The quantitative relationship between systolic anterior motion and the pressure gradient. *Circulation* 1984; **69**: 43–9.
8 Wigle ED, Adelman AG, Auger P *et al*. Mitral regurgitation in muscular subaortic stenosis. *Am J Cardiol* 1969; **24**: 698–706.
9 Grigg LE, Wigle ED, Williams WG, Daniel LB, Rakowski H. Transesophageal Doppler echocardiography in obstructive hypertrophic cardiomyopathy: Clarification of pathophysiology and importance in intraoperative decision making. *J Am Coll Cardiol* 1992; **20**: 45–52.
10 Yu EHC, Omran AS, Wigle ED, Williams WG, Siu SC, Rakowski H. Mitral regurgitation in hypertrophic obstructive cardiomyopathy: Relationship to obstruction and relief with myectomy. *J Am Coll Cardiol* 2000; **36**: 2219–24.
11 Sheikh KH, Pearce FB, Kisslo J. Use of Doppler echocardiography and amyl nitrite inhalation to characterize left ventricular outflow obstruction in hypertrophic cardiomyopathy. *Chest* 1997; **2**: 389–95.
12 Braunwald E, Ebert PA. Hemodynamic alterations in idiopathic hypertrophic subaortic stenosis induced by sympathomimetic drugs. *Am J Cardiol* 1962; **10**: 489–94.
13 Whalen RE, Cohen AI, Sumner RG, McIntosh HD. Demonstration of the dynamic nature of idiopathic hypertrophic subaortic stenosis. *Am J Cardiol* 1963; **11**: 8–17.
14 Brockenbrough EC, Braunwald E, Morrow AG. A hemodynamic technic for the detection of hypertrophic subaortic stenosis. *Circulation* 1961; **23**: 189–94.
15 Buda AJ, Mackenzie G, Wigle ED. The effect of negative intrathoracic pressure on the outflow tract gradient in muscular subaortic stenosis. *Circulation* 1981; **63**: 875–81.
16 Eriksson MJ, Sonnenberg B, Woo A *et al*. Long-term outcome in patients with apical hypertrophic cardiomyopathy. *J Am Coll Cardiol* 2002; **39**: 638–45.
17 Spirito P, Bellone P, Harris KM, Bernabo P, Bruzzi P, Maron BJ. Magnitude of left ventricular hypertrophy and risk of sudden death in hypertrophic cardiomyopathy. *New Engl J Med* 2000; **342**: 1778–85.

CHAPTER 6

Pathophysiology and Clinical Consequences of Atrial Fibrillation in Hypertrophic Cardiomyopathy

Iacopo Olivotto, MD, Barry J Maron, MD, and Franco Cecchi, MD

Atrial fibrillation (AF) represents the most common sustained arrhythmia as well as one of the most frequent reasons for hospitalization in patients with hypertrophic cardiomyopathy (HCM).[1-28] Although common and of obvious clinical relevance, AF has been largely overlooked in the HCM literature. Only recently, studies on community-based HCM populations have emphasized the high prevalence of AF in this disease and highlighted its potential impact on long-term prognosis in terms of cardiovascular mortality and functional disability.[4-6] This review focuses on recent advances regarding the clinical consequences of AF in HCM patients, and implications for management.

Left atrial function in HCM

During the cardiac cycle, atrial activity can be divided into *reservoir function*, by which venous return is stored during atrial relaxation; *conduit function*, by which the atrium acts as a passive chamber allowing flow from vein to ventricle during diastasis; and *atrial systole*, by which the atrium functions as a pump actively enhancing ventricular filling during the later part of ventricular diastole.[29,30] In HCM patients, and to a lesser extent in secondary left ventricular hypertrophy, left atrial (LA) passive emptying function is depressed, due to decreased left ventricular relaxation and compliance in early diastole.[31] Thus, left ventricular filling is largely dependent on atrial contraction,[30] which is potentiated in HCM by two principal mechanisms: (1) enhanced force of atrial systole against an increased afterload, by virtue of the Frank–Starling mechanism,[32,33] and (2) LA dilatation, which allows increased left atrial emptying volume during atrial contraction.[34] Therefore, atrial systolic function in HCM patients with diastolic dysfunction is often supernormal: in one study, atrial systole accounted for 31% of left ventricular filling in HCM patients, compared with 16% in normal controls, contributing more than 50% of filling in 15% of patients.[35] Under usual circumstances, increased LA contraction contributes effectively to the maintenance of left ventricular stroke volume during rest and exercise.[36] Such a favorable steady state may, however, change early in the course of evolving heart failure, when left atrial preload reserve reaches its limit, afterload mismatch ensues and LA ejection properties decline in response to further afterload increases.[36]

In addition, the possibility of a primary atrial myopathy in HCM has been postulated[9,36] but never defined. In a disease caused by sarcomere protein gene mutations, it is plausible to hypothesize some degree of involvement of the atrial myocardium. However, functional and morphological atrial abnormalities identified to date have usually been regarded as secondary to hemodynamic strain caused by ventricular dysfunction or mitral valve regurgitation,[9,36–40] and no specific pathological or ultrastructural alterations of the atria have been reported in HCM patients.[41,42] Nevertheless, the possibility of a coexisting primary dysfunction due to atrial myopathy merits further investigation in HCM (Table 6.1).

Pathophysiology of atrial fibrillation

The importance of active LA contribution to ventricular filling largely accounts for the negative hemodynamic consequences of AF in HCM patients. The acute onset of AF combines the abrupt loss of atrial systole and a mean rapid ventricular response rate:[4,9,13] these effects interact synergistically to further impair left ventricular filling, and may cause a sudden fall in cardiac output.[13] Consequently, AF is often associated with marked functional impairment in patients with HCM, and may be directly responsible for dramatic events, including acute pulmonary edema,[9,13] syncope,[24] myocardial ischemia[25,28] and even sudden death.[25–28] Presumably, the pre-existing degree of left ventricular diastolic impairment is a critical determinant of the adverse acute response to the onset of AF in individual patients.[1–4,9,32–33] However, a pre-existing impairment in ejection fraction and peak ejection rate have also been reported as predictive of acute clinical deterioration during AF.[14]

Even in HCM patients who do not experience dramatic clinical deterioration following AF onset, the arrhythmia frequently recurs, may eventually become chronic, and has the potential to jeopardize long-term clinical outcome, exercise tolerance and quality of life, often despite efforts aimed at the maintenance of sinus rhythm or the control of ventricular rate.[4–6] In one study, patients with AF were shown to have an almost 3-fold increase in the likelihood of progression to severe symptoms (NYHA class III–IV) at the end of a 9-year follow-up period, compared with HCM patients remaining in sinus rhythm.[4] The pathophysiologic mechanisms by which AF influences long-term clinical outcome are probably related to an increase in mean ventricular rate and reduced cardiac output on effort, bursts of myocardial ischemia, and thromboembolic complications including stroke.[4,8,9,13,17–22,49–53]

Nevertheless, the consequences of AF for the long-term prognosis of HCM show great heterogeneity among individual patients, and about one-third of patients may remain free of severe symptoms and thromboembolic complications.[4] Of note, the probability of a benign course is significantly reduced

Table 6.1 Evidence suggesting a primary atrial myopathy facilitating the occurrence of atrial fibrillation in patients with hypertrophic cardiomyopathy. LA = left atrial; MR = mitral regurgitation; AF = atrial fibrillation

Instrumental/clinical finding	Interpreted as secondary to	May also suggest	Reference
Reduced atrial ejection fraction	Afterload mismatch	Primary impairment of atrial myocyte contractility	Sanada et al. (1991)[36]
Prolonged P-wave duration	LA stretch/dilatation due to diastolic impairment and mitral regurgitation	Fragmented and prolonged atrial depolarization due to primary structural abnormalities	Cecchi et al. (1997)[7]
Onset of AF among patients with normal LA size (12% of all HCM patients with AF)	LA stretch due to diastolic impairment and mitral regurgitation	Predisposing effect to AF of specific mutations causing atrial myopathy	Olivotto et al. (2001)[4]
Familial occurrence of early onset AF	Specific hemodynamic alterations caused by the mutation causing early LA stretch	Predisposing effect to AF of specific mutations causing atrial myopathy	Gruver et al. (1999)[58]
Frequent LA dilatation in the absence of severe MR or diastolic dysfunction	Secondary to undetected hemodynamic stress	LA remodeling secondary to impaired myocyte contractility	Roberts and Roberts (1989)[41]
Increased calcium-antagonist receptors in atrial myocardium	Secondary to LA stretch/dilatation	Primary abnormalities in calcium fluxes through voltage-sensitive channels	Wagner et al. (1989)[37]

among patients developing chronic AF, suggesting that those efforts which target the maintenance of sinus rhythm may improve clinical outcome.[4,9]

Clinical and instrumental predictors

The potential substrates of AF in patients with HCM are numerous (Fig. 6.1). In clinical practice, several predictors of AF have been identified such as increasing age, left atrial dilatation, and functional limitation due to congestive symptoms (Table 6.2). Among these, left atrial dilatation has a particularly

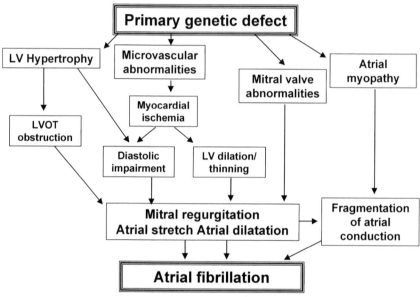

Fig. 6.1 Arrhythmogenic substrates and potential triggers for atrial fibrillation in hypertrophic cardiomyopathy. Hypothetical sequence of events leading from a primary genetic mutation to the development of atrial fibrillation via multiple pathophysiological processes and abnormalities known to occur in hypertrophic cardiomyopathy. Reproduced with permission from Olivotto *et al.* Clinical significance of atrial fibrillation in hypertrophic cardiomyopathy. *Curr Cardiol Rep* 2001; 3: 141–6.

Table 6.2 Predisposing factors and triggers of atrial fibrillation in patients with HCM. LV = left ventricular; MR = mitral regurgitation; NYHA = New York Heart Association; SVT = nonsustained episodes of supraventricular tachycardia

Associated with increased risk of AF	No significant influence on risk of developing AF	Not specifically assessed, possible association with AF
Left atrial size	Gender	Myocardial ischemia
Age	Maximum LV thickness	Autonomic dysfunction
NYHA class	Moderate/severe MR	Diastolic dysfunction
P-wave duration	LV outflow obstruction	Disease-causing mutation
SVT on Holter ECG		

strong independent predictive value for AF.[4,9] In addition, the degree of diastolic impairment may also represent an important predisposing factor to AF: [43–46,54] in its extreme manifestation (i.e. evolution to the restrictive end-stage phase) AF is a consistent feature of HCM (Fig. 6.2). Other pathophysiological abnormalities typical of HCM, such as myocardial ischemia and autonomic dysfunction, require further investigation with regard to their possible role as triggers for AF.[49–53,55–57] The possibility that the type of disease causing mutation may predispose to AF has also been suggested for families with early onset of the arrhythmia in many affected members.[58–60] Finally, other features of HCM, such as the magnitude of left ventricular hypertrophy and the presence of basal outflow obstruction, do not seem to be consistently associated with an increased likelihood for AF.[4,47,48]

For practical purposes, sufficiently accurate information regarding the likelihood of developing AF can be obtained in the individual patient by the combined assessment of left atrial dimensions and signal-averaged P-wave duration (Table 6.3), as well as the presence of supraventricular tachycardia on ambulatory (Holter) ECG.[7]

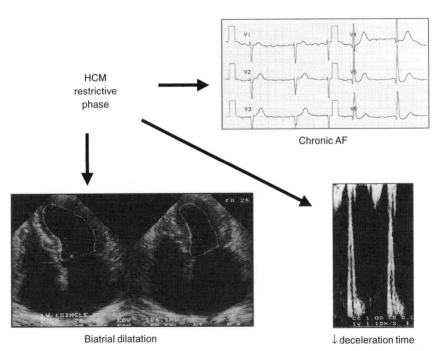

HCM restrictive phase

Chronic AF

Biatrial dilatation

↓ deceleration time

Fig. 6.2 Evolution of hypertrophic cardiomyopathy towards a restrictive phase in a 67-year-old patient with hypertrophic cardiomyopathy. The echocardiographic features include small left ventricular cavity, marked biatrial dilatation and a restrictive transmitral Doppler left ventricular filling pattern, typically associated with chronic atrial fibrillation.

Table 6.3 Sensitivity, specificity and predictive accuracy in assessing the risk for developing AF using signal-averaged P-wave duration in 110 patients with HCM. LA = left atrium. From Cecchi F *et al.* Risk for atrial fibrillation in patients with hypertrophic cardiomyopathy assessed by signal-averaged P-wave. *Heart* 1997; **78**: 44–9, with permission

	P-wave duration (ms)					
	≥ 120	≥ 130	≥ 140	≥ 145	≥ 150	≥ 140 + LA > 40 mm
Sensitivity (%)	95	63	56	39	29	44
Specificity (%)	42	59	83	88	94	93
Positive predictive accuracy (%)	49	48	66	67	75	78
Negative predictive accuracy (%)	94	73	76	71	69	73

Prevalence

The reported prevalence of AF in several HCM populations ranges from 10% to 28%.[1,2,5,6,8–10] In a recent study including 480 patients with HCM followed at two institutions for over 9 years, AF was documented in 22% of patients, with an incidence of 2% new cases per year.[4] Thus, HCM patients appear to have a 4- to 6-fold greater likelihood of developing AF when compared with the general population.[61–63]

AF prevalence increased progressively with age (Fig. 6.3) and was predominant in patients older than 60 years; mean age at onset of the arrhythmia was 54 years for paroxysmal AF and 57 years for chronic AF.[4] However, over one-third of patients with AF developed the arrhythmia before 50 years of age, and these patients were at greater risk of clinical deterioration and HCM-related death compared with patients with AF onset later in life.[4] Therefore, the management of early onset AF in younger patients with HCM, aimed at preventing

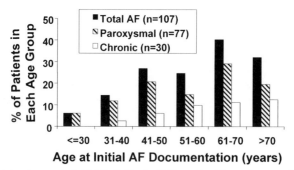

Fig. 6.3 Age at development of atrial fibrillation in 107 hypertrophic cardiomyopathy patients. Bars express the proportion of patients in each age group with paroxysmal or chronic atrial fibrillation. Patients evolving from paroxysmal to chronic atrial fibrillation are considered paroxysmal. Reproduced with permission from Olivotto *et al.* Impact of atrial fibrillation on the clinical course of hypertrophic cardiomyopathy. *Circulation* 2001; **104**: 2517–24.

complications over several subsequent decades of life, represents a clinical challenge.

Finally, in those patients with obstructive HCM undergoing surgical septal myectomy, postoperative AF occurred in approximately 30%.[16] Perioperative AF was associated with advanced age, preoperative palpitations, a prior history of AF, and relatively mild left ventricular hypertrophy.[16]

Cardiovascular mortality

Among the limited number of existing studies on AF in HCM populations, most report an adverse outcome associated with the arrhythmia.[4–6,9,13,23] The only exception is a study from a tertiary referral center which found no difference in survival between patients with and without AF, in spite of generally more severe clinical impairment and higher risk of thromboembolic complications in the AF group.[14] However, the low survival rates of the HCM patients in sinus rhythm who were used as controls may have had the effect of concealing an adverse effect of AF in this study.[14]

In the above-mentioned study of 480 patients with HCM followed for an average of 9 years, AF proved to be a key determinant of HCM-related outcome, and was associated with an almost 4-fold increase in cardiovascular mortality independent of other important clinical variables, such as age and NYHA functional class.[4] Annual HCM-related mortality was 3% in AF patients, compared with 1% among matched patients in sinus rhythm; among the AF patients, the prognosis was even more unfavorable in patients with onset of the arrhythmia at a younger age (≤50 years) (Fig. 6.4). In general, the impact of AF on outcome appears to be more profound in HCM patients than in the general population and in patients with other heart diseases.[63–65]

The overall risk of HCM-related mortality was not significantly related to the qualitative (paroxysmal versus chronic) or quantitative (number of paroxysmal episodes) manifestations of AF.[4] Nevertheless, patients developing chronic AF, compared with exclusively paroxysmal AF, showed a higher combined probability of HCM-related death, functional impairment and stroke.[4]

Of note, while associated with a marked increase in heart failure- and stroke-related death, AF did not appear to represent a consistent trigger of sudden and unexpected death in HCM patient populations.[4,9] On the other hand, a potential (although circumstantial) association between AF and sudden death in predisposed individuals is suggested by the observation that about 20% of those HCM patients who survived a documented cardiac arrest showed supraventricular arrhythmias (including AF) at the onset of symptoms preceding the collapse.[27] Indeed, AF with rapid ventricular conduction is capable of degenerating into ventricular fibrillation, due to a combination of electrophysiological instability and ischemia.[25,26,28] (Fig. 6.5).

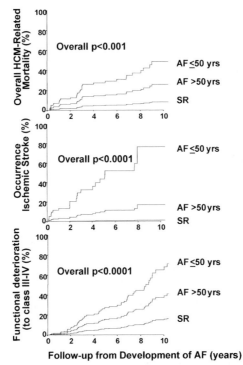

Fig. 6.4 Relation of early (<50 years; *n* = 39) *vs* late (>50 years; *n* = 68) development of AF to overall hypertrophic cardiomyopathy-related mortality (top panel), ischemic stroke (middle panel) and progression to NYHA class III–IV (bottom panel) compared with 133 matched hypertrophic cardiomyopathy patients in sinus rhythm (SR). Hazard plot based on multivariate Cox regression analysis including age, gender and NYHA functional class. Reproduced with permission from Olivotto *et al.* Impact of atrial fibrillation on the clinical course of hypertrophic cardiomyopathy. *Circulation* 2001; **104**: 2517–24.

Significance of outflow obstruction

The prevalence of AF does not differ among HCM patients with or without basal outflow obstruction.[4] Thus, despite the association of obstruction with significant degrees of mitral regurgitation[32,40,41] and its adverse effects on diastolic function,[33] the presence of obstruction *per se* does not imply an increased likelihood of developing AF. On the other hand, patients with obstruction appear to be particularly susceptible to the adverse hemodynamic consequences of AF, in that the combined presence of outflow obstruction at rest in HCM patients and AF more than doubles the risk for cardiovascular mortality, compared with nonobstructive patients.[4] Thus, HCM patients with left ventricular outflow obstruction appear to be highly dependent on active atrial contribution for left ventricular filling.[66] These observations may well account for the favorable changes in left atrial function following successful septal myectomy or percutaneous septal reduction.[32,33]

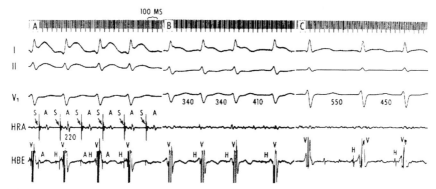

Fig. 6.5 Surface and intracardiac electrograms during atrial pacing in a 15-year-old boy with hypertrophic cardiomyopathy. (**A**) During right atrial pacing there is ST segment elevation in standard electrocardiographic leads I and II, and ST depression in lead V1. (**B**) ST segment changes in the surface electrocardiograms persist during atrial fibrillation. (**C**) After therapy with metoprolol and verapamil, the ventricular rate during atrial fibrillation has slowed and the ST segment changes no longer occur. A = atrial activation; H = His bundle potential; HBE = His bundle electrocardiogram; HRA = high right atrial electrocardiogram; S = stimulus artifact during atrial pacing; V = right ventricular activation. Reproduced from Stafford *et al*. Cardiac arrest in an adolescent with atrial fibrillation and hypertrophic cardiomyopathy. *J Am Coll Cardiol* 1986; **7**: 701-4, with permission from the American College of Cardiology Foundation.

Cardioembolic complications

Stroke and other cardioembolic events are well recognized causes of disability and death in HCM patients, and are strongly associated with AF.[4,8,17–23] A large study of 900 patients from four regional cohorts showed a 6% prevalence of stroke or other systemic embolic complications over a mean follow-up of 7 years.[19] Among HCM patients with AF, the risk of stroke was 8-fold greater than among those in sinus rhythm.[4,8,19–22] Thromboembolic events were slightly more common but not statistically different between patients with chronic or paroxysmal AF. Moreover, among patients with paroxysmal AF, risk was independent of the number of AF episodes.[4,19] Thus, patients with only a single AF paroxysm may be at risk for embolic complications just as are patients with multiple episodes or with long-standing AF. However, stroke was rarely the first clinical manifestation of AF in HCM.[19]

The primary determinant of cardioembolic events related to AF is undoubtedly slow and sluggish flow within the LA, which predisposes to clot formation.[67] However, this is probably not the only mechanism. Particularly in the elderly, or in patients in the end stage, AF may predispose patients to ischemic stroke by causing localized impairment of cerebral blood flow secondary to reduced cardiac output.[68] In addition, AF is associated with a hypercoagulable state, similar to that observed in patients with heart failure, probably mediated by an increase in catecholamine levels.[67] Such a hypercoagulable state has been documented in HCM patients by an increase in factors VIII:C and VIIIR:Ag and in platelet aggregation rate.[69,70] Taken together, these findings emphasize the necessity for early and adequate anticoagulation in HCM patients developing AF.

Clinical management

Prospective studies have not been performed to date addressing the optimal management of AF specifically in HCM patients. This circumstance is not uncommon in HCM, given its relatively rare occurrence in cardiologic practice and heterogeneous presentation.[1] As a consequence, current treatment strategies for AF in HCM patients following the acute onset and for long-term management are largely based on standard guidelines developed for patients with other cardiac conditions.[61,62,67]

In HCM patients with recent onset of AF, early reversal to sinus rhythm is desirable for its beneficial hemodynamic effects. Therefore, an aggressive approach to AF with pharmacological or electrical cardioversion in association with prophylactic anti-arrhythmic treatment (and anticoagulation) may prevent or delay AF-related complications. In a retrospective study on HCM patients with AF, long-term low-dose amiodarone treatment has been shown to have several advantages over conventional anti-arrhythmic treatment (such as digoxin, verapamil, β-blockers and class I agents), including a reduction in the number of cardioversion attempts and embolic complications, and longer intervals of sinus rhythm maintenance before AF recurrence.[14] Low-dose amiodarone treatment has been shown to be safe for long-term administration in HCM patients with ventricular arrhythmias.[71,72] The efficacy and safety of other class III agents, including sotalol and dofetilide, is still unknown in HCM patients.[62,73–75] Also, non-pharmacologic management of AF using implantable devices, such as multisite pacemakers and dual chamber defibrillators, has shown promising results but has not been systematically tested in HCM.[61,62,76]

In patients with persistent AF, in whom maintenance of sinus rhythm is not feasible, conservative strategies directed toward ventricular rate control represent a necessary alternative.[61,62,73,77] Results from the recently completed multicenter trial Atrial Fibrillation Follow-up Investigation of Rhythm Management (AFFIRM)[78] and other trials[79] suggest that optimal control of ventricular rate may be equivalent to sinus rhythm maintenance with regard to outcome. However, whether these therapeutic strategies are equivalent with regard to outcome in HCM is at present unresolved. Recent evidence suggests that (presumably due to the common occurrence of diastolic dysfunction and of the important role of atrial contraction) the maintenance of sinus rhythm may be preferable to cardioversion whenever obtainable (Fig. 6.6).[4]

In HCM patients who have developed persistent AF, adequate rate control can be obtained by aggressive management with β-adrenergic blocking agents, verapamil or diltiazem, or amiodarone, each alone or in combination. Digitalis, which is contraindicated in those patients with outflow obstruction, may be used in nonobstructive patients, particularly in the presence of systolic dysfunction and the end-stage phase.[80] However, in our experience digitalis is

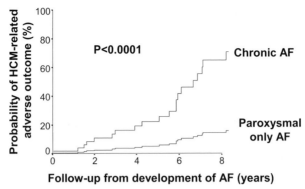

Fig. 6.6 Cumulative risk for adverse outcome in hypertrophic cardiomyopathy patients with exclusively paroxysmal (n = 45) and chronic atrial fibrillation (n = 62). Adverse outcome was defined as a combined end-point including hypertrophic cardiomyopathy-related death, progression to NYHA class III–IV or stroke. In this analysis, patients evolving from paroxysmal to chronic atrial fibrillation are considered chronic. Reproduced with permission from Olivotto *et al*. Impact of atrial fibrillation on the clinical course of hypertrophic cardiomyopathy. *Circulation* 2001; **104**: 2517–24.

often incapable of maintaining adequate rate control during exercise in HCM patients. In this regard, scrutiny of the chosen therapeutic regimen by Holter monitoring may be useful in assessing ventricular rate control during daily activities. In patients with persistently elevated ventricular rates associated with functional limitation, atrioventricular node ablation with rate-responsive pacemaker implantation has achieved effective rate control in many non-HCM patients[61,62] without adversely affecting long-term survival.[77]

Finally, both paroxysmal and chronic AF represent clear indications for oral anticoagulation.[1–4,8,61] Among 190 HCM patients with a history of AF followed at four institutions in Italy and the USA,[19] the cumulative incidence of systemic thromboembolism among non-anticoagulated AF patients was twice that of AF patients receiving warfarin (31% versus 15%; $P = 0.01$). Such observations are in agreement with a wide range of clinical studies on AF in patients with heart diseases other than HCM.[61,67] Thus, the threshold for initiation of anticoagulant treatment in HCM should be low, and independent of the number of documented AF episodes.[2,4,9] Nevertheless, such clinical decisions often need to be tailored in the individual patient with due consideration of the risk of hemorrhagic complications, lifestyle modification and expected compliance.[61,62]

Conclusions

AF is the most common sustained arrhythmia occurring in HCM patients and represents an independent risk factor for heart failure-related mortality, stroke and severe functional disability. Timely implementation of appropriate management strategies may effectively prevent long-term deterioration and acute complications of AF. However, studies dedicated to develop preventive and therapeutic guidelines for AF in HCM patients are still limited and many important issues remain to be resolved.

References

1 Maron BJ. Hypertrophic cardiomyopathy. *Lancet* 1997; **350**: 127–33.
2 Spirito P, Seidman CE, McKenna WJ, Maron BJ. The management of hypertrophic cardiomyopathy. *N Engl J Med* 1997; **336**: 775–85.
3 Wigle ED, Rakowski H, Kimball BP, Williams WG. Hypertrophic cardiomyopathy. Clinical spectrum and treatment. *Circulation* 1995; **92**: 1680–92.
4 Olivotto I, Cecchi F, Casey SA, Dolara A, Traverse JH, Maron BJ. Impact of atrial fibrillation on the clinical course of hypertrophic cardiomyopathy. *Circulation* 2001; **104**: 2517–24.
5 Cecchi F, Olivotto I, Montereggi A, Santoro G, Dolara A, Maron BJ. Hypertrophic cardiomyopathy in Tuscany: Clinical course and outcome in an unselected population. *J Am Coll Cardiol* 1995; **26**: 1529–36.
6 Maron BJ, Casey SA, Poliac L, Gohman TE, Almquist AK, Aeppli DM. Clinical course of hypertrophic cardiomyopathy in a regional United States cohort. *JAMA* 1999; **281**: 650–5.
7 Cecchi F, Montereggi A, Olivotto I, Marconi P, Dolara A, Maron BJ. Risk for atrial fibrillation in patients with hypertrophic cardiomyopathy assessed by signal-averaged P-wave. *Heart* 1997; **78**: 44–9.
8 Maron BJ, Olivotto I, Spirito P *et al.* Epidemiology of hypertrophic cardiomyopathy-related death: Revisited in a large non-referral based patient population. *Circulation* 2000; **102**: 858–64.
9 Olivotto I, Maron BJ, Cecchi F. Clinical significance of atrial fibrillation in hypertrophic cardiomyopathy. *Curr Cardiol Rep* 2001; **3**: 141–6
10 McKenna WJ. Arrhythmia and prognosis in hypertrophic cardiomyopathy. *Eur Heart J* 1983; **4** (Suppl. F): 225–34.
11 Savage DD, Seides SF, Maron BJ, Myers DJ, Epstein SE. Prevalence of arrhythmias during 24-hour electrocardiographic monitoring and exercise testing in patients with obstructive and nonobstructive hypertrophic cardiomyopathy. *Circulation* 1979; **59**: 866–75.
12 McKenna WJ, England D, Doi YL, Deanfield JE, Oakley C, Goodwin JF. Arrhythmia in hypertrophic cardiomyopathy: I – Influence on prognosis. *Br Heart J* 1981; **46**: 168–72.
13 Glancy DL, O'Brien KP, Gold HK, Epstein SE. Atrial fibrillation in patients with idiopathic hypertrophic subaortic stenosis. *Br Heart J* 1970; **32**: 652–9.
14 Robinson KC, Frenneaux MP, Stockins B, Karatasakis G, Poloniecki JD, McKenna WJ. Atrial fibrillation in hypertrophic cardiomyopathy: A longitudinal study. *J Am Coll Cardiol* 1990; **15**: 1279–85.
15 Greenspan AM. Hypertrophic cardiomyopathy and atrial fibrillation: A change of perspective. *J Am Coll Cardiol* 1990; **15**: 1286–7.
16 Ommen SR, Thomson HL, Nishimura RA, Tajik AJ, Schaff HV, Danielson GK. Clinical predictors and consequences of atrial fibrillation after surgical myectomy for obstructive hypertrophic cardiomyopathy. *Am J Cardiol* 2002; **89**: 242–4.
17 Furlan AJ, Craciun AR, Raju NR, Hart N. Cerebrovascular complications associated with idiopathic hypertrophic subaortic stenosis. *Stroke* 1984; **15**: 282–4.

18 Di Pasquale G, Andreoli A, Lusa AM *et al.* Cerebral embolic risk in hypertrophic cardiomyopathy. In: Baroldi G, Camerini F, Goodwin J, eds. *Advances in Cardiomyopathies.* Milan: Springer Verlag, 1990: 91–6.

19 Maron BJ, Olivotto I, Bellone P *et al.* Clinical profile of stroke in 900 patients with hypertrophic cardiomyopathy. *J Am Coll Cardiol* 2002; **39**: 301–7.

20 Higashikawa M, Nakamuri Y, Yoshida M, Kinoshita M. Incidence of ischemic strokes in hypertrophic cardiomyopathy is markedly increased if complicated by atrial fibrillation. *Jpn Circ J* 1997; **61**: 673–81.

21 Shigematsu Y, Hamada M, Mukai M, Matsuoka H, Sumimoto T, Hiwada K. Mechanism of atrial fibrillation and increased incidence of thromboembolism in patients with hypertrophic cardiomyopathy. *Jpn Circ J* 1995; **59**: 329–36.

22 Kogure S, Yamamoto Y, Yomono S, Hasegawa A, Suzaki T, Murata K. High risk of systemic embolism in hypertrophic cardiomyopathy. *Jpn Heart J* 1986; **27**: 475–80.

23 Doi Y, Kitaoka H. Hypertrophic cardiomyopathy in the elderly: Significance of atrial fibrillation. *J Cardiol* 2001; **37**. 133–8.

24 Brembilla-Perrot B, Terrier de La Chaise A, Beurrier D. Paroxysmal atrial fibrillation: Main cause of syncope in hypertrophic cardiomyopathy. *Arch Mal Coeur Vaiss* 1993; **86**: 1573–8.

25 Stafford WJ, Trohman RG, Bilsker M, Zaman L, Castellanos A, Myerburg RJ. Cardiac arrest in an adolescent with atrial fibrillation and hypertrophic cardiomyopathy. *J Am Coll Cardiol* 1986; **7**: 701–4.

26 Lopez Gil M, Arribas F, Cosio FG. Ventricular fibrillation induced by rapid atrial rates in patients with hypertrophic cardiomyopathy. *Europace* 2000; **2**: 327–32.

27 Cecchi F, Maron BJ, Epstein SE. Long-term outcome of patients with hypertrophic cardiomyopathy successfully resuscitated after cardiac arrest. *J Am Coll Cardiol* 1989; **13**: 1283–8.

28 Suzuki M, Hirayama T, Marumoto K, Okayama H, Iwata T. Paroxysmal atrial fibrillation as a cause of potentially lethal ventricular arrhythmia with myocardial ischemia in hypertrophic cardiomyopathy—a case report. *Angiology* 1998; **49**: 653–7.

29 Dernellis J, Stefanadis C, Toutouzas P. From science to bedside: The clinical role of atrial function. *Eur Heart J* 2000; **2** (Suppl. K): K48–57.

30 Daubert JC, Pavin D, Gras D *et al.* Importance of atrial contraction in hypertrophic obstructive cardiomyopathy: Implications for pacing. *J Interv Cardiol* 1996; **9**: 335–45.

31 Pitsavos C, Aggeli C, Stefanadis C, Toutouzas P. Non-invasive assessment of left atrial performance by echocardiographic modalities, *Eur Heart J* 2000; **2** (Suppl. K): K26–33.

32 Yu EH, Omran AS, Wigle ED *et al.* Mitral regurgitation in hypertrophic obstructive cardiomyopathy: Relationship to obstruction and relief with myectomy. *J Am Coll Cardiol* 2000; **36**: 2219–25.

33 Nagueh SF, Lakkis NM, Middleton KJ *et al.* Changes in left ventricular filling and left atrial function six months after nonsurgical septal reduction therapy for hypertrophic obstructive cardiomyopathy. *J Am Coll Cardiol* 1999; **34**: 1123–8.

34 Matsuda Y, Toma Y, Moritani K *et al.* Assessment of left atrial function in patients with hypertensive heart disease. *Hypertension* 1986; **8**: 779–85.

35 Bonow RO, Frederick TM, Bacharach SL *et al.* Atrial systole and left ventricular filling in patients with hypertrophic cardiomyopathy: Effect of verapamil. *Am J Cardiol* 1983; **51**: 1386–91.

36 Sanada H, Shimizu M, Shimizu K *et al.* Left atrial afterload mismatch in hypertrophic cardiomyopathy. *Am J Cardiol* 1991; **68**: 1049–54.

37 Wagner JA, Sax FL, Weisman HF *et al.* Calcium-antagonist receptors in the atrial tissue of patients with hypertrophic cardiomyopathy. *N Engl J Med* 1989; **320**: 755–61.

38 Wigle ED, Adelman AG, Auger P, Marquis Y. Mitral regurgitation in muscular subaortic stenosis. *Am J Cardiol* 1969; **24**: 698–706.

39 Kinoshita N, Nimura Y, Okamoto M, Miyatake K, Nagata S, Sakaribara H. Mitral regurgitation in hypertrophic cardiomyopathy: Noninvasive study by two-dimensional Doppler echocardiography. *Br Heart J* 1983; **49**: 574–83.

40 St. John Sutton MG, Tajik AJ, Gibson DG *et al.* Echocardiographic assessment of left ventricular filling and septal and posterior wall dynamics in idiopathic hypertrophic subaortic stenosis. *Circulation* 1978; **57**: 512–20.

41 Roberts CS, Roberts WC. Morphologic features. In: Zipes DP, Rowlands DJ, eds. *Progress in Cardiology*. Philadelphia: Lea & Febiger, 1989: 3–22.

42 Olsen EG. Anatomic and light microscopic characterization of hypertrophic obstructive and non obstructive cardiomyopathy. *Eur Heart J* 1983; **4** (Suppl. F): 1–8.

43 Maron BJ, Spirito P, Green KJ, Wesley YE, Bonow RO, Arce J. Noninvasive assessment of left ventricular diastolic function by pulsed Doppler echocardiography in patients with hypertrophic cardiomyopathy. *J Am Coll Cardiol* 1987; **10**: 733–42.

44 Hanrath P, Mathey DG, Siegert R, Bleifeld W. Left ventricular relaxation and filling pattern in different forms of left ventricular hypertrophy: An echocardiographic study. *Am J Cardiol* 1980; **45**: 15–23.

45 Spirito P, Maron BJ, Bonow RO. Noninvasive assessment of left ventricular diastolic function: Comparative analysis of Doppler echocardiographic and radionuclide angiographic techniques. *J Am Coll Cardiol* 1986; **7**: 518–26.

46 Losi MA, Betocchi S, Grimaldi M. Heterogeneity of left ventricular filling dynamics in hypertrophic cardiomyopathy. *Am J Cardiol* 1994; **73**: 987–90.

47 Spirito P, Lakatos E, Maron BJ. Degree of left ventricular hypertrophy in patients with hypertrophic cardiomyopathy and chronic atrial fibrillation. *Am J Cardiol* 1992; **69**: 1217–22.

48 Panza JA, Petrone RK, Fananapazir L, Maron BJ. Utility of continuous wave Doppler in noninvasive assessment of the left ventricular outflow tract pressure gradient in patients with hypertrophic cardiomyopathy. *J Am Coll Cardiol* 1992; **19**: 91–9.

49 Cannon RO, Rosing DR, Maron BJ *et al.* Myocardial ischemia in hypertrophic cardiomyopathy: Contribution of inadequate vasodilator reserve and elevated left ventricular filling pressures. *Circulation* 1985; **71**: 234–43.

50 O'Gara PT, Bonow RO, Maron BJ *et al.* Myocardial perfusion abnormalities in patients with hypertrophic cardiomyopathy: Assessment with thallium-201 emission computed tomography. *Circulation* 1987; **76**: 1214–23.

51 Maron BJ, Epstein SE, Roberts WC. Hypertrophic cardiomyopathy and transmural myocardial infarction without significant atherosclerosis of the extramural coronary arteries. *Am J Cardiol* 1979; **43**: 1086–102.

52 Pasternac A, Noble J, Streulens Y, Elie R, Henschke C, Bourassa MG. Pathophysiology of chest pain in patients with cardiomyopathies and normal coronary arteries. *Circulation* 1982; **65**: 778–89.

53 Camici P, Chiriatti G, Lorenzoni R *et al.* Coronary vasodilation is impaired in both hypertrophied and nonhypertrophied myocardium of patients with hypertrophic cardiomyopathy: A study with nitrogen-13 ammonia and positron emission tomography. *J Am Coll Cardiol* 1991; **17**: 879–86.

54 Yamaji K, Fujimoto S, Yutani C *et al*. Does the progression of myocardial fibrosis lead to atrial fibrillation in patients with hypertrophic cardiomyopathy? *Cardiovasc Pathol* 2001; **10**: 297–303.

55 Prasad K, Frenneaux MP. Sudden death in hypertrophic cardiomyopathy: Potential importance of altered autonomic control of vasculature. *Heart* 1998; **79**: 538–40.

56 Frenneaux MP, Counihan PJ, Caforio ALP, Chikamori T, McKenna WJ. Abnormal blood pressure response during exercise in hypertrophic cardiomyopathy. *Circulation* 1991; **82**: 1995–2002.

57 Brignole M, Gianfranchi L, Menozzi C *et al*. Role of autonomic reflexes in syncope associated with paroxysmal atrial fibrillation. *J Am Coll Cardiol* 1993; **22**: 1123–9.

58 Gruver EJ, Fatkin D, Dodds GA *et al*. Familial hypertrophic cardiomyopathy and atrial fibrillation caused by Arg663His beta-cardiac myosin heavy chain mutation. *Am J Cardiol* 1999; **83** (12A): 13H–18H.

59 Varnava A, Baboonian C, Davison F *et al*. New mutation of the cardiac troponin T gene causing familial hypertrophic cardiomyopathy without left ventricular hypertrophy. *Heart* 1999; **82**: 621A–624A.

60 Richard P, Charron P, Leclercq C *et al*. Homozygotes for a R869G mutation in the beta-myosin heavy chain gene have a severe form of familial hypertrophic cardiomyopathy. *J Mol Cell Cardiol* 2000; **32**: 1575–83.

61 Fuster V, Ryden LE, Asinger RW *et al*. ACC/AHA/ESC guidelines for the management of patients with atrial fibrillation: Executive summary a report of the American College of Cardiology/American Heart Association Task Force on Practice Guidelines and the European Society of Cardiology Committee for Practice Guidelines and Policy Conferences. *Circulation* 2003; **104**: 2118–50

62 Falk RH. Atrial fibrillation. *N Engl J Med* 2001; **344**: 1067–78.

63 Benjamin EJ, Wolf PA, D'Agostino RB, Silbershatz H, Kannel WB, Levy D. Impact of atrial fibrillation on the risk of death. The Framingham Heart Study. *Circulation* 1998; **98**: 946–52.

64 Middlekauff HR, Stevenson WG, Stevenson LW. Prognostic significance of atrial fibrillation in advanced heart failure. A study of 390 patients. *Circulation* 1991; **84**: 40–8.

65 Cameron A, Schwartz MJ, Kronmal RA, Kosinski AS. Prevalence and significance of atrial fibrillation in coronary artery disease (CASS Registry). *Am J Cardiol* 1988; **61**: 714–7.

66 Dernellis J, Tsiamis E, Stefanadis C *et al*. Effects of postural changes on left atrial function in patients with hypertrophic cardiomyopathy. *Am Heart J* 1998; **136**: 982–7.

67 Schlepper M. Identification of patients with atrial fibrillation at risk for thromboembolism. In: Olsson SB, Allessie MA, Campbell RWF, eds. *Atrial Fibrillation. Mechanisms and Therapeutic Strategies*. Armonk (NY): Futura Publishing, 1994: 15–24.

68 Lavy S, Stern S, Melamed E *et al*. Effect of chronic atrial fibrillation on regional cerebral blood flow. *Stroke* 1980; **1**: 35–8.

69 Longo G, Cecchi F, Grossi A *et al*. Coagulation and platelet function in hypertrophic cardiomyopathy. *Thromb Haemost* 1984; **51**: 299.

60 Yarom M, Lewis BS, Lijovetsky G *et al*. Platelet studies in patients with hypertrophic cardiomyopathy. *Cardiovasc Res* 1982; **16**: 324–30.

71 McKenna WJ, Oakley CM, Krikler DM, Goodwin JF. Improved survival with amiodarone in patients with hypertrophic cardiomyopathy and ventricular tachycardia. *Br Heart J* 1985; **53**: 412–16.

72 Cecchi F, Olivotto I, Montereggi A, Squillantini G, Dolara A, Maron BJ. Prognostic value of nonsustained ventricular tachycardia and efficacy of amiodarone treatment in an unselected patient population with hypertrophic cardiomyopathy. *Heart* 1998; **79**: 331–6.

73 Prystowski EN. Management of atrial fibrillation: Therapeutic options and clinical decisions. *Am J Cardiol* 2000; **85**: 3D–11D.

74 Reiffel JA. Drug choices in the treatment of atrial fibrillation. *Am J Cardiol* 2000; **85**: 12D–19D.

75 Tendera M, Wycisk A, Schneeweiss A, Polonski L, Wodniecki J. Effect of sotalol on arrhythmias and exercise tolerance in patients with hypertrophic cardiomyopathy. *Cardiology* 1993; **82**: 335–42.

76 Friedman PA, Dijkman B, Warman EN *et al.* Atrial therapies reduce atrial arrhythmia burden in defibrillator patients. *Circulation* 2001; **104**: 1023–28.

77 Ozcan C, Jahangir A, Friedman PA *et al.* Long-term survival after ablation of the atrioventricular node and implantation of a permanent pacemaker in patients with atrial fibrillation. *N Engl J Med* 2001; **344**: 1043–51.

78 Wyse DG, Waldo AL, DiMarco JP *et al.* Atrial Fibrillation Follow-up Investigation of Rhythm Management (AFFIRM) Investigators. A comparison of rate control and rhythm control in patients with atrial fibrillation. *N Engl J Med* 2002; **347**: 1825–33.

79 Saxonhouse SJ, Curtis AB. Risks and benefits of rate control versus maintenance of sinus rhythm. *Am J Cardiol* 2003; **91** (6A): 27–32.

80 Spirito P, Maron BJ, Bonow RO, Epstein SE. Occurrence and significance of progressive left ventricular wall thinning and relative cavity dilatation in patients with hypertrophic cardiomyopathy. *Am J Cardiol* 1987; **60**: 123–9.

CHAPTER 7

Other Modes of Disability or Death Including Stroke, and Treatment Strategies, in Hypertrophic Cardiomyopathy

Franco Cecchi, MD, Iacopo Olivotto, MD, and Barry J Maron, MD

Hypertrophic cardiomyopathy (HCM) was originally described as a rare and malignant disease resulting in the frequent occurrence of sudden death.[1-3] In the last decade, however, studies on community-based populations have changed our perception of the disease.[4-6] These studies have shown that HCM is not uncommon and is often compatible with normal life expectancy.[5] Moreover, while some patients die suddenly or experience cardiac arrest, about one-third develop dyspnea and other congestive symptoms, due to high intracavitary pressures, and evidence of heart failure (HF). These patients have a higher risk of suffering cardiovascular events, including atrial fibrillation (AF) and premature cardiovascular death.[4-6] Moreover, HF and AF are characterized by a higher prevalence of stroke and peripheral embolism.[7-9] Over long-term follow-up, HF and stroke constitute a common feature of the disease and account for a substantial proportion of HCM-related deaths in all age groups, with the exception of pediatric patients.[7] The role of AF, maximal left ventricular (LV) wall thickness, myocardial hypoperfusion and left ventricular outflow tract (LVOT) obstruction, as major determinants of HCM-related morbidity and mortality, have been emphasized recently.[9-12]

Epidemiology and clinical outcome

Selection bias and length of follow-up greatly influenced the results of outcome studies on HCM in the past. Data collected by tertiary referral centers included a large proportion of patients with moderate to severe functional limitation (up to more than 50%), often with severe LVOT obstruction. Consequently, their annual mortality rates were higher, in the range of 2–6%.[1-3] These cohorts did not reflect the overall population of patients with HCM, which is a relatively uncommon disease, with an estimated prevalence of about 0.2%. Data collected on a regional basis, mostly derived from community hospitals and outpatient clinics, show that only about 10% of patients have moderate to

Table 7.1 HCM-related annual mortality and cause of death in two multicenter studies.[6,7]
[†]n = 330; mean follow-up 9.4 years; [‡]n = 744; mean follow-up 8.0 years

	SPIC Study (Italy) Local community hospitals[†]	HCM centers[‡] Minneapolis, Florence, Genoa
Annual cardiovascular death rate	0.6%	1.4%
Sudden death	0.2%	0.7%
Heart failure	0.4%	0.5%
Stroke		0.2%

severe functional limitation at diagnosis and about 20% have LVOT obstruction. Studies based on these populations probably reflect more precisely the outcome of the disease after careful clinical management. Their annual mortality rates are usually lower, in the range of 0.6–1.4%[4–7] (Table 7.1).

HCM-related mortality

Recently, HCM mortality (age and cause of death) has been revisited in a relatively large nonreferral-based population.[7] The definition of HCM-related causes of death include HF as cardiac decompensation and a progressive disease course, stroke as a direct consequence of embolic cerebral events, mostly associated with atrial fibrillation, and sudden death as an unexpected sudden collapse occurring within 1 hour from the onset of symptoms, in patients with a previous stable or uneventful clinical course.

Sudden and unexpected death, which included patients resuscitated from cardiac arrest and those with appropriate implantable cardiac defibrillator discharges, accounted for about 50% of HCM-related deaths. While it was almost the only modality of death of those patients diagnosed at a young age, it was not confined to any age group (Fig. 7.1). HF deaths, including deaths of patients who had been transplanted, usually occurred after 45 years of age. Stroke deaths occurred mostly in older patients and were associated with HF and AF.

HCM-related morbidity

During follow-up a variety of cardiovascular events may occur. They often require hospital admission and greatly limit the quality of life of the patients. They include AF, syncope, episodes of acute HF or worsening of symptoms of chronic HF due to disease progression, stroke, ventricular arrhythmias and endocarditis (Table 7.2).

Atrial fibrillation

AF is the most common clinically occurring arrhythmia, and it may be expected in about 20–25% of patients; its consequences have been reported extensively[9] (Fig. 7.2). The incidence of episodes of acute HF, stroke and death

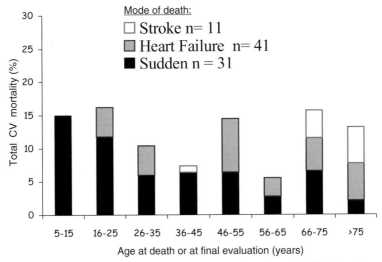

Fig. 7.1 Age distribution at the time of hypertrophic cardiomyopathy-related death, and cause of death in a multicenter study population (Minneapolis, Florence, Genoa)[7]

Table 7.2 Cumulative incidence of cardiovascular events in the SPIC study (Italy), a multicenter study of clinical outcome of hypertrophic cardiomyopathy patients diagnosed in community hospitals (n = 330; follow-up 9.4 years)[6]

Atrial fibrillation	24%
Disease progression (to NYHA FC III–IV)	16%
Acute heart failure	7%
End-stage heart failure	5%
Peripheral embolism/stroke	6%
Endocarditis	0.9%
Syncope	14%

due to HF is age-related, due to the progressive increase in the prevalence of AF in these age groups. AF with a high ventricular rate may precipitate myocardial ischemia and acute HF, which may be characterized by low cardiac output and severe hypotension in patients with myocardial hypoperfusion or hemodynamic instability. It may lead to death if sinus rhythm is not promptly restored.[9,13]

Congestive heart failure

About 15–20% of the patients may develop severe HF requiring hospitalization. In about one-third of such patients, acute HF due to abrupt worsening of mitral regurgitation, an ischemic event or rapid supraventricular tachyarrhythmias may occur, and may be the first clinical presentation of the disease. In the remaining patients clinical deterioration is more progressive, with increasing dyspnea, functional limitation, peripheral edema or pulmonary congestion,

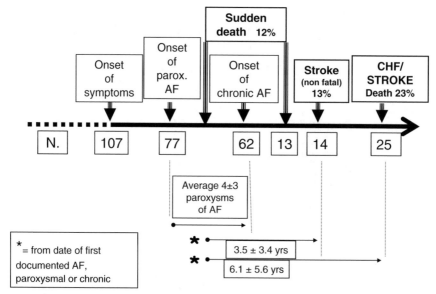

Fig. 7.2 Disease progression in 107 patients with hypertrophic cardiomyopathy and atrial fibrillation. At initial evaluation 30 patients had chronic atrial fibrillation. After paroxysmal atrial fibrillation developed in the 77 patients, chronic atrial fibrillation ensued after an average of four episodes of paroxysmal atrial fibrillation. Sudden death occurred in 13 patients (12%). Death due to congestive heart failure or stroke occurred in 25 patients (23%), after a mean of 6.1 years, and nonfatal stroke in 14 patients (13%), after a mean of 3.5 years since the first documented episode of atrial fibrillation. Only 10 patients (9%) had an uneventful course. Reprinted with permission from Cecchi F *et al.* (2003) What is the impact of atrial fibrillation in the clinical course of hypertrophic cardiomyopathy? In: Raviele A, ed. Cardiac Arrhythmias 2003: Proceedings of the 8th International Workshop on Cardiac Arrhythmias. Milan: Springer Verlag Italia, 2004.

due to low cardiac output. Severe LVOT obstruction associated with mitral regurgitation may be responsible for the symptoms, and rapid improvement can be observed in such patients when obstruction is relieved.[14] A minority of patients may develop severe mitral regurgitation because of abrupt chordal rupture, papillary muscle abnormality, or dysfunction due to ischemia[15] (Fig 7.3). In the remaining patients, progressive myocyte loss associated with wall thinning and a variable degree of myocardial fibrosis facilitates systolic and/or diastolic dysfunction, which may increase with time[16–18] (Fig. 7.4). LV remodelling may eventually lead to either the so-called end stage of the disease or the restrictive form;[17–20] the former is characterized by dilated atria and ventricles and global and/or segmental systolic dysfunction (Fig. 7.4), and the latter by a small left ventricle and enlarged atria and markedly restricted diastolic filling[17–20] (Fig. 7.4), eventually leading to heart transplantation or death.[16,17] Severe myocardial hypoperfusion, myocyte loss and progressive fibrosis might be responsible for wall thinning and the end stage.[10,17,21,22]

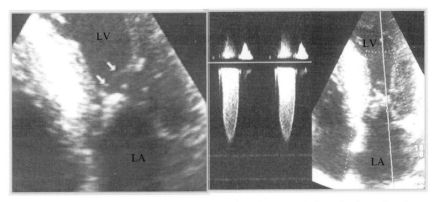

Fig. 7.3 Severe mitral regurgitation, due to abnormal papillary muscle insertion (arrow) on the anterior mitral leaflet in a patient with obstructive hypertrophic cardiomyopathy.

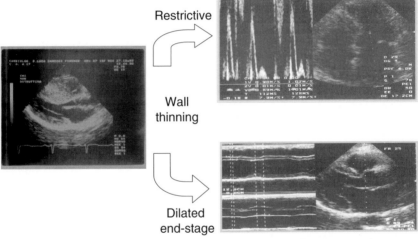

Fig. 7.4 Left ventricular remodeling in hypertrophic cardiomyopathy. Due to myocyte loss, progressive wall thinning may occur and lead either to a restrictive stage phase, with progressive biatrial dilation, a small left ventricular chamber and a restrictive filling pattern of mitral inflow with pulsed Doppler, or to a dilated end-stage phase, with a mildly dilated left ventricle and left atrium, low ejection fraction and impaired cardiac output.

Stroke

Stroke and other peripheral embolic events may be relatively frequent complications, with a cumulative incidence of about 5–6% of patients and an average annual incidence less than 1%, which progressively increases after 50 years of age.[8,21–22] Therefore, stroke usually occurs in older women, in the presence of AF (both paroxysmal or chronic) after an average of 6 years following the first episode of AF[9] (Fig. 7.2). Patients with AF showed an 8-fold increase in the risk of ischemic stroke (presumably of cardioembolic origin in most patients) compared with control patients in sinus rhythm.[9] While noncerebral peripheral embolism may be treated promptly, ischemic stroke due to cerebral embolism may have catastrophic consequences and is a major cause of disability and death in HCM.

Syncope

Syncope is frequently reported in HCM, with a prevalence of 10–20%. Repeated syncopal episodes, in particular in the young, are considered a risk factor for sudden death.[1-4] Careful investigation of the circumstances in which syncope occurs is needed. It may be of vasovagal origin, but may also depend on sinus node dysfunction or transient atrioventricular block. Syncope on effort is less common and outflow obstruction was initially thought to be the cause. However, about 20% of HCM patients with syncope show an abnormal blood pressure response during exercise and some of these patients also develop severe hypotension, which may be responsible for syncope.[25]

Endocarditis

Endocarditis is a rare complication, largely confined to patients with LVOT obstruction, with an annual incidence of 0.1–0.9%.[6,26] It may lead to variable degrees of valve incompetence, further complicating the clinical picture in HCM. In order to avoid this important complication, careful antibiotic prophylaxis is mandatory.

Risk factors and predictors of adverse prognosis

While sudden death remains largely unpredictable, AF, HF and its complications, including stroke, can be anticipated to a large extent, and often prevented or delayed with appropriate management (Table 7.3). The most important predictors of subsequent clinical deterioration and congestive heart failure are left atrial dilation and AF, severe LV hypertrophy, LVOT obstruction, moderate or severe functional limitation (NYHA classes III–IV), systolic and diastolic dysfunction, intramyocardial hypoperfusion, and impairment in coronary vascular reserve.[1,2,4,10]

Treatment strategies

Although in the last decade the understanding of HCM has greatly increased, treatment strategies are limited by the lack of randomized studies and are mostly based on empirical choice. The aim of therapy should be the reduction of symptoms and modifiable risk factors, notably left atrial dilation and AF, in order to avoid disease progression and the occurrence of HF and stroke. Drug therapy will usually be required for long periods, if not for ever.

Table 7.3 Risk factors for heart failure and stroke in hypertrophic cardiomyopathy. LVOT = left ventricular outflow tract

Heart failure	Stroke
Older ages	Older ages
History of heart failure	Heart failure
Atrial fibrillation	Atrial fibrillation
Left atrial dilation	Left atrial dilation
LVOT obstruction	LVOT obstruction
Severe mitral regurgitation	Female gender
Maximum left ventricle wall thickness	
Low peak oxygen consumption	
Systolic and diastolic dysfunction	
Myocardial hypoperfusion	
Malignant genetic mutations	

As myocardial ischemia can be precipitated by an elevated heart rate,[13] heart rate control with limitation of maximal heart rate is likely to be beneficial in most patients. Nevertheless, no data are available on the effect of reducing myocardial ischemia with drugs that lower oxygen consumption and heart rate. Heart rate trends may be documented by ambulatory monitoring and may be of great importance for accurate drug titration. Moreover, such monitoring may show episodes of sinoatrial block or chronotropic incompetence, either due to sinus node dysfunction or the effect of β-blocking drugs and/or amiodarone, and can be the cause of severe functional limitation. Accurate drug titration or DDDR (dual-chamber paced, dual-chamber sensed, dual response to sensing, rate modulation) pacing should be considered in overcoming this latter problem.

Clinical evaluation
Careful assessment of HF risk factors and functional limitation is mandatory for clinical decision-making, and before starting treatment. At the initial visit a noninvasive protocol usually includes careful family and personal histories, standard 12-lead ECG, 48-hour ambulatory ECG monitoring, two-dimensional Doppler echocardiography to define segmental LV wall thickness, systolic thickening and kinetics, atrial and ventricular chamber dimension, LV and left atrial ejection fraction, diastolic function parameters such as isovolumic relaxation time and deceleration time, end-systolic LVOT area, mitral valve leaflet length, the presence of systolic anterior motion of mitral valve and transvalvular flow velocity, and LVOT peak gradient in the basal state and after provocation (derived by continuous-wave Doppler velocity in the outflow tract). In our experience dobutamine stress echocardiography should not be routinely used for LVOT obstruction evaluation because of the high likelihood of false-positive results. The cardiopulmonary exercise test, with continuous monitoring

of blood pressure, ECG and oxygen consumption, should also be part of the clinical assessment. Its safety and usefulness have been reported.[25]

Invasive tests, such as coronary angiography, are usually required to rule out coexistent coronary artery disease. Laboratory genetic analysis is still regarded as a research tool. The assessment of myocardial blood flow and coronary vasodilator reserve, after dipyridamole infusion by PET, may detect hypoperfusion and reduced coronary vasodilator reserve, which is a predictor of long-term adverse outcome.[10,21]

Patients with no symptoms or risk factors

The subgroup of patients without symptoms or risk factors for HF have low risk for progressive symptoms or premature death from HF or stroke.[4-6] There are no data regarding the usefulness of prophylactic therapy, either with β-blocking or calcium channel-blocking drugs, in avoiding such disease progression or clinical manifestations in HCM patients.

Patients with no or mild symptoms (functional class I or II) and risk factors for HF

This subgroup comprises the vast majority of patients currently followed by community cardiologists or at referral institutions. Individual patients have a variable but substantial risk of disease progression during their clinical course, including premature HCM-related mortality. Empiric therapy may have a beneficial effect on symptoms and disease course in most patients. The relief of outflow obstruction and mitral regurgitation and restoration of sinus rhythm is usually followed by amelioration of symptoms and a net reduction of functional limitation. The reduction of risk factors for HF, including left atrial dilation, supraventricular and ventricular arrhythmias, or systolic and diastolic dysfunction may delay LV remodeling and lower the probability of cardiovascular events and death. Therapeutic protocols based on isolated or combined drug treatment, DC cardioversion and the surgical or nonsurgical relief of obstruction, are widely available (Table 7.4).

Patients with moderate-severe symptoms (functional class III–IV), and the end-stage phase

Treatment in this subgroup aims to improve symptoms by the correction of hemodynamic abnormalities, including high intracavitary pressures and fluid retention, and by achieving optimal heart rate control. LVOT obstruction with associated mitral regurgitation may be treated either surgically, with classical LV myotomy–myectomy or with percutaneous transcoronary septal myocardial ablation. Valve replacement may be needed for severe mitral regurgitation due to intrinsic valve diseases.

Conclusions

Forty years after the first clinical report, the epidemiology and clinical course

Table 7.4 Drug treatment options. ICD = implantable cardiac defibrillator

---

Angina, mild dyspnea, mild outflow obstruction
β-Blockers (nadolol 20–240 mg)
Calcium channel blockers (diltiazem 120–300 mg, verapamil 160–480 mg)
Amiodarone (100–300 mg)
Disopyramide (250–750 mg)
Oral anticoagulation (in the presence of paroxysmal AF or left atrial diameter >50 mm)

Arrhythmias
Atrial fibrillation
   Acute onset: propafenone (i.v.), DC cardioversion
   Prophylaxis: amiodarone, sotalol, nadolol
   Oral anticoagulation following onset of AF (also paroxysmal)
Ventricular ectopics/nonsustained runs of VT
   Amiodarone, sotalol, low-dose amiodarone + β-blockers
   ICD (for high-risk patients)
Sustained ventricular tachycardia/ventricular fibrillation
   ICD (+ amiodarone/sotalol/low-dose amiodarone + nadolol)
   Radiofrequency ablation (for SVT)
Sinoatrial/atrioventricular block
   DDDR pacing (ICD?)

Heart failure and end-stage phase
Diuretics
Amiodarone, β-blockers
Digoxin, calcium channel blockers (for AF heart rate control)
ACE inhibitors, angiotensin receptor inhibitors
Nitrates
Oral anticoagulation
Pacing (ICD)
Heart transplantation

---

of HCM are now well described. A detailed risk profile, based largely on non-invasive tests, can be obtained in many patients with HCM. Clinical decision-making should be based on the individual risk profile for the occurrence of AF, HF and stroke. Although the efficacy of treatment strategies has not been assessed by randomized studies, the amelioration of symptoms and avoidance of disease progression and major cardiovascular events eventually leading to HF and stroke is feasible in a substantial proportion of patients.

References

1 Maron BJ. Hypertrophic cardiomyopathy. *Lancet* 1997; **350**: 127–33.
2 Spirito P, Seidman CE, McKenna WJ, Maron BJ. The management of hypertrophic cardio-myopathy. *N Engl J Med* 1997; **336**: 775–85.
3 McKenna WJ, England D, Doi YL *et al.* Arrhythmia in hypertrophic cardiomyopathy: I – Influence on prognosis. *Br Heart J* 1981; **46**: 168–72.

4 Cecchi F, Olivotto I, Montereggi A, Santoro G, Dolara A, Maron BJ. Hypertrophic cardiomyopathy in Tuscany: Clinical course and outcome in an unselected population. *J Am Coll Cardiol* 1995; **26**: 1529–36.

5 Maron BJ, Casey SA, Poliac L, Gohman TE, Almquist AK, Aeppli DM. Clinical course of hypertrophic cardiomyopathy in a Regional United States Cohort. *JAMA* 1999; **281**: 650–5.

6 Cecchi F, Olivotto I, Lazzeroni E *et al.* Decorso clinico della cardiomiopatia ipertrofica in una popolazione non selezionata. L'esperienza dello Studio Policentrico Italiano Cardiomiopatie (SPIC). *G Ital Cardiol* 1997; **27**: 1133–43.

7 Maron BJ, Olivotto I, Spirito P *et al.* Epidemiology of hypertrophic cardiomyopathy-related death: Revisited in a large non-referral based patient population. *Circulation* 2000; **102**; 858–64.

8 Maron BJ, Olivotto I, Bellone P *et al.* Clinical profile of stroke in 900 patients with hypertrophic cardiomyopathy. *J Am Coll Cardiol* 2002; **39**: 301–7.

9 Olivotto I, Cecchi F, Casey AS, Dolara A, Traverse JH, Maron BJ. Impact of atrial fibrillation on the clinical course of hypertrophic cardiomyopathy. *Circulation* 2001; **104**: 2517–24.

10 Cecchi F, Olivotto I, Gistri R *et al.* Coronary microvascular dysfunction and prognosis in hypertrophic cardiomyopathy. *N Engl J Med* 2003; **349**: 1027–35.

11 Spirito P, Bellone P, Harris KM, Bernabo P, Bruzzi P, Maron BJ. Magnitude of left ventricular hypertrophy and risk of sudden death in hypertrophic cardiomyopathy. *N Engl J Med* 2001; **344**: 63–5.

12 Maron MS, Olivotto S, Betocchi S *et al.* Effect of left ventricular outflow tract obstruction on clinical outcome in hypertrophic cardiomyopathy. *N Eng J Med* 2003; **348**: 295–303.

13 Stafford WJ, Trohman RG, Bilsker M *et al.* Cardiac arrest in an adolescent with atrial fibrillation and hypertrophic cardiomyopathy. *J Am Coll Cardiol* 1986; **7**: 701–4.

14 Yu EH, Omran AS, Wigle ED *et al.* Mitral regurgitation in hypertrophic obstructive cardiomyopathy: Relationship to obstruction and relief with myectomy. *J Am Coll Cardiol* 2000; **36**: 2219–25.

15 Klues HG, Roberts WC, Maron BJ. Morphological determinants of echocardiographic patterns of mitral valve systolic anterior motion in obstructive hypertrophic cardiomyopathy. *Circulation* 1993; **87**: 1570–9.

16 Ten Cate FJ, Roelandt J. Progression to left ventricular dilatation in patients with hypertrophic obstructive cardiomyopathy. *Am Heart J* 1979; **97**: 762–5.

17 Spirito P, Maron BJ, Bonow RO *et al.* Occurrence and significance of progressive left ventricular wall thinning and relative cavity dilatation in hypertrophic cardiomyopathy. *Am J Cardiol* 1987; **59**: 123–9.

18 Maron BJ, Spirito P. Implications of left ventricular remodeling in hypertrophic cardiomyopathy. *Am J Cardiol* 1998; **81**: 1339–44.

19 Appleton CP, Hatle LK, Popp RL. Demonstration of restrictive ventricular physiology by Doppler echocardiography. *J Am Coll Cardiol* 1988; **11**: 757–68.

20 Appleton CP, Hatle LK, Popp RL. Relationship of transmitral flow velocity patterns to left ventricular diastolic function: New insights from a combined hemodynamic and Doppler echocardiography study. *J Am Coll Cardiol* 1988; **12**: 426–40.

21 Lorenzoni R, Gistri R, Cecchi F *et al.* Coronary vasodilator reserve is impaired in patients with hypertrophic cardiomyopathy and left ventricular dysfunction. *Am Heart J* 1998; **136**: 972–81.

22 Cannon RO, Rosing DR, Maron BJ *et al.* Myocardial ischemia in hypertrophic cardio-myopathy: Contribution of inadequate vasodilator reserve and elevated left ventricular filling pressures. *Circulation* 1985; 71: 234–43.

23 Furlan AJ, Craciun AR, Raju NR *et al.* Cerebrovascular complications associated with idiopathic hypertrophic subaortic stenosis. *Stroke* 1984; **15**: 282–4.

24 Higashikawa M, Nakamuri Y, Yoshida M *et al.* Incidence of ischemic strokes in hypertrophic cardiomyopathy is markedly increased if complicated by atrial fibrillation. *Jpn Circ J* 1997; **61**: 673–81.

25 Olivotto I, Maron BJ, Montereggi A, Mazzuoli F, Dolara A, Cecchi F. Prognostic value of systemic blood pressure response during exercise in a community-based patient population with hypertrophic cardiomyopathy. *Am Coll Cardiol* 1999; **33**: 2044–51.

26 Spirito P, Rapezzi C, Bellone P *et al.* Infective endocarditis in hypertrophic cardiomyopathy: Prevalence, incidence, and indications for antibiotic prophylaxis. *Circulation* 1999; **99**: 2132–7.

27 Cecchi F, Olivotto I. What is the impact of atrial fibrillation in the clinical course of hypertrophic cardiomyopathy? In: Raviele A, ed. *Cardiac Arrhythmias 2003: Proceedings of the 8th International Workshop on Cardiac Arrhythmias.* Heidelberg: Springer Verlag, 2003.

CHAPTER 8

Disturbed Vascular Control in Hypertrophic Cardiomyopathy: Mechanisms and Clinical Significance

Ross Campbell, BSc, Jayne A. Morris-Thurgood, PhD, and Michael P. Frenneaux, FRCP, FRACP

Hypertrophic cardiomyopathy (HCM) is an inherited disease with marked phenotypic variability that includes the extent of hypertrophy, the presence and severity of symptoms, and the natural history of the disease.[1] The early literature, derived from large tertiary referral centres, suggested that it was an uncommon disease and emphasized the high risk of sudden cardiac death in these patients—up to approximately 6% per year in adolescents and young adults in whom the diagnosis had been made in childhood.[2] However, it has become clear that the patients seen in these tertiary centres represent the tip of a much larger iceberg. Recent studies suggest that HCM may in fact be a relatively common inherited disorder with a prevalence, determined by echocardiographic screening of the population, of 0.2%.[1] The corollary is that, overall, HCM may be rather less malignant than we have previously thought.[3] Nevertheless, sudden cardiac death (SCD) is an important consequence of the disease and, tragically, often occurs as its first manifestation in previously asymptomatic young individuals. HCM is one of the most common causes of SCD in young adults. The annual incidence of SCD in young adults is between 1 and 5 per 100 000 population, HCM accounting for approximately 7% of such cases.[4]

There has therefore been considerable attention focused on identifying high- *vs* low-risk individuals with HCM in order to appropriately target therapies, such as automatic implantable cardioverter–difibrillators and amiodarone. Currently it is believed that SCD usually requires the presence of both a substrate and a trigger or triggers. Various triggers may potentially precipitate SCD, including profound hypotension, which, perhaps by inducing myocardial ischaemia, may cause malignant tachy- or bradyarrhythmias. In this review we will present evidence that disturbed reflex control of the vasculature is a frequent abnormality in patients with HCM. This abnormal control may result in sudden inappropriate vasodilatation, resulting in episodes of hypotension, which may in turn be responsible for recurrent syncope and act as a trigger for SCD.

Almost 50% of SCDs in HCM patients occur during or soon after exercise. A small study of beta-blocker therapy published in 1970 noted exercise hypotension in some patients,[5] but the significance of this observation was largely ignored for two decades. It is now apparent that abnormal blood pressure responses on exercise are seen in a substantial proportion of patients with HCM and confer an increased risk of SCD.

Hemodynamic changes occurring during exercise in healthy individuals

In order to understand the abnormalities of vascular function occurring during exercise in some patients with HCM, it is important to appreciate the normal physiological responses to exercise in health.

During maximal treadmill exercise, profound hemodynamic changes occur which maximize blood flow to exercising skeletal muscle. Cardiac output increases approximately 4-fold in healthy untrained subjects, but substantially more in athletes. This is due to both an increase in heart rate (approximately 2.5- to 3-fold in young adults) and an increase in stroke volume.[6,7] The latter is achieved by an increase in contractility and by the use of the Frank–Starling mechanism [i.e. an increase in left ventricular (LV) end-diastolic volume],[8] a consequence of profound (neurally mediated) constriction of splenic and intestinal veins which shifts blood volume into the central compartment.[9,10] Systemic vascular resistance falls approximately 2.5-fold during maximal exercise, and mean blood pressure increases by approximately 50%.

The fall in systemic vascular resistance during exercise is the composite of two very different responses in exercising *vs* nonexercising vascular beds. There is profound vasodilation in exercising vascular beds—thus leg blood flow may increase up to 20-fold. This is thought to be due to local metabolic factors, including adenosine, augmented by shear-related nitric oxide release. In contrast, there is marked constriction of vessels in nonexercising regions (such as the forearm, intestine and kidney).[11–15] This results from a complex interplay of opposing vasoconstrictor and vasodilator neural and neurohumoral influences, which are summarized in Fig. 8.1. Cortical influences (the 'central command reflex')[13,16] and input from skeletal muscle ergo- and metaboreceptors[11,15–17] both promote (vasoconstrictor) sympathetic outflow from the brainstem. In the later stages of exercise, plasma levels of circulating vasoconstrictors, such as arginine vasopressin, angiotensin II and endothelin, rise substantially and may also contribute to the vasoconstriction.[18–20] These vasoconstrictor influences may also be partially attenuated by neural input from arterial baroreceptors (due to increased arterial stretch) and from mechanosensitive receptors in the atria and left ventricle.[21]

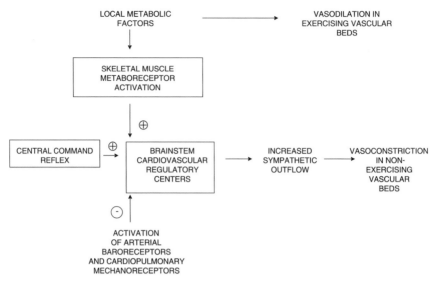

Fig. 8.1 Schematic illustration of the neural influences on vascular responses to exercise.

Abnormal blood pressure responses during exercise in HCM patients

It is now clear that a substantial proportion of patients with HCM have abnormal blood pressure responses (ABPR) during maximal treadmill exercise. This was first described by Edwards and colleagues in 1970 in a small study,[5] and subsequently confirmed by us in a consecutive series of 129 patients (mean age 41 years) with HCM attending a large tertiary referral centre.[22] We have defined ABPR as either a failure of systolic BP to rise by >20 mm Hg during maximal treadmill exercise, or as a fall of >20 mm Hg at peak exercise compared with before exercise or with a value recorded earlier in exercise. According to these criteria, we observed ABPR in approximately one-third of patients. In a study of 126 patients attending a community-based hospital (mean age 42 years), ABPR was observed in 22% of patients.[23]

Role of abnormal vascular control mechanisms

ABPR may be due to inadequate cardiac output response and/or to an exaggerated fall in systemic vascular resistance. We performed invasive hemodynamic studies in 14 HCM patients with normal exercise blood pressure responses and 14 with ABPR. In this highly selected study population, the increase in cardiac output was marginally (but significantly) higher in the ABPR group, and by implication, ABPR was due to an exaggerated fall in systemic vascular resistance during exercise.[22]

In a subsequent study of 103 consecutive patients with HCM we examined the vascular response in a nonexercising vascular bed (the forearm) during supine cycle exercise and the blood pressure response during maximal treadmill exercise. Forearm vascular resistance (FVR) was measured using mercury in Silastic strain gauge plethysmography. As noted above, there is normally an increase in FVR during leg exercise. In contrast, in over a third of the patients with HCM, FVR failed to increase or paradoxically fell during exercise. This abnormal pattern was strongly associated with ABPR during maximal treadmill exercise[12] (Fig. 8.2).

These data indicate that the primary cause of ABPR may, in most cases, be an exaggerated fall in systemic vascular resistance due to vasodilatation or to a failure of vasoconstriction in nonexercising vascular beds. It should be noted, however, that a 'normal' left ventricle might be expected to increase cardiac output to a greater extent in the face of a fall in systemic vascular resistance than was seen in HCM patients. Consistent with this, we have shown that patients with vasovagal syncope frequently demonstrate an abnormal fall in FVR during cycle exercise, yet ABPR was relatively uncommon.[14] Several factors may conspire to limit the ability to increase the cardiac output in response to the exaggerated fall in systemic vascular resistance in HCM patients. Although we found no association between ABPR and resting outflow tract obstruction, this does not exclude dynamic outflow tract obstruction as an important mechanism. Indeed, recent studies report normalization of ABPR following alcohol septal ablation.[24] However, as discussed below, other mechanisms might contribute to this. It was noted earlier that the normal increase in stroke volume during exercise results in part from an increase in left ventricular end-diastolic volume. We have shown that patients with HCM frequently exhibit a failure of splenic venoconstriction during exercise (presumably via a mechanism similar to that responsible for the failure of resistance vessel constriction).[25] This, together with the diastolic dysfunction which characterizes the disease, may markedly limit the ability to increase cardiac output in some patients.

In our subsequent clinical experience we certainly encountered some patients in whom cardiac output limitation was the dominant mechanism of ABPR during exercise, but in the majority an exaggerated fall in systemic vascular resistance was the dominant mechanism. This has not, however, been a universal finding of other groups. Systolic dysfunction has been documented in some HCM patients during exercise and during dobutamine stress.[26–28] One recent study argued that a failure of cardiac output augmentation may be the dominant mechanism of ABPR during exercise. In this study, the cardiac output response to exercise was evaluated using the nuclear VEST, which is a nonimaging gamma camera. In contrast to the findings of our invasive hemodynamic study, HCM patients with ABPR had significantly lower cardiac output responses than patients with normal blood pressure responses.[29] However, caution should be exercised. Despite exercising for almost 8 minutes on a Bruce protocol (estimated $\dot{V}O_2$max at least 20 ml/kg/min), their cardiac

NORMAL
Rest

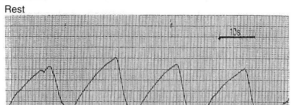

Exercise

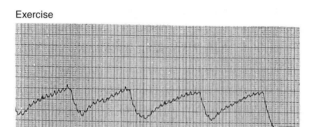

HYPOTENSIVE HCM
Rest

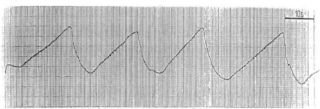

Exercise

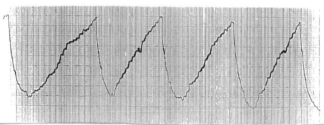

Fig. 8.2 Forearm plethysmography tracings from two patients, one with a normal blood pressure response on exercise (NBPR) and the other with an abnormal blood pressure response on exercise (ABPR). The slope of the upstroke is proportional to forearm blood flow (FBF). In the patient with NBPR the slope becomes less during exercise, indicating a fall in FBF due to vasoconstriction. In contrast, in the patient with ABPR the slope becomes steeper during exercise, indicating an increase in FBR due to vasodilation.

output increased using this measure by only 50%, which would be expected to be associated with a $\dot{V}O_2$max of less than 10 ml/kg/min. The validity of the nuclear VEST technique as a measure of cardiac output during exercise must therefore be questioned.

Prognostic significance of ABPR during maximal treadmill exercise

Several studies have now shown that the presence of ABPR during maximal treadmill exercise carries with it an increased risk of SCD. One hundred and sixty-one consecutive patients with HCM aged less than 40 years (mean age 27 years) who were attending a tertiary cardiomyopathy referral center were followed for a mean of 44 months. Sixty (37%) demonstrated ABPR at the initial assessment. During the follow-up period SCD occurred in 9/60 patients with ABPR vs 3/101 with a normal blood pressure response ($P < 0.009$). During this relatively brief follow-up period the positive predictive accuracy of ABPR for SCD was therefore low (15%), but the presence of a normal blood pressure response was highly reassuring (negative predictive accuracy 97%).[30] In a community-based hospital series of 126 consecutive patients who were rather older (mean age 42 years), ABPR was observed in 22%. During a mean follow-up period of approximately 5 years there were nine HCM-related deaths (three SCD and six heart failure); four of these subjects had ABPR. ABPR had a low positive predictive accuracy (14%) and a normal blood pressure response had high negative predictive accuracy (95%) for cardiovascular death.[23] A large Japanese series also supports a link between ABPR during exercise and increased risk of SCD. Three hundred and nine consecutive patients in whom HCM was diagnosed between 1971 and 1994 were followed for an average of nearly 10 years. During follow-up there were 28 SCDs. Two factors were found to be independent predictors of SCD on multivariate analysis: a flat blood pressure response during exercise ($P = 0.006$), and (in contrast to most studies), a high resting left ventricular outflow tract gradient ($P = 0.003$).[31]

Abnormal vascular control mechanisms in HCM: potential mechanisms

It was noted earlier that, in healthy subjects during exercise, central command and skeletal muscle metaboreceptor inputs increase (vasoconstrictor) sympathetic outflow from the brainstem. This overcomes the opposing effects of activation of arterial baroreceptors (by increased arterial pulsatile stretch) and of activation of stretch-sensitive left ventricular and atrial receptors. In 1973, Mark and colleagues reported that exercise syncope in patients with aortic stenosis was associated with an abnormal fall in forearm vascular resistance during leg exercise (similar to that seen in HCM patients), and that this reverted to a normal response following successful aortic valve replacement.[32] In another study in anesthetized dogs, this group showed that inflation of a balloon in the left ventricle caused a fall in skeletal muscle vascular resistance, whereas infla-tion of the balloon in the left atrium had no effect.[33] They concluded that the abnormal exercise vascular response seen in patients with aortic stenosis was most likely a result of enhanced activation of stretch-sensitive left ventricular receptors (mechanoreceptors), due to increased left ventricular wall stress. The latter could be attributed to increased intracavitary pressures resulting from the aortic stenosis.

The parallels between these findings in aortic stenosis and the abnormal vascular responses leading to ABPR during exercise in HCM are clear, but the role of left ventricular mechanoreceptors in generating the abnormal vascular responses in HCM is inferential rather than proven. Increased left ventricular wall stresses might be expected to occur in HCM patients for at least three reasons. The first reason is the presence of left ventricular outflow tract obstruction. Whilst we did not show a relation between the presence or magnitude of resting left ventricular outflow tract obstruction and ABPR dur-ing exercise, this does not exclude a role for dynamic obstruction, via either its effects on cardiac output or on left ventricular wall stress and therefore left ventricular mechanoreceptor firing. As noted earlier, recent reports suggest that alcohol septal ablation can normalize ABPR during exercise.[24] Secondly, the presence of patchy myocyte disarray and/or fibrosis may cause markedly heterogeneous physical properties of the myocardium with localized areas of greatly increased wall stress. Thirdly, the presence of subendocardial isch-emia[28] may cause abnormal left ventricular wall stresses. Consistent with this, we have shown that abnormal vasodilation during exercise (presumably due to LV mechanoreceptor activation), may also be an important mechanism of exercise hypotension in patients with ischemic heart disease.[34]

There is, however, further evidence pointing to dysfunction of left ventricu-lar mechanoreceptors in patients with HCM. Central blood volume unloading, such as occurs when blood pools in the pelvic and lower limb veins on assum-ing an upright posture, normally causes reflex compensatory adjustments which result in an increase in systemic vascular resistance, venoconstriction, and a modest increase in heart rate. In health, these adjustments ensure that the fall in blood pressure is small and brief. The initial fall in cardiac chamber size and blood pressure results in reduced afferent input from cardiopulmo-nary and arterial baroreceptors respectively, which results in increased sym-pathetic outflow from the brainstem. Lesser degrees of central blood volume unloading which are insufficient to reduce blood pressure can be induced by application of lower-body negative pressure (which pools blood in the pelvic and lower limb veins). A marked increase in FVR is evident despite the absence of any fall in blood pressure. Available evidence suggests that this response is predominantly mediated via inactivation of left ventricular mechanoreceptors.[35] We showed that an abnormal forearm vascular response to application of subhypotensive lower-body negative pressure was frequently seen in patients with HCM. In these patients FVR failed to increase or para-doxically fell. There was no evidence of an abnormality of central or efferent mechanisms. Furthermore, the function of carotid baroreceptors was assessed and was shown to be normal.[36] We considered that the most likely interpretation of these observations was a failure of the normal inactivation (and in some cases paradoxical activation) of left ventricular mechanoreceptors during central blood volume unloading in these patients. The mechanism of this abnormality is unclear but heterogeneous strain changes associated with the patchy myocyte disarray and fibrosis may provide a substrate.

Potential role of natriuretic peptides in the ABPR during exercise

Patients with HCM typically have raised plasma levels of the natriuretic peptides ANP (atrial natriuretic peptide) and BNP (B-type natriuretic peptide). The increase in plasma ANP is mainly determined by diastolic function, whereas the increase in BNP is mainly determined by outflow tract obstruction.[37] Whereas in healthy subjects the plasma levels of natriuretic peptides do not significantly increase on exercise, in some cardiac disease states, including congestive heart failure, there may be a marked increase.[38] In patients with hypertension, the increase in plasma BNP during exercise was 6- to 7-fold greater than in healthy controls, presumably because of a greater increase in left ventricular end diastolic pressure.[39] In patients with hypertensive left ventricular hypertrophy this phenomenon was even more marked.[40] Patients with HCM typically also demonstrate marked increases in left ventricular end diastolic pressure during exercise.[41] An augmented increase in plasma natriuretic peptides might therefore be expected in patients with HCM, but this remains to be determined. Natriuretic peptides have vasorelaxant effects on vascular smooth muscle acting via the particulate guanylate cyclase pathway.[42] Such an increase in natriuretic peptides might theoretically contribute to the abnormal vascular responses to exercise seen in patients with HCM. In addition, natriuretic peptides have been shown to have sympatholytic effects that act at various points in the reflex pathways, including centrally and via activation of cardiac vagal afferents.[43] Increased local production of BNP within the left ventricle during exercise might therefore potentially contribute to the putative left ventricular mechanoreceptor activation, providing a unifying hypothesis.

Autonomic control of heart rate and heart period variability in HCM

Thus far we have focused on abnormalities of reflex control of the vasculature in patients with HCM. Input from arterial and cardiopulmonary mechanoreceptors is also important in the control of heart rate (or more correctly, heart period). Reduced baroreflex sensitivity and heart rate variability have been shown to be potent adverse prognostic markers in patients who have suffered myocardial infarction[44] and in patients with chronic heart failure.[45] This may in part arise from the effects of the associated sympathetic activation and vagal withdrawal on the susceptibility to ventricular arrhythmia.[46]

Heart rate may be assessed by frequency domain and by time domain techniques. Frequency domain techniques identify very low frequency, low frequency (LF) and high frequency (HF) components. Changes in HF and LF variability are often (controversially) used to assess changes in cardiac autonomic tone. The HF component corresponds to the respiratory frequency and is predominantly due to respiratory-related changes in vagal efferent activity. The mechanism of LF variability has been particularly controversial, but appears to predominantly reflect baroreflex modulation of heart rate in response to spontaneous changes in blood pressure.[47] Fei and colleagues reported reduced LF variability in unmedicated HCM patients compared with controls (implying impaired baroreflex modulation), but preserved HF variability.[48] In another study, LF variability was reduced in patients with 'obstructive' HCM, but not in those with 'nonobstructive' HCM, compared with controls. Furthermore, patients with obstruction demonstrated a failure of the normal increase (or reversal) of LF variability during upright tilt.[49] In another study employing time domain indices, reduced heart rate variability also correlated with the degree of subaortic obstruction.[50]

In contrast to the above studies, others have identified a specific impairment of vagal modulation of heart rate. Counihan and colleagues reported increased overall heart rate variability but reduced 'vagal' measures (HF variability in the frequency domain and pNN5O in the time domain) in HCM patients with an adverse family history. These abnormalities did not add to the established risk factors in determining the risk of SCD, however.[51] Gilligan and colleagues also implied reduced vagal activity in HCM patients *vs* controls on the basis of reduced heart rate responses to deep breathing and to the Valsalva manoeuvre.[52]

Abnormal vascular control: a mechanism for recurrent syncope?

Recurrent syncope is a relatively frequent symptom in patients with HCM, and, at least in younger patients, carries an increased risk of SCD, particularly when combined with other risk factors.[53,54] Multiple mechanisms may be responsible, including arrhythmia and dynamic left ventricular outflow tract obstruction, yet despite extensive investigation the cause is not identified in the majority of patients.[55,56] We recently assessed a highly selected series of 18 HCM patients with recurrent syncope for which no cause had been identified despite extensive investigation and 11 HCM patients with no such history. Beat-by-beat blood pressure waveforms were recorded using a Portapres system during a 24-hour period. Recurrent abrupt spontaneous episodes of hypotension without associated reflex tachycardia were observed in eight of the patients with a history of syncope but none of those without such a history. Symptom diaries revealed that 60% of these episodes were temporally associated with an episode of impaired consciousness. Using a validated transfer function, we were able to show that systemic vascular resistance fell markedly during these episodes, whereas cardiac output did not change. It is noteworthy that many of these episodes of hypotension occurred during minor activity or at rest. Thus, abrupt vasodilatation may be responsible for some cases of syncope both on exercise and at rest.

The combination of vasodilatation with associated hypotension without a reflex tachycardia has much in common with vasovagal syncope. Upright tilt testing is commonly used as a diagnostic test in such patients. In the above study, vasovagal tilt test responses occurred with similar frequency in patients with and without a history of recurrent syncope and in those with and without episodic hypotension during ambulatory monitoring. This is consistent with an earlier report by Sneddon and colleagues in which vasovagal responses were observed in 22% of 46 HCM patients, but this response was not associated with a history of recurrent syncope.[57] These data suggest that the episodic hypotension we have observed may have a different physiological basis to vasovagal reactions occurring during upright tilt. In contrast, Gilligan and colleagues reported a high incidence of both classic vasovagal reactions (nine of 36 patients) and transient episodes of hypotension not amounting to classic vasovagal responses (10 of 36 patients) in HCM. One or other of these patterns was observed in 86% of patients with a history of recurrent syncope *vs* 26% of those without such a history and 22% of controls ($P = 0.001$).[58] However, the significance of such transient episodes of hypotension is uncertain.

A recent study by Manganelli and colleagues which employed the nuclear VEST suggested that a hypotensive response to upright tilt in HCM patients with a history of recurrent syncope was due to a fall in cardiac output associated with a compensatory increase in systemic vascular resistance.[59] This response was not seen in HCM patients without a history of recurrent syncope, and contrasted with a progressive fall in systemic vascular resistance in association with hypotension seen in patients with a classical history of vasovagal syncope. The authors argue that, at least in some cases, syncope may be a consequence of the preload dependence of the stiff left ventricle in these patients.

How may abnormal reflex control of vascular tone act as a trigger for SCD?

Whilst it is clear that ABPR during maximal treadmill exercise confers an increased risk of SCD in patients aged less than 40 years, a cause–effect relation rather than an association is not proven. Nevertheless, such a mechanism is plausible, as outlined below.

Hypotension may potentially act as a trigger for SCD, but requires an appropriate substrate; if this were not so, vasovagal syncope would be associated with an increased risk of SCD. The extensive myocyte disarray and fibrosis which characterizes the disease may represent this substrate, conferring an increased risk of ventricular arrhythmia. Patients with HCM are prone to

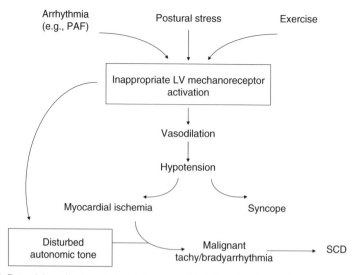

Fig. 8.3 Potential mechanisms by which inappropriate left ventricular mechanoreceptor activation may cause syncope or trigger sudden cardiac death in patients with hypertrophic cardiomyopathy.

myocardial ischemia, due to increased myocardial oxygen demand (as a result of LV hypertrophy), reduced transcoronary perfusion gradient (as a result of increased left ventricular end diastolic pressure), thickening of small vessels and possibly systolic obliteration of septal perforator vessels. Hypotension may therefore precipitate myocardial ischemia in patients with HCM. The combination of myocardial ischemia and abrupt changes in autonomic efferent activity to the heart may potentially precipitate arrhythmia (either malignant tachyarrhythmia or bradycardia) (Fig. 8.3). Furthermore, two studies in small groups of HCM patients using positron emission tomography have suggested that in these patients there was impaired neuronal reuptake of catecholamines in areas of hypersomal myocardium. This may result in increased local catecholamine levels, which are likely to be exaggerated during abrupt increases in sympathetic outflow.[60,61]

Summary

Abnormal reflex control of vascular tone is frequently seen in patients with HCM. Over 30% of patients demonstrate ABPR during maximal treadmill exercise. In most cases this is due to an exaggerated fall in systemic vascular resistance. In a large prospective study in HCM patients aged less than 40 years, ABPR was shown to be a marker of increased risk of sudden cardiac death, with high negative predictive accuracy (97%) but low positive predictive accuracy (15%) during 44 months (mean) of follow-up. Subsequent work from the St George's group has emphasized the importance of multiple risk factors (including ABPR as one component). Sudden episodes of hypotension (EHy) also occur during everyday life in patients with HCM, and may occur during minor activity and even at rest. In a small study these episodes were shown to be due to a sudden fall in systemic vascular resistance with maintenance of cardiac output. Abnormal reflex control of vascular resistance may potentially be an important cause of syncope in HCM. The mechanism of this abnormal reflex control of the vasculature is unproven. In patients with EHy, baroreflex control of heart rate (BRS) was impaired compared with those without such episodes. Furthermore, HCM patients frequently demonstrate impaired forearm vascular constriction (or even vasodilation) during application of subhypotensive lower body negative pressure (LBNP). The vasoconstrictor response to LBNP is thought to be mediated principally by stretch-sensitive LV mechanoreceptors. ABPR and EHy may therefore be due to inappropriate firing of left ventricular mechanoreceptors related to local increases in wall strain due to the patchy nature of myocyte disarray.

Acknowledgment

All authors are supported by the British Heart Foundation.

References

1 Maron BJ, Gardin JM, Flack JM, Gidding SS, Kurosaki TT, Bild DE. Prevalence of hypertrophic cardiomyopathy in a general population of young adults. Echocardiographic analysis of 4111 subjects in the CARDIA Study. Coronary Artery Risk Development in (Young) Adults. *Circulation* 1995; **92**: 785–9.

2 McKenna W, Deanfield J, Faruqui A, England D, Oakley C, Goodwin J. Prognosis in hypertrophic cardiomyopathy: Role of age and clinical, electrocardiographic and hemodynamic features. *Am J Cardiol* 1981; **47**: 532–8.

3 Maron BJ, Casey SA, Poliac LC, Gohman TE, Almquist AK, Aeppli DM. Clinical course of hypertrophic cardiomyopathy in a regional United States cohort. *JAMA* 1999; **281**: 650–5.

4 Wren C, O'Sullivan JJ, Wright C. Sudden death in children and adolescents. *Heart* 2000; **83**: 410–13.

5 Edwards RH, Kristinsson A, Warrell DA, Goodwin JF. Effects of propranolol on response to exercise in hypertrophic obstructive cardiomyopathy. *Br Heart J* 1970; **32**: 219–25.

6 Poliner LR, Dehmer GJ, Lewis SE, Parkey RW, Blomqvist CG, Willerson JT. Left ventricular performance in normal subjects: A comparison of the responses to exercise in the upright and supine positions. *Circulation* 1980; **62**: 528–34.

7 Shepherd JT. Circulatory response to exercise in health. *Circulation* 1987; **76** (6 Pt 2): VI3–10.

8 Stratton JR, Levy WC, Cerqueira MD, Schwartz RS, Abrass IB. Cardiovascular responses to exercise. Effects of aging and exercise training in healthy men. *Circulation* 1994; **89**: 1648–55.

9 Flamm SD, Taki J, Moore R *et al.* Redistribution of regional and organ blood volume and effect on cardiac function in relation to upright exercise intensity in healthy human subjects. *Circulation* 1990; **81**: 1550–9.

10 Thomson HL, Atherton JJ, Khafagi FA, Frenneaux MP. Failure of reflex venoconstriction during exercise in patients with vasovagal syncope. *Circulation* 1996; **93**: 953–9.

11 Alam M, Smirk FH. Observations in man upon a blood pressure raising reflex arising from the voluntary muscles. *J Physiol* 1937; **89**: 372–83.

12 Counihan PJ, Frenneaux MP, Webb DJ, McKenna WJ. Abnormal vascular responses to supine exercise in hypertrophic cardiomyopathy. *Circulation* 1991; **84**: 686–96.

13 Mitchell JH, Reeves DR Jr, Rogers HB, Secher NH, Victor RG. Autonomic blockade and cardiovascular responses to static exercise in partially curarized man. *J Physiol (Lond)* 1989; **413**: 433–45.

14 Thomson HL, Lele SS, Atherton JJ, Wright KN, Stafford W, Frenneaux MP. Abnormal forearm vascular responses during dynamic leg exercise in patients with vasovagal syncope. *Circulation* 1995; **92**: 2204–9.

15 Victor RG, Bertocci LA, Pryor SL, Nunnally RL. Sympathetic nerve discharge is coupled to muscle cell pH during exercise in humans [published erratum appears in *J Clin Invest* 1988; **82**: 2181]. *J Clin Invest* 1988; **82**: 1301–5.

16 Mitchell JH. Cardiovascular control during exercise: Central and reflex neural mechanisms. *Am J Cardiol* 1985; **55**: 34–41D.

17 Piepoli M, Clark AL, Volterrani M, Adamopoulos S, Sleight P, Coats AJ. Contribution of muscle afferents to the hemodynamic, autonomic, and ventilatory responses to exercise in patients with chronic heart failure: Effects of physical training. *Circulation* 1996; **93**: 940–52.

18 Freund BJ, Claybaugh JR, Dice MS, Hashiro GM. Hormonal and vascular fluid responses to maximal exercise in trained and untrained males. *J Appl Physiol* 1987; **63**: 669–75.

19 Inder WJ, Hellemans J, Swanney MP, Prickett TC, Donald RA. Prolonged exercise increases peripheral plasma ACTH, CRH, and AVP in male athletes. *J Appl Physiol* 1998; **85**: 835–41.

20 Kinugawa T, Ogino K, Miyakoda H *et al.* Responses of catecholamines, renin–angiotensin system, and atrial natriuretic peptide to exercise in untrained men and women. *Gen Pharmacol* 1997; **28**: 225–8.

21 Haywood GA, Counihan PJ, Sneddon JF, Jennison SH, Bashir Y, McKenna WJ. Increased renal and forearm vasoconstriction in response to exercise after heart transplantation. *Br Heart J* 1993; **70**: 247–51.

22 Frenneaux MP, Counihan PJ, Caforio AL, Chikamori T, McKenna WJ. Abnormal blood pressure response during exercise in hypertrophic cardiomyopathy [see comments]. *Circulation* 1990; **82**: 1995–2002.

23 Olivotto I, Maron BJ, Montereggi A, Mazzuoli F, Dolara A, Cecchi F. Prognostic value of systemic blood pressure response during exercise in a community-based patient population with hypertrophic cardiomyopathy. *J Am Coll Cardiol* 1999; **33**: 2044–51.

24 Kim JJ, Lee CW, Park SW *et al.* Improvement in exercise capacity and exercise blood pressure response after transcoronary alcohol ablation therapy of septal hypertrophy in hypertrophic cardiomyopathy. *Am J Cardiol* 1999; **83**: 1220–3.

25 Thomson HL, Morris-Thurgood J, Atherton J, McKenna WJ, Frenneaux MP. Reflex responses of venous capacitance vessels in patients with hypertrophic cardiomyopathy [see comments]. *Clin Sci (Colch)* 1998; **94**: 339–46.

26 Okeie K, Shimizu M, Yoshio H *et al.* Left ventricular systolic dysfunction during exercise and dobutamine stress in patients with hypertrophic cardiomyopathy. *J Am Coll Cardiol* 2000; **36**: 856–63.

27 Shimizu M, Ino H, Okeie K *et al.* Systolic dysfunction and blood pressure responses to supine exercise in patients with hypertrophic cardiomyopathy. *Jpn Circ J* 2001; **65**: 325–9.

28 Yoshida N, Ikeda H, Wada T *et al*. Exercise-induced abnormal blood pressure responses are related to subendocardial ischemia in hypertrophic cardiomyopathy. *J Am Coll Cardiol* 1998; **32**: 1938–42.

29 Ciampi Q, Betocchi S, Lombardi R *et al*. Hemodynamic determinants of exercise-induced abnormal blood pressure response in hypertrophic cardiomyopathy. *J Am Coll Cardiol* 2002; **40**: 278–84.

30 Sadoul N, Prasad K, Elliott PM, Bannerjee S, Frenneaux MP, McKenna WJ. Prospective prognostic assessment of blood pressure response during exercise in patients with hypertrophic cardiomyopathy. *Circulation* 1997; **96**: 2987–91.

31 Maki S, Ikeda H, Muro A *et al*. Predictors of sudden cardiac death in hypertrophic cardiomyopathy. *Am J Cardiol* 1998; **82**: 774–8.

32 Mark AL, Kioschos JM, Abboud FM, Heistad DD, Schmid PG. Abnormal vascular responses to exercise in patients with aortic stenosis. *J Clin Invest* 1973; **52**: 1138–46.

33 Mark AL, Abboud FM, Schmid PG, Heistad DD. Reflex vascular responses to left ventricular outflow obstruction and activation of ventricular baroreceptors in dogs. *J Clin Invest* 1973; **52**: 1147–53.

34 Lele SS, Scalia G, Thomson H *et al*. Mechanism of exercise hypotension in patients with ischemic heart disease. Role of neurocardiogenically mediated vasodilation. *Circulation* 1994; **90**: 2701–9.

35 Eckberg DL, Sleight P. *Human Baroreflexes in Health and Disease*. New York: Oxford University Press, 1992.

36 Thomson HL, Morris-Thurgood J, Atherton J, Frenneaux M. Reduced cardiopulmonary baroreflex sensitivity in patients with hypertrophic cardiomyopathy. *J Am Coll Cardiol* 1998; **31**: 1377–82.

37 Briguori C, Betocchi S, Manganelli F *et al*. Determinants and clinical significance of natriuretic peptides and hypertrophic cardiomyopathy. *Eur Heart J* 2001; **22**: 1328–36.

38 Steele IC, McDowell G, Moore A *et al*. Responses of atrial natriuretic peptide and brain natriuretic peptide to exercise in patients with chronic heart failure and normal control subjects. *Eur J Clin Invest* 1997; **27**: 270–6.

39 Tanaka M, Ishizaka Y, Ishiyama Y *et al*. Exercise-induced secretion of brain natriuretic peptide in essential hypertension and normal subjects. *Hypertens Res* 1995; **18**: 159–66.

40 Kohno M, Yasunari K, Yokokawa K *et al*. Plasma brain natriuretic peptide during ergometric exercise in hypertensive patients with left ventricular hypertrophy. *Metabolism* 1996; **45**: 1326–9.

41 Lele SS, Thomson HL, Seo H, Belenkie I, McKenna WJ, Frenneaux MP. Exercise capacity in hypertrophic cardiomyopathy. Role of stroke volume limitation, heart rate, and diastolic filling characteristics. *Circulation* 1995; **92**: 2886–94.

42 Winquist RJ, Faison EP, Waldman SA, Schwartz K, Murad F, Rapoport RM. Atrial natriuretic factor elicits an endothelium-independent relaxation and activates particulate guanylate cyclase in vascular smooth muscle. *Proc Natl Acad Sci USA* 1984; **81**: 7661–4.

43 Abramson BL, Ando S, Notarius CF, Rongen GA, Floras JS. Effect of atrial natriuretic peptide on muscle sympathetic activity and its reflex control in human heart failure. *Circulation* 1999; **99**: 1810–5.

44 La Rovere MT, Bigger JT Jr, Marcus FI, Mortara A, Schwartz PJ. Baroreflex sensitivity and heart-rate variability in prediction of total cardiac mortality after myocardial infarction. ATRAMI (Autonomic Tone and Reflexes After Myocardial Infarction) Investigators [see comments]. *Lancet* 1998; **351**: 478–84.

45 Mortara A, La Rovere MT, Pinna GD *et al.* Arterial baroreflex modulation of heart rate in chronic heart failure: Clinical and hemodynamic correlates and prognostic implications. *Circulation* 1997; **96**: 3450–8.

46 Schwartz PJ, La Rovere MT, Vanoli E. Autonomic nervous system and sudden cardiac death. Experimental basis and clinical observations for post-myocardial infarction risk stratification. *Circulation* 1992; **85** (1 Suppl.): I77–91.

47 Sleight P, La Rovere MT, Mortara A *et al.* Physiology and pathophysiology of heart rate and blood pressure variability in humans: Is power spectral analysis largely an index of baroreflex gain? [see comments] [published erratum appears in *Clin Sci (Colch)* 1995; **88**: 733]. *Clin Sci (Colch)* 1995; **88**: 103–9.

48 Fei L, Slade AK, Prasad K, Malik M, McKenna WJ, Camm AJ. Is there increased sympathetic activity in patients with hypertrophic cardiomyopathy? *J Am Coll Cardiol* 1995; **26**: 472–80.

49 Limbruno U, Strata G, Zucchi R *et al.* Altered autonomic cardiac control in hypertrophic cardiomyopathy. Role of outflow tract obstruction and myocardial hypertrophy. *Eur Heart J* 1998; **19**: 146–53.

50 Doven O, Sayin T, Guldal M, Karaoguz R, Oral D. Heart rate variability in hypertrophic obstructive cardiomyopathy: Association with functional classification and left ventricular outflow gradients. *Int J Cardiol* 2001; **77**: 281–6.

51 Counihan PJ, Fei L, Bashir Y, Farrell TG, Haywood GA, McKenna WJ. Assessment of heart rate variability in hypertrophic cardiomyopathy. Association with clinical and prognostic features. *Circulation* 1993; **88**: 1682–90.

52 Gilligan DM, Chan WL, Sbarouni E, Nihoyannopoulos P, Oakley CM. Autonomic function in hypertrophic cardiomyopathy. *Br Heart J* 1993; **69**: 525–9.

53 Elliott PM, Poloniecki J, Dickie S *et al.* Sudden death in hypertrophic cardiomyopathy: Identification of high risk patients. *J Am Coll Cardiol* 2000; **36**: 2212–18.

54 Maron BJ, Bonow RO, Cannon RO III, Leon MB, Epstein SE. Hypertrophic cardiomyopathy. Interrelations of clinical manifestations, pathophysiology, and therapy (1). *N Engl J Med* 1987; **316**: 780–9.

55 McKenna WJ, Elliott PM. Hypertrophic cardiomyopathy. In: Topol EJ, ed. *Textbook of Cardiovascular Medicine.* Philadelphia: Lippincott-Raven, 1998: 745–68.

56 Spirito P, Seidman CE, McKenna WJ, Maron BJ. The management of hypertrophic cardiomyopathy. *N Engl J Med* 1997; **336**: 775–85.

57 Sneddon JF, Slade A, Seo H, Camm AJ, McKenna WJ. Assessment of the diagnostic value of head-up tilt testing in the evaluation of syncope in hypertrophic cardiomyopathy. *Am J Cardiol* 1994; **73**: 601–4.

58 Gilligan DM, Nihoyannopoulos P, Chan WL, Oakley CM. Investigation of a hemodynamic basis for syncope in hypertrophic cardiomyopathy. Use of a head-up tilt test. *Circulation* 1992; **85**: 2140–8.

59 Manganelli F, Betocchi S, Ciampi Q *et al.* Comparison of hemodynamic adaptation to orthostatic stress in patients with hypertrophic cardiomyopathy with or without syncope and in vasovagal syncope. *Am J Cardiol* 2002; **89**: 1405–10.

60 Li ST, Tack CJ, Fananapazir L, Goldstein DS. Myocardial perfusion and sympathetic innervation in patients with hypertrophic cardiomyopathy. *J Am Coll Cardiol* 2000; **35**: 1867–73.

61 Schafers M, Dutka D, Rhodes CG *et al.* Myocardial presynaptic and postsynaptic autonomic dysfunction in hypertrophic cardiomyopathy. *Circ Res* 1998; **82**: 57–62.

CHAPTER 9

Clinical Significance of Diastolic Dysfunction and the Effect of Therapeutic Interventions

Sandro Betocchi, MD and Raffaella Lombardi, MD

Patients with hypertrophic cardiomyopathy (HCM) present with a variety of symptoms, the most common being dyspnea, which can be found in about nine out of ten symptomatic patients.[1] Dyspnea can be the consequence of impaired systolic function (systolic heart failure) or of elevated left ventricular (LV) diastolic pressure, stemming from diastolic dysfunction. Patients with HCM exhibit typically normal systolic LV performance, with the exception of a small percentage of patients with LV dilatation and impaired systolic function (the so called end-stage form of HCM). As a consequence, most patients with HCM complain of dyspnea because of diastolic dysfunction.

The term diastole encompasses two entities that are completely different from a pathophysiological standpoint: active diastole (isovolumetric relaxation and early filling) and passive diastole (late filling and atrial contribution to filling). Active diastole is an energy-consuming process which is strictly linked to inotropic properties of myocardium and depends on intracellular calcium handling; it can be acutely changed by interventions and drugs. Passive diastole is influenced by several factors, the most important being LV wall composition, namely hypertrophy, cellular disarray, and interstitial fibrosis. The impact of LV geometry on passive diastolic function has not been sufficiently elucidated. Pericardial constraint plays a major role only in LV dilatation, but not in the nondilated form of HCM. Diastolic dysfunction may occur if any of these entities is altered.[2]

Active diastole

Isovolumetric relaxation is almost invariably altered in HCM, as about 90% of symptomatic patients exhibit a prolongation in the time constant of isovolumetric relaxation.[2] The mechanisms underlying this impairment are complex. Besides an intrinsic alteration of the relaxation properties of an individual myocyte, additional factors that involve the left ventricle as a whole play a relevant role.

Pathophysiology

Several years ago, Gwathmey and co-workers studied the mechanical behavior of muscle strips from patients with HCM.[3] They found that the diastolic tension at rest (i.e. the remaining tension at the end of relaxation) was higher in HCM than in normals, and that such tension rose with increasing rate of stimulation: for stimulation rates of 0.1 Hz (i.e. 6 contractions/min), the resting tension was approximately normal, but it was elevated for rates of 1 Hz (60 contractions/min), and further rose sharply for rates of 2 Hz (120 contractions/min). In other words, diastolic tension is elevated in HCM even at normal heart rates, and high heart rates are deleterious. This phenomenon was amplified by increasing Ca^{++} concentrations. The interpretation of this finding is that the affinity of contractile proteins for Ca^{++} is altered in HCM and fast heart rates do not allow Ca^{++} to be taken up sufficiently from the sarcoplasmic reticulum; this hypothesis has been confirmed in transgenic animals with HCM due to a α-myosin heavy chain mutation[4] as well as in men with α-tropomyosin mutation.[5] Gwathmey's interesting paper analyzes also the effects of verapamil, a drug commonly used in the treatment of symptoms in patients with HCM: at therapeutic concentrations, verapamil did not normalize resting tension in HCM, and it took much higher levels (never achieved in clinical practice) to actually bring resting tension back to the normal range. The authors than asked themselves why verapamil was effective in the clinical setting but not *in vitro*, and concluded that this was due to the reduction in heart rate achieved with verapamil long-term treatment.[3] In light of this interpretation, one can understand why β-blockers, which are intrinsically detrimental to isovolumetric relaxation, prove clinically useful in HCM.

Physiologically, isovolumetric relaxation should be almost completed when the mitral valve opens and filling begins. The LV pressure we measure during the filling phase of diastole is the sum of two components: the residual pressure resulting from isovolumetric relaxation that extends beyond mitral valve opening, and the pressure that builds up from the LV filling (Fig. 9.1, left panel). Early in diastole, measured pressure is mostly affected by the decaying relaxation pressure; later, its weight is negligible and almost all of the measured pressure is accounted for by the pressure resulting from filling. When isovolumetric relaxation is impaired and prolonged, as is the case in HCM, the relaxation pressure extends throughout diastole, and is relevant also toward the end of diastole (Fig. 9.1, right panel); as a consequence, diastolic pressure rises throughout diastole. This increase in diastolic pressure results in symptoms (dyspnea, reduced exercise tolerance).

There is an additional factor that impairs relaxation. It is known from experiments in animals as well as in man that asynchrony prolongs isovolumetric relaxation.[6] This mechanism plays a role in HCM, as asynchrony of contraction and relaxation is often present.[2] In addition, a left bundle branch block often develops in these patients, contributing to asynchrony and the consequent impairment in isovolumetric relaxation.

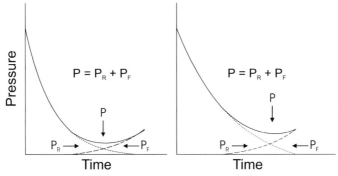

Fig. 9.1 Schematic representation of left ventricular pressure–time relationships with normal (left panel) and prolonged (right panel) isovolumetric relaxation. The measured pressure (P) is indicated by a solid line; the pressure resulting from decaying left ventricular tension during isovolumetric relaxation (P_R) is indicated by a dotted line; the pressure resulting from left ventricle filling (P_F) is indicated by a dashed line. Measured pressure is the sum of the latter two components: if isovolumetric relaxation is normal, late diastolic pressure reflects passive left ventricular properties as it coincides with P_F; in contrast, if isovolumetric relaxation is prolonged late diastolic pressure contains a sizeable component of residual P_R.

Left ventricular hypertrophy is a determinant of diastolic dysfunction, as it affects both isovolumetric relaxation and passive filling. It is noteworthy, though, that patients with the HCM genotype and a normal phenotype (i.e. without significant hypertrophy) exhibit alterations in active diastolic function.[7] Although hypertrophy affects both phases of diastole, it is more relevant for passive diastolic function and its role will be discussed below.

It has been known for a long time that ischemia impairs isovolumetric relaxation. In HCM, ischemia occurs frequently even with normal epicardial coronary arteries, as a consequence of hypertrophy, increased subendocardial coronary resistance (due to increased LV diastolic pressures), and increased oxygen consumption. Little is known, however, about the relevance of ischemia to diastolic dysfunction in HCM, mostly because of the difficulty of assessing ischemia in these patients.

LV outflow tract obstruction is present in up to one-third of patients with HCM and might affect isovolumetric relaxation: in the physiology laboratory, an afterload increase is associated with changes in the relaxation properties; such changes, however, depend on the time when the additional load is imposed upon the muscle. Long ago, Gaasch and colleagues showed that an additional load slows relaxation when it occurs early in systole (contraction load), whereas it improves relaxation when imposed in late systole (relaxation load).[9] LV outflow tract obstruction is an additional load that takes place at mid-systole, and its timing can vary, so that it can either be considered a contraction or a relaxation load. It is therefore not surprising that patients with LV outflow tract gradient exhibit, as a group, alterations in isovolumetric relaxation similar to those occurring in patients without obstruction, as the two effects even out.[2] In contrast, alcohol septal ablation, a procedure that reduces the LV outflow tract gradient, may improve diastolic function.[10]

Clinical and therapeutic implications

The goal of treatment in HCM is twofold: to prevent sudden death and to reduce or abolish symptoms. Since diastolic dysfunction is a determinant of symptoms, several attempts have been made to improve isovolumetric relaxation, in the hope of influencing symptoms.

A milestone in the therapy of HCM was the use of β-blockers. These drugs are mostly effective in patients with LV outflow tract obstruction, but can improve symptoms also in nonobstructive patients.[8] As isovolumetric relaxation is improved by β-agonists,[11] β-blockers are detrimental. However, they are somehow effective in the clinical scenario, so their beneficial effects on symptoms caused by diastolic dysfunction, such as dyspnea, must be due to their bradycardia effect.

An array of studies has focused on calcium channel blockers, a family of drugs that have the potential to be the treatment of choice for alteration in isovolumetric relaxation. There is solid evidence that drugs of the phenylalkylamine family, such as verapamil and possibly gallopamil, improve early diastolic filling[12] and symptoms[13] in patients with HCM. Benzothiazepines, such as diltiazem, are also effective in the acute setting, as they improve isovolumetric relaxation and early filling velocity.[14] In contrast, drugs of the dihydropyridine family, such as nifedipine, have controversial effects on diastolic function in HCM[15,16] and are certainly contraindicated in obstructive HCM, because the vasodilation they induce can increase LV outflow tract obstruction; in nonobstructive patients their effects probably depend on the serum concentration achieved.[17]

Dihydropyridines have little or no use in the treatment of HCM; in clinical practice, verapamil and, to a lesser extent, diltiazem are the calcium channel blockers most commonly used. Although none of the treatments used in HCM is evidence-based *sensu strictu*, there is consensus that, in most patients, verapamil reduces symptoms and improves exercise tolerance. A study by Bonow and co-workers provides a *caveat*: exercise tolerance improves in only those HCM patients in whom an improvement in diastolic function can be ascertained.[18] If we extrapolate *in vitro* data, we should conclude that verapamil treatment is effective on diastolic function inasmuch as it is effective in reducing heart rate.[3]

There is no way of improving asynchrony in HCM: while this issue has been addressed in patients with congestive heart failure, no attempts have been made to resynchronize cardiac mechanics in HCM. A treatment for obstruction gained momentum a few years ago but seems to have faded away: dual-chamber (DDD) pacing. It reduces LV outflow tract obstruction while increasing asynchrony and, hence, worsening isovolumetric relaxation.[19,20] This probably explains in part the disappointing clinical results.[21] Long-term DDD pacing affects asynchrony and diastolic properties in HCM while decreasing obstruction. However, the results differ according to the degree of diastolic dysfunction: patients with minimal dysfunction do not benefit from DDD pacing, as the beneficial effects of gradient reduction are shadowed by the negative impact on diastolic function. In contrast, patients with diastolic dysfunction benefit from gradient reduction without experiencing any worsening in diastolic function.[22]

Passive diastole

If one examines a gross anatomy specimen from a heart with HCM, it comes as no surprise that LV distensibility (i.e. passive diastolic properties) is markedly altered. Whether LV hypertrophy is the major determinant of passive diastolic dysfunction is a controversial issue, as there are reports showing that diastolic dysfunction can occur in segments with minimal hypertrophy,[23] and it has been proved that active diastolic function can be impaired in the presence of a normal phenotype.[7] However, in most cases passive diastolic function is abnormal in the presence of hypertrophy and increased interstitial fibrosis.

Pathophysiology

Hypertrophic cardiomyopathy is an autosomal dominant disease. Mutations occur in genes encoding proteins of the sarcomere (structural or regulatory). These mutations impair the sarcomeric function and probably activate a compensatory mechanism responsible for the typical anatomic features of this disease: hypertrophy, muscle fiber disarray, and interstitial fibrosis.[1,24] Marian hypothesized that, despite preserved global LV systolic function, the decreased contractility at the myocyte and molecular levels in HCM leads to increased mechanical stretch and, hence, cellular stress, thus activating the local release of some cytokines and growth factors.[25] This hypothesis is supported by various studies showing that TGF-β1, IGF-1, TNF-α, and endothelin 1 are up-regulated in HCM, as in pressure-overload hypertrophy.[26-28] Thus, as in secondary hypertrophy, factors responsible for myocyte hypertrophy are also responsible for fibroblast proliferation: the outcome of this process is LV hypertrophy and increased interstitial fibrosis.

Whether this hypothetical mechanism will prove correct or not, there is no question that interstitial fibrosis is increased in HCM. Shirani and colleagues, in an autopsy study, showed that in children and young adults with HCM and sudden cardiac death (not in the end stage), the amount of cardiac matrix collagen was 8-fold greater than in normal controls and 3-fold greater than in patients with systemic hypertension.[29] This study was carefully designed so as to exclude areas of discrete fibrosis, which can be considered a reparative process to injury such as ischemia and has little role in the impairment of passive diastolic function. Furthermore, these authors showed that the matrix collagen compartment expanded during growth.[29] In a similar morphological study, Varnava and colleagues showed that the magnitude of hypertrophy (as maximal wall thickness) correlates with the severity of fibrosis and disarray.[30]

Furthermore, they found that, while disarray was present at an early age and diminished with time, interstitial fibrosis increased with age. For this reason, these authors suggested that disarray is the primary response to the mutated gene, while fibrosis and hypertrophy are later, secondary responses.[30]

To assess the impact of fibrosis on diastolic dysfunction, we have analyzed myocardial collagen metabolism in patients with HCM by a noninvasive biochemical method:[31] briefly, we measured serum concentrations of peptides derived from the synthesis and degradation of collagen I and III, and of the enzymes involved in collagen degradation (matrix metalloproteinase 1 or collagenase, and its tissue inhibitor). In patients with HCM and diastolic dysfunction, collagen I synthesis is increased compared with degradation; furthermore, collagenase activity is suppressed (Fig. 9.2).[32] These findings indicate that HCM patients with diastolic dysfunction tend to accumulate collagen, and suggest that collagen accumulation causes passive diastolic dysfunction.

The association of hypertrophy, disarray, and increased interstitial fibrosis leads to a stiffer LV wall: this implies that the diastolic pressure–volume relationship moves leftward and slightly upward compared with the normal state (Fig. 9.3). These mechanisms occur in order for diastolic pressures to be within an acceptable range (i.e. associated with minimal symptoms); as a consequence of this leftward shift, LV volumes are smaller. When cardiac output has to increase (such as during exercise) end-diastolic volume increases, but this implies a marked elevation in diastolic pressure. This is the mechanism by which exercise intolerance takes place in patients with HCM and normal systolic function. A small LV volume is typically a sign of diastolic dysfunction in HCM (restrictive physiology) and is associated with a higher New York Heart

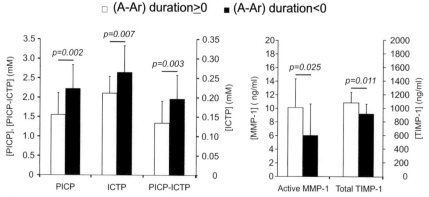

Fig. 9.2 Serum concentration of peptides deriving from synthesis (procollagen I C-terminal peptide, PICP) and degradation of collagen I (collagen I C-terminal telopeptide, ICTP), and their difference (left panel): a larger difference in patients with passive diastolic dysfunction [(A–Ar) duration <0] indicates that the collagen molecules synthesized outnumber the degraded molecules (i.e. collagen accumulates). Collagenase activity is suppressed, further suggesting collagen accumulation (right panel).

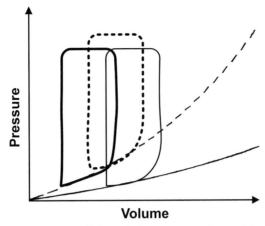

Fig. 9.3 Schematic representation of left ventricular pressure–volume relationships with normal distensibility (thin solid lines) and increased stiffness (dashed lines and thick solid line). If distensibility is decreased, the pressure–volume loop shifts leftward and slightly upward (thick solid line). When cardiac output has to increase, left ventricular volume increases and the loop is shifted rightward and markedly upward (thick dashed line).

Association functional class.[33] The effect of altered passive diastolic properties on exercise tolerance is shown by an inverse relationship between an estimate of LV end-diastolic pressure and exercise tolerance, as assessed by maximal oxygen consumption during exercise.[34]

Clinical and therapeutic implications

The treatment of symptoms due to passive diastolic dysfunction is very difficult. There is no evidence-based therapy, and attempts are merely empirical and driven by the pathophysiology. A reasonable way to reduce LV diastolic pressures and, hence, improve exercise tolerance is the use of diuretics. They reduce circulating blood volume and, as a consequence, the left ventricle fills less and its pressure–volume loop shifts leftward, thus moving to a portion of the pressure–volume relationship where diastolic pressures are lower (Fig. 9.3). There are inherent risks in this treatment in HCM, however. If filling pressures are decreased too much, LV filling (which is heavily dependent on the filling pressure) is inadequate; this implies a fall in cardiac output with subsequent symptoms of fatigue, lightheadedness, dizziness, and possibly presyncope.

Recently, Weber and co-workers[35] have put forward the new concept of cardioreparation. The idea underlying this concept is that the composition of the LV wall is the determinant of passive diastolic dysfunction, and that a therapy that could normalize LV wall composition would improve diastolic function. This has been accomplished in patients with secondary hypertrophy, such as patients with aortic stenosis following valve replacement,[36] as well as in patients with hypertension and LV hypertrophy.[37–39]

In patients with HCM, this possibility has never been tested. While it has been suggested that LV hypertrophy can, to a certain extent, decrease following reduction in LV outflow tract obstruction,[10] the clinical significance of this finding is unresolved. As outlined above, it has been suggested that myocyte hypertrophy and disarray and increased interstitial collagen synthesis are secondary to the increased release of trophic and mitotic factors, so one can speculate that the inhibition of the effects of these factors in the heart would lead to the reduction of cardiac hypertrophy and fibrosis and would therefore improve diastolic dysfunction.[25] Recently, several studies have been published on the possible cardioprotective role in HCM of two classes of drugs (antagonists of the renin–angiotensin–aldosterone system and statins) that at the present time are considered unconventional therapy for this disease.[40–42] Lim and colleagues showed that treatment with losartan in a transgenic mouse model of HCM reduces the expression of TGF-β1 (a known mediator of the profibrotic effect of angiotensin II)[43] and reverses myocardial fibrosis.[40] Patel and co-workers showed that treatment with simvastatin in a transgenic rabbit model of HCM, induces regression of cardiac hypertrophy and a decrease in interstitial fibrosis, and improves diastolic function.[41] Recent preliminary data from the same group show that treatment with spironolactone causes regression of both fibrosis and disarray.[42]

These findings, in addition to supporting the hypothesis that interstitial fibrosis is secondary and can be reversed in HCM, suggest that there are new categories of drugs that could represent novel options for the treatment and prevention of cardiac hypertrophy, fibrosis, and passive diastolic dysfunction in HCM. Because of the effects on load of AT1 (angiotensin II type 1 receptor)-blocking drugs, this treatment should be confined to nonobstructive patients. It should be pointed out, however, that this hypothesis, based on animal experiments, awaits confirmation in patients with HCM and, to date, should only be considered as an intriguing possibility for the future therapy of patients with HCM.

Conclusions

The treatment of diastolic dysfunction is conceptually difficult in HCM and lacks solid evidence based on controlled, large-scale studies, and consequently the medical treatment of diastolic dysfunction may vary among those investigators who deal with HCM patients most frequently. However, Fig. 9.4 shows a tentative pathophysiological approach to the treatment of diastolic dysfunction in HCM.

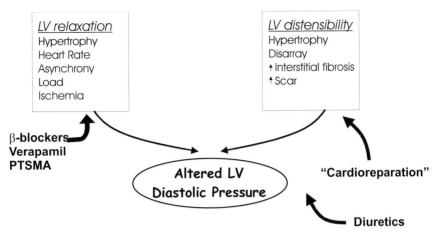

Fig. 9.4 Scheme of pathophysiology-driven treatment of diastolic dysfunction in hypertrophic cardiomyopathy. A reduction in heart rate, achieved by the use of β-blockers and calcium antagonists, is beneficial as it reduces diastolic pressures. Calcium antagonists have also a direct effect on isovolumetric relaxation. Diuretics also are able to reduce diastolic pressures. Whether drugs such as spironolactone and ACE inhibitors (or angiotensin II type 1 receptor blockers) have a beneficial effect on left ventricular hypertrophy and interstitial fibrosis requires investigation.

References

1 Maron BJ, Bonow RO, Cannon RO, III, Leon MB, Epstein SE. Hypertrophic cardiomyopathy: Interrelation of clinical manifestation, pathophysiology, and therapy. *N Engl J Med* 1987; **316**: 780–844.

2 Betocchi S, Hess OM, Losi MA, Nonogi H, Krayenbuehl HP. Regional left ventricular mechanics in hypertrophic cardiomyopathy. *Circulation* 1993; **88**: 2206–10.

3 Gwathmey JK, Warren SE, Briggs GM *et al*. Diastolic dysfunction in hypertrophic cardiomyopathy. Effect on active force generation during systole. *J Clin Invest* 1991; **87**: 1023–31.

4 Georgakopoulos D, Christie ME, Giewat M, Seidman CM, Seidman JG, Kass DA. The pathogenesis of familial hypertrophic cardiomyopathy: Early and evolving effects from an α-cardiac myosin heavy chain missense mutation. *Nat Med* 1999; **5**: 327–30.

5 Karibe A, Tobacman LS, Strand J *et al*. Hypertrophic cardiomyopathy caused by a novel α-tropomyosin mutation (V95A) is associated with mild cardiac phenotype, abnormal calcium binding to troponin, abnormal myosin cycling, and poor prognosis. *Circulation* 2001; **103**: 65–71.

6 Betocchi S, Piscione F, Villari B *et al*. Effects of induced asynchrony on left ventricular diastolic function in patients with coronary artery disease. *J Am Coll Cardiol* 1993; **21**: 1124–31.

7 Nagueh SF, Bachinski LL, Meyer D *et al*. Tissue Doppler imaging consistently detects myocardial abnormalities in patients with hypertrophic cardiomyopathy and provides a novel means for an early diagnosis before and independently of hypertrophy. *Circulation* 2001; **104**: 128–30.

8 Elliott PM, McKenna WJ. Hypertrophic cardiomyopathy. In: Crawford MH, DiMarco JP, eds. *Cardiology*. London: Mosby, 2001: 5.12.1–12.

9 Gaasch WH, Blaunstein AS, Andrias CW, Donahue RP, Avitall B. Myocardial relaxation. II. Hemodynamic determinants of rate of left ventricular isovolumic pressure decline. *Am J Physiol* 1980; **239**: H1–6.

10 Nagueh SF, Lakkis NM, Middleton KJ *et al.* Changes in left ventricular diastolic function 6 months after nonsurgical septal reduction therapy for hypertrophic obstructive cardiomyopathy. *Circulation* 1999; **99**: 344–7.

11 Udelson JE, Cannon RO III, Bacharach SL, Rumble TF, Bonow RO. β-Adrenergic stimulation with isoproterenol enhances left ventricular diastolic performance in hypertrophic cardiomyopathy despite potentiation of myocardial ischemia. Comparison with atrial pacing. *Circulation* 1989; **79**: 371–82.

12 Bonow RO, Rosing DR, Bacharach SL *et al.* Effects of verapamil on left ventricular systolic function and diastolic filling in patients with hypertrophic cardiomyopathy. *Circulation* 1981; **64**: 787–96.

13 Rosing DR, Kent KM, Maron BJ, Epstein SE. Verapamil therapy: A new approach to the pharmacologic treatment of hypertrophic cardiomyopathy. II. Effects on exercise capacity and symptomatic status. *Circulation* 1979; **60**: 1208–13.

14 Betocchi S, Piscione F, Losi MA *et al.* Effects of diltiazem on left ventricular systolic and diastolic function in hypertrophic cardiomyopathy. *Am J Cardiol* 1996; **78**: 451–7.

15 Betocchi S, Cannon RO, Watson RM *et al.* Effects of sublingual nifedipine on hemodynamics and on systolic and diastolic function in patients with hypertrophic cardiomyopathy. *Circulation* 1985; **72**: 1001–7.

16 Paulus WJ, Lorell BH, Craig WE, Wynne J, Murgo JP, Grossman W. Comparison of the effects of nitroprusside and nifedipine on diastolic properties in patients with hypertrophic cardiomyopathy: Altered left ventricular loading or improved muscle relaxation? *J Am Coll Cardiol* 1983; **2**: 879–86.

17 Betocchi S, Bonow RO, Cannon RO III *et al.* Relation between serum nifedipine concentration and hemodynamic effects in nonobstructive hypertrophic cardiomyopathy. *Am J Cardiol* 1988; **61**: 830–5.

18 Bonow RO, Dilsizian V, Rosing DR, Maron BJ, Bacharach SL, Green MV. Verapamil-induced improvement in left ventricular diastolic filling and increased exercise tolerance in patients with hypertrophic cardiomyopathy. *Circulation* 1985; **72**: 853–64.

19 Nishimura RA, Hayes DL, Ilstrup DM, Holmes DR, Tajik JA. Effect of dual-chamber pacing on systolic and diastolic function in patients with hypertrophic cardiomyopathy: Acute Doppler echocardiographic and catheterization hemodynamic study. *J Am Coll Cardiol* 1996; **27**: 421–30.

20 Betocchi S, Losi MA, Piscione F *et al.* Effects of dual-chamber pacing in hypertrophic cardiomyopathy on left ventricular outflow tract obstruction and on diastolic function. *Am J Cardiol* 1996; **77**: 498–504.

21 Maron BJ, Nishimura RA, McKenna WJ, Rakowski H, Josephson ME, Kieval RS for the M-PATHY Study Investigators. Assessment of permanent dual-chamber pacing as a treatment for drug-refractory symptomatic patients with obstructive hypertrophic cardiomyopathy (M-PATHY). *Circulation* 1999; **99**: 2927–33.

22 Betocchi S, Elliott PM, Briguori C *et al.* Dual chamber pacing in hypertrophic cardiomyopathy: Long-term effects on diastolic function. *Pacing Clin Electrophysiol* 2002; **25**: 1433–40.

23 Spirito P, Maron BJ. Relation between extent of left ventricular hypertrophy and diastolic filling abnormalities in hypertrophic cardiomyopathy. *J Am Coll Cardiol* 1990; **15**: 808–13.

24 Bonne G, Carrier L, Richard P, Hainque B, Schwartz K. Familiar hypertrophic cardiomyopathy. From mutation to functional defects. *Circ Res* 1998; **83**: 580–93.

25 Marian AJ. Pathogenesis of diverse clinical and pathological phenotypes in hypertrophic cardiomyopathy. *Lancet* 2000; **355**: 58–60.

26 Li RK, Li G, Mickle DAG *et al.* Overexpression of transforming growth factor-β1 and insulin-like growth factor-I in patients with idiopathic hypertrophic cardiomyopathy. *Circulation* 1997; **96**: 874–81.

27 Patel R, Lim DS, Reddy D *et al.* Variants of trophic factors and expression of cardiac hypertrophy in patients with hypertrophic cardiomyopathy. *J Mol Cell Cardiol* 2000; **32**: 2369–77.

28 Hasegawa K, Fujiwara H, Koshiji M *et al.* Endothelin-1 and its receptor in hypertrophic cardiomyopathy. *Hypertension* 1996; **27**: 259–64.

29 Shirani J, Pick R, Roberts WC, Maron BJ. Morphology and significance of the left ventricular collagen network in young patients with hypertrophic cardiomyopathy and sudden cardiac death. *J Am Coll Cardiol* 2000; **35**: 36–44.

30 Varnava AM, Elliott PM, Sharma S, McKenna WJ, Davies MJ. Hypertrophic cardiomyopathy: The interrelation of disarray, fibrosis, and small vessel disease. *Heart* 2000; **84**: 476–82.

31 Laviades C, Varo N, Fernandez J *et al.* Abnormalities of the extracellular degradation of collagen type I in essential hypertension. *Circulation* 1998; **98**: 535–8.

32 Lombardi R, Betocchi S, Losi MA *et al.* Myocardial collagen turnover in hypertrophic cardiomyopathy. *Circulation* 2003; **108**: 1455–60

33 Manganelli F, Betocchi S, Losi MA *et al.* Influence of left ventricular cavity size on clinical presentation in hypertrophic cardiomyopathy. *Am J Cardiol* 1999; **83**: 547–52.

34 Briguori C, Betocchi S, Romano M *et al.* Exercise capacity in hypertrophic cardiomyopathy depends on left ventricular diastolic function. *Am J Cardiol* 1999; **84**: 309–15.

35 Weber KT, Brilla CG, Campbell SE, Reddy HK. Myocardial fibrosis and the concept of cardioprotection and cardioreparation. *J Hypertens* 1992; **10**: S87–94.

36 Villari B, Vassalli G, Monrad ES, Chiariello M, Turina M, Hess OM. Normalization of diastolic dysfunction in aortic stenosis late after valve replacement. *Circulation* 1995; **91**: 2353–8.

37 Brilla CG, Funck RC, Rupp H. Lisinopril-mediated regression of myocardial fibrosis in patients with hypertensive heart disease. *Circulation* 2000; **102**: 1388–93.

38 Lopez B, Querejeta R, Varo N *et al.* Usefulness of serum carboxy-terminal propeptide of procollagen type I in assessment of the cardioreparative ability of antihypertensive treatment in hypertensive patients. *Circulation* 2001; **104**: 286–91.

39 Diez J, Querejeta R, Lopez B, Gonzales A, Larman M, Martinez Ubago JL. Losartan-dependent regression of myocardial fibrosis is associated with reduction of left ventricular chamber stiffness in hypertensive patients. *Circulation* 2002; **105**: 2512–7.

40 Lim DS, Lutucuta S, Bachireddy P *et al.* Angiotensin II blockade reverses myocardial fibrosis in a transgenic mouse model of human hypertrophic cardiomyopathy. *Circulation* 2001; **103**: 789–91.

41 Patel R, Nagueh SF, Tsybouleva N *et al.* Simvastatin induces regression of cardiac hypertrophy and fibrosis and improves cardiac function in a transgenic rabbit model of human hypertrophic cardiomyopathy. *Circulation* 2001; **104**: 317–24.

42 Patel R, Nemoto S, DeFreitas G *et al.* Spironolactone reverses myocyte disarray and interstitial fibrosis in the cardiac troponin T transgenic mouse model of hypertrophic cardiomyopathy [abstract]. *J Am Coll Cardiol* 2002; **39**: 156A.

43 Kawano H, Do YS, Kawano Y *et al.* Angiotensin II has multiple profibrotic effects in human cardiac fibroblasts. *Circulation* 2000; **101**: 1130–7.

CHAPTER 10

Value of Exercise Testing in Assessing Clinical State and Prognosis in Hypertrophic Cardiomyopathy

Sanjay Sharma, MRCP, MD

Hypertrophic cardiomyopathy (HCM) is a complex genetic disease of cardiac sarcomeric contractile proteins[1–5] characterized by left ventricular hypertrophy (LVH), myocardial disarray, functional limitation and increased risk of sudden death. Pathophysiologic manifestations of the disorder include hyperdynamic systolic contraction, impaired relaxation (diastolic dysfunction), myocardial ischemia and arrhythmias. In approximately 30% of cases, abnormal elongation of mitral valve leaflets and consequent anterior papillary muscle displacement result in systolic anterior movement of the mitral valve apparatus, causing left ventricular outflow obstruction.[6–9]

A proportion of HCM patients remain entirely asymptomatic and are diagnosed incidentally. However, symptoms are present in as many as 70% and include chest pain, exertional dyspnea, palpitation and syncope.[6,7,9] Chest pain and dyspnea often result in reduced exercise tolerance and functional capacity. In a small minority, sudden death may be the first manifestation of the condition.[9–12]

Once the diagnosis of HCM is established, investigations are directed at assessing functional capacity and identifying patients at increased risk of sudden death, and exercise stress testing has an important role in both purposes (Table 10.1).

Exercise testing in HCM is generally safe in expert hands, provided the exercise room is equipped with appropriate cardiopulmonary resuscitation

Table 10.1 Role of cardiopulmonary exercise in hypertrophic cardiomyopathy

Assessment of functional capacity
Identification of determinants of functional capacity
Evaluation of the mechanisms of exercise limitation
Evaluation of efficacy of therapies
Differentiation from other forms of left ventricular hypertrophy
Risk stratification for sudden death

apparatus. In our experience over the last 10 years there has only been one potentially fatal event in over 3000 tests in which exercise-induced sustained ventricular tachycardia occurred and was successfully terminated with electrical cardioversion. Conventional exercise testing may be supplemented by simultaneous respiratory gas exchange analysis (cardiopulmonary exercise testing) which involves measurement of the peak oxygen consumption $(p\dot{V}O_2)$.[13] Peak oxygen consumption is the product of peak exercise cardiac output and the systemic arteriovenous difference. It is reduced in patients with cardiopulmonary disease and is the most commonly used marker of functional capacity in heart failure. Predicted values are available enabling highly objective assessment of exercise capacity in patients with HCM. In addition, $p\dot{V}O_2$ measurement during exercise has provided an understanding of the pathophysiological determinants of exercise capacity in HCM and played an important role in differentiating HCM with mild morphological changes from other conditions, such as physiologic hypertrophy ('athlete's heart').

Also, exercise stress testing has an important role in the risk stratification of patients with HCM. Measurement of the blood pressure profile during exercise identifies HCM patients with an abnormal vascular response, which is a recognized risk factor for sudden death.[14]

Assessment of functional capacity and myocardial ischemia

Functional capacity

Patients with HCM often report exercise limitation and decreased functional capacity, although the precise mechanism may be difficult to define in each individual.[6–9] Presently, the most common method for assessing functional capacity is the New York Heart Association (NYHA) classification. Although this is much more practical than objective exercise testing, it has certain important shortcomings. A patient's perception of 'normal' exercise capacity may relate to a sedentary life and so he/she may be labeled incorrectly as 'asymptomatic', whereas in reality the patient has a diminished functional capacity. This is underscored by two large studies assessing the clinical course of HCM, in which 91% of 277 patients[15] and 76% of 202 patients[16] respectively were asymptomatic or had mild symptoms based on NYHA classification, whereas studies using cardiopulmonary exercise have found that the vast majority of patients with HCM have low $p\dot{V}O_2$.[17,18] Our own experience of 135 consecutive HCM patients demonstrated a low $p\dot{V}O_2$ (<80% of the maximal predicted value) in 98% of cases (Fig. 10.1)[18] irrespective of NYHA functional class, the magnitude of LVH or the presence of a pressure gradient across the left ventricular outflow tract. Indeed, 70% of our patients in NYHA functional class I had an abnormally low $p\dot{V}O_2$.[18] Although $p\dot{V}O_2$ correlates with NYHA,[17,18] there is considerable variability within any given functional class and significant overlap in $p\dot{V}O_2$ measurements between patients in NYHA classes I, II and III (Fig. 10.2).[18] These

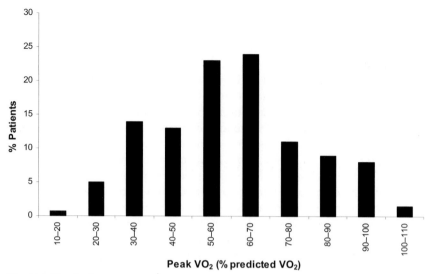

Fig. 10.1 The distribution of peak $\dot{V}O_2$ in a cohort of 135 hypertrophic cardiomyopathy patients.

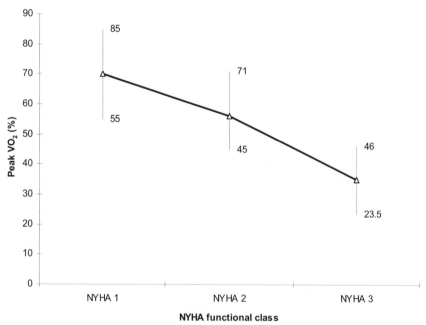

Fig. 10.2 Relationship between New York Heart Association functional class and peak oxygen consumption.

findings suggest that, in any given individual, $p\dot{V}O_2$ may be a superior index of functional capacity compared with NYHA class.

Myocardial ischemia

Noninvasive exercise testing is not useful in identifying myocardial ischemia in HCM, probably due to the contaminating effects of marked LVH. Most patients with HCM have an abnormal resting ECG with significant ST-segment and T-wave abnormalities,[1,6,7,19–21] complicating interpretation during exercise.

Mechanisms of functional limitation

Cardiopulmonary exercise testing has provided a better understanding of the role of both central and peripheral mechanisms causing exercise limitation in HCM. Studies carried out in HCM patients have shown that $p\dot{V}O_2$ is clearly related to peak cardiac output.[22,23] Peak cardiac output is governed by the ability to augment stroke volume, which in turn is determined by left ventricular filling pressures.[23,24] Diastolic dysfunction leading to poor left ventricular filling is thought to occur as a result of myocardial hypertrophy, fibrosis and disarray.[23,24] Myocardial ischemia and mechanical left ventricular outflow tract obstruction may also impede stroke volume augmentation.[25] Abnormal vascular responses during exercise may also divert blood flow from the skeletal muscle vascular bed to the splanchnic circulation, causing early metabolic acidosis and functional incapacity.[26] The potential role of peripheral mechanisms is discussed below.

Determinants of functional capacity

The pathophysiology of functional limitation in HCM is complex. With the help of cardiopulmonary exercise testing, certain potential determinants of functional capacity can be identified.

Left ventricular hypertrophy

LVH is the primary feature of HCM and is regarded by many as a surrogate marker of disease severity. It is now well recognized that severe LVH is an independent marker of increased risk of sudden death in HCM.[27,28] In contrast, previous work in HCM has failed to show any relationship between the severity of hypertrophy and any $p\dot{V}O_2$ value.[18] We conducted a study of over 500 HCM patients and showed no correlation between LVH and exercise capacity.[29] This result confirms that LVH alone is not an important determinant of functional capacity in HCM. Other variables, such as myocardial disarray, fibrosis and microvascular ischemia (which are not easily measured in quantitative terms), probably have a more significant impact on functional capacity.

Left ventricular outflow tract obstruction

Dynamic outflow tract obstruction at rest is present in 25–30% of HCM pa-

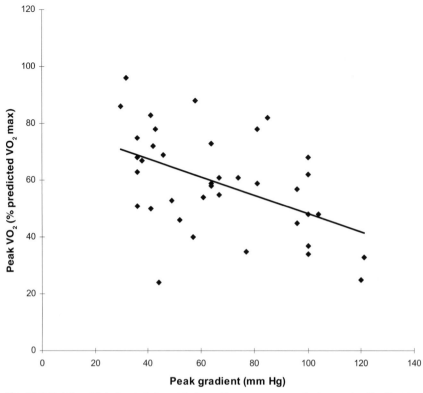

Fig. 10.3 Relationship between left ventricular outflow pressure gradient, measured by Doppler echocardiography, and peak oxygen consumption.

tients.[1–6,9] Although impaired functional capacity in obstructive HCM has been attributed to mechanical obstruction, the exact significance of the left ventricular outflow gradient in determining functional capacity and clinical outcome has been a subject of controversy for several years.[1,7,30] Our own experience showing an inverse relationship between left ventricular outflow tract pressure gradient and $p\dot{V}O_2$ suggests that mechanical outflow obstruction has pathophysiological consequences (Fig. 10.3).[18] A recent study addressing the long-term effect of basal left ventricular outflow tract obstruction in HCM has helped clarify the issue by demonstrating a strong association between mechanical outflow obstruction and progression to heart failure. The same study has also revealed that left ventricular outflow obstruction in patients with HCM is associated with an increased risk of sudden death and stroke.[31] These findings imply that abolition of the outflow tract gradient and normalization of left ventricular pressures using pharmacological or mechanical means may provide symptomatic benefit and prevent sudden death. Indeed, there are reports confirming improvements in $p\dot{V}O_2$ and exercise following transcoronary septal ablation[32,33] and surgical myectomy.[34] The effect of abolition of mechanical outflow obstruction in preventing sudden death remains to be evaluated.

Diastolic dysfunction

Numerous invasive and noninvasive studies assessing the relationship between diastolic function and exercise capacity have been conducted in HCM. Invasive studies during exercise have shown an inverse correlation between time to peak filling at peak exercise and cardiopulmonary indices, suggesting that left ventricular compliance during exercise is related to $p\dot{V}O_2$ and peak cardiac output.[24] In contrast, noninvasive measures of diastolic function at rest by means of mitral inflow Doppler measurements are discordant with the invasive studies.[18,35] This is not surprising as left ventricular compliance may be greatly altered during exercise compared with the resting state. A change in posture may also affect ventricular compliance, and this may be of relevance when comparing studies at rest (supine position) and during exercise (upright position).

Chronotropic incompetence

Chronotropic incompetence is defined as the inability to achieve 80% or more of the predicted maximal heart rate during peak exercise. Since cardiac output is the product of stroke volume and heart rate, chronotropic incompetence would be expected to reduce functional capacity in patients with impaired augmentation of stroke volume. Chronotropic incompetence affects 25% of HCM patients, even when assessed off negative chronotropic drugs. Patients with chronotropic incompetence tend to be in NYHA class III or IV and have low $p\dot{V}O_2$.[18] We conducted a multivariate analysis in a large series of HCM patients and found chronotropic incompetence to be an independent predictor of exercise limitation.[36] This point raises the potential therapeutic role of cardiac pacing in such patients to improve functional capacity.

Peripheral mechanisms

Patients with HCM have certain abnormalities that are seen during cardiopulmonary exercise and suggest the involvement of peripheral mechanisms in exercise limitation.[18] A low $\dot{V}O_2$/work rate ratio occurring from the beginning of exercise in HCM patients indicates a measure of inefficiency of exercise, i.e. a high work load is carried out to achieve a certain level of $\dot{V}O_2$. This pattern is similar, albeit not as severe, to that seen in individuals with primary skeletal muscle abnormalities or mitochondrial myopathies,[13] and in patients with conditions associated with poor blood flow to skeletal muscle.[13] Histological and histochemical studies in HCM patients with β-myosin heavy chain mutations have revealed reduced density and abnormal architecture of skeletal muscle mitochondria.[37] This, in turn, may represent a reduced capacity for oxidative metabolism and premature lactic acidosis. This is supported by the observation of an abnormally low anaerobic threshold in the majority of HCM patients during cardiopulmonary exercise testing.[17,18] In addition, approximately 30% of HCM patients exhibit abnormal vascular responses during exercise. Patients with abnormal vascular responses have low $p\dot{V}O_2$, supporting the proposition that there is an inappropriate increase in the perfusion of nonexercising vascular beds at the expense of exercising skeletal muscle blood flow;[38] such wasted perfusion may explain the observed low $p\dot{V}O_2$.

Diagnosis and differentiation of HCM from other forms of LVH

In most cases of HCM the clinical diagnosis is confirmed with echocardiography. However, molecular genetic studies in patients with HCM have demonstrated the absence of overt LVH. Therefore, in the context of a family history of HCM, the presence of cardiovascular symptoms and/or ECG changes may be taken as evidence of gene inheritance.[39] A signification proportion of such patients also have low $p\dot{V}O_2$ and abnormal vascular responses during exercise, supporting the possibility of HCM. In the absence of widespread availability of genotyping for HCM, a low $p\dot{V}O_2$ and abnormal blood pressure response during exercise in first-degree relatives may identify those who have inherited the disease but have morphologically mild disease characterized by nonspecific ECG abnormalities and the absence of conventional diagnostic echocardiographic abnormalities.

Although LVH is the primary feature of HCM, there are other conditions, both physiological and pathological, which are also characterized by LVH and can occasionally cause diagnostic confusion (Fig. 10.4). Cardiopulmonary exercise testing can assist in such cases, in which differentiation may be difficult. The majority of the other conditions associated with LVH are easily differentiated from HCM. Noonan's syndrome, storage disorders such as amyloidosis and Fabry's disease, and Friedreich's ataxia are occasionally associated with

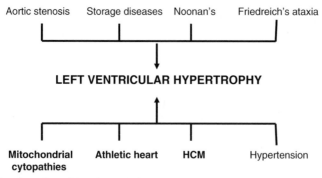

Fig. 10.4 A variety of conditions feature left ventricular hypertrophy and should be considered in the differential diagnosis of hypertrophic cardiomyopathy. Cardiopulmonary exercise testing may assist in differentiating hypertrophic cardiomyopathy from athlete's heart and mitochondrial cytopathies.

typical phenotypic features. LVH as a result of hypertension is usually identified following high blood pressure readings or a previous history of hypertension. Similarly, aortic stenosis is clinically obvious in most cases and can be confirmed using echocardiography.

Mitochondrial disorders

It is recognized that mitochondrial cytopathies are associated with LVH and severe exercise limitation[9,40] as well as other abnormalities, such as retinitis pigmentosa, diabetes, deafness and skeletal muscle myopathies.[9] ECG and echocardiography are not always helpful in discriminating between HCM and mitochondrial cytopathies. Cardiopulmonary exercise testing offers a means of differential diagnosis as these patients have a defect in the peripheral uptake and utilization of oxygen in the face of a normal cardiac output.[13] There is a strong predisposition to premature metabolic acidosis due to a low capacity for oxidative phosphorylation. This manifests itself with a very low $p\dot{V}O_2$, which is out of proportion to the degree of cardiomyopathy. In addition, a very low anaerobic threshold and a flat oxygen pulse curve are hallmarks of these patients. The low anaerobic threshold reflects early onset of lactic acidemia, whereas the failure of the oxygen pulse to rise with exercise is probably the result of reduced peripheral oxygen extraction. Furthermore, the marked metabolic acidosis in these patients with mitochondrial cytopathies triggers an increased respiratory drive that is reflected in early onset of an increased minute ventilation (VE) and $VE/\dot{V}CO_2$ ratio. In summary, mitochondrial disease affecting the heart and skeletal muscle should be considered as a differential diagnosis in all patients with mild LVH who present with severe exercise limitation even in the absence of extracardiac abnormalities. A very low $p\dot{V}O_2$ and anaerobic threshold and a high $VE/\dot{V}CO_2$ aids in differentiating patients with mitochondrial cytopathies from HCM.

Athlete's heart

Regular intensive physical exercise can cause mild increases in left ventricular wall thickness.[41] Although the degree of LVH documented in athletes is less than the hypertrophy usually observed in HCM, a significant proportion of HCM patients possess mild hypertrophy with a left ventricular wall thickness in the range of 12–15 mm and a very few remain at significant risk of sudden death.[4,42,43] Differential diagnosis in this 'gray zone' can prove challenging even for the most experienced clinician. The distinction between physiological athlete's heart and pathological hypertrophy is of paramount importance as the commonest cause of sudden death in young athletes is HCM.[44–46] In addition, a sizeable proportion of sudden deaths in HCM occurs either during or after physical exertion.[46]

An erroneous diagnosis of 'athlete's heart' in a patient with HCM can potentially jeopardize a young life. Conversely, an erroneous diagnosis of HCM will result in unnecessary disqualification from competitive sport, which may have profound social, psychological and financial consequences for an athlete.

A number of clinical and echocardiographic features may be of assistance in diagnosing HCM.[47,48] The ECG may not be as useful in differentiating HCM from athlete's, particularly in adult athletes, because deep T-wave inversions and ST-segment depression (common in HCM)[19,20] may be observed in up to 10% of elite athletes.[49] Detraining is a potential way to resolve the dilemma as physiologic LVH shows regression after 3 months of refraining from strenuous physical exercise,[50] but has limitations since competitive athletes are extremely reluctant to detrain for obvious reasons. The response to detraining is also variable, making interpretation of any changes difficult. In individuals in the gray zone, cardiopulmonary exercise testing provides a definitive and simple method of differentiating athlete's heart from HCM. In our experience only 1.5% of individuals with HCM have a $p\dot{V}O_2$ exceeding predicted values, and it is extremely unusual for an individual with HCM to achieve a $p\dot{V}O_2$ exceeding 120% of the predicted maximum or an absolute value of 45 ml/kg/min on a cycle ergometer.[18] In contrast, elite athletes commonly have $p\dot{V}O_2$ values in the range of 55–70 ml/kg/min and usually exceed predicted values by as much as 50%. Based on these observations and our own study comparing elite athletes with LVH and athletes with genetically proven HCM and mild LVH, we concluded that a $p\dot{V}O_2$ greater than 50 ml/kg/min or greater than 120% of the predicted peak value fully discriminates between the two entities (Fig. 10.5).[51]

Risk stratification for sudden death

Hypertrophic cardiomyopathy is associated with an increased risk of sudden death and is the commonest cause of sudden cardiac death in adolescents and young adults below the age of 35 years.[1] The incidence of sudden death is

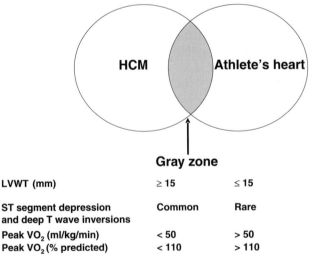

	HCM	Athlete's heart
LVWT (mm)	≥ 15	≤ 15
ST segment depression and deep T wave inversions	Common	Rare
Peak VO$_2$ (ml/kg/min)	< 50	> 50
Peak VO$_2$ (% predicted)	< 110	> 110

Fig 10.5 Role of cardiopulmonary exercise testing in the differential diagnosis of the 'gray zone' between hypertrophic cardiomyopathy and athlete's heart.

Table 10.2 Risk markers for sudden death in HCM

Survivor of sudden cardiac death
Prior sustained ventricular tachycardia
History of syncope
Family history of sudden death
Nonsustained ventricular tachycardia on ECG Holter monitoring
Abnormal blood pressure response during exercise testing
Severe diffuse left ventricular hypertrophy (left ventricular wall thickness ≥30 mm)
Left ventricular outflow obstruction

estimated at 3% per annum in tertiary referral center patients[52,53] and 1% per annum in nontertiary referral center patients.[15,16] Markers of a high risk of sudden death in HCM are summarized in Table 10.2.

Exercise testing plays a key role in the evaluation of prognosis in HCM, as blood pressure measurement during exercise can help identify those at high risk of sudden death. A failure of systolic blood pressure to rise to at least 20 mm Hg from rest to peak exercise, a progressive fall in blood pressure during exercise, or, an initial rise in systolic blood pressure followed by a drop of 20 mm Hg are regarded as abnormal blood pressure responses and a risk factor for sudden death.[14] The exact mechanism responsible for these abnormal vascular responses is unresolved but mechanoreceptors have been implicated.[26] Activation of these receptors has also been implicated in syncope associated with aortic stenosis and ischemic cardiomyopathy. It has been suggested that these receptors are activated by distortion and stretching of the ventricular myocardium, providing higher centers with information on the contractile state of the heart. The regional myocyte disarray and fibrosis seen in HCM may lead to areas of increased wall stress, which may activate ventricular mechanoreceptors during exercise. The inappropriate vasodilatation and hypotension may lead to cardiac ischemia and the possibility of development of arrhythmias. Almost 33% of patients with HCM have an abnormal blood pressure response, but, as for all other conventional risk markers for sudden death, the positive predictive value is low (<25%).[14] The need for prophylactic therapy against sudden cardiac death should therefore be determined by the presence of at least one other conventional risk marker in addition to an abnormal blood pressure response.[9] The importance of accurate risk stratification in HCM is underscored by the proven efficacy of prophylactic interventions such as implantable cardioverter–defibrillators.[51] Furthermore, the high negative predictive value of 97% means that the absence of an abnormal blood pressure response is potentially useful in providing reassurance to patients in the absence of other risk markers for sudden cardiac death.

Conclusions

Cardiopulmonary exercise testing is useful in the management of HCM. Its most important role is in the assessment of functional capacity. It is also of value in the diagnosis, risk stratification and differentiation of HCM from other forms of LVH. Furthermore, cardiopulmonary exercise testing has provided valuable information regarding the determinants of functional capacity and has helped to unravel some of the mechanisms of exercise limitation in HCM.

References

1 Spirito P, Seidman CE, McKenna WJ, Maron BJ. The management of hypertrophic cardiomyopathy. *N Engl J Med* 1997; **336**: 775–85.

2 Mogensen J, Klausen IC, Pedersen AK *et al.* α-Cardiac actin is a novel disease gene in familial hypertrophic cardiomyopathy. *J Clin Invest* 1999; **103**: R39–43.

3 Kimura A, Harada H, Park J-E *et al.* Mutations in the cardiac troponin I gene associated with hypertrophic cardiomyopathy. *Nat Genet* 1996; **13**: 63–9.

4 Thierfelder L, Watkins H, MacRae C *et al.* α-Tropomyosin and cardiac troponin T mutations cause familial hypertrophic cardiomyopathy: A disease of the sarcomere. *Cell* 1994; **77**: 701–12.

5 Watkins H, Conner D, Thierfelder L *et al.* Mutation in the cardiac myosin binding protein-C gene on chromosome 11 cause familial hypertrophic cardiomyopathy. *Nat Genet* 1995; **11**: 434–7.

6 Frank S, Braunwald E. Idiopathic hypertrophic subaortic stenosis: Clinical analysis of 126 patients with emphasis on the natural history. *Circulation* 1968; **37**: 759–88.

7 Maron BJ, Bonow RO, Canon RO III, Leon MB, Epstein SE. Hypertrophic cardiomyopathy: Interrelations of clinical manifestations, pathophysiology and therapy. *N Engl J Med* 1987; **316**: 780–9, 844–52.

8 Braunwald E, Morrow AG, Cornelli WP, Aygen MM, Hilbish TF. Idiopathic hypertrophic subaortic stenosis: Clinical, haemodynamic and angiographic manifestations. *Am J Med* 1960; **29**: 924–45.

9 McKenna WJ, Elliott PM. Hypertrophic cardiomyopathy. In: Topol EJ, ed. *Comprehensive Cardiovascular Medicine.* Philadelphia: Lipincott-Raven, 1998: 775–98.

10 McKenna WJ, Deanfield JE. Hypertrophic cardiomyopathy: An important cause of sudden death. *Arch Dis Child* 1984; **59**: 971–95.

11 Spirito P, Chiarella F, Carratino L, Zoni-Berisso M, Bellotti P, Vecchio C. Clinical course and prognosis of hypertrophic cardiomyopathy in an outpatients population. *N Engl J Med* 1989; **320**: 749–55.

12 McKenna WJ, Franklin RCG, Nihoyannopoulos P, Robinson KC, Deinfield JE. Arrhythmia and prognosis in infants, children and adolescents with hypertrophic cardiomyopathy. *J Am Coll Cardiol* 1988; **11**: 147–53.

13 Wasserman K, Hansen JE, Sue D, Whipp B. *Principles of Exercise Testing and Interpretation.* Philadelphia: Lea & Febiger, 1987: 27–45.

14 Sadoul N, Prasad K, Elliott PM, Bannerjee S, Frenneaux MP, McKenna WJ. Prospective prognostic assessment of blood pressure response during exercise in patients with hypertrophic cardiomyopathy. *Circulation* 1997; **96**: 2987–91.

15 Maron BJ, Casey SA, Poliac LC *et al.* Clinical course of hypertrophic cardiomyopathy in a regional United States cohort. *JAMA* 1999; **281**: 651–5.

16 Cecchi F, Olivotto I, Montereggi A *et al.* Hypertrophic cardiomyopathy in Tuscany: Clinical course and outcome in an unselected regional population. *J Am Coll Cardiol* 1995; **26**: 1529–36.

17 Jones S, Elliott PM, Sharma S, McKenna WJ, Whipp BJ. Cardiopulmonary responses to exercise in patients with hypertrophic cardiomyopathy. *Heart* 1998; **80**: 60–7.

18 Sharma S, Elliott PM, Whyte G *et al.* Utility of cardiopulmonary exercise in the assessment of clinical determinants of functional capacity in hypertrophic cardiomyopathy. *Am J Cardiol* 2000; **86**: 162–8.

19 Savage DD, Seides SF, Clark CE *et al.* Electrocardiographic findings in patients with obstructive and non-obstructive hypertrophic cardiomyopathy. *Circulation* 1978; **58**: 402–9.

20 Maron BJ, Wolfson JK, Ciro E, Spirito P. Relation of electrocardiographic abnormalities and patterns of left ventricular hypertrophy identified by 2-dimensional echocardiography in patients with hypertrophic cardiomyopathy. *Am J Cardiol* 1983; **51**: 189–94.

21 Elliott PM, Kaski JC, Prasad K *et al.* Chest pain during daily life in patients with hypertrophic cardiomyopathy: An ambulatory electrocardiographic study. *Eur Heart J* 1996; **17**: 1056–64.

22 Frenneaux MP, Porter A, Caforio ALP, Odawara, Counihan PJ, McKenna WJ. Determinants of exercise capacity in hypertrophic cardiomyopathy. *J Am Coll Cardiol* 1989; **13**: 1521–6.

23 Chikamori T, Counihan PJ, Doi YL *et al.* Mechanisms of exercise limitation in hypertrophic cardiomyopathy. *J Am Coll Cardiol* 1992; **19**: 507–12.

24 Lele SS, Thomson HL, Seo H, Belenkie I, McKenna WJ, Frenneaux MP. Exercise capacity in hypertrophic cardiomyopathy. Role of stroke volume limitation, heart rate and diastolic filling characteristics. *Circulation* 1995; **92**: 2886–94.

25 Maron BJ, Epstein SE. Clinical significance and therapeutic implications of left ventricular outflow tract pressure gradient in hypertrophic cardiomyopathy. *Am J Cardiol* 1986; **58**: 1093–6.

26 Counihan PJ, Frenneaux MP, Webb DJ, McKenna WJ. Abnormal vascular responses to supine exercise in hypertrophic cardiomyopathy. *Circulation* 1991; **84**: 686–96.

27 Spirito P, Bellone P, Harris KM, Bernabo P, Bruzzi P, Maron BJ. Magnitude of left ventricular hypertrophy and risk of sudden death in hypertrophic cardiomyopathy. *N Engl J Med* 2000; **342**: 1778–85.

28 Elliott PM, Gimeno Blanes JR, Mahon NG, Poloniecki JD, McKenna WJ. Relation between severity of left ventricular hypertrophy and prognosis in patients with hypertrophic cardiomyopathy. *Lancet* 2001; **357**: 420–4.

29 Firoozi S, Sharma S, Varma C, Virdee MS, Elliott PM, McKenna WJ. Is LVH a determinant of exercise capacity in hypertrophic cardiomyopathy? [abstract] *Heart* 2001; **85** (Suppl. I): P31.

30 Sugrue DD, McKenna WJ, Dickie S *et al.* Relation between left ventricular gradient and relative stroke volume ejected in early and late systole in hypertrophic cardiomyopathy: Assessment with radionuclide cineangiography. *Br Heart J* 1984; **52**: 602–9.

31 Maron MS, Olivotto I, Betocchi S *et al.* Effect of left ventricular outflow tract obstruction on clinical outcome in hypertrophic cardiomyopathy. *N Engl J Med* 2003; **348**: 295–303.

32 Ruzyllo W, Chojnowska L, Demkow M *et al.* Left ventricular outflow tract gradient decrease with non-surgical myocardial reduction improves exercise capacity in patients with hypertrophic cardiomyopathy. *Eur Heart J* 2000; **21**: 770–7.

33 Ziemssen P, Faber L, Schlichting J *et al.* Percutaneous septal ablation in patients with hypertrophic obstructive cardiomyopathy results in improvement of exercise capacity [abstract]. *J Am Coll Cardiol* 2000; **35**: 182A.

34 Redwood DR, Goldstein RE, Hirshfeld J *et al.* Exercise performance after septal myotomy and myectomy in patients with obstructive hypertrophic cardiomyopathy. *Am J Cardiol* 1979; **44**: 215–20.

35 Nihoyannopoulos P, Karatasakis G, Frenneaux M, McKenna WJ, Oakley CM. Diastolic function in hypertrophic cardiomyopathy: Relation to exercise capacity. *J Am Coll Cardiol* 1992; **19**: 536–40.

36 Sharma S, Elliott PM, Whyte G *et al.* Chronotropic incompetence is an important determinant of functional limitation in hypertrophic cardiomyopathy [abstract]. *Eur Heart J* 1999; **20**: 624.

37 Cuda G, Fananapazir L, Zhu W-S, Sellers J, Epstein ND. Skeletal muscle expression and abnormal function of β-myosin in hypertrophic cardiomyopathy. *J Clin Invest* 1993; **91**: 2861–5.

38 Counihan PJ, Frenneaux MP, Webb DJ, McKenna WJ. Abnormal vascular responses to supine exercise in hypertrophic cardiomyopathy. *Circulation* 1991; **84**: 686–96.

39 McKenna WJ, Spirito P, Desnos M, Dubourg O, Komajda M. Experience from clinical genetics in hypertrophic cardiomyopathy: Proposal for new diagnostic criteria in adult members of affected families. *Heart* 1997; **77**: 130–2.

40 Anan R, Nakagawa M, Miyata M *et al.* Cardiac involvement in mitochondrial diseases: A study on 17 patients with documented mitochondrial DNA defects. *Circulation* 1995; **91**: 955–61.

41 Pellicia A, Maron BJ, Spataro A, Proschan M, Spirito P. The upper limit of physiologic cardiac hypertrophy in highly trained elite athletes. *N Engl J Med* 1991; **324**: 295–301.

42 McKenna WJ, Stewart JT, Nihoyannopoulos P, McCinty F, Davies MJ. Hypertrophic cardiomyopathy without hypertrophy. *Br Heart J* 1990; **63**: 287–90.

43 Maron BJ, Kragel AH, Roberts WC. Sudden death in hypertrophic cardiomyopathy with normal left ventricular mass. *Br Heart J* 1990; **63**: 308–10.

44 Maron BJ, Roberts WC, McAllister HA, Rosing DR, Epstein SE. Sudden death in young athletes. *Circulation* 1980; **62**: 218–29.

45 Maron BJ, Epstein SE, Roberts WC. Causes of sudden death in competitive athletes. *J Am Coll Cardiol* 1986; **7**: 204–14.

46 Maron BJ, Shirani J, Poliac LC, Mathenge R, Roberts WC, Mueller FO. Sudden death in young competitive athletes. Clinical, demographic and pathological profiles. *JAMA* 1996; **276**: 199–204.

47 Maron BJ, Pellicia A, Spirito P. Cardiac disease in young trained athletes. Insights into methods for distinguishing athletes heart from structural heart disease, with particular emphasis on hypertrophic cardiomyopathy. *Circulation* 1995; **91**: 1596–601.

48 Lewis JF, Spirito P, Pellicia A, Maron BJ. Usefulness of Doppler echocardiographic assessment of diastolic filling in distinguishing 'athlete's heart' from hypertrophic cardiomyopathy. *Br Heart J* 1992; **68**: 296–300.

49 Pelliccia A, Maron BJ, Culasso F *et al.* Clinical significance of abnormal electrocardiographic patterns in trained athletes. *Circulation* 2000; **102**: 278–84.

50 Maron B, Pelliccia A, Sparato A, Granata M. Reduction in left ventricular wall thickness after deconditioning in highly trained Olympic athletes. *Br Heart J* 1993; **69**: 125–8.

51 Sharma S, Elliott PM, Whyte G *et al.* Utility of metabolic exercise testing in distinguishing hypertrophic cardiomyopathy from physiologic left ventricular hypertrophy in athletes. *J Am Coll Cardiol* 2000; 36: 864–70.

52 McKenna WJ, Deanfield J, Faruqui A, England D, Oakley CM, Goodwin JF. Prognosis in hypertrophic cardiomyopathy: Role of age, and clinical, electrocardiographic and hemodynamic features. *Am J Cardiol* 1981; **47**: 532–8.

53 McKenna WJ, Franklin RCG, Nihoyannopoulos P *et al.* Arrhythmia and prognosis in infants, children and adolescents with hypertrophic cardiomyopathy. *J Am Coll Cardiol* 1988; **11**: 147–53.

54 Maron BJ, Shen W-K, Link MS *et al.* Efficacy of implantable cardioverter-defibrillators for the prevention of sudden death in patients with hypertrophic cardiomyopathy. *N Engl J Med* 2000; **342**: 365–73.

CHAPTER 11

Pathophysiology and Significance of Myocardial Ischemia in Hypertrophic Cardiomyopathy

Rajesh Thaman, MBBS, MRCP, Bhavesh Sachdev, MBBS, MRCP, and Perry M. Elliott, MBBS, MD, MRCP

Hypertrophic cardiomyopathy (HCM) is a genetically determined myocardial disorder caused in the majority of cases by inherited mutations in genes that encode cardiac sarcomeric proteins. The pathological consequences include myocyte and myofibrillar disarray, myocardial fibrosis and small vessel disease.[1] These in turn, result in a complex disturbance of left ventricular pump function and electrical stability. Up to 30% of patients with the disease complain of typical angina symptoms during daily activities. Pathological and clinical evidence suggests that myocardial ischemia may be responsible; there are also limited data suggesting that myocardial ischemia can be a trigger for ventricular arrhythmia.[2,3] However, the clinical evaluation of myocardial ischemia in patients with HCM remains problematic. This chapter examines the evidence for myocardial ischemia in HCM and discusses its significance with particular reference to its role in disease progression and sudden death.

Pathophysiology of myocardial ischemia in HCM

Myocardial ischemia is the result of inadequate oxygen delivery arising as a consequence of an absolute or relative reduction in myocardial blood flow. This in turn has biochemical consequences that impair energy homeostasis within myocardial cells, and disrupt normal myocardial electrical–mechanical function. Several aspects of the pathophysiology of HCM may cause or predispose to the development of myocardial ischemia.

Microvascular changes

Experimentally induced myocardial hypertrophy is associated with a reduction in myocardial capillary density.[4] Similar structural changes within the coronary microcirculation have been described in HCM, together with an inverse relationship between the degree of hypertrophy and capillary density.[5] Autopsy studies in patients with HCM have also demonstrated intramural arterioles with abnormally thick walls caused by medial hypertrophy and increased collagen deposition.[6–8] They are found predominantly within the

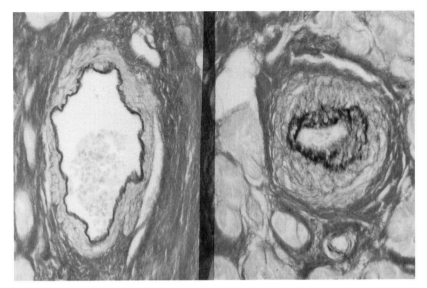

Fig. 11.1 Sections through two intramural coronary blood vessels demonstrating normal anatomy (left panel) and medial thickening in a patient with hypertrophic cardiomyopathy (right panel). Reproduced with permission from Kaski JC, ed. *Chest Pain with Normal Coronary Angiograms. Pathogenesis, Diagnosis and Management.* Kluwer Academic Publishers, © 1999: 281–91.

subendocardium of the hypertrophied septum and are found at equal frequency in patients with and without outflow tract obstruction (Fig. 11.1). The cause and significance of these small vessel abnormalities are uncertain. Similar small vessel changes occur in other cardiovascular diseases, such as aortic stenosis, hypertension and dilated cardiomyopathy, but they are usually less extensive. It has been suggested that abnormal intramural vessels are more numerous in regions of extensive myocardial scarring and in patients with end-stage ventricular dilatation.[6,8] However, other studies have shown that small vessel abnormalities occur throughout the myocardium.[9]

Several studies have reported evidence for a more generalized vascular defect affecting arterioles in HCM. For example, impaired coronary vasodilator reserve has been shown to occur in association with attenuated forearm vasodilatation after intra-arterial infusion of sodium nitroprusside.[10] In the same study there was no correlation between septal thickness and coronary vasodilator reserve or peripheral vascular response, suggesting that the underlying mechanism is independent of the severity of hypertrophy.

Left ventricular hypertrophy

Left ventricular hypertrophy increases the vulnerability of the myocardium to ischemia even in the presence of an anatomically normal coronary circulation, by increasing total myocardial oxygen demand.[11,12] This is exacerbated by the asymmetric nature of the hypertrophy, which results in asynchronous and incoordinate ventricular contraction and relaxation. This reduces cardiac efficiency and may generate high intramyocardial pressures in both systole and diastole, thereby reducing local coronary flow. At the microscopic level, myocyte hypertrophy and an excess of fibrillar collagen increase extravascular compressive forces.[13] Oxygen demand is also increased by the loss of normal myocyte-to-myocyte orientation and the abnormal intercellular connections that characterize HCM, resulting in inefficient myocardial contraction.

Left ventricular outflow tract obstruction

Left ventricular outflow tract obstruction occurs in approximately 25% of individuals with HCM. It might be anticipated that the increased intraventricular pressures associated with obstruction might cause subendocardial hypoperfusion and ischemia by increasing end-diastolic pressures and wall tension. However, most studies have failed to show a direct relation between angina and the degree of left ventricular outflow tract gradient at rest. Nevertheless, the fact that symptomatic improvement[14] and a reduction in reversible thallium-201 perfusion defects[15] occur following successful surgical septal reduction suggests that obstruction may cause myocardial ischemia, at least in patients with moderate to severe obstruction.

Large vessels

Although most patients with HCM and chest pain have angiographically normal or dilated epicardial vessels, the systolic compression of epicardial coronary vessels and septal perforator arteries[16,17] is well recognized. The effect of systolic compression on coronary blood flow, however, is unknown because the majority of myocardial flow occurs in diastole, when these vessels are widely patent. It may, however, explain the dramatic systolic flow reversal observed during intracoronary and transesophageal Doppler studies of proximal coronary vessel blood flow.[18]

Biochemical evidence for myocardial ischemia in HCM

Coronary sinus lactate extraction has been used widely as a metabolic marker of myocardial ischemia in a variety of cardiovascular diseases. Several papers have reported reduced lactate consumption (implying anaerobic metabolism) during pacing in association with ST-segment depression, reductions in coronary sinus blood flow and elevated left ventricular end-diastolic pressure in patients with HCM.[19] Reversible thallium perfusion defects have also been reported in patients with net lactate production during rapid cardiac pacing[20] (Fig. 11.2a). However, coronary sinus lactate concentration is determined by a number of other factors unrelated to myocardial ischemia, including substrate availability and adrenergic stimulation.[21,22] Other potential limitations of this technique include susceptibility to sampling errors and difficulty in detecting rapid changes in coronary venous metabolite concentration.[23,24]

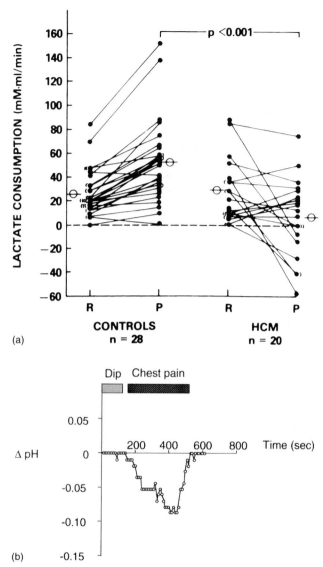

Fig. 11.2 (a) Individual values for lactate consumption in control subjects and in patients with hypertrophic cardiomyopathy measured at rest (R) and peak pacing (P). Patients below the dashed line have net lactate production. Reproduced with permission from Cannon *et al.* Myocardial ischemia in patients with hypertrophic cardiomyopathy: contribution of inadequate vasodilator reserve and elevated left ventricular filling pressures. *Circulation* 1985; **71**: 234–3. (b) Change in coronary sinus pH following dipyridamole infusion in a patient with hypertrophic cardiomyopathy. Reproduced from Elliott *et al.* Changes in coronary sinus pH during dipyridamole stress in patients with hypertrophic cardiomyopathy. *Heart* 1996; **75**: 179–83, with permission from the BMJ Publishing Group.

Some of the problems associated with lactate estimation may be overcome by continuous measurement of coronary sinus pH and oxygen saturation. The advantages of this technique include continuous monitoring, a rapid response and independence from changes in coronary sinus blood flow. Both techniques, however, share the disadvantage of being unable to detect ischemia in parts of the myocardium not drained by the coronary sinus.

In a small study of 11 patients with HCM, dipyridamole infusion was shown to cause chest pain together with a substantial decline in coronary sinus pH[25] (Fig. 11.2b). Maximal pH changes during coronary sinus sampling correlated with neither left ventricular cavity dimensions nor wall thickness. No association was detected between coronary sinus pH changes and reversible thallium perfusion defects, ST-segment depression or maximal oxygen consumption during exercise.

Conventional markers of myocardial ischemia in HCM

Although invasive coronary sinus studies have confirmed the presence of myocardial ischemia in patients with HCM, they are an impractical method for screening patients in routine clinical practice. The same noninvasive techniques that are used to detect myocardial ischemia in patients with coronary artery disease (radionuclide perfusion imaging, ST-segment analysis) have also been evaluated in HCM. However, as the following discussion shows, their interpretation can be problematic.

Electrocardiographic monitoring

ST-segment depression in patients with HCM is described during exercise[17,26] and immediately preceding syncope and cardiac arrest.[3] It is also common during 48-hour ambulatory monitoring[27] (Fig. 11.3). However, the significance of electrocardiographic ST-segment changes during exercise and Holter remains uncertain, as most studies show little if any correlation with exercise capacity or symptoms attributable to myocardial ischemia. Moreover, there is no significant relation between ST changes during exercise and lactate production.[22] In young patients, ST-segment changes during ambulatory monitoring have been associated with a history of typical exertional angina and dyspnea. More recently, a study of 79 patients followed for over 72 months showed that dipyridamole-induced ST-segment depression was predictive of an unfavourable outcome with a higher likelihood of future cardiac events; specifically, these were unstable angina, left ventricular and atrial dilatation, atrial fibrillation, and syncope.[28] Collectively, these data suggest that, while ST-segment changes may be a nonspecific marker of disease severity, they have insufficient sensitivity and specificity for the purpose of screening for myocardial ischemia in patients with HCM.

Single photon perfusion imaging

Studies using planar and single photon emission computed tomography thal-

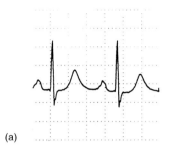

(a)

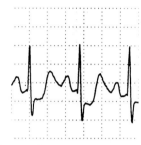

(b)

Fig. 11.3 Ambulatory electrocardiograms from a 45-year-old patient with hypertrophic cardio-myopathy at rest (a) and during an episode of chest pain (b). Reproduced from Elliott *et al.* Chest pain during daily life in patients with hypertrophic cardiomyopathy: an ambulatory electrocardiographic study. *Eur Heart J* 1996; **17**: 1056–64, with permission from the European Society of Cardiology.

lium-201 scintigraphy (SPECT) have shown that regional perfusion defects occur in 50–60% of patients with HCM[29–31] (Fig. 11.4).

Fixed defects have been identified with greatest frequency in the anteroseptal region of the left ventricle, followed by the inferior, lateral and posteroseptal areas.[29] Fixed defects are associated with larger left ventricular end-diastolic and end-systolic dimensions, increased left atrial size, reduced fractional shortening and lower peak exercise oxygen consumption.[27,29] This is consistent with the hypothesis that fixed perfusion abnormalities in patients with HCM represent areas of myocardial fibrosis.[29,30]

Associations with reversible defects have been more elusive and only one study to date has demonstrated a correlation between the presence of angina and reversible myocardial scintigrams.[32] This lack of correlation between reversible defects and symptoms has been explained by the suggestion that HCM is associated with a high prevalence of 'silent' ischemia or noncardiac chest pain. This hypothesis is supported by the findings in a study demonstrating that 'reversible' thallium-201 perfusion abnormalities are associated with lactate production but not symptoms during pacing stress.[16] However, other studies have failed to show an association between thallium-201 defects

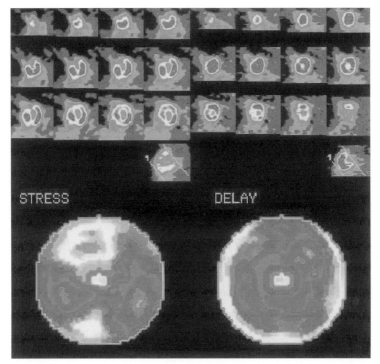

Fig. 11.4 Dipyridamole thallium-201 scan from a 19-year-old female patient. This figure demonstrates a reversible perfusion defect in the anterioseptal and inferior segment of the left ventricle during dipyridamole infusion.

and lactate production,[33] and it is possible that the disparity between symptomatic status and reversible perfusion defects may also relate to the intrinsic limitations of single photon imaging. For example, thallium-201 perfusion defects result from relative differences in myocardial thallium-201 uptake, and it is possible that a homogeneous reduction in coronary microvascular flow might not be detected by qualitative analysis of thallium-201 perfusion images.[34] Secondly, the limited resolution of conventional thallium scanning might preclude reliable detection of subendocardial hypoperfusion in some patients with HCM. Regional differences in tracer concentration secondary to factors such as variable myocardial thickness are also more likely in HCM.

Several workers have suggested that the sensitivity of thallium-201 imaging is improved by measuring thallium-201 washout. One study showed that the mean total thallium-201 washout was lower in patients with chest pain, with a modest inverse correlation with maximal left ventricular wall thickness.[29] Patients with nonsustained ventricular tachycardia (NSVT) during 48-hour ambulatory monitoring were also shown to have lower thallium-201 washout than patients without NSVT. However, there was considerable overlap in values for total washout in patients with and without ischemic symptoms, and

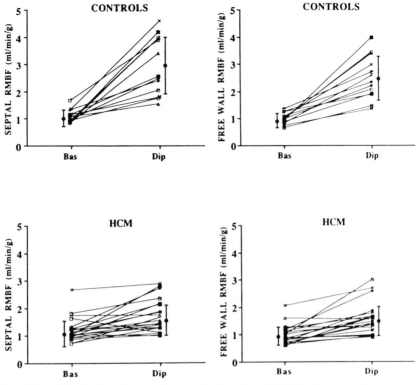

Fig. 11.5 Individual values of regional myocardial blood flow (RMBF) in the interventricular septum and free left ventricular wall at baseline (Bas) and following dipyridamole infusion (Dip) in control subjects and patients with hypertrophic cardiomyopathy. Reproduced from Camici P *et al.* Coronary vasodilatation is impaired in both hypertrophied and non-hypertrophied myocardium of patients with hypertrophic cardiomyopathy: A study with nitrogen-13 ammonia and positron emission tomography. *J Am Coll Cardiol* 1991; **17**: 879–86, with permission from the American College of Cardiology Foundation.

the potential influence of other technical and physiological factors on myocardial thallium-201 clearance[35] means that the value of this additional analysis in the management of patients with HCM is probably limited.

Positron emission tomography

Positron emission tomography (PET) is theoretically superior to conventional single photon imaging in that it has better spatial resolution and can quantify regional myocardial tissue flow. Studies using nitrogen-13 ammonia and dynamic positron emission tomography[36,37] have demonstrated that coronary blood flow per unit of left ventricular mass is inappropriately reduced both at rest and during pacing in association with metabolic evidence for ischemia. During dipyridamole-induced coronary microvascular vasodilatation, a reduction in coronary vasodilator reserve has been observed both in hypertrophied and nonhypertrophied regions of myocardium[36] (Fig. 11.5). The reduction in vasodilator reserve may be more pronounced in patients with a history of chest pain and ST-segment depression.[36] PET has also demonstrated subendocardial hypoperfusion after dipyridamole infusion across the septum of patients with asymmetrical septal hypertrophy ('subendocardial steal').[38]

PET has been used to investigate the relationship between myocardial blood flow and myocardial glucose utilization using fluorine-18 labelled deoxyglucose (FDG).[39,40] In the fasting state, high levels of serum free fatty acids suppress myocardial glucose metabolism, except in areas of myocardial ischemia, where there is enhanced anaerobic glycolysis. FDG is exchanged across cellular membranes in proportion to glucose, but is both a poor substrate for glycolysis and is relatively impermeable to cell membranes. It therefore becomes 'trapped' in areas of increased glucose uptake. Studies in HCM have shown patterns of FDG uptake suggestive of both myocardial ischemia and apparently selective abnormalities of glucose metabolism, independent of coronary flow.[41]

Significance of myocardial ischemia in HCM

Although the link between ischemia and symptoms has been difficult to establish in HCM, the weight of circumstantial evidence suggests that ischemia is important in the pathophysiology of the disease. Given the magnitude of ischemia observed in metabolic studies, it seems inconceivable that myocardial ischemia does not contribute to the exertional symptoms experienced by patients with HCM. It is also likely that recurrent episodes of ischemia may lead to myocardial fibrosis and scarring and, as a consequence, contribute to progressive systolic and diastolic left ventricular dysfunction. The role that myocardial ischemia plays in the mechanisms underlying sudden death is still uncertain. The precise substrate for arrhythmia in HCM remains unknown, but myocyte disarray and fibrosis theoretically create the necessary conditions for disordered impulse conduction. Recent evidence has shown that marked 'fractionation' of paced ventricular electrocardiograms is present in some patients with HCM and a history of ventricular fibrillation,[42] and it is reasonable to suppose that this is exacerbated by changes in cell membrane potentials caused by myocardial ischemia.

Clinical evidence that ischemia may trigger fatal ventricular arrhythmia comes from observational data linking sudden death with moderate to severe exertion[43] and the demonstration of ST-segment depression prior to ventricular fibrillation.[2,3] In a study of 23 young individuals with HCM, a positive correlation was detected between reversible thallium-201 defects and patients with a history of cardiac arrest or syncope.[44] In contrast, a larger prospective study failed to show any relation between sudden death and reversible defects.[29] When patients with a history of ventricular fibrillation and syncope were considered separately in the larger study, there was an association with fixed but

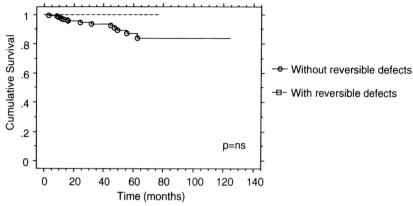

Fig. 11.6 Kaplan–Meier survival plot demonstrating cumulative survival in patients with and without reversible thallium-201 perfusion defects. Reproduced from Yamada *et al.* Relation of thallium-201 perfusion abnormalities to clinical and prognostic markers in hypertrophic cardiomyopathy. *Eur Heart J* 1998; **19**: 500–7, with permission from the European Society of Cardiology.

not reversible defects (Fig. 11.6). These apparently disparate findings might be explained by the different stresses used in the two studies (exercise and dipyridamole respectively) and the characteristics of the patient populations. However, the fact that none of the patients that died suddenly in the larger prospective study had a reversible defect suggests that thallium scintigraphy is not useful in clinical risk stratification.

Future evaluation of ischemia in HCM

In order to solve the conundrum of myocardial ischemia in HCM, new strategies for the identification of myocardial ischemia in patients with HCM are required. Because of the heterogeneity of the disorder, large numbers of patients have to be studied and thus any investigation into the impact of myocardial ischemia on natural history should employ predominantly noninvasive techniques that can be repeatedly applied in the outpatient setting. One such easily applied investigation includes levels of plasma brain naturetic peptides (BNP), which have recently been found to be elevated in patients with HCM and exercise-induced myocardial perfusion defects.[45] However, further work is required in order to validate its use as a marker for ischemia. At present, one of the most promising techniques is PET, as this can provide a quantitative measurement of global and regional myocardial blood flow as well as an assessment of myocardial metabolism. The downside to using PET relates to its limited availability, its high cost, and the small risk of radionuclide exposure. Magnetic resonance imaging may provide an alternative as its excellent spatial resolution and rapidly improving temporal resolution makes it possible to measure myocardial contractile performance in any plane as well as 'real-time' myocardial perfusion imaging, both at rest and during pharmacological stress.

References

1 Davies MJ, McKenna WJ. Hypertropic cardiomyopathy: Pathology and pathogenesis. *Histopathology* 1995; **26**: 493–500.

2 Stafford WJ, Trohman RG, Bilsker M, Zaman L, Castellanos A, Myerburg RJ. Cardiac arrest in an adolescent with atrial fibrillation and hypertrophic cardiomyopathy. *J Am Coll Cardiol* 1986; **7**: 710–4.

3 Nicod P, Polikar R, Peterson KL. Hypertrophic cardiomyopathy and sudden death. *N Engl J Med* 1988; **318**: 1255–7.

4 Tomanek RJ, Palmer RJ, Pfeiffer GL, Schreiber KL, Eastham CL, Marcus ML. Morphometry of canine coronary arteries, arterioles and capillaries during hypertension and left ventricular hypertrophy. *Circ Res* 1986; **58**: 38–46.

5 Krams R, Kofflard MJ, Duncker DJ, Von Birgelen C, Carlier S, Serruys PW. Decreased coronary flow reserve in hypertrophic cardiomyopathy is related to remodelling of the coronary microcirculation. *Brief Rapid Communications* 1997; **10**: 230–1.

6 Maron BJ, Wolfson JK, Epstein SE, Roberts WC. Intramural ('small vessel') coronary artery disease in hypertrophic cardiomyopathy. *J Am Coll Cardiol* 1986; **8**: 545–57.

7 Maron BJ, Epstein SE, Roberts WC. Hypertrophic cardiomyopathy and transmural myocardial infarction without significant atherosclerosis of extramural coronary arteries. *Am J Cardiol* 1979; **43**: 1086–102.

8 Tanaka M, Fujiwara H, Onodera T *et al.* Quantitative analysis of narrowing of intramyocardial small arteries in normal hearts, hypertensive hearts, and hearts with hypertrophic cardiomyopathy. *Circulation* 1987; **75**: 1130–9.

9 Varnava AM, Elliott PM, Sharma S, McKenna WJ, Davies MJ. Hypertrophic cardiomyopathy: The interrelation of disarray, fibrosis, and small vessel disease. *Heart* 2000; **84**: 476–82.

10 Pedrinelli R, Spessot M, Chiriatti G *et al.* Evidence for a systemic defect of resistance-sized arterioles in hypertrophic cardiomyopathy. *Coron Artery Dis* 1993; **4**: 67–72.

11 O'Gorman DJ, Sheridan DJ. Abnormalities of the coronary circulation associated with left ventricular hypertrophy. *Clin Sci* 1991; **81**: 703–13.

12 Scheler S, Motz W, Strauer BE. Transient myocardial ischemia in hypertensives: The missing link with left ventricular hypertrophy. *Eur Heart J* 1992; **13** (Suppl. D): 62–5.

13 Shirani J, Pick R, Roberts WC, Maron BJ. Morphology and significance of the left ventricular collagen network in young patients with hypertrophic cardiomyopathy and sudden cardiac death. *J Am Coll Cardiol* 2000; **35**: 36–44.

14 Wigle ED, Sasson Z, Henderson MA *et al.* Hypertrophic cardiomyopathy: The importance of the site and extent of hypertrophy: A review. *Prog Cardiovasc Dis* 1985; **28**: 1–83.

15 Canon RO 3rd, Dilsizian V, O'Gara PT *et al.* Impact of surgical relief of outflow obstruction on thallium perfusion abnormalities in hypertrophic cardiomyopathy. *Circulation* 1992; **85**: 1039–45.

16 Brugada P, Bar FW, de Zwaan C, Green M, Wellens HJ. 'Sawfish' systolic narrowing of the left anterior descending artery: An angiographic sign of hypertrophic cardiomyopathy. *Circulation* 1982; **66**: 800–3.

17 Pichard AD, Mellor J, Teicholz LE, Lipnik S, Gorlin R, Herman MV. Septal perforation compression (narrowing) in idiopathic hypertrophic subaortic stenosis. *Am J Cardiol* 1977; **40**: 310–14.

18 Akasaka T, Yoshikawa J, Yoshida K, Maeda K, Takagi T, Miyake S. Phasic coronary flow characteristics in patients with hypertrophic cardiomyopathy: A study by coronary Doppler catheter. *J Am Soc Echocardiogr* 1994; **7**: 9–19.

19 Cannon RO, Dilsizian V, O'Gara P *et al.* Myocardial metabolic, haemodynamic, and electrocardiographic significance of reversible thallium-201 abnormalities in hypertrophic cardiomyopathy. *Circulation* 1991; **83**: 1660–7.

20 Cannon RO, Rosing DR, Maron BJ *et al.* Myocardial ischemia in patients with hypertrophic cardiomyopathy: Contribution of inadequate vasodilator reserve and elevated left ventricular filling pressures. *Circulation* 1985; **71**: 234–43.

21 Camici P, Marraccini P, Lorenzoni R *et al.* Metabolic markers of stress induced myocardial ischemia. *Circulation* 1991; **83** (5 Suppl.): III8–13.

22 Gertz EW, Wisneski JA, Neese R, Houser A, Korte R, Bristow JD. Myocardial lactate extraction: Multi-determined metabolic function. *Circulation* 1980; **61**: 256–6.

23 Crake T, Crean PA, Shapiro LM, Rickards AF, Poole-Wilson PA. Coronary sinus pH during percutaneous transluminal angioplasty: Early development of acidosis during myocardial ischaemia in man. *Br Heart J* 1987; **58**: 110–15.

24 Cobbe SM, Poole-Wilson PA. Continuous coronary sinus and arterial pH monitoring during pacing induced ischaemia in coronary artery disease. *Br Heart J* 1982; **47**: 369–74.

25 Elliott PM, Rosano GMC, Gill JS, Poole-Wilson PA, Kaski JC, McKenna WJ. Changes in coronary sinus pH during dipyridamole stress in patients with hypertrophic cardiomyopathy. *Heart* 1996; **75**: 179–83.

26 Pasternac A, Noble J, Streulens Y, Elie R, Henschke C, Bourassa MG. Pathophysiology of chest pain in patients with cardiomyopathies and normal coronary arteriograms. *Circulation* 1982; **65**: 778–89.

27 Elliott PM, Kaski JC, Prasad K *et al.* Chest pain during daily life in patients with hypertrophic cardiomyopathy: An ambulatory electrocardiographic study. *Eur Heart J* 1996; **17**: 1056–64.

28 Lazzeroni E, Picano E, Morozzi L *et al.* Dipyridamole-induced ischaemia as a prognostic marker of future adverse events in adult patients with hypertrophic cardiomyopathy. Echo Persantine Italian Cooperative (EPIC) Study group, Subproject Hypertrophic Cardiomyopathy. *Circulation* 1997; **96**: 4268–72.

29 Yamada M, Elliott PM, Gane J, Britten A, Kaski JC, McKenna WJ. Relation of thallium-201 perfusion abnormalities to clinical and prognostic markers in hypertrophic cardiomyopathy. *Eur Heart J* 1998; **19**: 500–7.

30 O'Gara PT, Bonow RO, Maron BJ *et al.* Myocardial perfusion abnormalities in patients with hypertrophic cardiomyopathy: Assessment with thallium-201 emission computed tomography. *Circulation* 1987; **76**: 1214–23.

31 Takata J, Counihan PJ, Gane JN *et al.* Regional thallium-201 washout and myocardial hypertrophy in hypertrophic cardiomyopathy and its relation to exertional chest pain. *Am J Cardiol* 1993; **72**: 211–17.

32 Pitcher D, Wainright R, Maisey M, Curry P, Sowton E. Assessment of chest pain in hypertrophic cardiomyopathy using thallium-201 myocardial scintigraphy. *Br Heart J* 1980; **44**: 650–6.

33 Hanrath P, Montz R, Mathey D *et al.* Correlation between myocardial thallium-201 kinetics, myocardial lactate metabolism and coronary angiographic findings in hypertrophic cardiomyopathy. *Z Kardiol* 1980; **69**: 353–9.

34 Maddahi J, Abdulla A, Garia EV, Swan HJC, Berman DS. Noninvasive identification of left main and triple vessel coronary artery disease: Improved accuracy using quantitative analysis of regional myocardial stress distribution and washout of thallium-201. *J Am Coll Cardiol* 1986; **7**: 53–6.

35 Hoffman JI. Transmural myocardial perfusion. *Prog Cardiovasc Dis* 1987; **29**: 429–64.

36 Camici P, Chiriatti G, Lorenzoni R *et al.* Coronary vasodilatation is impaired in both hypertrophied and non-hypertrophied myocardium of patients with hypertrophic cardiomyopathy: A study with nitrogen-13 ammonia and positron emission tomography. *J Am Coll Cardiol* 1991; **17**: 879–86.

37 Camici P, Cecchi F, Gistri R *et al.* Dipyridamole induced subendocardial underperfusion in hypertrophic cardiomyopathy assessed by positron-emission tomography. *Coron Artery Dis* 1991; **2**: 837–41.

38 Choudhury L, Elliott P, Rimoldi O *et al.* Transmural myocardial blood flow distribution in hypertrophic cardiomyopathy and effect of treatment. *Basic Res Cardiol* 1999; **94**: 49–59.

39 Nienaber CA, Gambhir SS, Moddy FV *et al.* Regional myocardial blood flow and glucose utilization in symptomatic patients with hypertrophic cardiomyopathy. *Circulation* 1993; **87**: 1580–90.

40 Grover-McKay M, Schwaiger M, Krivokapich J, Perloff JK, Phelps ME, Schelbert HR. Regional myocardial blood flow and metabolism at rest in mildly symptomatic patients with hypertrophic cardiomyopathy. *J Am Coll Cardiol* 1989; **13**: 317–24.

41 Gould KL. Myocardial metabolism by positron emission tomography in hypertrophic cardiomyopathy. *J Am Coll Cardiol* 1989; **13**: 325–6.

42 Saumarez RC, Camm AJ, Panagos A *et al.* Ventricular fibrillation in hypertrophic cardiomyopathy is associated with increased fractionation of paced right ventricular electrocardiograms. *Circulation* 1992; **86**: 467–74.

43 Maron BJ, Roberts WC, Epstein SE. Sudden death in hypertrophic cardiomyopathy: A profile of 78 patients. *Circulation* 1982; **65**: 1388–94.

44 Dilsizian V, Bonow RO, Epstein SE, Fananapazir L. Myocardial ischemia detected by thallium scintigraphy is frequently related to cardiac arrest and syncope in young patients with hypertrophic cardiomyopathy. *J Am Coll Cardiol* 1993; **22**: 796–804.

45 Nakamura T, Sakamoto K, Tetsuhiro Y *et al.* Increased plasma brain naturetic peptide level as a guide for silent myocardial ischemia in patients with non-obstructive hypertrophic cardiomyopathy. *J Am Coll Cardiol* 2002; **39**: 1657–63.

CHAPTER 12

Hypertrophic Cardiomyopathy in Japan: Clinical, Morphologic and Genetic Expression

Yoshinori Doi, MD, PhD, Hiroaki Kitaoka, MD, Nobuhiko Hitomi, MD, Naohito Yamasaki, MD, Yoshihisa Matsumura, MD, Takashi Furuno, MD, and Barry J. Maron, MD

Hypertrophic cardiomyopathy (HCM) is a primary disease of cardiac muscle that is characterized by a hypertrophied, nondilated left ventricle unassociated with other cardiac diseases.[1,2] Left ventricular hypertrophy, particularly asymmetric septal hypertrophy (ASH), is the most characteristic feature of HCM. Morphologic expression regarding the site and extent of left ventricular hypertrophy can often be heterogeneous.[3,4] The apical form of HCM, in which left ventricular wall thickening is confined to the region of the left ventricular apex below papillary muscle level, was first reported by Sakamoto and colleagues in 1976[5] and subsequently by Yamaguchi and colleagues in 1979.[6] Since its original description in Japan, apical HCM has received considerable attention and a number of studies have been published from Japan as well as from centers outside of Japan.[7–17] However, some controversy and confusion seem to persist regarding the morphologic and clinical expression and natural history of apical HCM.[18,19] The purpose of this chapter is to present our experience and to review published data in order to provide the most up-to-date information, which may help clarify some of the issues regarding this particular subset of HCM.

Apical hypertrophy was originally reported from Japan as a subset of nonobstructive HCM in which hypertrophy is limited to the apical region of the left ventricle. This morphologic variety of HCM is characterized by a striking electrocardiographic pattern of 'giant negative T waves (GNT)', defined as ≥10 mm deep, in addition to tall R waves in the left precordial leads, associated with an angiographic 'spade-shaped deformation of the left ventricular cavity' at end-diastole that indicates hypertrophy localized to the left ventricular apex[5,6] (Fig. 12.1). Subsequently, apical HCM has been reported from centers outside of Japan, although characteristic electrocardiographic and angiographic features are not often observed in these Western patients.[14–16] Moreover, in these patients hypertrophy appears more diffuse, with extension of hypertrophy beyond the apical region and not confined to the apex. Because of such differences in morphologic expression, there is still some controversy and confu-

Apical HCM

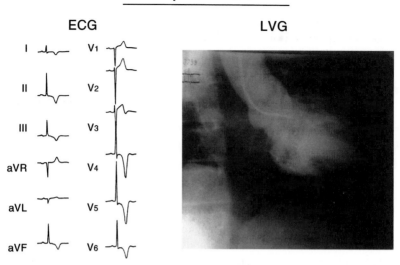

Fig. 12.1 A representative patient with apical hypertrophic cardiomyopathy, showing a striking electrocardiographic pattern of giant negative T waves (GNT) and an angiographic spade-shaped deformation of the left ventricle at end-diastole.

sion regarding the precise nature of this condition. It has been suggested that, although such variations might be related to differences in patient selection, genetic, racial, or environmental factors could also account for them.[9,18]

In Japan, the prevalence of apical HCM has been reported to be 13–25%, so it constitutes a significant segment of the overall HCM patient population.[6,7,20] Apical HCM is a clinically benign and nonfamilial disease that is identified predominantly in older men and is commonly associated with mild systemic hypertension. Most of these patients are asymptomatic and usually have a good long-term prognosis.[6,7] These clinical features in Japanese patients again differ significantly from those in most Western patients with apical HCM (Table 12.1).

Table 12.1 Apical hypertrophic cardiomyopathy

	Japanese	Western
Prevalence	13–25%	1–3%
Symptoms	None	None or severe
Family history	Rare	Infrequent or frequent
Gender	Male	Male > female
Giant negative T waves	All	Rare or common
Apical hypertrophy	Below papillary muscle level	More extensive

Definition and morphologic considerations

Differences among investigators with regard to the diagnostic method and the morphologic definition of apical HCM have contributed to the confusion regarding the diagnosis of this subset of HCM. This is probably because there is no generally agreed morphologic definition of apical HCM. In their original report of apical hypertrophy, Sakamoto and colleagues described localized hypertrophy confined to the most distal region of the left ventricle below papillary muscle level.[5] Therefore, the basal ventricular septum and the posterior wall show normal thickness in the parasternal short-axis and long-axis views by two-dimensional echocardiography.[5] Such isolated distal hypertrophy can be imaged only in apical views. On the other hand, apical HCM reported from centers outside of Japan are usually characterized by more extensive and diffuse hypertrophy, often beyond the true ventricular apex.[14–16]

When the diagnosis is based on angiographic demonstration of the spade-shaped left ventricular configuration, Koga and colleagues suggested that there are two forms of apical HCM; the Japanese form (spade-shaped) and the Western form (nonspade-shaped).[9,10] In their 152 patients with HCM, 29 patients showed apical hypertrophy without basal septal hypertrophy (spade-shaped) and 26 patients showed distal asymmetric septal hypertrophy particularly in the apical region (apical ASH, nonspade-shaped). There were also 20 patients with spade-shaped left ventricular configuration associated with basal and apical ASH (spade-like ASH). When 29 patients with a spade-shaped left ventricle (apical hypertrophy) were compared with 26 patients with a nonspade-shaped left ventricle (apical ASH), the clinical expression was significantly different. The patients with apical hypertrophy were older (53 ± 7 *vs* 32 ± 13 years) and males were predominant. A family history of HCM was uncommon and the GNT was frequently present (93%). Most of the patients were asymptomatic. These clinical features are similar to the original descriptions by Sakamoto and colleagues[5] and Yamaguchi and colleagues.[6] In contrast, patients with apical ASH were young (32 ± 13 years) and showed frequent prevalence of a family history of HCM (74%). The GNT was rare (4%) and 31% of the patients were severely symptomatic (New York Heart Association functional class III–IV). Koga and colleagues[9,10] then classified those patients with apical ASH (nonspade-shaped) as the Western form, which was thought to be a part of the broad disease spectrum of HCM. It was also postulated that the Japanese form of (pure) apical hypertrophy might constitute a separate disease entity.[9]

Patients with apical and basal septal hypertrophy can easily be confused with patients with 'pure' apical HCM, since the GNT may be present in addition to the angiographic spade-shaped deformation of the left ventricle. Moreover, patients with distal asymmetric septal hypertrophy (apical ASH in Koga's series) can also be confused with patients with pure apical HCM. Indeed, patients reported as having apical HCM from centers outside of Japan often show more extensive septal hypertrophy that is not confined to the apical segment. Therefore, in order to avoid confusion regarding the morphologic

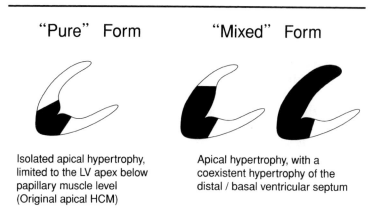

"Pure" Form

Isolated apical hypertrophy,
limited to the LV apex below
papillary muscle level
(Original apical HCM)

"Mixed" Form

Apical hypertrophy, with a
coexistent hypertrophy of the
distal / basal ventricular septum

Fig. 12.2 Morphologic definition of apical hypertrophic cardiomyopathy (HCM). In the 'pure' form there is isolated apical hypertrophy confined to the most distal apical segments well below the papillary muscles (original apical HCM). In the 'mixed' form there is more extensive apical hypertrophy, with coexistent hypertrophy of the distal and/or basal ventricular septum. Abbreviations as in Fig. 12.3.

definition, we suggest the use of terms such as 'pure' and 'mixed', as previously used by Maron[18] and Eriksson and colleagues.[21]

In our opinion, the term 'apical HCM' should be used for those patients with isolated apical hypertrophy confined to the most distal region of the left ventricular apex, well below papillary muscle level (pure apical HCM). Patients with apical hypertrophy and coexistent hypertrophy of the distal ventricular septum and occasionally the basal septum should be dealt with separately as the 'mixed' form (Fig. 12.2). It is likely that they are a part of the common disease spectrum of HCM, as suggested by Louie and Maron[15] and Koga and colleagues.[9]

Genetic expression

HCM is a familial cardiac disease with heterogeneous clinical and morphologic expression, caused by mutations in several genes that encode proteins of the cardiac sarcomere. Therefore, HCM is now described as a disease of the sarcomere.[2] The most common causes of HCM are mutations of the β-myosin heavy chain (βMyHC), cardiac myosin binding protein C (MyBP-C) and cardiac troponin T (cTnT). Although several genotype–phenotype correlation studies suggest that mutations affect the phenotypic expression of HCM, particularly the magnitude of left ventricular hypertrophy and the risk of sudden death, mutations in fact exhibit variable clinical and morphologic expression.[1,2,22]

Molecular genetic analysis in apical HCM may have several obstacles. Familial occurrence is usually uncommon in patients with pure apical HCM.

Some confusion regarding the precise morphologic definition of apical HCM may also make genotype–phenotype correlation difficult. Nevertheless, there have been several gene mutations reported in patients with apical HCM. Kimura and colleagues reported that three of 36 patients with apical HCM had mutations in the cardiac troponin I (cTnI) gene; in particular, Arg162Trp, Gly203Ser and Lys183del mutations were found in patients with apical HCM, although these same mutations have also been reported in their patients with typical HCM forms.[23] MyBP-C gene mutations in three patients with apical HCM and βMyHC gene mutation (Lys935Glu) in one patient with apical HCM were also reported, although again these mutations were also found in their patients with typical HCM.[22,23] Anan and colleagues recently reported that three individuals with a Phe110Ile mutation in the cTnT gene showed apical hypertrophy.[24] These three patients appeared to have pure form of apical HCM and two of them had a GNT. Forissier and colleagues described a family with an Arg92Leu mutation in the cTnT gene.[25] One individual showed apical hypertrophy without a GNT. It is not clear whether this patient had pure apical HCM or the mixed form, although the three other individuals in the same family showed other types of left ventricular hypertrophy.

Prevalence

The prevalence of apical HCM in Japan was previously estimated to be about 25%.[6,7] Subsequently, results from a multicenter HCM registry (786 patients) indicated that 13% of patients had apical HCM. Therefore, apical HCM constitutes a significant segment of the overall patient population with HCM in Japan. On the other hand, the number of patients reported from centers outside of Japan is relatively small. Thus, patients with pure apical HCM seem to be relatively uncommon except in Japan.[18] In their morphologic observations in 600 patients with HCM from two referral centers, Klues and colleagues found that only 1% of their patients had a pattern of wall thickening confined to the most apical region of the left ventricle.[4] The reason for this difference in prevalence is not known, although it may possibly be related to differences in the definition of apical HCM. Also, these patients are a highly selected hospital-based referral population and may not have included a representative proportion of asymptomatic patients. A recent report by Eriksson and colleagues indicates 7% prevalence of apical HCM in their cohort from a large tertiary referral center.[21]

Therefore, we directly compared regional cohorts of adult patients with HCM (≥18 years) from Japan (Kochi; $n = 100$) and the USA (Minneapolis; $n = 361$), using the same disease criteria.[26] Apical HCM was defined as wall thickening confined to the region of the left ventricular apex below papillary muscle level, without any coexistent hypertrophy of the distal or basal ventricular septum (pure apical HCM). The Japanese and American patients were similar clinically and did not differ significantly with regard to the severity of symptoms and outflow obstruction. The Japanese and American patients showed the same maximum left ventricular wall thickness but differed significantly in the distribution of left ventricular hypertrophy, the Japanese patients more frequently showing the apical form of HCM (15 *vs* 3%). GNT was more common in Japanese patients with apical HCM (64 *vs* 30%). Both Japanese and American patients with apical HCM had no or mild symptoms. Therefore, although the clinical expression of HCM is generally similar among Japanese and American patients, the apical form of HCM was five times more common in an unselected regional Japanese population. It is possible that specific sarcomeric gene mutations may predispose to this morphologic expression of HCM. However, differences in patient selection in the two countries could, in part, account for such variations, since asymptomatic apical HCM with GNT may be detected in the healthy population in Japan, related to the practice of screening large segments of the adult working population for heart disease with electrocardiography.[27]

Clinical expression: GNT

GNT is usually defined as ≥10 mm deep inversion in the lateral precordial leads. It is one of the most characteristic clinical features in patients with apical HCM in some reports from Japan. Except for reports by Webb and colleagues[17] and Eriksson and colleagues,[21] in which just over 50% had the GNT, most of the patients with apical HCM reported from outside of Japan have not shown this striking T-wave inversion. These patients, with apical HCM, showed a relatively diffuse distribution of hypertrophy with extension of the hypertrophy beyond the apical segments without an angiographic spade-shaped appearance of the left ventricle.[14–16] On the other hand, in our experience there are some patients with diffuse apical hypertrophy beyond the true left ventricular apex who may at times show a GNT together with an angiographic spade-shaped deformity of the left ventricle.[26] Not only the presence of apical hypertrophy but also the magnitude and site of apical hypertrophy may be important for the development of the GNT. In this context, Suzuki and colleagues evaluated the localization of apical hypertrophy using magnetic resonance imaging in 40 patients;[12,13] 26 patients showed a GNT and 14 patients showed mildly negative T waves.

GNT can also be found in patients with typical HCM. Alfonso and colleagues studied 83 patients with typical HCM.[28] Patients with a GNT showed a more distal distribution of left ventricular hypertrophy (which was more severe than in those without a GNT), were somewhat older, and showed greater precordial voltages.

Therefore, GNT can be found in most patients with pure apical HCM as well as in some patients with a mixed form of hypertrophy. The GNT may also be present in some patients with typical HCM. Recognition that the GNT can be present in a variety of patients may clarify some of the confusion regarding the definition of apical HCM and the clinical significance of the GNT (Fig. 12.3).

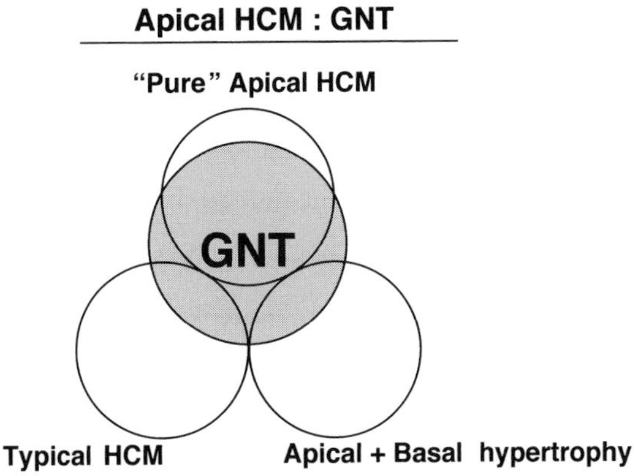

Fig. 12.3 Giant negative T waves (GNT) can be found in most patients with pure apical hypertrophic cardiomyopathy (HCM). It may also be present in some patients with apical and distal/basal hypertrophy (the mixed form) and in some patients with typical HCM.

Clinical course

The experience reported from Japan suggests a benign clinical course in patients with apical HCM. However, Koga and colleagues reported long-term changes of the GNT in 29 patients with apical HCM.[29] Fifteen of 21 patients (71%) who were followed for more than 10 years showed disappearance of the GNT. Thirty-eight per cent of the patients showed loss of the tall R wave. Progression of myocardial changes in the apex was suspected. Also, two patients developed typical morphologic features of ASH. On the other hand, Sakamoto recently reported the long-term prognosis of 126 patients with apical HCM.[30,31] The mean follow-up period was 13 years (1–29 years) and age at diagnosis was 52.4 years. There were no HCM-related deaths and most patients remained in a stable condition without significant symptoms. A few patients experienced clinical deterioration: there was a discrete apical aneurysm in one patient and atrial fibrillation in four patients. Also, Eriksson and colleagues reported the long-term outcome in 105 patients with apical HCM (89 with pure and 16 with mixed forms).[21] Apical HCM in these North American patients showed a generally benign prognosis, although one-third of the patients experienced some cardiovascular complications, such as myocardial infarction and arrhythmias. Therefore, most of the patients with pure apical HCM appear to have a good clinical course and may remain in a stable condition without symptoms for long periods of time. There are some patients who may experience loss of the GNT.[29] Progression to typical morphologic features of HCM, as well as complications such as a discrete apical aneurysm and arrhythmias, can occur at times, although it seems relatively uncommon.[8,21,26,31] (Fig. 12.4).

On the basis of the published data (as well as our own experience), it can be postulated that pure apical HCM is probably at the mild end of the broad clinical and morphologic spectrum of HCM. However, until more data are as-

Apical HCM: Clinical Course

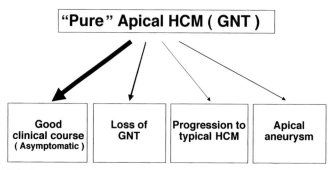

Fig. 12.4 Clinical course of pure apical hypertrophic cardiomyopathy. Most patients have an excellent prognosis. However, some patients may have an unusual clinical course. Abbreviations as in Fig. 12.1.

sembled, it is advised to separate this pure apical HCM from the mixed form with extension of the hypertrophy beyond the apical segments. Further studies, including systematic genetic analysis, are needed to determine the exact nature and clinical significance of apical hypertrophy and its relation to the overall disease spectrum of HCM.

References

1 Maron BJ. Hypertrophic cardiomyopathy. *Lancet* 1997; **350**: 127–33.
2 Spirito P, Seidman CE, McKenna WJ *et al.* The management of hypertrophic cardiomyopathy. *N Engl J Med* 1997; **336**: 775–85.
3 Shapiro LM, McKenna WJ. Distribution of left ventricular hypertrophy in hypertrophic cardiomyopathy: A two-dimensional echocardiographic study. *J Am Coll Cardiol* 1983; **2**: 437–44.
4 Klues HG, Schiffers A, Maron BJ. Phenotypic spectrum and patterns of left ventricular hypertrophy in hypertrophic cardiomyopathy: Morphologic observations and significance as assessed by two-dimensional echocardiography in 600 patients. *J Am Coll Cardiol* 1995; **26**: 1699–708.
5 Sakamoto T, Tei C, Murayama M *et al.* Giant T wave inversion as a manifestation of asymmetrical apical hypertrophy (AAH) of the left ventricle: Echocardiographic and ultrasono-cardiotomographic study. *Jpn Heart J* 1976; **17**: 611–29.
6 Yamaguchi H, Ishimura T, Nishiyama S *et al.* Hypertrophic nonobstructive cardiomyopathy with giant negative T waves (apical hypertrophy): Ventriculographic and echocardiographic features in 30 patients. *Am J Cardiol* 1979; **44**: 401–12.
7 Koga Y, Itaya K, Toshima H. Prognosis in hypertrophic cardiomyopathy. *Am Heart J* 1984; **108**: 351–9.
8 Ishiwata S, Nishiyama S, Nakanishi S *et al.* Two types of left ventricular wall motion abnormalities with distinct clinical features in patients with hypertrophic cardiomyopathy. *Eur Heart J* 1993; **14**: 1629–39.

9 Koga Y, Nohara M, Miyazaki Y *et al.* Two forms of apical hypertrophic cardiomyopathy: Japanese and Western forms. In: Toshima H, Maron BJ, eds. *Cardiomyopathy Update 2: Hypertrophic Cardiomyopathy.* Tokyo: University of Tokyo Press, 1988: 293–308.

10 Koga Y, Takahashi H, Ifuku M *et al.* Hypertrophic cardiomyopathy with ventricular septal hypertrophy localized to the apical region of the left ventricle (apical ASH). [In Japanese]. *J Cardiogr* 1984; **14**: 301–10.

11 Chikamori T, Doi Y, Akizawa M *et al.* Comparison of clinical, morphological, and prognostic features in hypertrophic cardiomyopathy between Japanese and western patients. *Clin Cardiol* 1992; **15**: 833–7.

12 Suzuki J, Watanabe F, Takenaka K *et al.* New subtype of apical hypertrophic cardiomyopathy identified with nuclear magnetic resonance imaging as an underlying cause of markedly inverted T waves. *J Am Coll Cardiol* 1993; **22**: 1175–81.

13 Suzuki J, Shimamoto R, Nishikawa J *et al.* Morphological onset and early diagnosis in apical hypertrophic cardiomyopathy: A long term analysis with nuclear magnetic resonance imaging. *J Am Coll Cardiol* 1999; **33**: 146–51.

14 Maron BJ, Bonow RO, Seshagiri TNR *et al.* Hypertrophic cardiomyopathy with ventricular septal hypertrophy localized to the apical region of the left ventricle (apical hypertrophic cardiomyopathy). *Am J Cardiol* 1982; **49**: 1838–48.

15 Louie EK, Maron BJ. Apical hypertrophic cardiomyopathy: Clinical and two-dimensional echocardiographic assessment. *Ann Intern Med* 1987; **106**: 663–70.

16 Keren G, Belhassen B, Sherez J *et al.* Apical hypertrophic cardiomyopathy: Evaluation by noninvasive and invasive techniques in 23 patients. *Circulation* 1985; **71**: 45–56.

17 Webb JG, Sasson Z, Rakowski H *et al.* Apical hypertrophic cardiomyopathy: Clinical follow-up and diagnostic correlates. *J Am Coll Cardiol* 1990; **15**: 83–90.

18 Maron BJ. Apical hypertrophic cardiomyopathy: The continuing saga. *J Am Coll Cardiol* 1990; **15**: 91–3.

19 Maron BJ. The giant negative T wave revisited … in hypertrophic cardiomyopathy. *J Am Coll Cardiol* 1990; **15**: 972–3.

20 Doi Y, Kitaoka H. Hypertrophic cardiomyopathy in the elderly: Significance of atrial fibrillation. *J Cardiol* 2001; **37** (Suppl. I): 133–8.

21 Eriksson MJ, Sonnenberg B, Woo A *et al.* Long-term outcome in patients with apical hypertrophic cardiomyopathy. *J Am Coll Cardiol* 2002; **39**: 638–45.

22 Kimura A. Mutations in genes for sarcomeric proteins. [In Japanese]. *Nippon Rinsho* 2000; **58**: 117–22.

23 Kimura A, Harada H, Park J-E *et al.* Mutations in the cardiac troponin I gene associated with hypertrophic cardiomyopathy. *Nat Genet* 1997; **16**: 379–82.

24 Anan R, Shono H, Kisanuki A *et al.* Patients with familial hypertrophic cardiomyopathy caused by a Phe110Ile missense mutation in the cardiac troponin T gene have variable cardiac morphologies and a favorable prognosis. *Circulation* 1998; **98**: 391–7.

25 Forissier J-F, Carrier L, Farza H *et al.* Codon 102 of the cardiac troponin T gene is a putative hot spot for mutations in familial hypertrophic cardiomyopathy. *Circulation* 1996; **94**: 3069–73.

26 Kitaoka H, Doi Y, Casey SA *et al.* Comparison of prevalence of apical hypertrophic cardiomyopathy in Japan and the United States. *Am J Cardiol* 2003; **92**: II83–6.

27 Hada Y, Sakamoto T, Amano K *et al.* Prevalence of hypertrophic cardiomyopathy in a population of adult Japanese workers as detected by echocardiographic screening. *Am J Cardiol* 1987; **59**: 183–4.

28 Alfonso F, Nihoyannopoulos P, Stewart J *et al.* Clinical significance of giant negative T waves in hypertrophic cardiomyopathy. *J Am Coll Cardiol* 1990; **15**: 965–71.

29 Koga Y, Katoh A, Matsuyama K *et al.* Disappearance of giant negative T waves in patients with the Japanese form of apical hypertrophy. *J Am Coll Cardiol* 1995; **26**: 1672–8.

30 Sakamoto T, Suzuki J. Apical hypertrophic cardiomyopathy. [In Japanese]. *Nippon Rinsho* 2000; **58**: 93–101.

31 Sakamoto T. Apical hypertrophic cardiomyopathy (apical hypertrophy): An overview. *J Cardiol* 2001; **37**: (Suppl. I): 161–78.

CHAPTER 13

Prevalence, Prevention and Treatment of Infective Endocarditis in Hypertrophic Cardiomyopathy

Paolo Spirito, MD, Marco Piccininno, MD, and Camillo Autore, MD

Infective endocarditis is a recognized complication of hypertrophic cardiomy-opathy (HCM) and is associated with substantial morbidity and mortality.[1–3] The vegetations are most commonly located on the anterior mitral leaflet, at the point where the mitral valve comes into contact with the septal endocar-dium during dynamic obstruction to left ventricular outflow (Fig. 13.1).[1–3] In a minority of patients the vegetations develop on the aortic cusps, probably be-cause the surface of the cusps is damaged by the high velocity and turbulence of blood flow during left ventricular outflow obstruction.[1–3]

Prevalence, incidence, and prevention of endocarditis

Infective endocarditis is uncommon in HCM. The frequency of the infection was recently investigated in a population of more than 800 HCM patients.[3] In the overall study population, the prevalence of endocarditis was 0.4% and the incidence 0.1 per 100 person-years. However, endocarditis was confined to patients with left ventricular outflow obstruction under basal conditions. The incidence of endocarditis in the patients with outflow obstruction was 0.4 per 100 person-years, and the cumulative risk at 10 years was 4.3%. The likelihood of developing the infection was also related to left atrial size. In patients with both outflow obstruction and a markedly dilated left atrium (≥50 mm), the incidence of endocarditis increased to 0.9 per 100 person-years. This associa-tion between risk of endocarditis and atrial size could be explained by the fact that a large left atrium may reflect, in part, long-standing and severe outflow obstruction with mitral regurgitation.

In the same study, the functional profile was ascertained for each of the 33 HCM patients with infective endocarditis reported in the literature during the previous 20 years.[1,2,4–13] Each had the obstructive form of the disease. There-fore, endocarditis in HCM appears to be virtually confined to patients with outflow obstruction under basal conditions, and the risk is highest in patients with both outflow obstruction and marked left atrial dilatation. Consequently, antibiotic prophylaxis for infective endocarditis should be routinely recom-

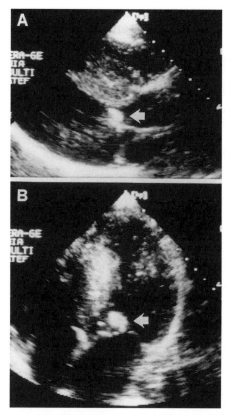

Fig. 13.1 Two-dimensional echocardiographic stop-frames in a patient with hypertrophic cardio-myopathy and infective endocarditis. A large vegetation (arrows) attached to the anterior mitral leaflet is visualized in the long-axis (A) and four-chamber views (B). Reprinted with permission from Spirito P, Rapezzi C, Bellone P *et al*. Infective endocarditis in hypertrophic cardiomyopathy. Prevalence, incidence, and indications for antibiotic prophylaxis. *Circulation* 1999; **99**: 2132–7.

mended only in patients with the obstructive form of the disease.[3] Prophylactic antibiotic regimens are reported in Table 13.1 and are based on the recommendations of the American Heart Association for the prevention of bacterial endocarditis.[14] Streptococci and staphylococci seem to be the bacteria most commonly responsible for infective endocarditis in HCM.[1–3,5,7,9,11]

Clinical consequences of infective endocarditis

In HCM, diastolic function is usually impaired, left ventricular cavity is small and ventricular volume cannot increase adequately in response to valve regurgitation.[15,16] Therefore, in patients with HCM, the severe valve incompetence often associated with infective endocarditis usually leads to a marked decrease in cardiac output, an increase in end-diastolic pressure,

Table 13.1 Antibiotic prophylactic regimens for prevention of bacterial endocarditis in patients with hypertrophic cardiomyopathy, based on the recommendations of the American Heart Association.[14]

Procedures	Standard regimen
Dental, oral, respiratory tract, esophageal, gastrointestinal, genitourinary	Adults: amoxicillin 2.0 g orally 1 h before procedure, or ampicillin 2.0 g i.m./i.v.* within 30 min before procedure
	In patients allergic to penicillin
Dental, oral, respiratory tract, esophageal	Adults: clindamycin 600 mg or cephalexin 2.0 g or clarithromycin 500 mg orally 1 h before procedure; or i.m./i.v.*, clindamycin 600 mg or cefazolin 1.0 g within 30 min before procedure Children: clindamycin 20 mg/kg or cephalexin 50 mg/kg or clarithromycin 25 mg/kg orally 1 h before procedure; or i.m./i.v.*, clindamycin 20 mg/kg or cefazolin 25 mg/kg within 30 min before procedure
Gastrointestinal, genitourinary	Adults: vancomycin 1.0 g i.v. over 1–2 h; complete infusion within 30 min of starting the procedure Children: vancomycin 20 mg/kg i.v. over 1–2 h; complete infusion within 30 min of starting the procedure

*I.m./i.v. regimens are reported for patients who are unable to take oral medications.

and important symptoms of heart failure.[1–3] Rupture of the chordae tendineae and/or perforation of the mitral leaflets or aortic cusps may precipitate acute, massive valve regurgitation with pulmonary edema and death (Fig. 13.2).[1–3] Systemic embolism, paravalvular abscess and valve aneurysm are other potential consequences of infective endocarditis.[1,2] It should be underlined, however, that most of the literature on infective endocarditis in HCM is based on case reports and autopsy observations.[2,4–13] Therefore, the literature is inevitably skewed toward patients with the most unfavorable clinical course. In the only large clinical survey of infective endocarditis in HCM, about half of the patients who developed endocarditis had a relatively benign clinical course and did not require cardiac surgery.[3] Therefore, infective endocarditis in HCM is not invariably associated with an unfavorable prognosis.

Surgical therapy

The surgical management of HCM patients with endocarditis has not been specifically addressed in the literature. However, on the basis of general clinical experience, when infection is not in an active phase and the morphology of the damaged valve permits, valve repair (associated with septal myotomy–myectomy) is preferable to valve replacement in patients with obstructive HCM and mitral valve endocarditis. Such a surgical approach may result in

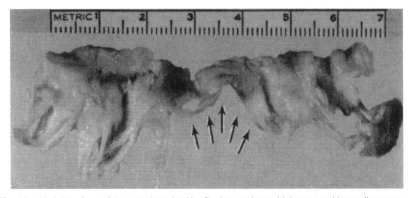

Fig. 13.2 Atrial surface of the anterior mitral leaflet in a patient with hypertrophic cardiomyopathy and infective endocarditis. The arrows indicate the area where cordae tendineae are missing (ruptured) and a portion of the leaflet is absent (destroyed by the infection). Reprinted with permission from the American College of Cardiology, *J Am Coll Cardiol* 1992; **19**: 365–71.

similar or even superior hemodynamic benefit in terms of reduction or abolition of mitral valve regurgitation and the outflow gradient, while avoiding the potential complications generally associated with a cardiac valve prosthesis.[17–19] In patients with outflow obstruction and endocarditis of the aortic valve who require valve replacement, surgery should also include myotomy–myectomy when the general clinical condition allows.

References

1 Alessandri N, Pannarale G, Del Monte F *et al*. Hypertrophic obstructive cardiomyopathy and infective endocarditis: A report of seven cases and a review of the literature. *Eur Heart J* 1990; **11**: 1041–8.

2 Roberts WC, Kishel JC, McIntosh CL *et al*. Severe mitral or aortic valve regurgitation, or both, requiring valve replacement for infective endocarditis complicating hypertrophic cardiomyopathy. *J Am Coll Cardiol* 1992; **19**: 365–71.

3 Spirito P, Rapezzi C, Bellone P *et al*. Infective endocarditis in hypertrophic cardiomyopathy. Prevalence, incidence, and indications for antibiotic prophylaxis. *Circulation* 1999; **99**: 2132–7.

4 Wang K, Gobel FL, Gleason DF. Bacterial endocarditis in idiopathic hypertrophic subaortic stenosis. *Am Heart J* 1975; **89**: 359–65.

5 Robbins N, Szilagyi G, Tanowitz HB *et al*. Infective endocarditis caused by *Streptococcus mutans*. A complication of idiopathic hypertrophic subaortic stenosis. *Arch Intern Med* 1977; **137**: 1171–4.

6 Pitcher D, Mary D. *Listeria monocytogenes* endocarditis in hypertrophic cardiomyopathy. *BMJ* 1978; **15**: 961.

7 Greenland P, Murphy GW. Acute valvular insufficiency complicating hypertrophic obstructive cardiomyopathy. *Chest* 1979; **75**: 182–3.

8 LeJemtel TH, Factor SM, Koenigsberg M *et al.* Mural vegetations at the site of endocardial trauma in infective endocarditis complicating idiopathic hypertrophic subaortic stenosis. *Am J Cardiol* 1979; **44**: 569–74.

9 Chagnac A, Rudniki C, Loebel H *et al* Infectious endocarditis in idiopathic hypertrophic subaortic stenosis: Report of three cases and review of the literature. *Chest* 1982; **81**: 346–9.

10 Ah Fat LN, Patel BR, Pickens S. *Actinobacillus actinomycetemcomitans* endocarditis in hypertrophic obstructive cardiomyopathy. *J Infect* 1983; **6**: 81–4.

11 Ovsyshecher IA, Zimlichman R. Infective endocarditis in hypertrophic cardiomyopathy secondary to amiodarone treatment. *Chest* 1983; **83**: 833.

12 Malouf J, Nasrallah A, Daghir I, Harake M, Mufarrij A. *Candida tropicalis* endocarditis in idiopathic hypertrophic subaortic stenosis. *Chest* 1984; **86**: 508.

13 Stulz P, Zimmerli W, Mihatsch J, Gradel E. Recurrent infective endocarditis in idiopathic hypertrophic subaortic stenosis. *Thorac Cardiovasc Surg* 1989; **37**: 99–102.

14 Dajani AS, Taubert KA, Wilson W *et al.* Prevention of bacterial endocarditis. Recommendations by the American Heart Association. *JAMA* 1997; **277**: 1794–801.

15 Maron BJ, Bonow RO, Cannon RO III *et al.* Hypertrophic cardiomyopathy: Interrelations of clinical manifestations, pathophysiology, and therapy. *N Engl J Med* 1987; **316**: 780–9, 844–52.

16 Wigle ED, Rakowski H, Kimball BP *et al.* Hypertrophic cardiomyopathy. Clinical spectrum and treatment. *Circulation* 1995; **92**: 1680–92.

17 Cooley DA, Leachman RD, Hallman GL *et al.* Idiopathic hypertrophic subaortic stenosis: Surgical treatment including mitral valve replacement. *Arch Surg* 1971; **103**: 606–9.

18 McIntosh CL, Maron BJ. Current operative treatment of obstructive hypertrophic cardiomyopathy. *Circulation* 1988; **78**: 487–95.

19 Spirito P, Seidman CE, McKenna WJ *et al.* The management of hypertrophic cardiomyopathy. *N Engl J Med* 1997; **336**: 775–85.

CHAPTER 14

Pharmacologic Treatment of Symptomatic Hypertrophic Cardiomyopathy

Mark V. Sherrid, MD and Ivan Barac, MD

There are five considerations in the treatment plan of patients with newly diagnosed hypertrophic cardiomyopathy (HCM). Risk stratification is essential to assess the likelihood of sudden death; in selected patients at higher risk prophylactic implanted defibrillator may be recommended. Prophylaxis against endocarditis is recommended for patients with obstruction. Patients are counseled to avoid competitive athletics and extremes of strenuous exertion and to obtain screening of first-degree relatives with echocardiography and ECG.[1-3]

Medical therapy of HCM is individualized to relieve the symptoms of exercise intolerance and angina (or possibly syncope). Understanding of pathophysiology forms the basis for medical treatment.[3-13]

Pathophysiology of heart failure symptoms

Patients typically have left ventricular (LV) diastolic dysfunction due to increased chamber stiffness and impaired relaxation. Increased chamber stiffness is due to structural abnormalities, hypertrophy and myofiber disarray, often with interstitial and perivascular fibrosis.[8] Early ventricular relaxation is also impaired due to a variety of functional causes: (1) inactivation-dependent mechanisms due to increased intracellular calcium, prolonged activation of contractile proteins, increased number of calcium channels, and ischemia; (2) load-dependent factors, such as afterload and gradient; and (3) nonuniform/asynchronous relaxation.[9] Besides increased LV diastolic filling pressures, diastolic dysfunction prevents increase in exercise stroke volume and cardiac output, which may correlate best with functional impairment.[10]

Myocardial ischemia was first convincingly shown by pacing-induced coronary sinus lactate production.[11] Decrease in coronary flow reserve, shown by a variety of invasive and noninvasive modalities, is an important contributor to ischemia and chest pain.[11,12] Limited flow reserve is likely to have several causes. Nonatherosclerotic narrowing of the intramural coronary arteries has been shown.[13] Evidence of intramural coronary narrowing has been found at multiple levels: in the septal perforators, in the small intramural arteries and in the preterminal resistance arterioles. Dynamic coronary circulation is also abnormal in HCM with impaired vasomotion and endothelial dysfunction.[14] These abnormalities lead to a high prevalence of scintigraphic perfusion abnormalities, which are observed in more than 50% of patients.[12,15] Syncope may have diverse etiologies, including intraventricular obstruction, ventricular arrhythmias, atrial arrhythmias, heart block and inappropriate vasodilatation.

Pharmacologic treatment in the absence of obstruction

Verapamil is the most often-used medication in patients without outflow obstruction. There are features of HCM that make the application of calcium channel blockers appealing. On the cellular level, HCM patients have increased action potential duration, increased calcium transients and relative calcium overload, which contribute to impaired relaxation and poor tolerance of tachycardia.[9] This is attenuated by verapamil (and exacerbated by digoxin).[16] *In vitro,* agents that alter calcium influx through the L-type channels may blunt the hypertrophic response of cardiomyocytes.[17]

Verapamil was first introduced for HCM by Kaltenbach and colleagues in 1978.[18] In the first study, of 22 adult patients treated with oral verapamil (mean dose of 480 mg/day and mean duration of treatment 15 months) symptom relief occurred in 11 patients, including five in whom the LV outflow tract (LVOT) gradient decreased. Side-effects were mild and it was concluded that verapamil appeared to be more effective and better tolerated than β-blockers. Numerous clinical studies followed.[19–31] In various studies verapamil improved symptoms by one or more New York Heart Association (NYHA) classes in 60% of patients after 14 months of treatment,[23] in 43% after 25 months[24] and in 57% after 40 months.[31] Exercise duration increased in the majority of patients, by an average of 53%.[23] This effect was sustained at 1 year[21,23,24] and 2 years and decreased after verapamil withdrawal.[21] Hopf and Kaltenbach[29] reported results of more than 10 years of follow-up on verapamil (average dose 515 mg/day): the annual mortality was 2% and exercise tolerance improved in 84% of patients.[29] Gregor and colleagues,[31] however, reported less durable effects, diminishing to equivocal benefit after 4 months. Most investigators have found an increase in treadmill exercise time on verapamil.[20–24] However, using bicycle exercise neither an increase in exercise time nor maximum oxygen consumption could be demonstrated.[25]

Acute and subacute hemodynamic effects of verapamil in HCM have been studied extensively in order to elucidate the mechanisms of its beneficial and adverse effects.[19–21,26–29,32–37] A limitation has been that almost all investigations have included both obstructed and nonobstructed patients.[18–24,28,29] Since LV relaxation improves when systolic overload is relieved, the direct effect of verapamil on diastolic dysfunction is difficult to prove in patients with dynamic gradients. There is some evidence that verapamil's clinical benefit in mild to moderately obstructed patients may be through its beneficial effects on diastole.[21,26]

There have been several studies of the acute effect of intravenous verapamil in the catheterization laboratory using Millar catheters to measure LV diastolic pressures.[26,32–35,37] Bonow and colleagues[26,37] found improved early diastolic parameters—the constant of relaxation τ decreased and isovolumetric relaxation time and time to peak filling rate shortened, which led to an increase in peak filling rate and more effective diastole. Hess and colleagues found improved relaxation but no benefit in diastolic chamber stiffness.[34] Tendera and colleagues found a fall in LV end-diastolic pressure and an improved chamber compliance pressure–volume relationship.[32] In contrast TenCate and colleagues[35] found a significant rise in diastolic pressure (from 21 to 23 mm Hg) and no improvement in any measure of diastolic function. Kass and colleagues[33] reported a rise in end-diastolic pressure from 19 to 21.6 mm Hg using Millar catheters and no change in τ or improvement in chamber compliance.

Using radionuclide angiography, Bonow and others found that verapamil decreased regional nonuniformity of relaxation and improved relaxation synchronicity.[27,37] Enhanced peak LV filling was due to enhanced early synchrony after drug, and correlated with increased exercise capacity.[21,26,27] This beneficial effect and its correlation with improved exercise capacity have been observed by others.[36] The effect was sustained in most studies and disappeared after drug was withdrawn.[28]

Symptoms of angina due to ischemia in HCM (in the absence of atherosclerotic coronary artery disease) are generally treated with verapamil, which improves scintigraphic evidence of ischemia. In a study of 29 patients, about 50% had exercise perfusion defects. Verapamil improved exercise perfusion in more than 70%[15] (Fig 14.1) This improvement has been confirmed by others.[38] The usual dose is 360 mg/day as tolerated. Doppler echocardiographic studies of coronary blood flow have shown benefit; i.e. decreases in peak coronary diastolic flow velocity and flow resistance index at rest, as well as correction of abnormal vasomotor response to pacing, sustained handgrip and cold exposure.[14,39]

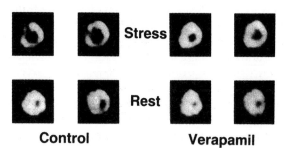

Fig. 14.1 Short-axis tomograms obtained immediately after maximal treadmill exercise (top) and after 3 hours of rest (bottom) in an 18-year-old asymptomatic man with hypertrophic cardiomyopathy. Under control conditions (left), reversible septal and inferoposterior perfusion defects develop during exercise and are improved at rest. There is also apparent cavity dilatation induced by exercise. During oral verapamil (right), myocardial perfusion and apparent cavity dilatation are improved during exercise. Reproduced with permission from Udelson *et al.* Verapamil prevents silent myocardial perfusion abnormalities during exercise in asymptomatic patients with hypertrophic cardiomyopathy. *Circulation* 1989; **79**: 1052–60.

The effect of verapamil on LV hypertrophy varied in several studies, with no convincing effect shown.[18,24,40] Endomyocardial biopsy specimens of 38 patients with HCM showed no changes in progression of hypertrophy or fibrosis.[41]

β-Blockers are also commonly used in nonobstructive HCM. The rationale is to decrease heart rate and increase filling time. Diuretics are given for refractory dyspnea or for the occasional patient with edema. Care must be taken to avoid over-diuresis.

Other calcium channel blockers have been tested. Nifedipine has not shown convincing benefit and may worsen symptoms and gradient.[24,42] In an acute hemodynamic study, Betocchi and colleagues showed that diltiazem decreased τ and increased peak filling rate, thus improving relaxation while not changing gradient or chamber stiffness.[43] Systemic resistance and blood pressure fell and the authors warned about the possibility of an increase in LVOT gradient and LV diastolic pressures.

In obstructed patients, disopyramide improves diastolic function and reduces LV filling pressures.[44–46] In contrast, in nonobstructive HCM filling pressures rise after the administration of disopyramide.[46] Thus, at present there is no definite role for disopyramide for symptom relief in nonobstructive HCM.

Significance of outflow obstruction

All the symptoms of HCM may occur in the absence of intraventricular obstruction, which occurs only in roughly one-fourth of patients.[1–3] However, the addition of LV outflow tract obstruction worsens symptoms[47] and increases mortality.[48] Obstruction increases systolic LV pressure and systolic wall tension and myocardial work. With high gradients, afterload due to obstruction overcomes LV contractility. Thus, in patients with LVOT gradients greater than 60 mm Hg, a sudden drop in mid-systolic LV ejection velocity is observed, which is due to the sudden imposition of afterload caused by mitral–septal contact.[49] Coronary perfusion pressure decreases since aortic diastolic pressure falls while LV diastolic pressure rises. Pacing produced ischemia and secondary anaerobic metabolism are documented, reversed by successful myectomy.[11] Systolic anterior motion (SAM) causes mitral regurgitation, in which functional deformation of the mitral valve causes incomplete coaptation.

Treatment is tailored to whether or not a patient has obstruction, with resting gradients greater than 30 mm Hg considered significant. Provocation with Valsalva's maneuver, exercise or the postprandial state may cause a rise in gradient and transfer a patient previously diagnosed as nonobstructive to obstructive.

Mechanism of outflow obstruction

SAM with mitral–septal contact is the usual mechanism for LV outflow obstruction. Obstructed patients have anatomic features that predispose to systolic mitral–septal contact. The mitral valve leaflets are relatively long and residual portions of leaflets extend past the coaptation point and protrude into the outflow tract. Most importantly, the mitral valve is situated anteriorly in the left ventricular cavity.[4] This is due to anterior displacement of the papillary muscles, which are often bound by muscular connections to the anterior wall.[4] This anterior displacement puts the mitral valve into the flow stream of LV ejection, subjecting the mitral valve to the hemodynamic force of ejection flow.[4–7]

Recent data have shown that although Venturi forces are necessarily present in the outflow tract, it is drag (the pushing force of flow) that is the dominant force which initiates the anterior motion, pushing the protruding mitral leaflet into the septum.[4–7] Drag is the component of force on a body that is in the direction of the flow—examples are the familiar force of rushing water or the wind. SAM has been referred to as 'anteriorly directed mitral prolapse,' which is an apt analogy since in both conditions large mitral leaflets are displaced from their normal positions by the pushing force of flow, resulting in mitral regurgitation.[7]

After mitral–septal contact, the pressure gradient across the protruding mitral leaflet further narrows the orifice, initiating an amplifying feedback loop in which obstruction begets more obstruction.[5–7,49] Overall, obstruction due to mitral–septal contact is best described as a time-dependent, amplifying feedback loop that is triggered by flow drag.[4–7,49]

Pharmacologic treatment of obstruction

Most symptomatic patients with obstructive HCM can be managed successfully with medication.[1–3] However, not infrequently patients will present on medications that have the potential to increase obstruction, such as vasodilators or positive inotropes, which should be discontinued. Common vasodilators include angiotensin-converting enzyme (ACE) inhibitors and receptor blockers, nifedipine, amlodipine, hydralazine, long- and short-acting nitrates, and α-blockers (usually given for prostatism). Positive inotropes include digoxin, dopamine and dobutamine.

β-Blockers

Patients with outflow obstruction are generally treated first with β-blocking agents. Though useful in mild and moderate obstruction, they are usually not effective for gradient reduction or symptom relief in patients with high resting gradients. However, β-blockade blunts the exercise-related rise in gradient.[50,51] β-Blockers potently slow heart rate, both at rest and with exertion, which may improve filling and ischemia. However, excessive slowing of exercise heart rate may have adverse consequences in HCM, since patients rely on a rise in heart rate to increase cardiac output and stroke volume.[10] Also, often HCM patients are already limited by chronotropic incompetence before medication,[52] and high doses of β-blockers may exacerbate or cause fatigue and worsen exercise tolerance. The potential to worsen exercise capacity has been shown with nadolol: 13 of 16 patients showed a decrease of more than 10% in peak exercise oxygen consumption.[25]

There are no data showing a particular benefit of one β-blocker over the others. To promote patient compliance, sustained release preparations of metoprolol or atenolol are most often used. The dose is titrated until the resting heart rate falls to 60 beats/min. We generally do not maximize β-blockade, as has been reported in the pediatric HCM population;[53] adults tolerate massive doses of β-blockade poorly.

β-Blockers may be beneficial to acutely ill patients who have high resting adrenergic tone and very high gradients. In acutely ill hospitalized patients with acute life-threatening heart failure, intravenous metoprolol or esmolol can be used. On-line blood pressure and acute echocardiographic monitoring are essential in a monitored setting. Metoprolol 5 mg intravenously over 2 minutes may be repeated every 5 minutes for total of 15 mg, and often results in immediate improvement in both gradient and symptoms. Administering a β-blocker intravenously to a patient in acute congestive heart failure may seem counterintuitive, but it is frequently life-saving. The best pharmacologic agent to support blood pressure in patients in shock due to obstruction is phenyl- ephrine. If dopamine or dobutamine are given in error this may exacerbate hypotension and heart failure and can result in death.

For patients with refractory obstruction and symptoms after β-blockade another drug is tried. There is regional heterogeneity in the selection of the second drug trial. The most frequent approach is to substitute verapamil for the β-blocker. We and others support the alternative strategy of adding disopyramide to β-blockade.[2,6,54,55]

Verapamil

After Kaltenbach's initial report,[18] Rosing and colleagues[19] showed a 48% decrease in pressure gradient after intravenous verapamil administration. Systemic vascular resistance consistently decreased, as did LVOT gradient, both at rest and with provocation.[19,26] With oral administration, exercise treadmill time increased by 26%.[22,23]

Verapamil has been widely evaluated in obstructive HCM[19–24,32,34] and similar decreases in gradient have been observed by others.[26,30,32,37] However, the pressure gradient has been noted to remain unchanged in the small subset of patients with a fall in systemic pressure.[20,26] Years of clinical use have confirmed the beneficial effect of verapamil on symptoms and exercise tolerance in selected patients, but the impact on survival is unresolved. The magnitude of symptom relief with verapamil is similar to the effect of β-adrenergic blocking agents.

However, verapamil has been associated with cardiac complications.[56] In a large prospective study of 227 patients with HCM, verapamil was discontinued due to side-effects in 7%; of these, 59% occurred in the first month and all but one in the first 6 months. Side-effects included pulmonary congestion, hypotension, junctional rhythm or Mobitz type I block, edema and constipation.

There were seven cardiac deaths: four from pulmonary edema and three from sudden cardiac death. Most patients with pulmonary congestion had substantial symptoms and baseline LVOT gradients higher than 50 mm Hg.[24]

Electrophysiologic side-effects may include sinus bradycardia with junctional escape rhythm (11%), Mobitz type I atrioventricular block (3%), sinus arrest (2%), Mobitz II (1%) and, rarely, complete heart block.[56] Other case-reports have confirmed the relationship between verapamil treatment and syncope or complete heart block.

The hemodynamic side-effects may occur in individual obstructed patients because the vasodilating effects of verapamil may outweigh its negative inotropic effects.[56] Rarely, a worsening LVOT gradient may occur and increase pulmonary capillary wedge pressure. Risk factors for these adverse consequences are rapid intravenous or oral titration, combination with quinidine, marked gradient, and elevated pulmonary capillary wedge pressure. Sudden cardiac death is likely due to vasodilatation/hypotension-triggered sympathetic stimulation. Because of these side-effects, Epstein and Rosing[19,56] offered contraindications for verapamil use: (1) combined high pulmonary capillary wedge pressure and LV outflow pressure gradient; (2) a history of paroxysmal nocturnal dyspnea/orthopnea with high pressure gradient; (3) sick sinus syndrome without pacemaker; and (4) atrioventricular nodal disease without pacemaker. Also, caution is necessary with a prolonged PR interval, and concomitant quinidine should be avoided. Lorell[57] reiterates these cautions. These are important limitations since one would want to administer verapamil to medically refractory patients who would otherwise require septal myectomy or other interventions. Therefore, verapamil is best reserved for those patients with both mild or moderate symptoms and modest outflow gradients.

Disopyramide

This negative inotropic drug is effective in lowering outflow gradients and improving symptoms, even in patients with high degrees of resting obstruction.[44-46,58-64] The usual starting dose is 400–600 mg/day, using the controlled release preparation to allow twice-a-day administration. It is often offered to medically refractory patients who would otherwise require septal myectomy or other interventions.

Disopyramide was introduced by investigators from Toronto who first administered it intravenously in the catheterization laboratory, demonstrating marked and consistent gradient reduction.[44,45] It was subsequently shown to be effective with oral administration.[58,59,61,63] Disopyramide increased treadmill exercise time and was more effective then propranolol.[59]

Disopyramide is a type I anti-arrhythmic drug with potent negative inotropic effects.[65] It acts by not only blocking sodium channels but also by lowering intracellular calcium.[66] In normals it decreases LV fractional shortening by about 30%;[65] in contrast, propranolol has little effect on resting ejection fraction in normals. The advantage of disopyramide may rest on its more effective reduction in ejection acceleration, as discussed below. In obstructive HCM, despite the decrease in systolic function, LV end-diastolic pressure also falls, due to relief of obstruction and its attendant systolic load.[44-46] Improvement in coronary vasodilator reserve with disopyramide has been shown in obstructive HCM, using intracoronary Doppler ultrasound.[62] Others have shown a beneficial effect of disopyramide on the balance of myocardial oxygen supply and demand in obstructive HCM. After disopyramide administration, resting coronary flow (measured with intracoronary Doppler) was unchanged; LV work, measured from pressure–volume loops, decreased, indicating an improvement in the supply–demand balance.[64]

There is a dose–response correlation in which higher disopyramide dosage and serum levels correlate with lower gradients,[58,60] and reduction in gradient has been observed with levels lower than those required for anti-arrhythmic therapy. Serum disopyramide levels can be monitored in patients to assess compliance and assure systemic levels,[58] and documentation is useful in patients with renal failure since the drug has renal excretion. Vagolytic side-effects, including dry mouth and exacerbation of prostatism, limit disopyramide administration. Therefore, disopyramide should not be initiated in patients with prostatism, narrow-angle glaucoma or impaired systolic LV function. Pro-arrhythmic ventricular tachycardia has not been reported with disopyramide given to patients with obstructive HCM. Disopyramide is most often used in combination with a β-blocker, which offers the advantage of slowing the exercise heart rate and decreasing sympathetic-mediated increase in gradient.[61]

There is an adverse pro-arrhythmic drug interaction between macrolide antibiotics and disopyramide.[67] Another antibiotic family should be selected to treat infections which occur during disopyramide therapy. Other anti-arrhythmic drugs should not be given in combination with disopyramide.

Recently we reported a retrospective study of 118 obstructed HCM patients, mean age 47 years, treated at 4 HCM centers and followed for an average of 4.2 years.[54] The mean maximal dose of disopyramide was 432 mg/day and 97% also received β-blockade. We compared these patients with 373 obstructed patients treated at the same institutions but without disopyramide. Patients who received disopyramide had higher gradients and more advanced symptoms than those not treated with disopyramide. After 4 years, two-thirds of the patients were still taking disopyramide but one-third required major nonpharmacologic interventions, (surgery, alcohol ablation or pacemaker) for the management of symptoms and refractory gradient. Most recent gradient on disopyramide was 42 ± 28 mm Hg, significantly lower than the baseline gradient of 74 ± 36 mm Hg, a 43% reduction ($P < 0.0001$). Also, when patients who received intervention to lower the gradient (such as septal myectomy or alcohol septal ablation) were removed from this analysis, gradient still declined by 43% ($P < 0.0001$) (Fig. 14.2). NYHA class improved on disopyramide, from a mean of 2.3 to 1.8 ($P < 0.002$). Comparing the disopyramide and control patients, annual rate of all-cause cardiac death and transplantation trended lower in the disopyramide group (1.4 vs 2.6%, $P = 0.07$) (Fig. 14.3).

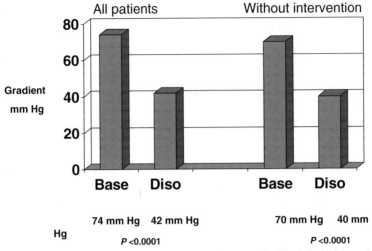

Fig. 14.2 Echocardiographic gradient reduction after disopyramide (Diso). (Left) Comparison in all 118 patients, before and after disopyramide. (Right) Comparison in patients not treated with mechanical intervention.

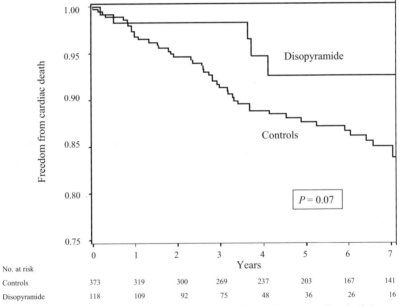

Fig. 14.3 Kaplan–Meier mortality curve showing freedom from all-cause cardiac death in patients treated with and without disopyramide.

There were five HCM-related sudden cardiac deaths that occurred in association with disopyramide, occurring a mean of more than 4 years after initial administration. The annual rate of sudden death was lower in the disopyramide patients (1.0 *vs* 1.8%, $P = 0.08$), but did not achieve statistical significance.

All deaths also trended lower (2.8 *vs* 3.8%, *P* = 0.10). There was no sustained ventricular tachycardia with disopyramide.

The most common cause of drug discontinuation was lack of effectiveness. Dry mouth caused discontinuation in 4% and prostatism in 2%. From this study it was concluded that disopyramide produces a long-lasting, favorable reduction of gradient and a parallel improvement in symptoms. With disopyramide, two-thirds of the obstructed patients were treated medically without need for other interventions for more than 4 years. One-third of the patients required intervention for relief of refractory symptoms. There was no excess in sudden cardiac death, ventricular tachycardia, or atrial fibrillation associated with disopyramide use. Some investigators regard disopyramide as the most efficacious medication for relieving outflow obstruction in HCM[2,6,54,55] and recommend that a therapeutic trial of disopyramide in conjunction with a β-blocker should be considered before proceeding to major nonpharmacologic interventions.

Comparisons of drug efficacy

Comparative studies of verapamil and β-blockers have yielded variable results.[25,68] Verapamil was generally better tolerated than β-blockers with a trend toward better symptom control and exercise tolerance. There has been no consistent benefit in mortality reported.

Pollick compared oral disopyramide and propranolol.[59] Patients showed longer exercise time with disopyramide than with propranolol. There are no comparisons of verapamil and disopyramide available. Some investigators believe disopyramide may be a better choice for patients who do not respond to β-blockade as it offers a more predictable response and has fewer side-effects.

Drug combinations

Other than the safe combination of disopyramide and β-blockade,[61] there are few data to support the use of drug combinations in HCM.[42] The combination of β-blockade and verapamil often causes profound bradycardia. On occasion, we have successfully added a low dose of verapamil to the combination of disopyramide and β-blocker (most often after a dual chamber pacemaker has been placed).

The class Ia anti-arrhythmic cibenzoline has been reported to reduce outflow gradients in HCM.[69] LV fractional shortening decreased by 27%, similar in magnitude to the reduction observed with disopyramide. This anti-arrhythmic does not have the vagolytic side-effects of disopyramide (but is not available in the USA).

Most asymptomatic patients are not afforded medical therapy because no drug has been shown in a randomized trial to improve the natural history of HCM or decrease mortality. However, a recent study reporting increased mortality associated with outflow obstruction[48] may prompt more aggressive medical treatment in mildly symptomatic patients with significant obstruction. Ostman-Smith and colleagues[53] reported mortality benefit in a nonrandomized study of children with very high-dose propranolol; children and adults often experience side-effects from very high-dose β-blockers.

Mechanism of benefit of negative inotropes

We have recently studied how negative inotropes reduce or abolish LVOT obstruction.[6] We studied 11 symptomatic patients with echocardiography before and after elimination of marked obstruction. Successful medical treatment of obstruction slows acceleration of LV ejection, measured at a point 2.5 cm apical to the mitral valve and 1 cm from the septum. Mean acceleration to peak velocity in the LV at this point was decreased by 34%, while peak velocity was unchanged. Before treatment, velocity peaked in the first half of the systolic ejection period; after successful treatment it peaked in the second half. Such decreased acceleration is observed easily by visual inspection of pulsed Doppler tracings from apical views of the left ventricle (Fig. 14.4). In contrast, the position of the mitral valve coaptation point relative to the ventricular septum was unchanged after treatment.

Since the force of flow drag is directly related to the square of velocity, even small decreases in initial ejection velocity lead to larger decreases in the initial pushing force on the leaflet.[5] The decrease in force on the leaflet appears to delay SAM (the trigger of obstruction), causing the mitral valve to contact the septum later in the systolic ejection period. This leaves less time in systole for the feedback loop to narrow the orifice, reducing the final pressure difference. Thus, delay in SAM leads to delay of the feedback loop, leaving it less time to act and ultimately yielding a lower pressure gradient[6] (Fig. 14.5). Implicit in this notion is the countertraction of the chordae and papillary muscles, which resist SAM. Any reduction in pushing forces favors the restraining forces of the mitral subvalvular apparatus.

Doppler examinations of LV acceleration can aid the clinician in managing patients who are obstructed and symptomatic after medical treatment. In these patients it is often difficult to decide whether to increase medications or to recommend intervention (such as septal myectomy). If LV acceleration is not significantly slowed by medical treatment, medications can be increased or added. If acceleration in the LV has slowed but there is still significant obstruction, medication alone may not be adequate to eliminate obstruction. These patients will probably require intervention.[6]

Significance of provocable gradients

LVOT gradients may vary spontaneously from day to day or even from minute to minute. Circumstances of daily life can increase the gradient, including the postprandial state, ethanol ingestion, erect posture and physiologic exercise. Indeed, we search aggressively for obstruction in symptomatic patients because there are relatively few effective treatments for symptomatic nonobstructive HCM. Maneuvers we routinely use to provoke obstruction are Valsalva, intense exercise, and postprandial state (that is, we often perform echocardiography after the patient has eaten a moderate-sized meal). Echocardiograms performed after the patient has eaten assess patients when physiologically at their worst. If symptoms are predominantly exercise-related and

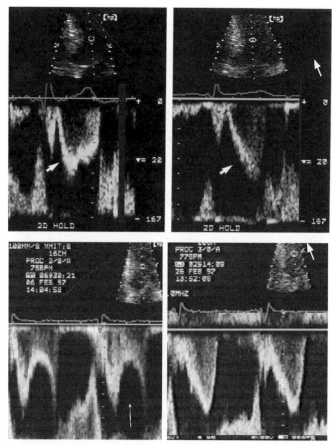

Fig. 14.4 Comparison of left ventricular pulsed Doppler tracings before treatment (left panels) and after successful medical treatment with β-blockade and disopyramide (right panels) in two patients, A (top) and B (bottom). The sample volume is 2.5 cm apical of the mitral valve coaptation point. In patient A (top panels), before treatment, ejection acceleration was rapid (arrowhead) and velocity peaked in the first half of systolic. After treatment, ejection acceleration was slowed (arrowhead) and velocity peaked in the second half of a systole. Systolic anterior mitral motion was delayed and a 96 mm Hg gradient was eliminated. Note that though acceleration slowed, peak velocity remained virtually unchanged. This contrast highlights the importance of acceleration and the timing of ejection in successful medical therapy. The velocity calibration is identical in both panels. The scale is 20 cm/s between the white marks. In patient B (bottom panels), after treatment and gradient abolition, ejection acceleration was slowed (arrowheads) and velocity peaked in the second half of a systole. The thin longer arrow points to the drop in mid-systolic left ventricular ejection velocity that is typically seen in patients with gradients greater than 60 mm Hg. This is caused by the sudden imposition of afterload caused by the gradient and a mismatch between left ventricular contractility and afterload. It has been termed the 'lobster claw abnormality' because of its typical appearance.[49] This abnormality is no longer present after relief of obstruction. Reproduced in part with permission from Sherrid *et al*. The mechanism of negative inotropes in obstructive hypertrophic cardiomyopathy. *Circulation* 1998; **97**: 41–7.

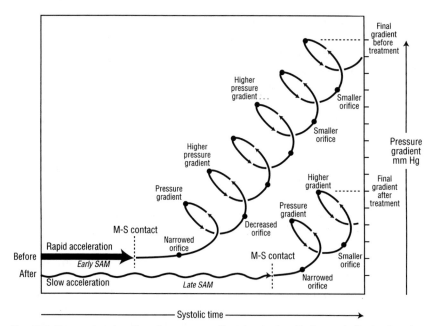

Fig. 14.5 Proposed explanation of pressure gradient development before and after treatment of obstruction. (Upper tracing) Before treatment, rapid left ventricular acceleration apical of the mitral valve, shown as a horizontal thick arrow, triggers early systolic anterior motion and early mitral–septal contact. Once mitral–septal contact occurs, a narrowed orifice develops and a pressure difference results. The pressure difference forces the leaflet against the septum, which decreases the orifice size and further increases the pressure difference. An amplifying feedback loop is established, shown as a rising spiral. The longer the leaflet is in contact with the septum the higher the pressure gradient. (Lower tracing) After treatment, negative inotropes slow early systolic acceleration (shown as a horizontal wavy arrow) and may thereby decrease the force on the mitral leaflet, delaying systolic anterior motion. Mitral–septal contact occurs later, leaving less time in systole for the feedback loop to narrow the orifice. This reduces the final pressure difference. In addition, delaying systolic anterior motion may allow more time for papillary muscle shortening to provide countertraction. In the figure, for clarity, the 'before' arrow is positioned above the 'after' arrow, although at the beginning of systole they both actually begin with a pressure gradient of 0 mm Hg. M-S contact = mitral–septal contact; SAM = systolic anterior motion. Reproduced with permission, from Sherrid et al. The mechanism of negative inotropes in obstructive hypertrophic cardiomyopathy. Circulation 1998; **97**: 41–7.

if the gradient is low, we perform exercise echocardiography. After symptom-limited exercise, the sonographer first records the continuous-wave Doppler gradient from the apical views and then records wall motion, and also color Doppler for mitral regurgitation. Maneuvers used to provoke gradients in HCM, such as amyl nitrite inhalation and dobutamine infusion, are much less physiologic than standard exercise. We feel less secure in attributing symptoms to obstruction provoked with these maneuvers.

General drug strategies

The process of finding the right drug to reduce outflow obstruction can be time-consuming and frustrating for the symptomatic patient and physician alike. The physician seeks to give the smallest dose of the drug(s) that works. So drugs are generally introduced with gradually increasing dosage and echocardiograms are performed after each dosage change or with the addition of a new drug. This strategy can result in prolonged hospital stays, repeated office visits and multiple echos, and is also expensive.

To facilitate the rapid elimination of outflow obstruction, we have evolved a system of acute drug testing with repeat echocardiograms over 3 days. Patients are treated using a clinical protocol of acute drug testing with the goal of rapid gradient elimination on sequential Doppler echocardiography.[6] Intravenous metoprolol (15 mg administered over 10 minutes) is used first, unless contraindicated. If the Doppler gradient is reduced within 30 minutes to less than 30 mm Hg, oral β-blockers are continued as sole therapy. If a gradient of 30 mm Hg or greater persists, oral disopyramide is administered on the same day. We administer disopyramide 250 mg as an oral loading dose and then repeat the echocardiogram 2.5 hours later.[58] In patients with a contraindication to disopyramide, oral verapamil is begun at 240–360 mg/day in divided doses. Patients who respond to disopyramide with a gradient less than 30 mm Hg are continued on oral disopyramide controlled release (CR) 250 mg every 12 hours and metoprolol to bring the resting heart rate to 55–60 beats/min. Patients with gradients greater than 30 mm Hg after the first dose are treated with disopyramide CR 250–300 mg every 12 h and metoprolol for 3 days. Patients who do not respond to this regimen with gradients greater than 36 mm Hg and who remain symptomatic generally will require intervention. A schematic of this treatment plan is shown in Fig. 14.6.

Most symptomatic patients respond to medication with symptom relief and gradient reduction.[1–3,55] Patients refractory to β-blockade will often respond to disopyramide. Patients should be treated with disopyramide before considering them medically refractory and before proceeding to intervention. In an illustrative case, abolition of a 96 mm Hg gradient followed intravenous disopyramide, while no change occurred following intravenous propranolol;[70] this is consistent with the systematic comparison of the two drugs by Pollick[59] and our routine use.[6]

Midcavity obstruction

Patients with midventricular obstruction have hypertrophy with hyperkinetic LV wall motion. Midcavity obstruction may be due to an anomalous papillary muscle inserting in the base of the mitral valve or to systolic apposition of the ventricular walls. Hypertrophied papillary muscles often play a role in muscular obstruction at this level. Obstruction can trap blood in a small apical cavity. Occasionally, the apex can infarct, with resulting aneurysm (with scar formation and sometimes thrombus) and ventricular arrhythmia (monomorphic ventricular tachycardia). Medical treatment of midventricular obstruction is with negative inotropes (similar to HCM with SAM and mitral–septal con-

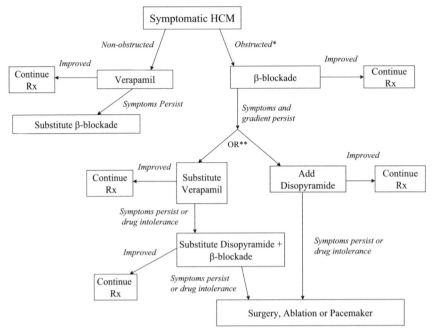

Fig. 14.6 Proposed algorithm for medical therapy of symptomatic hypertrophic cardiomyopathy. See text for description of dosing and medication details. *Patients are considered for medical therapy of obstruction if they have a gradient greater than 30 mm Hg at rest or after provocation with the Valsalva maneuver or exercise. The criterion of 30 mm Hg may prompt medical therapy; surgical or ablation intervention is usually reserved for patients who fail medical therapy but have gradients at rest or after provocation greater than 50 mm Hg. **Either verapamil or disopyramide may be selected as the second-line agent. Verapamil is generally substituted for β-blockade, while disopyramide is added to β-blockade. The differences between these agents are detailed in the text.

tact), using β-blockade, verapamil or disopyramide. A proposed algorithm for the medical treatment of symptomatic HCM patients is presented in Fig. 14.6.

Treatment of coexistent systemic hypertension

Since the prevalence of systemic hypertension can approach 40% in the elderly population, it would be expected that hypertension and HCM would coexist in a sizeable number of patients. This poses diagnostic and therapeutic problems. From a diagnostic point of view it is sometimes difficult to assess if LV hypertrophy is primary or secondary to the hypertension. The presence of SAM with obstruction, a family history of HCM, particularly small LV cavity size, or extreme LV hypertrophy associated with mild hypertension may aid in this distinction.[71]

In patients with hypertension and LVOT obstruction, either at rest or after provocation, vasodilating drugs are contraindicated because they worsen obstruction and symptoms and can even lead to cardiovascular collapse. Rather, control of hypertension in these patients rests with β-blockers or verapamil and the judicious use of thiazide diuretics. The centrally acting agent clonidine is also useful and may be administered at night to avoid daytime sedation. In patients without a provocable gradient, angiotensin inhibition or blockade can be safely used.

Treatment of end-stage HCM

A small minority of HCM patients progress to LV systolic dysfunction with low ejection fraction.[1] Dyspnea and exercise intolerance worsens in these patients, who often deteriorate relatively rapidly and have high mortality from heart failure. Medical treatment must be adjusted in these patients from negative inotropes to ACE inhibitors, digoxin, diuretics and β-blockers. Transplantation is a viable option for NYHA class IV patients.

Prevention of hypertrophy and fibrosis

No pharmacologic agent has yet been shown to improve hypertrophy or fibrosis, the distinctive pathologic features in patients with HCM. In the future this could possibly be approached by either preventing expression in subjects known to carry an HCM genotype or by inducing LV regression in those already exhibiting the phenotype. ACE inhibitors reduce hypertrophy in patients with hypertensive heart disease, and since the DD genotype for the ACE polymorphism has been shown to be associated with increased hypertrophy in HCM, there has been some interest in whether ACE inhibition might decrease hypertrophy in HCM patients. However, as yet there have been no published trials using ACE inhibitors in HCM. A persistent concern about the use of ACE inhibitors has been their potential for increasing LV outflow obstruction (under resting or provocable conditions) in susceptible patients. Consequently, ACE inhibitors are not part of the routine care of HCM patients at this time. Transgenic mouse models have offered possible routes to the prevention and regression of hypertrophy and fibrosis.[72–74]

References

1 Maron BJ. Hypertrophic cardiomyopathy: A systematic review. *JAMA* 2002; **287**: 1308–20.

2 Wigle ED, Rakowski H, Kimball BP, William WG. Hypertrophic cardiomyopathy – clinical spectrum and treatment. *Circulation* 1995; **92**: 1680–92.

3 Spirito P, Seidman CE, McKenna WJ, Maron BJ. The management of hypertrophic cardiomyopathy. *N Engl J Med* 1997; **336**: 775–85.

4 Jiang L, Levine RA, King ME, Weyman AE. An integrated mechanism for SAM of the mitral valve in hypertrophic cardiomyopathy based on echocardiographic observations. *Am Heart J* 1987; **113**: 633–44.

5 Sherrid MV, Chu CK, DeLia E, Mogtader A, Dwyer Jr. EM. An echocardiographic study of the fluid mechanics of obstruction in hypertrophic cardiomyopathy. *J Am Coll Cardiol* 1993; **22**: 816–25.

6 Sherrid MV, Pearle G, Gunsburg D. The mechanism of negative inotropes in obstructive hypertrophic cardiomyopathy. *Circulation* 1998; **97**: 41–7.

7 Sherrid M, Gunsburg DZ, Moldenhauer S, Pearle G. Systolic anterior motion begins at low left ventricular outflow tract velocity in obstructive hypertrophic cardiomyopathy. *J Am Coll Cardiol* 2000; **36**: 1344–54.

8 Shirani J, Pick R, Roberts WC, Maron BJ. Morphology and significance of the left ventricular collagen network in young patients with hypertrophic cardiomyopathy and sudden cardiac death. *J Am Coll Cardiol* 2000; **5**: 36–44.

9 Bonow RO. Left ventricular diastolic function in hypertrophic cardiomyopathy. *Herz* 1991; **16**: 13–21.

10 Lele SS, Thomson HL, Seo H, Belenkie I, McKenna WJ, Frenneaux MP. Exercise capacity in hypertrophic cardiomyopathy. Role of stroke volume limitation, heart rate and diastolic filling characteristics. *Circulation* 1995; **92**: 2886–94.

11 Cannon RO, Rosing DR, Maron BJ. Myocardial ischemia in patients with hypertrophic cardiomyopathy: Contribution of inadequate vasodilator reserve and elevated left ventricular filling pressures. *Circulation* 1985; **71**: 234–43.

12 Dilsiziam V, Bonow RO, Epstein SE, Fananapazir L. Myocardial ischemia detected by thallium scintigraphy is frequently related to cardiac arrest and syncope in young patients with hypertrophic cardiomyopathy. *J Am Coll Cardiol* 1993; **22**: 796–80.

13 Maron BJ, Wolfson JK, Epstein SE, Roberts WC. Intramural ('small vessel') coronary artery disease in hypertrophic cardiomyopathy. *J Am Coll Cardiol* 1986; **8**: 545–57.

14 Petkow DP, Krzanowski M, Nizankowski R, Szczeklik A, Dubiel JS. Effect of verapamil on systolic and diastolic coronary blood flow velocity in asymptomatic and mildly symptomatic patients with hypertrophic cardiomyopathy. *Heart* 2000; **83**: 262–6.

15 Udelson JE, Bonow RO, O'Gara PT *et al.* Verapamil prevents silent myocardial perfusion abnormalities during exercise in asymptomatic patients with hypertrophic cardiomyopathy. *Circulation* 1989; **79**: 1052–60.

16 Gwathmey JK, Warren SE, Briggs GM *et al.* Diastolic dysfunction in hypertrophic cardiomyopathy. Effect on active force generation during systole. *J Clin Invest* 1991; **87**: 1023–31.

17 Lubic SP, Giacomini KM, Giacomini JC. The effects of modulation of calcium influx through the voltage-sensitive calcium channel on cardiomyocyte hypertrophy. *J Mol Cell Cardiol* 1995; **27**: 917–25.

18 Kaltenbach M, Hopf R, Kober G, Bussmann WD, Keller M, Petersen Y. Treatment of hypertrophic obstructive cardiomyopathy with verapamil. *Br Heart J* 1979; **42**: 35–42.

19 Rosing DR, Kent KM, Borer JS, Seides SF, Maron BJ, Epstein SE. Verapamil therapy: A new approach to the pharmacologic treatment of hypertrophic cardiomyopathy. I. Hemodynamic effects. *Circulation* 1979; **60**: 1201–7.

20 Hanrath P, Schluter M, Sonntag F, Diemert J, Bleifeld W. Influence of verapamil therapy on left ventricular performance at rest and during exercise in hypertrophic cardiomyopathy. *Am J Cardiol* 1983; **52**: 544–8.

21 Bonow RO, Dilsizian V, Rosing DR, Maron BJ, Bacharach SL, Green MV. Verapamil-induced improvement in left ventricular diastolic filling and increased exercise tolerance in patients with hypertrophic cardiomyopathy: Short- and long-term effects. *Circulation* 1985; **72**: 853–64.

22 Rosing DR, Kent KM, Maron BJ, Epstein SE. Verapamil therapy: A new approach to the pharmacologic treatment of hypertrophic cardiomyopathy. II. Effects on exercise capacity and symptomatic status. *Circulation* 1979; **60**: 1208–13.

23 Rosing DR, Condit JR, Maron BJ *et al*. Verapamil therapy: A new approach to the pharmacologic treatment of hypertrophic cardiomyopathy: III. Effects of long-term administration. *Am J Cardiol* 1981; **48**: 545–53.

24 Rosing DR, Idanpaan-Heikkila U, Maron BJ, Bonow RO, Epstein SE. Use of calcium-channel blocking drugs in hypertrophic cardiomyopathy. *Am J Cardiol* 1985; **55**: 185B–195B.

25 Gilligan DM, Chan WL, Joshi J *et al*. A double-blind, placebo-controlled crossover trial of nadolol and verapamil in mild and moderately symptomatic hypertrophic cardiomyopathy. *J Am Coll Cardiol* 1993; **21**: 1672–9.

26 Bonow RO, Rosing DR, Epstein SE. The acute and chronic effects of verapamil on left ventricular function in patients with hypertrophic cardiomyopathy. *Eur Heart J* 1983; **4** (Suppl. F): 57–65.

27 Bonow RO, Vitale DF, Maron BJ, Bacharach SL, Frederick TM, Green MV. Regional left ventricular asynchrony and impaired global left ventricular filling in hypertrophic cardiomyopathy: Effect of verapamil. *J Am Coll Cardiol* 1987; **9**: 1108–16.

28 Hartmann A, Schnell J, Hopf R, Kneissl G. Persisting effect of Ca(2+)-channel blockers on left ventricular function in hypertrophic cardiomyopathy after 14 years' treatment. *Angiology* 1996; **47**: 765–73.

29 Hopf R, Kaltenbach M. Ten year results and survival of patients with hypertrophic cardiomyopathy treated with calcium antagonists. *Z Kardiol* 1987; **76**: 137–44.

30 Spicer RL, Rocchini AP, Crowley DC, Rosenthal A. Chronic verapamil therapy in pediatric and young adult patients with hypertrophic cardiomyopathy. *Am J Cardiol* 1984; **53**: 1614–9.

31 Gregor P, Widimsky P, Cervenka V, Visek V, Sladkova T, Dvorak J. Use of verapamil in the treatment of hypertrophic cardiomyopathy. *Cor Vasa* 1986; **28**: 404–12.

32 Tendera M, Polonski L, Kozielska E. Left ventricular end-diastolic pressure–volume relationships in hypertrophic cardiomyopathy. Changes induced by verapamil. *Chest* 1983; **84**: 54–7.

33 Kass DA, Wolff MR, Ting CT *et al*. Diastolic compliance of hypertrophied ventricle is not acutely altered by pharmacologic agents influencing active processes. *Ann Intern Med* 1993; **119**: 466–73.

34 Hess OM, Grimm J, Krayenbuehl HP. Diastolic function in hypertrophic cardiomyopathy: Effects of propranolol and verapamil on diastolic stiffness. *Eur Heart J* 1983; **4**: 47–56.

35 TenCate FJ, Serruys PW, Mey S, Roelandt J. Effects of short-term administration of verapamil on left ventricular relaxation and filling dynamics measured by a combined hemodynamic-ultrasonic technique in patients with hypertrophic cardiomyopathy. *Circulation* 1983; **68**: 1274–9.

36 Tendera M, Schneeweiss A, Bartoszewski A, Polonski L, Wodniecki J, Salamon A. The acute response of left ventricular filling dynamics to intravenous verapamil predicts the changes in exercise tolerance after oral verapamil therapy in patients with hypertrophic cardiomyopathy. *Eur Heart J* 1993; **14**: 410–15.

37 Bonow RO, Ostrow HG, Rosing DR *et al*. Effects of verapamil on left ventricular systolic and diastolic function in patients with hypertrophic cardiomyopathy: Pressure–volume analysis with a nonimaging scintillation probe. *Circulation* 1983; **68**: 1062–73.

38 Taniguchi Y, Sugihara H, Ohtsuki K *et al*. Effect of verapamil on myocardial ischemia in patients with hypertrophic cardiomyopathy: Evaluation by exercise thallium-201 SPECT. *J Cardiol* 1994; **24**: 45–51.

39 Dimitrow PP, Krzanowski M, Grodecki J *et al.* Verapamil improves the pacing-induced vasodilatation in symptomatic patients with hypertrophic cardiomyopathy. *Int J Cardiol* 2002; **83**: 239–47.

40 Curtius JM, Stoecker J, Loesse B, Welslau R, Scholz D. Changes of the degree of hypertrophy in hypertrophic obstructive cardiomyopathy under medical and surgical treatment. *Cardiology* 1989; **76**: 255–63.

41 Kunkel B, Schneider M, Eisenmenger A, Bergmann B, Hopf R, Kaltenbach M. Myocardial biopsy in patients with hypertrophic cardiomyopathy: Correlations between morphologic and clinical parameters and development of myocardial hypertrophy under medical therapy. *Z Kardiol* 1987; **76**: 33–8.

42 Hopf R, Thomas J, Klepzig H, Kaltenbach M. Treatment of hypertrophic cardiomyopathy with nifedipine and propranolol in combination. *Z Kardiol* 1987; **76**: 469–78.

43 Betocchi S, Piscione F, Losi MA *et al.* Effects of diltiazem on left ventricular systolic and diastolic function in hypertrophic cardiomyopathy. *Am J Cardiol* 1996; **78**: 451–7.

44 Pollick C. Muscular subaortic stenosis: Hemodynamic and clinical improvement after disopyramide. *N Engl J Med* 1982; **307**: 997–9.

45 Pollick C, Kimball B, Henderson M, Wigle ED. Disopyramide in hypertrophic cardiomyopathy. I. Hemodynamic assessment after intravenous administration. *Am J Cardiol* 1988; **62**: 1248–51.

46 Matsubara H, Nakatani S, Nagata S *et al.* Salutary effect of disopyramide on left ventricular diastolic function in hypertrophic obstructive cardiomyopathy. *J Am Coll Cardiol* 1995; **26**: 768–75.

47 Wigle D, Sasson Z, Henderson MA *et al.* Hypertrophic cardiomyopathy. The importance of the site and the extent of hypertrophy. A review. *Progr Cardiovasc Dis* 1985; **28**: 1–83.

48 Maron MS, Olivotto I, Betocchi S *et al.* Effect of left ventricular outflow tract obstruction on clinical outcome in hypertrophic cardiomyopathy. *N Engl J Med* 2003; **348**: 295–303.

49 Sherrid MV, Gunsburg DZ, Pearle G. Midsystolic drop in left ventricular ejection velocity in obstructive hypertrophic cardiomyopathy. The lobster claw abnormality. *J Am Soc Echocardiogr* 1997; **10**: 707–12.

50 Harrison DC, Braunwald E, Glick G, Mason DT, Chidsey CA, Ross J Jr. Effects of beta adrenergic blockade on the circulation with particular reference to observations in patients with hypertrophic subaortic stenosis. *Circulation* 1964; **29**: 84–98.

51 Goodwin JF, Shah PM, Oakley CM, Cohen J, Yipintsoi T, Pocock W. The clinical pharmacology of hypertrophic obstructive cardiomyopathy. In: Wolstenholme GEW, O'Conner M, eds. *Cardiomyopathies*. Boston, MA: Little Brown, 1964: 189–213.

52 Sharma S, Elliott P, Whyte G *et al.* Utility of cardiopulmonary exercise in the assessment of clinical determinants of functional capacity in hypertrophic cardiomyopathy. *Am J Cardiol* 2000; **86**: 162–8.

53 Ostman-Smith I, Wettrell G, Riesenfeld T. A cohort study of childhood hypertrophic cardiomyopathy: Improved survival following high-dose beta-adrenoceptor antagonist treatment. *J Am Coll Cardiol* 1999; **34**: 1813–22.

54 Sherrid MV, Barac I, Maron B *et al.* A multicenter study of the safety and efficacy of disopyramide for treating symptomatic obstructive hypertrophic cardiomyopathy [abstract]. *J Am Coll Cardiol* 2003; (Suppl. A): 170A.

55 McKenna WJ, Behr ER. Hypertrophic cardiomyopathy: Management, risk stratification, and prevention of sudden death. *Heart* 2002; **87**: 169–76.

56 Epstein SE, Rosing DR. Verapamil: Its potential for causing serious complications in patients with hypertrophic cardiomyopathy. *Circulation* 1981; **64**: 437–41.

57 Lorell BH. Use of calcium channel blockers in hypertrophic cardiomyopathy. *Am J Med* 1985; **78**: 43–54.

58 Sherrid M, Delia E, Dwyer E. Oral disopyramide therapy for obstructive hypertrophic cardiomyopathy. *Am J Cardiol* 1988; **62**: 1085–8.

59 Pollick C. Disopyramide in hypertrophic cardiomyopathy. Noninvasive assessment after oral administration. *Am J Cardiol* 1988; **62**: 1252–5.

60 Kimball BP, Bui S, Wigle ED. Acute dose–response effects of intravenous disopyramide in hypertrophic obstructive cardiomyopathy. *Am Heart J* 1993; **125**: 1691–7.

61 Cokkinos DV, Salpeas D, Ioannou NE, Christoulas S. Combination of disopyramide and propranolol in hypertrophic cardiomyopathy. *Can J Cardiol* 1989; **5**: 33–6.

62 Hongo M, Nakatsuka T, Takenaka H *et al.* Effects of intravenous disopyramide on coronary hemodynamics and vasodilator reserve in hypertrophic obstructive cardiomyopathy. *Cardiology* 1996; **87**: 6–11.

63 Duncan WJ, Tyrrell MJ, Bharadwaj BB. Disopyramide as a negative inotrope in obstructive cardiomyopathy in children. *Can J Cardiol* 1991; **7**: 81–6.

64 Niki K, Sugawara M, Asano R *et al.* Disopyramide improves the balance between myocardial oxygen supply and demand in patients with hypertrophic obstructive cardiomyopathy. *Heart Vessels* 1997; **12**: 111–18.

65 Pollick C, Giacomini KM, Blaschke TF *et al.* The cardiac effects of d- and l-disopyramide in normal subjects: A noninvasive study. *Circulation* 1982; **66**: 447–53.

66 Sakai Y, Sekiya S, Inazu M, Homma I, Honda H, Irino O. Evidence that the Na+–Ca2+ exchange system is related to the antiarrhythmic action of disopyramide. *Gen Pharmacol* 1989; **20**: 105–9.

67 Ragosta M, Weihl AC, Rosenfeld LE. Potentially fatal interaction between erythromycin and disopyramide. *Am J Med* 1989; **86**: 465–6.

68 Kober G, Hopf R, Biamino G *et al.* Long-term treatment of hypertrophic cardiomyopathy with verapamil or propranolol in matched pairs of patients: Results of a multicenter study. *Z Kardiol* 1987; **76**: 113–18.

69 Hamada M, Shigematsu Y, Ikeda S *et al.* Class Ia antiarrhythmic drug cibenzoline: A new approach to the medical treatment of hypertrophic obstructive cardiomyopathy. *Circulation* 1997; **96**: 1520–4.

70 Tokudome T, Mizushige K, Ueda T, Sakamoto S, Matsuo H. Effect of disopyramide on left ventricular pressure gradient in hypertrophic obstructive cardiomyopathy in comparison with propranolol – a case report. *Angiology* 1999; **50**: 331–5.

71 Topol EJ, Traill TA, Fortuin NJ. Hypertensive hypertrophic cardiomyopathy of the elderly. *N Engl J Med* 1985; **312**: 277–83.

72 Sussman MA, Lim HW, Gude N *et al.* Prevention of cardiac hypertrophy in mice by calcineurin inhibition. *Science* 1998; **281**: 1690–3.

73 Lim DS, Lutucuta S, Bachireddy P *et al.* Angiotensin II blockade reverses myocardial fibrosis in a transgenic mouse model of human hypertrophic cardiomyopathy. *Circulation* 2001; **103**: 789–91.

74 Patel R, Nagueh SF, Tsybouleva N *et al.* Simvastatin induces regression of cardiac hypertrophy and fibrosis and improves cardiac function in a transgenic rabbit model of human hypertrophic cardiomyopathy. *Circulation* 2001; **104**: 317–24.

CHAPTER 15

Obstructive Hypertrophic Cardiomyopathy: Results of Septal Myectomy

Joseph A. Dearani, MD and Gordon K. Danielson, MD

Introduction

Hypertrophic cardiomyopathy (HCM), a primary myocardial disease due to distinct genetic mutations, is characterized by inappropriate hypertrophy of the myocardium and is associated with various clinical presentations ranging from complete absence of symptoms to sudden unexpected death. Ventricular morphologies can vary widely, as shown in Fig. 15.1. There is a subgroup of pa-

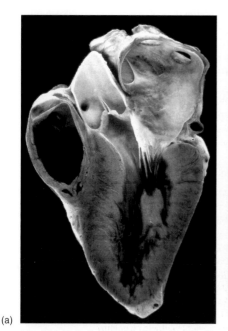
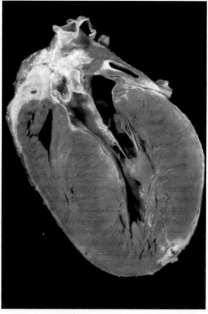

(a)   (b)

Fig. 15.1 Pathologic specimens of localized basal septal hypertrophy type in hypertrophic cardiomyopathy (a) and diffuse type (b). (Courtesy of William D. Edwards, MD.)

tients who develop severe limiting symptoms of dyspnea, angina, or syncope, or a combination of these, due primarily to dynamic obstruction of the left ventricular outflow tract and associated mitral regurgitation. The established medical therapy for patients with obstructive HCM has been a trial of large doses of β-blockers, calcium channel inhibitors, or disopyramide, either alone or in combination. Operation has been recommended for those symptomatic patients with fixed or inducible left ventricular outflow tract (LVOT) gradients who are intolerant of or unresponsive to these medications.[1]

History of surgical treatment

Surgical awareness of obstructive HCM began in the late 1950s. The first surgical procedures proposed for relief of left ventricular outflow tract obstruction (LVOTO) involved simple incision in the basal septal bulge, sometimes deepened with the surgeon's finger (myotomy), or excision of muscle under direct visualization (myectomy).[2–6] Cleland probably described the first procedure for surgical treatment of LVOTO, in which he performed a limited transaortic septal myectomy.[2] Since that time, many different surgical procedures have been described (Table 15.1). Historically, surgical exposure of the septum has been obtained through the aorta, left ventricle, right ventricle, or left atrium. To preserve conduction tissue in the septum, the surgeon can remove tissue only in a specific location in the septum. Decrease in left ventricular outflow gradient is accomplished not only by physical enlargement of the outflow tract but also by interruption of the pathophysiological sequence of events [primarily systolic anterior motion (SAM) of the anterior mitral leaflet] that cause the outflow gradient.[1] Complete relief of LVOTO by septal myectomy also results in correction of mitral regurgitation caused by SAM. Any residual mitral regurgitation due to ruptured chordae, mitral valve prolapse, or annular dilatation can usually be corrected by mitral valve repair and annuloplasty.

Table 15.1 Surgical techniques for outflow obstruction in hypertrophic cardiomyopathy

Surgeon	Year	Procedure
Cleland	1958	Transaortic septal myectomy
Morrow	1960	Transaortic myotomy/myectomy
Kirklin	1961	Transaortic/transventricular myectomy
Lillehei	1963	Transatrial myectomy, detachment of mitral valve
Johnson	1964	Transatrial mitral valve replacement, myectomy
Cooley	1967	Trans-right ventricle septal myectomy
Stinson	1968	Cardiac transplantation
Cooley	1970	Mitral valve replacement without myectomy
Rastan, Konno	1975	Aortoventriculoplasty
Bernhard, Cooley	1976	Apicoaortic conduit
Vouhé	1984	Trans-right ventricle myectomy
Alvarez-Diaz	1984	Trans-right ventricle myectomy, patch

Replacement of the mitral valve with a low-profile mitral valve prosthesis—once proposed as an alternative to septal myectomy—also obliterates the left ventricular outflow gradient and improves symptoms. The major disadvantage of this procedure is that one disease process is replaced with another, such as problems of durability, infection, thromboembolism, and anticoagulation, that is associated with prosthetic valves. Mitral valve replacement is now reserved for patients with primary mitral valve disease (such as myxomatous degeneration) associated with severe mitral regurgitation. Other surgical approaches that have been proposed to treat obstructive HCM include classic or modified Konno–Rastan aortoventriculoplasty, apicoaortic conduit, and cardiac transplantation; these approaches are now reserved for selected indications.

Transaortic septal myectomy is currently considered to be the most appropriate surgical treatment for patients with obstructive HCM and severe symptoms unresponsive to medical therapy.[7-24] However, there is a significant learning curve for this procedure, and early surgical experience was associated with complications of complete heart block, ventricular septal defect, injury to the aortic or mitral valves, and incomplete relief of obstruction. Current surgical results are vastly improved, although the reported experience in North America is limited to a few centers.

Surgical technique

Over the last three decades, our technique of septal myectomy has evolved from the classic Morrow myotomy and myectomy (Fig. 15.2A) to a more extended left ventricular septal myectomy (Fig. 15.2B).

Intraoperative transesophageal echocardiography (TEE) is performed after induction of general anesthesia, with particular attention to the cardiac anatomy, mitral valve function, and thickness of the ventricular septum. Exposure is gained through a median sternotomy and pressures are measured in all four cardiac chambers and aorta. If the right ventricular pressure is elevated, pulmonary arterial pressure is also measured to evaluate possible right ventricular outflow tract obstruction or pulmonary hypertension. If the LVOT gradient is low (<30 mm Hg) because of the conditions under anesthesia, provocation with an isoproterenol infusion is performed. Documentation of the LVOT gradient is important so that a comparison can be made with post-myectomy measurements (Figs 15.3 and 15.4). Standard cardiopulmonary bypass with moderate hypothermia (30–34°C) is used and the left heart is vented. Myocardial protection, especially important because of the severe ventricular hypertrophy, is begun with a generous infusion of cold blood cardioplegia into the aortic root followed by additional doses given selectively into the left and right coronary ostia every 20 minutes. Topical cooling with ice-slush saline is also applied, and an insulting pad is placed behind the left ventricle during the more complex procedures. A transverse aortotomy is made, carried rightward toward the noncoronary sinus and down to the aortic annulus, and retracted

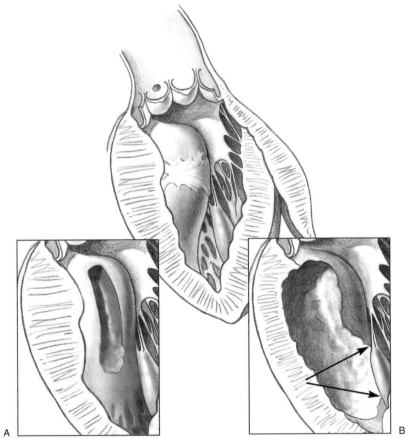

Fig. 15.2 Diagram showing two operative approaches for performing septal myectomy in obstructive hypertrophic cardiomyopathy. Typical outflow tract morphology with predominant basal septal hypertrophy and subaortic obstruction due primarily to systolic anterior motion of the mitral valve (center panel). Endocardial thickeneing at the line of apposition of the anterior mitral leaflet to the septum (friction lesion) is shown (center panel). (**A**) A standard rectangular myectomy trough (Morrow procedure) is created from 1 cm below the aortic valve apically to a point beyond the line of mitral–septal contact and intraventricular obstruction, allowing relief of the outflow tract gradient and preservation of sinus rhythm. (**B**) In the presence of muscular midcavity obstruction due to anomalous papillary muscles with direct insertion into the mitral valve or to extensive diffuse septal hypertrophy extending to the bases of the papillary muscles, a much more substantial myectomy is performed by combining the standard operation with an extended midventricular resection. The apical portion of the myectomy trough is much wider and includes the distal third of the right side of the septum.

with pledgeted sutures. The aortic valve commissures are suspended with pledgeted sutures to maximize exposure of the hypertrophied septum and anterior mitral leaflet. Inspection of the anatomy is performed with identification of the line of apposition of the anterior mitral leaflet to the septum (friction lesion). Optimal visualization of the ventricular septum is facilitated by

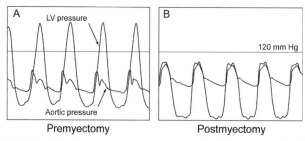

Fig. 15.3 An example of simultaneous measurements obtained intraoperatively of LV and aortic pressures before (**A**) and after (**B**) septal myectomy. A reference line of 120 mm Hg is shown. The premyectomy LV outflow tract gradient was approximately 80 mm Hg and was completely abolished after a successful myectomy.

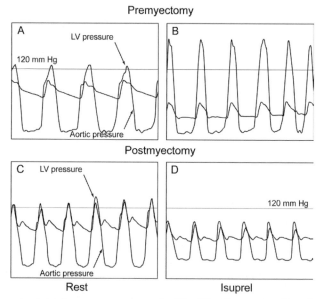

Fig. 15.4 An example of simultaneous measurements of the LV outflow tract gradient obtained intraoperatively. Note the significant increase in the premyectomy gradient (**A**) after infusion of isoproterenol (Isuprel) (**B**). The gradient was abolished after successful myectomy (**C, D**).

posterior displacement of the left ventricle with a sponge forceps. In addition, a small rake retractor can be used to engage the distal septum so that it can be pulled cephalad toward the aortic annulus.

The classical portion of the resection is begun by making two parallel longitudinal incisions in the septum, the first beneath the nadir of the right coronary cusp and the second beneath the commissure between the right and the left coronary cusps. These incisions are connected superiorly with a third incision 1.0 cm below the aortic valve, and a deep wedge of septal tissue is resected (Fig. 15.2A). Care is taken to carry the incision apically beyond the point of mitral–septal contact (marked by the fibrous friction lesion). This classical resection is then extended in several ways, beginning with continued resection leftward toward the mitral valve annulus and apically to the bases of the papillary muscles. The apical third of the right side of the septum is then resected, effectively making a much wider trough at the apex than the base (a laboratory flask-like configuration as shown in Fig. 15.2B). For midventricular obstruction due to hypertrophied papillary muscles or muscle bundles, additional resection is made around the bases of the papillary muscles. All areas of papillary muscle fusion to the septum or ventricular free wall are divided, and anomalous chordal structures and fibrous attachments of the mitral leaflets to the ventricular septum are divided or excised. The resected area is deepened with a rongeur. Instruments commonly used for this procedure are shown in Fig. 15.5. The adequacy and distal extent of resection are evaluated by direct inspection and digital palpation. The most common reason for residual gradients is inadequate septectomy at the midventricular level. In general, one can visualize the bases of the papillary muscles while looking through the aortic root after the myectomy has been completed. The outflow tract is irrigated to remove any particulate debris and the aortic and mitral valves are inspected to insure that there has been no injury to them. After the patient is weaned from cardiopulmonary bypass, pressures are remeasured in the left ventricle and aorta and TEE evaluation is repeated. TEE can quantify and localize any residual gradient and exclude an iatrogenic ventricular septal defect. If successful

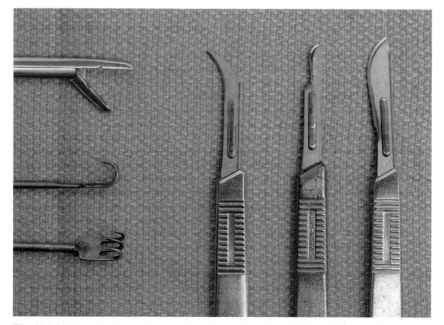

Fig. 15.5 Instruments commonly used during surgical myectomy. The use of some or all of these instruments is made at the discretion and preference of the operating surgeon.

myectomy has been performed, there will be little or no residual gradient and little or no SAM. In general, we would resume cardiopulmonary bypass for re-resection if the gradient was greater than 15–20 mm Hg. Transthoracic echo-cardiographic evaluation is routinely performed prior to hospital discharge.

Surgical results

In 1988, we reviewed an early 15-year experience with 115 Mayo Clinic patients who underwent operation for obstructive HCM from 1972 through 1987.[8] Patient ages ranged from 1 to 83 years (mean, 45 years). Methods of relief of LVOTO were septal myectomy ($n = 109$), mitral valve replacement ($n = 4$), and myectomy plus mitral valve replacement ($n = 2$). Concomitant procedures included coronary artery bypass ($n = 19$) and aortic valve replacement ($n = 9$). Mean peak systolic gradients from left ventricle to aorta decreased from 70 ± 38 to 9 ± 11 mm Hg. There were six hospital deaths, for an overall operative risk of 5.2%; only one death occurred among 83 patients less than age 65 years (operative risk 1.2%), and five deaths occurred in 32 older patients (operative risk, 15.6%; $P = 0.008$ for the difference between age groups). For patients who had septal myectomy alone, including all ages, the operative risk was 2.5%.

Follow-up ranged up to 16 years (mean, 5 years) and 5-year actuarial survival rate, including hospital deaths, was 84 ± 4%. The 5-year survival rate was decreased in patients who had combined valve or coronary artery procedures in addition to myectomy (69 vs 91%, $P < 0.005$) and in patients aged 65 years or older (54 vs 93%, $P < 0.005$). Preoperative symptoms were relieved in 57 of 75 patients (76%) with dyspnea, 49 of 59 patients (83%) with angina, and 22 of 23 patients (96%) with syncope. This early experience convincingly showed that operation was effective in relieving symptoms in patients with the obstructive form of HCM.

A subsequent review was made of 65 additional patients who had septal myectomy with or without concomitant cardiac procedures between 1986 and 1992.[13] Patient ages ranged from 20 to 70 years. Specific symptoms and overall functional status were evaluated before surgery and at the end of the first postoperative year. Subsequent long-term follow-up was also obtained. The extent of postoperative improvement was measured by the presence and severity of persistent symptoms, overall New York Heart Association (NYHA) functional class, and patient self-perceptions of overall improvement. Before operation, 95% were in NYHA functional class III or IV, 95% had dyspnea, 62% had angina, 63% had near-syncope, and 23% had syncope. There was no early mortality among the 45 patients who underwent isolated septal myectomy; the overall early mortality rate was 4.6%. At the 1-year postoperative evaluation, 89% of survivors were in NYHA functional class I or II, and 47% reported that they had 100% improvement. Significant improvement was observed in 67% of patients with dyspnea, 90% with angina, 86% with near-syncope, and 100% with syncope (Fig. 15.6). The 5-year survival rate was 92%. These results reaf-

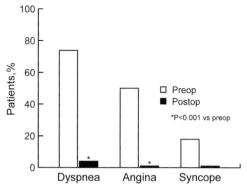

Fig. 15.6 Symptom-specific improvement of dyspnea, angina, and syncope in patients undergoing myectomy for obstructive hypertrophic cardiomyopathy.

firmed the efficacy of myectomy for treatment of obstructive HCM in symptomatic adult patients.

In total, from September 1972 to August 2002, 291 patients had septal myectomy for obstructive HCM on the authors' surgical services. A retrospective review of the first 199 patients to September 2000 was made. Ages ranged from 2 months to 80 years (median, 45 years). Preoperative NYHA class was III/IV in 120 patients (60%). Mitral valve regurgitation was moderate to severe in 108 patients (54%). Median resting LVOT gradient was 85 mm Hg (Fig. 15.7). Ninety patients (45%) required additional cardiac procedures, including division of abnormal mitral papillary muscle attachments ($n = 20$), mitral valve replacement ($n = 5$), and other procedures ($n = 65$). Median intraoperative postmyectomy LVOT gradient was 4 mm Hg. Postoperative mitral regurgitation was moderate in 16 patients (8%). Permanent heart block occurred in two patients (1%). No early deaths occurred in the 109 patients undergoing isolated myectomy. There were three early deaths in patients undergoing associated

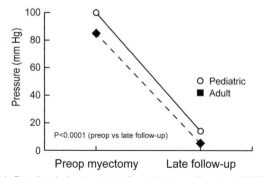

Fig. 15.7 Change in Doppler-derived resting left ventricular outflow tract (LVOT) gradient after septal myectomy in children and adults. There was a significant reduction in LVOT gradient in both groups ($P < 0.0001$).

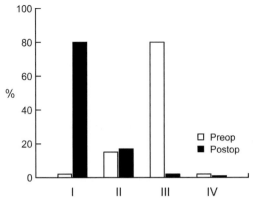

Fig. 15.8 Change in New York Heart Association (NYHA) functional classification before and after septal myectomy. There was a significant improvement in functional class following myectomy, with the majority of patients in class I or II.

cardiac procedures (overall early mortality, 1.5%). Follow-up in 178 patients (91%) ranged up to 23 years (median, 4 years). Overall survival was 91 ± 3% at 5 years and 83 ± 4% at 10 years. Median resting LVOT gradient on follow-up echocardiography in 121 patients (68%) was 5 mm Hg (Fig. 15.7). Follow-up NYHA class was I/II in 127 patients (81%) (Fig. 15.8). Other centers have reported similar early and late results.[7,10,12,14–22]

Obstructive HCM in children

There is also an important role for surgery in pediatric patients with obstructive HCM, although operation is technically more challenging because of the smaller structures and more delicate tissues. The prognosis for symptomatic pediatric patients with obstructive HCM has been shown to be much less favorable than for symptomatic adults.[25,26] In order to determine if surgical relief of LVOTO has a positive influence on this poor prognosis, we reviewed 25 consecutive pediatric patients on our hospital service who underwent septal myectomy between April 1975 and May 1995.[11] Ages ranged from 2 months to 20 years (mean, 11.2 years). Seventeen patients had moderate to severe mitral valve insufficiency. Medical therapy had failed in all patients and one patient had undergone dual-chamber pacemaker implantation without improvement. LVOT gradients ranged from 50 to 154 mm Hg (mean 100 ± 25) (Fig. 15.7).

Concomitant cardiac procedures included mitral valve repair ($n = 2$), automatic implantable cardioverter–defibrillator implantation ($n = 1$), and closure of atrial septal defect ($n = 1$). Intraoperative premyectomy LVOT gradients ranged from 20 to 117 mm Hg (mean 60 ± 26) and postmyectomy gradients ranged from 0 to 20 mm Hg (mean 7 ± 6). Postmyectomy mitral insufficiency was reduced to a regurgitant fraction of 0–12% and no patient required mitral valve replacement. One patient required a pacemaker because of complete heart block; on subsequent follow-up sinus rhythm had returned. There was no early mortality and no instance of aortic or mitral valve injury or iatrogenic ventricular septal defect. Follow-up ranged from 10 months to 20 years (mean 6.4 years), and there were no late deaths. Postoperative LVOT gradients by echocardiography averaged 14 mm Hg (Fig. 15.7) with a median of 5 mm Hg. All patients but one were in NYHA class I or II.

Subsequent to this review (June 1995 to April 2003), 31 additional pediatric patients have undergone septal myectomy with no early mortality and no complications, such as ventricular septal defect or complete heart block, and no need for mitral valve replacement. At late follow-up ($n = 56$), eight patients required reoperation, including repeat myectomy, heart transplantation (5 and 6 years after myectomy), mitral valve repair, mitral or aortic valve replacement, and Konno–Rastan procedure. Two late deaths occurred, one from chronic rejection after heart transplantation; the other death was sudden, 8 years after myectomy (in the latter patient the most recent echocardiogram showed no evidence of LVOTO).

We have concluded that extended septal myectomy is a safe and effective means of relieving cardiac symptoms and LVOTO in pediatric as well as adult patients with severe obstructive HCM unresponsive to medical management. For pediatric patients especially, late survivorship compares very favorably with the natural history of the disease in this age group, in which the annual mortality rate has been reported to be as high as 6% in symptomatic patients evaluated in tertiary referral centers.[26]

Obstructive HCM with papillary muscle abnormalities

Classical septal myectomy effectively abolishes LVOTO, SAM, and associated mitral regurgitation and yields excellent late results. However, some symptomatic patients with obstructive HCM have associated anomalies of the mitral subvalvular apparatus which, if unrecognized and untreated, can lead to intraoperative death or incomplete or only temporary relief of obstruction.[23,24,27–30] Perhaps the most important of these anomalies is anomalous papillary muscle insertion directly into the anterior mitral leaflet, an entity which has been well documented by Klues and associates[28] (Fig. 15.9A). Mitral valve replacement has been advocated by some as the best surgical solution for this anomaly in HCM; however, excellent relief of LVOTO with preservation of the mitral valve may be possible by performance of an extended septal myectomy.[23,30] Other anomalies of mitral subvalvular apparatus include extensive fusion of papillary muscles with the ventricular septum or left ventricular free wall, abnormal chordae tendineae (false cords) which attach to the ventricular septum or free wall, and accessory papillary muscles, all of which may tether the mitral leaflets towards the septum and produce LVOTO (Fig. 15.9 A, B, C). Additional mechanisms of dynamic LVOTO, which are not necessarily related to papillary muscle anomalies, include midventricular obstruction secondary

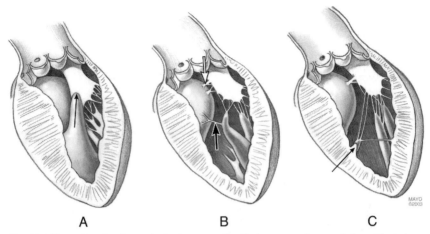

A   B   C

Fig. 15.9 Examples of various mitral valve anomalies that can occur in association with obstructive hypertrophic cardiomyopathy. These include direct insertion of the head of the papillary muscle into the leading edge of the anterior mitral leaflet (**A**, arrow), and extensive fusion of the base of the papillary muscle to the septum. Other anomalies include accessory chordal or fibrous attachments between the lateral edge (as opposed to the leading edge) of the anterior leaflet and the septum (**B**, white arrow) or between a papillary muscle and the septum (**B**, black arrow) or lateral free wall, or accessory papillary muscle(s) with attachments to the anterior mitral leaflet (**C**, arrow). All chordal attachments to the leading edge of the anterior leaflet need to be preserved.

to severely hypertrophied papillary muscles or other muscle bundles, and exaggerated anterior displacement of the anterolateral papillary muscle.[31,32]

Increasing awareness of the importance of anomalies of the mitral subvalvular apparatus and improved ability to visualize subvalvular structures by means of optical magnification and fiberoptic lighting have led to their increased identification and successful surgical treatment.[23,28–30] We recently reported the results of 56 patients who had obstructive HCM associated with an anomalous subvalvular mitral apparatus.[23] Eighty-two per cent were in functional class III or IV preoperatively. All patients underwent an extended septal myectomy as described above, with concomitant resection of anomalous chordae and relief of papillary muscle fusion (Fig. 15.10). There were no early deaths and no patients required mitral valve replacement. Mean pressure gradients decreased from 70 ± 28 to 5 ± 8 mm Hg. Freedom from reoperation at 5 years was 95%, and 98% of patients were in functional class I or II.

Reoperation after septal myectomy

While it is well recognized that successful septal myectomy provides excellent early and late outcomes for the vast majority of patients with severe obstructive HCM, a few patients may have recurrent or persistent LVOTO after septal

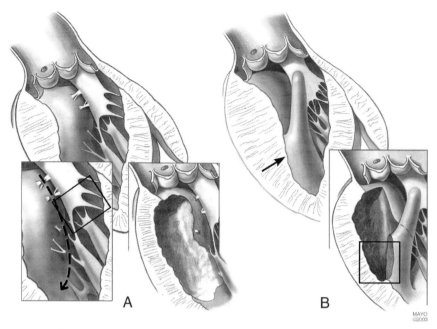

Fig. 15.10 Surgical approaches to the treatment of mitral valve anomalies. The general principle is to divide all attachments that exist between the lateral edge of the anterior leaflet and the septum and to divide all attachments between the papillary muscle(s) and septum (**A**, dotted arrow). It is important to maintain intact all chordal attachments to the leading edge of the anterior leaflet (**A**, box). The presence of a direct papillary muscle insertion into the anterior leaflet may be accompanied by fusion of the papillary muscle to the septum (**B**, arrow). Surgical myectomy is performed in the extended fashion, as previously described, and in addition the papillary muscle is incised off the septum down to its base (**B**, box).

myectomy. Reoperation may be required and may include repeat myectomy or mitral valve replacement. We recently reviewed 610 septal myectomies performed at our institution from 1975 to July 2003.[24] Thirteen (2.1%) were repeat myectomies for residual or recurrent LVOTO after classic myectomies performed at our institution ($n = 6$) or elsewhere ($n = 7$). The patients had a mean age of 32 ± 22 years; six patients were less than 16 years of age. Mechanisms for obstruction included midventricular obstruction, anomalous mitral subvalvular apparatus, and incomplete subaortic resection at the initial operation. Successful repeat myectomy was performed in all cases. Iatrogenic ventricular septal defect occurred in one patient and was successfully repaired. The requirement for reoperation after septal myectomy will undoubtedly be reduced by more contemporary surgical techniques that include a more extensive myectomy, relief of papillary muscle abnormalities, and the use of intraoperative evaluation by TEE.

Comment

From the pathophysiological standpoint, septal myectomy improves cardiac output, decreases mitral regurgitation, enhances myocardial blood flow by decreasing left ventricular afterload and intracavitary pressure, improves diastolic function, favorably affects myocardial oxygen consumption and metabolism, and decreases left ventricular end-diastolic pressure, consistent with an improvement in overall diastolic filling of the heart.[33] Surgery is not regarded as curative, but is performed to achieve improved quality of life and functional (exercise) capacity. While definitive data are lacking, some evidence in retrospective nonrandomized studies suggests that surgical relief of LVOTO in severely symptomatic patients may reduce long-term mortality and possibly the risk of sudden death (Fig. 15.11).[8–11,17,22,26]

Dual-chamber pacing and percutaneous transluminal alcohol septal ablation have recently been advocated for treatment of obstructive HCM. Their comparative merits versus septal myectomy continue to be evaluated. These techniques have been effective in selected patients, but are not appropriate for children, for those in whom fixed obstruction is present instead of obstructive HCM,[34] for patients in whom LVOTO is due to papillary muscle anomalies,[23,24] or for patients with unfavorable septal artery anatomy.

Concomitant cardiac valve replacement, myocardial revascularization, and other major cardiac procedures performed at the time of surgery for obstructive HCM necessarily increase the operative mortality (although only modestly, in current experience, for patients less than 65 years of age). Accordingly, comparisons of results of myectomy with newer nonsurgical treatment alter-

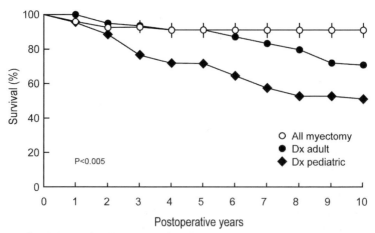

Fig. 15.11 Survival curve for all patients undergoing isolated septal myectomy in our series (open circles), including operative mortality, compared with survival curves for symptomatic patients followed in a tertiary referral institution with diagnosis in childhood (diamond) or adulthood (closed circle).[26] The survival in the myectomy group was significantly better than that in the nonsurgical group for adults and especially for children ($P < 0.005$).

natives (especially with regard to mortality) should be made only to those patients undergoing isolated obstructive HCM surgery. As experience increases and lengthens with newer alternatives to surgery, the results can be compared with the more than 40 years of experience with septal myectomy.

Summary

Septal myectomy effectively relieves LVOTO and cardiac symptoms in both adults and children with obstructive HCM. Abnormal attachments of the papillary muscles and chordae and other cardiac lesions can be repaired at the same time as myectomy. Operation can also relieve LVOTO in those patients thought to have obstructive HCM but who are subsequently found at surgery to have some form of fixed obstruction. Septal myectomy is also effective in those patients who have not improved after dual-chamber pacemaker implantation or alcohol septal ablation.

The operative mortality rate for isolated septal myectomy in both children and adults is low (0–2.5%). Surgical mortality, morbidity, and results continue to improve with the more recent surgical experience. Median echocardiographic LVOT gradients at rest on late follow-up can be as low as 5 mm Hg, and therefore relief of obstruction appears to be permanent. Symptomatic improvement with myectomy is gratifying; 90% of patients improve by at least one functional class and most retain this improvement on late follow-up. Late survivorship compares very favorably with the natural history of nonoperated patients with symptomatic obstructive HCM. These results serve as a basis for comparison with newer nonsurgical catheter-based alternatives.

References

1 Nishimura RA, Giuliani ER, Brandenburg RO, Danielson GK. Hypertrophic Cardiomyopathy. In: Giuliani ER, Gersh BJ, McGoon MD, Hayes DL, Schaff HV, eds. *Myocardial Disease: Mayo Clinic Practice of Cardiology,* 3rd edn, Chapter 20. St. Louis (MO): Mosby-Year Book, 1996: 689–711.

2 Goodwin JF, Hollman A, Cleland WP, Teare D. Obstructive cardiomyopathy simulating aortic stenosis. *Br Heart J* 1960; **22**: 403–14.

3 Kirklin JW, Ellis FH Jr. Surgical relief of diffuse subvalvular aortic stenosis. *Circulation* 1961; **24**: 739–42.

4 Morrow AG, Brockenbrough EC. Surgical treatment of idiopathic hypertrophic subaortic stenosis: Technique and hemodynamic results of subaortic ventriculomyotomy. *Ann Surg* 1961; **154**: 181–9.

5 Wigle ED, Heimbecker RO, Gunton EW. Idiopathic ventricular septal hypertrophy causing muscular subaortic stenosis. *Circulation* 1962; **26**: 325–40.

6 Kelly DT, Barratt-Boyes BG, Lowe JB. Results of surgery and hemodynamic observations in muscular subaortic stenosis. *J Thorac Cardiovasc Surg* 1966; **51**: 353–65.

7 McIntosh CL, Maron BJ. Current operative treatment of obstructive hypertrophic cardiomyopathy. *Circulation* 1988; **78**: 487–95.

8 Mohr R, Schaff HV, Danielson GK, Puga FJ, Pluth JR, Tajik AJ. The outcome of surgical treatment of hypertrophic obstructive cardiomyopathy: Experience over 15 years. *J Thorac Cardiovasc Surg* 1989; **97**: 666–74.

9 Mohr R, Schaff HV, Puga FJ, Danielson GK. Results of operation for hypertrophic obstructive cardiomyopathy in children and adults less than 40 years of age. *Circulation* 1989; **80** (Suppl. 1): 191–6.

10 Williams WG, Rebeyka IM. Surgical intervention and support for cardiomyopathies of childhood. *Prog Pediatr Cardiol* 1992; **1**: 61–71.

11 Theodoro DA, Danielson GK, Feldt RH, Anderson BJ. Hypertrophic obstructive cardiomyopathy in pediatric patients: Results of surgical treatment. *J Thorac Cardiovasc Surg* 1996; **112**: 1589–99.

12 Schulte HD, Bircks WH, Loesse B, Godehardt EAJ, Schwartzkopff B. Prognosis of patients with hypertrophic obstructive cardiomyopathy after transaortic myectomy. *J Thorac Cardiovasc Surg* 1993; **106**: 709–17.

13 McCully RB, Nishimura RA, Tajik AJ, Schaff HV, Danielson GK. Extent of clinical improvement after surgical treatment of hypertrophic obstructive cardiomyopathy. *Circulation* 1996; **94**: 467–71.

14 Wigle ED, Rakowski H, Kimball BP *et al.* Hypertrophic cardiomyopathy: Clinical spectrum and treatment. *Circulation* 1995; **92**: 1680–92.

15 Schulte HD, Borisov K, Gams E, Gramsch-Zabel H, Schwartzkopff B. Management of symptomatic hypertrophic obstructive cardiomyopathy – long-term results after surgical therapy. *J Thorac Cardiovasc Surg* 1999; **47**: 213–18.

16 Robbins RC, Stinson EB. Long-term results of left ventricular myotomy and myectomy for obstructive hypertrophic cardiomyopathy. *J Thorac Cardiovasc Surg* 1996; **111**: 586–94.

17 Williams WG, Wigle ED, Rakowski H, Smallhorn J, LeBlanc J, Trusler GA. Results of surgery for hypertrophic obstructive cardiomyopathy. *Circulation* 1987; **76**: V104–8.

18 Cohn LH, Trehan H, Collins JJ Jr. Long-term follow-up of patients undergoing myotomy/myectomy for obstructive hypertrophic cardiomyopathy. *Am J Cardiol* 1992; **70**: 657–60.

19 Heric B, Lytle BW, Miller DP, Rosenkranz ER, Lever HM, Cosgrove DM. Surgical management of hypertrophic obstructive cardiomyopathy. Early and late results. *J Thorac Cardiovasc Surg* 1995; **110**: 195–206.

20 McIntosh CL, Maron BJ, Cannon RO III, Klues HG. Initial results of combined anterior mitral leaflet plication and ventricular septal myotomy–myectomy for relief of left ventricular outflow tract obstruction in patients with hypertrophic cardiomyopathy. *Circulation* 1992: **86**: II60–7.

21 Krajcer Z, Leachman RD, Cooley DA, Coronado R. Septal myotomy–myomectomy versus mitral valve replacement in hypertrophic cardiomyopathy. Ten-year follow-up in 185 patients. *Circulation* 1989; **80**: I57–64.

22 Merrill WH, Friesinger GC, Graham TP Jr *et al.* Long-lasting improvement after septal myectomy for hypertrophic obstructive cardiomyopathy. Experience over 15 years. *J Thorac Cardiovasc Surg* 1989; **97**: 666–74.

23 Minakata K, Dearani JA, Nishimura RA, Maron BJ, Danielson GK. Extended septal myectomy for hypertrophic obstructive cardiomyopathy with anomalous mitral papillary muscles or chordae. *J Thorac Cardiovasc Surg.* (In press.)

24 Minakata K, Dearani JA, Schaff HV, O'Leary PW, Ommen SR, Danielson GK. Mechanisms for left ventricular outflow tract obstruction after initial septal myectomy for obstructive hypertrophic cardiomyopathy. *Ann Thorac Surg* (submitted).

25 Maron BJ, Roberts WC, Edwards JE, McAllister HA, Foley DD, Epstein SE. Sudden death in patients with hypertrophic cardiomyopathy: Characterization of 26 patients without functional limitation. *Am J Cardiol* 1978; **41**: 803–10.

26 McKenna W, Deanfield J, Faruqui A, England D, Oakley C, Goodwin J. Prognosis in hypertrophic cardiomyopathy: Role of age and clinical, electrocardiographic and hemodynamic features. *Am J Cardiol* 1981; **47**: 532–8.

27 Cape EG, Simons D, Jimoh A, Weyman AE, Yoganathan AP, Levine RA. Chordal geometry determines the shape and extent of systolic anterior mitral motion: In vitro studies. *J Am Coll Cardiol* 1989; **13**: 1438–48.

28 Klues HG, Roberts WC, Maron BJ. Anomalous insertion of papillary muscle directly into anterior mitral leaflet in hypertrophic cardiomyopathy: Significance in producing left ventricular outflow obstruction. *Circulation* 1991; **84**: 1188–97.

29 Schoendube FA, Klues HG, Reith S, Flachskampf FA, Hanrath P, Messmer BJ. Long-term clinical and echocardiographic follow-up after surgical correction of hypertrophic obstructive cardiomyopathy with extended myectomy and reconstruction of the subvalvular mitral apparatus. *Circulation* 1995; **92** (Suppl. II): II122–7.

30 Maron BJ, Nishimura RA, Danielson GK. Pitfalls in clinical recognition and a novel operative approach for hypertrophic cardiomyopathy with severe outflow obstruction due to anomalous papillary muscle. *Circulation* 1998; **98**: 2505–8.

31 Klues HG, Maron BJ, Dollar AL, Roberts WC. Diversity of structural mitral valve alterations in hypertrophic cardiomyopathy. *Circulation* 1992; **85**: 1651–60.

32 Reis RL, Bolton MR, King JF, Pugh DM, Dunn MI, Mason DT. Anterior-superior displacement of papillary muscles producing obstruction and mitral regurgitation in idiopathic hypertrophic subaortic stenosis—operative relief by posterior-superior realignment of papillary muscles following ventricular septal myectomy. *Circulation* 1974; **50** (2 Suppl.): II181–8.

33 Cannon RO III, McIntosh CL, Schenke WH, Maron BJ, Bonow RO, Epstein SE. Effect of surgical reduction in left ventricular outflow obstruction on hemodynamics, coronary flow, and myocardial metabolism in hypertrophic cardiomyopathy. *Circulation* 1989; **79**: 766–75.

34 Bruce CJ, Nishimura RA, Tajik AJ, Schaff HV, Danielson GK. Fixed left ventricular outflow tract obstruction in presumed hypertrophic obstructive cardiomyopathy: Implications for therapy. *Ann Thorac Surg* 1999; **68**: 100–4.

CHAPTER 16

United States Perspectives on the Role of Dual-Chamber Pacing in Patients with Hypertrophic Cardiomyopathy

Paul Sorajja, MD, Steve R. Ommen, MD, and Rick A. Nishimura, MD

The use of dual-chamber pacing for symptomatic relief in obstructive hypertrophic cardiomyopathy has been met with great enthusiasm and some controversy over the past decade. Underlying this interest is the less invasive nature of this modality in comparison with surgical myotomy–myectomy, and the highly beneficial results that were observed in early, nonrandomized studies.[1-4] However, subsequent investigations have raised concerns over the precise role of dual-chamber pacing in patients with obstructive hypertrophic cardiomyopathy.[5] The application of dual-chamber pacing to these patients therefore requires careful consideration of both its technical aspects and hemodynamic effects and previous trials of its clinical utility.

Physiology and pathophysiology

Dual-chamber pacing decreases the dynamic left ventricular outflow tract obstruction through pre-excitation of the interventricular septum. This intervention reduces the inward motion of the septum during systole, thereby impeding left ventricular outflow tract narrowing, which otherwise accentuates systolic anterior motion of the mitral valve. To achieve these ends, the pacing electrode needs to be positioned at the right ventricular apex and the atrioventricular interval is optimized to ensure full ventricular capture.[6] The atrioventricular interval must not be set to 'short' as this can lead to significant falls in cardiac output and systemic pressure (Fig. 16.1). Dual-chamber pacing as opposed to single-chamber ventricular pacing is preferred because patients with hypertrophic cardiomyopathy often do not tolerate the loss of atrioventricular synchrony.

With proper techniques, dual-chamber pacing acutely leads to a 30–60% reduction of the left ventricular outflow tract (LVOT) gradient without systemic compromise.[1-4] Some investigators also have noted favorable long-term ventricular remodeling, which theoretically may result from the alteration of

HOCM Pacing Study

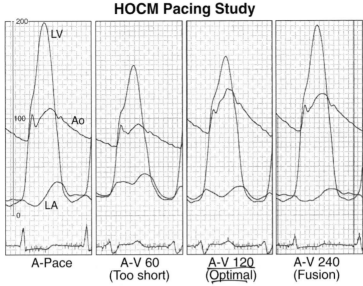

| A-Pace | A-V 60 (Too short) | A-V 120 (Optimal) | A-V 240 (Fusion) |

Fig. 16.1 High-fidelity pressure tracings demonstrating the hemodynamic effects of different pacing parameters in hypertrophic cardiomyopathy. (Far left) Baseline state (atrial pacing, A-Pace). (Middle left) Pacing at the atrioventricular (A-V) interval of 60 ms, which was too short and resulted in elevation in left atrial (LA) pressure and a decline in ascending aortic (Ao) pressure. (Middle right) Pacing at the optimal A-V interval, resulting in amelioration of the left ventricular outflow tract gradient. (Far right) Pacing at the A-V interval of 240 ms, which was too long and resulted in fusion of the native QRS complex and suboptimal left ventricular outflow tract gradient reduction. Reproduced from Symanski *et al.* The use of pacemakers in the treatment of cardiomyopathies. *Curr Probl Cardiol* 1996; 21: 385–443, with permission from Elsevier.

stress–strain relationships during regional septal activation.[4] Using positron emission tomography studies of patients with hypertrophic cardiomyopathy and angina, ventricular pacing resulted in the induction of more homogeneous blood flow.[7] The cause of this alteration is unknown, but may arise in part from changes in cardiac workload, epicardial coronary artery compression, or both. Though regression of myocardial hypertrophy with dual-chamber pacing also has been reported, interpretation of this observation has been difficult because of conflicting data.[4,8]

There has been concern that worsening of diastolic dysfunction may occur with permanent pacing. The vast majority of patients with hypertrophic cardiomyopathy suffer from diastolic dysfunction, which is due to a complex interplay of altered ventricular loading conditions, ventricular nonuniformity, and myocardial ischemia. Dual-chamber pacing may enhance the nonuniformity of ventricular contraction and relaxation by altering regional myocardial activation. In separate investigations, elevation of left ventricular filling pressures, prolongation of τ (the time constant of relaxation), and decline in cardiac output have been observed during pacing in comparison with measurements taken during sinus rhythm (Fig. 16.2).[9,10] The major cause of left

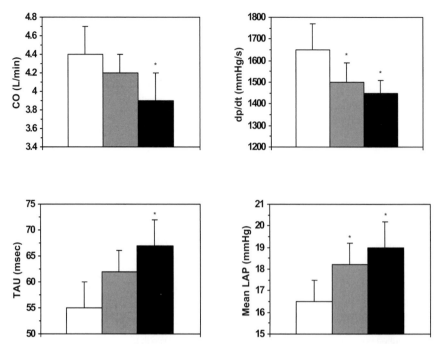

Fig. 16.2 Systolic and diastolic function during dual-chamber pacing in hypertrophic cardiomy-opathy. Variables of systolic function [cardiac output (CO) and peak positive dp/dt] and diastolic function [time constant of relaxation (TAU) and mean left atrial pressure (LAP)] were examined during normal sinus rhythm (open bar), DDD pacing at an atrioventricular delay of 60 ms (shaded bar), and DDD pacing at the optimal A-V interval (solid bar) in 29 patients. From Nishimura *et al*. Effect of dual-chamber pacing on systolic and diastolic function in patients with hypertrophic cardiomyopathy. *J Am Coll Cardiol* 1996; **27**: 421–30. Reproduced with permission from the American College of Cardiology Foundation.

atrial pressure elevation is an atrioventricular interval that is inappropriately short and does not permit complete pre-excitation of the ventricle. Thus, atrial contraction is not completed at the time of ventricular contraction and mitral valve closure, and results in both elevation of atrial pressure and inadequate ventricular filling. For patients with extremely short native PR intervals, drug therapy or even radiofrequency ablation of the atrioventricular node has been used to optimize ventricular capture. In those patients who achieve complete pre-excitation with an efficient atrioventricular delay and a drop in gradient, however, the left atrial pressure will decrease due to the beneficial effect on the contraction load of the ventricle.

Clinical studies

Early studies of pacing in hypertrophic cardiomyopathy consisted of small, observational reports that documented clinical benefits with dual-chamber pacing.[1-4] These reports cited alleviation of the LVOT gradient, modest improvements in exercise tolerance, and relief of dyspnea, angina, and syncope. The largest of these studies was from the National Institutes of Health, which examined 84 patients over a mean follow-up of 2.3 years.[4] Symptomatic relief occurred in 89% of patients with complete abolition in 33%. Mean New York Heart Association (NYHA) class (mean ± SD) decreased significantly from 3.2 ± 0.5 to 1.6 ± 0.6. Dual-chamber pacing also was associated with an objective increase in exercise duration (mean ± SD, 8.8 ± 3.3 min) in comparison with observations in normal sinus rhythm (6.3 ± 2.3 min). Additionally, over one-third of patients discontinued cardioactive medications. The therapeutic benefits of pacing were attributed to reductions in the LVOT gradient (96 ± 41 mm Hg at baseline; 27 ± 31 mm Hg at follow-up). These striking observations spurred great interest in the use of dual-chamber pacing for hypertrophic cardiomyopathy patients, leading to the need for clinical trials to confirm these benefits.

Randomized trials
Mayo Clinic study
Beginning in 1993, we at the Mayo Clinic directly examined the degree of benefit afforded to hypertrophic cardiomyopathy patients by quantifying their quality of life and exercise capacity in a randomized fashion during active pacing (DDD mode) and during placebo (AAI pacing at 30 beats/min).[5,11] All patients had severe, refractory symptoms, and either a resting LVOT gradient of ≥30 mm Hg or a provoked gradient of ≥50 mm Hg. Nineteen patients were blindly randomized into either treatment arm for 2–3 months, and then crossed over into the opposite study arm for an additional 2–3 months.

In the Mayo Clinic study, 63% of patients reported symptomatic improvement during DDD pacing. However, symptomatic improvement also occurred in 42% of patients during AAI mode, raising the concept of a placebo effect due to pacemaker implantation itself. Moreover, although DDD pacing resulted in a higher exercise duration (6.9 ± 2.2 min) than at baseline (5.7 ± 2.7 min), this increase was not statistically different from that observed during AAI pacing (6.3 ± 2.3 min). These findings suggest that other factors (e.g. training effects of repeated exercise testing) may be responsible for an increase in exercise duration on follow-up treadmill tests. Similar observations were made in the Pacing in Hypertrophic Obstructive Cardiomyopathy (PIC) study, which also was a randomized, placebo-controlled trial of dual-chamber pacing.[12] In this study, DDD pacing was associated with symptomatic improvement, but 28% also had subjective improvement with AAI pacing. Of note, quality-of-life measures were higher in those randomized to DDD initially than in the second treatment period in the PIC study.

M-PATHY trial
The M-PATHY trial is the most recent investigation of dual-chamber pacing in hypertrophic cardiomyopathy.[13] This study enrolled 48 patients from 14 centers in the USA, Canada, and the UK. All patients had severe, refractory

symptoms and a LVOT gradient of 50 mm Hg or more. The study population comprised 26 women and 22 men with a mean ± SD age of 53 ± 17 years (range, 22–83 years). As in the Mayo Clinic and PIC studies, M-PATHY randomized patients to 12 weeks of either DDD or AAI pacing followed by cross-over into the opposite treatment arm. In addition, patients were allowed to remain in DDD pacing for an additional 6 months under unblinded clinical observation. Functional assessment consisted of symptomatic evaluation, completion of the Minnesota quality-of-life questionnaire, measurement of the LVOT gradient, and exercise testing with peak myocardial oxygen consumption ($M\dot{V}O_2$) determinations. Particular care was taken to blind physicians during assessment by having one observer monitor the electrocardiogram (i.e. unblinded) while a second observer monitored and encouraged the patient to provide maximal effort during treadmill exercise (i.e. blinded).

In the M-PATHY trial, DDD pacing led to significant reductions in the LVOT gradient at 3 months (48 ± 33 mm Hg) and 12 months (48 ± 32 mm Hg) in comparison with baseline values (82 ± 33 mm Hg). DDD pacing also resulted in significant symptomatic relief compared with the baseline state. However, NYHA functional class and quality-of-life scores also were improved with AAI pacing and were no different than during DDD pacing at either the 3-month or the 12-month follow-up. Increased exercise duration (10.7 ± 4 min with DDD pacing after 3 months *vs* 9.2 ± 4 min at baseline, $P < 0.05$) and peak myocardial oxygen consumption (16.7 ± 4 with DDD pacing after 3 months *vs* 16.2 ± 5 ml/min/kg at baseline) were observed with DDD pacing compared with baseline. However, there was no statistical difference in either exercise duration or peak myocardial oxygen consumption during DDD pacing when compared with AAI pacing (exercise duration 10.6 ± 3 min, peak myocardial oxygen consumption 16.6 ± 5 ml/min/kg). Continuous DDD pacing for an additional 6 months did not result in a longer exercise duration (10.8 ± 4 min) or peak myocardial oxygen consumption (16.7 ± 4 ml/min/kg) compared with the findings after an initial 3 months of DDD pacing. Thus, there was no overall advantage of DDD pacing over placebo in both subjective and objective measures of functional capacity, despite a significant reduction in the LVOT gradient.

The M-PATHY trial did identify a subgroup of responders based upon an improvement in functional class and an increase of more than 10% in treadmill time. However, there were only 6 of 48 (12%) who met these criteria.

Long-term follow-up

Thirty-six Mayo Clinic patients have undergone pacemaker implantation as part of the original Mayo Clinic study or the M-PATHY trial. We have obtained a longer follow-up of these patients, with a median (± SD) follow-up duration at last contact of 59 ± 27 months. One patient died of unknown causes. Fifteen patients (41%) have had sustained symptomatic improvement with DDD pacing. In four patients (11%), worsening of symptoms led to discontinuation of pacing. Sixteen patients (44%) with refractory symptoms have required surgical myotomy–myectomy or percutaneous septal myocardial alcohol ablation, which resulted in complete relief in these patients.

Fourteen patients have continued with DDD pacing and undergone exercise testing in follow-up after 1 year. There was a significant increase in exercise duration from 7.7 ± 3.6 min at baseline to 10.4 ± 2.2 minutes at the end of follow-up. However, as in the short-term studies, this increase in the final exercise duration during long-term DDD pacing was not different from that observed during AAI pacing (9.5 ± 2.9 minutes). There was no difference between baseline values of peak myocardial oxygen consumption and DDD pacing after 1 year (Fig. 16.3).

Identifying hypertrophic cardiomyopathy patients who benefited either subjectively or objectively from dual-chamber pacing is difficult. In our Mayo Clinic patients, those who had severe exercise limitation ($M\dot{V}O_2$ less than 15 ml/kg/min; $n = 8$) had a greater improvement in $M\dot{V}O_2$ (3.2 ± 0.8 ml/kg/min) than patients who were not as limited (0.1 ± 1.1 ml/kg/min; $P = 0.04$). A similar observation in elderly hypertrophic cardiomyopathy patients has been made by other investigators, suggesting that markedly limited patients might respond better to dual-chamber pacing than individuals with less impairment.[12] However, only three of the eight patients with a peak myocardial oxygen consumption of less than 15 ml/kg/min reported an improvement in symptoms, illustrating the discrepancy that may occur between the subjective and objective findings. Among all patients in the Mayo Clinic experience, there was no difference in absolute or relative LVOT gradient reduction between patients who received benefit and those who did not. This finding, which has been shown in other studies,[12,13] raises the question of the actual physiologic benefit of this therapeutic modality.

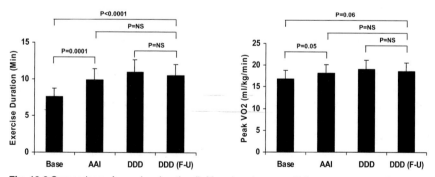

Fig. 16.3 Comparison of exercise duration (left) and peak myocardial oxygen consumption (right) in hypertrophic cardiomyopathy patients at baseline (Base) after 3 months of placebo or AAI pacing, after 3 months of DDD pacing, and after continuous DDD pacing [DDD (F-U)]. In both panels, group data with mean and SE at each period are shown on the left-hand side while plots of the changes in individual patients are shown on the right-hand side.

Dual-chamber pacing versus surgery

Surgical myotomy–myectomy remains the time-honored intervention for patients with hypertrophic cardiomyopathy and drug-refractory symptoms. Surgery achieves a reduction in the LVOT gradient of 90% or more, leading to symptom alleviation in nearly all patients, more than one-half of patients having complete relief. Candidates for surgery are those with drug-refractory symptoms and hypertrophy that is amenable to resection through a transaortic approach. Perioperative mortality in experienced centers is less than 2%, but is even lower among younger patients.[14]

At the Mayo Clinic, we have compared the results of dual-chamber pacing with results of surgery in patients with hypertrophic cardiomyopathy.[15] This study observed greater reduction of the LVOT gradient with surgery compared with dual-chamber pacing. Surgical myectomy will usually result in a LVOT gradient that is either less than 10 mm Hg or completely abolished, as opposed to dual-chamber pacing, which results in a gradient usually greater than 25–30 mm Hg. There were greater improvements in subjective (NYHA class) and objective (exercise duration and peak myocardial oxygen uptake) measures of functional capacity in patients who underwent surgery than in patients who received dual-chamber pacing (Fig. 16.4). While the retrospective nature of these comparisons may limit their interpretation, the superiority of surgery for the amelioration of symptoms due to obstructive hypertrophic cardiomyopathy, in a larger proportion of patients, remains in little doubt among many clinicians.

Perspectives

Early observational trials of dual-chamber pacing in hypertrophic cardiomyopathy generated great enthusiasm by reporting symptomatic improvement in both subjective and objective measures. Clinicians and patients alike were attracted to the relatively less invasive nature of pacing in contrast to surgical myotomy–myectomy. However, prospective randomized studies have raised questions about the actual benefits of pacing in these patients. It is clear that dual-chamber pacing will result in an overall modest decrease in the LVOT gradient. However, a decrease in gradient is not necessarily indicative of symptomatic improvement. While patients who received active treatment (DDD pacing) had improvements in quality of life and exercise capacity in these trials, similar results occurred in placebo-treated patients (back-up AAI pacing). Overall, there really has been little significant difference in the objective exercise results of patients who undergo DDD pacing compared with a control arm.

Nonetheless, there remains a small subset of hypertrophic cardiomyopathy patients whose symptoms are relieved, gradient is reduced, and exercise tolerance is improved by continuous dual-chamber pacing. The challenge faced by the clinician lies in the ability to identify such patients, as studies have been unable to reliably separate responders from nonresponders. There is no

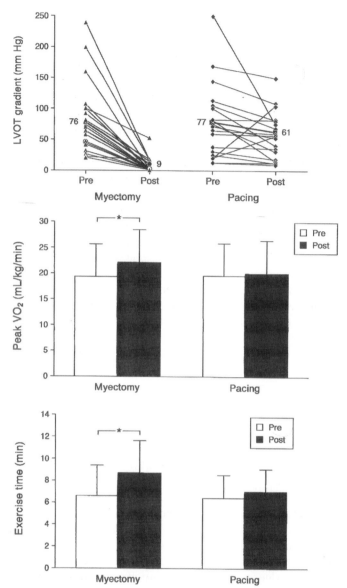

Fig. 16.4 Comparison of surgical myotomy–myectomy and dual-chamber pacing. (Top) Change in Doppler-derived resting left ventricular outflow tract gradient for patients before and after surgery (left) and pacing (right). (Middle) Surgery (left) resulted in a significant increase in exercise time (*P < 0.05), whereas pacing (right) did not. (Bottom) Surgery (left) resulted in a significant increase in peak myocardial oxygen consumption, whereas pacing (right) did not. Open bars = before treatment; solid bars = after treatment. From Ommen *et al.* Comparison of dual-chamber pacing versus septal myectomy for the treatment of patients with hypertrophic obstructive cardiomyopathy: A comparison of objective hemodynamic and exercise end points. *J Am Coll Cardiol* 1999; **34**: 191–6. Reproduced with permission from the American College of Cardiology Foundation.

established relation between the long-term clinical benefit from dual-chamber pacing and temporary (or permanent) reduction of the LVOT gradient, baseline symptoms, or other clinical variables. At the present time, there must be clear understanding by both clinicians and patients that prospective identification of pacing responders is not yet possible. Investigations are needed to identify these responders on a morphologic or perhaps a genetic basis.

Until we can predict those who will respond to dual-chamber pacing, this therapeutic modality may be an acceptable first therapy in those patients with high perioperative risks, such as elderly patients with significant comorbidities. The modest improvements in functional capacity afforded by dual-chamber pacing may satisfy these patients and the risk in this subgroup is likely to be less than with either surgery or septal ablation. Patients should be made aware of placebo effects that have been documented in several large clinical trials and that a significant number of patients still require surgery for symptomatic relief despite permanent pacing. In younger patients and those who desire a more active lifestyle, however, both subjective and objective measures are improved to a greater extent with surgical septal myotomy–myectomy. Randomized trials comparing all therapeutic modalities are required to establish the ultimate role of these treatments for the patient with severely symptomatic hypertrophic cardiomyopathy.

References

1 McDonald K, McWilliams E, O'Keefe B *et al.* Functional assessment of patients treated with permanent dual chamber pacing as a primary treatment for hypertrophic cardiomyopathy. *Eur Heart J* 1988; **9**: 893–8.

2 Jeanrenaud X, Goy J-J, Kappenberger L. Effects of dual-chamber pacing in hypertrophic obstructive cardiomyopathy. *Lancet* 1992; **339**: 1318–23.

3 Fananapazir L, Cannon RO, Tripodi D *et al.* Impact of dual-chamber permanent pacing in patients with obstructive hypertrophic cardiomyopathy with symptoms refractory to verapamil and b-adrenergic blocker therapy. *Circulation* 1992; **85**: 2149–61.

4 Fananapazir L, Epstein ND, Curiel RV *et al.* Long-term results of dual-chamber (DDD) pacing in obstructive hypertrophic cardiomyopathy: Evidence for progressive symptomatic and hemodynamic improvement and reduction of left ventricular hypertrophy. *Circulation* 1994; **90**: 2731–42.

5 Nishimura RA, Trusty JM, Hayes DL *et al.* Dual-chamber pacing for hypertrophic cardiomyopathy: A randomized, double-blind, crossover trial. *J Am Coll Cardiol* 1997; **29**: 435–41.

6 Jeanrenaud X, Schlapfer J, Fromer M *et al.* Dual chamber pacing in hypertrophic obstructive cardiomyopathy: Beneficial effect of atrioventricular junction ablation for optimal left ventricular capture and filling. *Pacing Clin Electrophysiol* 1997; **20**: 293–300.

7 Posma JL, Blanksma PK, van der Wall EE. Redistribution of myocardial perfusion during permanent dual chamber pacing in symptomatic nonobstructive hypertrophic cardiomyopathy: A quantitative positron emission tomography study. *Heart* 1996; **75**: 522–4.

8 Iliou MC, Laverne TL, Hernigou A *et al.* Left ventricular remodeling by long-term dual chamber pacing in hypertrophic obstructive cardiomyopathy. *Circulation* 1996; **94** (Suppl. I): I-361A.

9 Betocchi S, Losi M-A, Piscione F *et al.* Effects of dual chamber pacing in hypertrophic cardiomyopathy on left ventricular outflow tract obstruction and on diastolic function. *Am J Cardiol* 1996; **77**: 498–502.

10 Nishimura RA, Hayes DL, Ilstrup DM *et al.* Effects of dual-chamber pacing on systolic and diastolic function in patients with hypertrophic cardiomyopathy. *J Am Coll Cardiol* 1996; **27**: 421–30.

11 Erwin JP III, Nishimura RA, Lloyd MA, Tajik AJ. Dual chamber pacing for patients with hypertrophic obstructive cardiomyopathy: a clinical perspective in 2000. *Mayo Clin Proc* 2000; **75**: 173–80.

12 Kappenberger L, Linde C, Daubert C *et al.* Pacing in hypertrophic obstructive cardiomyopathy: a randomized crossover study. *Eur Heart J* 1997; **18**: 1249–56.

13 Maron BJ, Nishimura RA, McKenna WJ *et al.* Assessment of permanent dual-chamber pacing as a treatment for drug-refractory symptomatic patients with obstructive hypertrophic cardiomyopathy (M-PATHY). *Circulation* 1999; **99**: 2927–33.

14 McCully RB, Nishimura RA, Tajik AJ *et al.* Extent of clinical improvement after surgical treatment of hypertrophic obstructive cardiomyopathy. *Circulation* 1996; **94**: 467–71.

15 Ommen SR, Nishimura RA, Squires RW, Schaff HV, Danielson GK, Tajik AJ. Comparison of dual-chamber pacing versus septal myectomy for the treatment of patients with hypertrophic obstructive cardiomyopathy. *J Am Coll Cardiol* 1999; **34**: 191–6.

CHAPTER 17

Dual-Chamber Pacing for Hypertrophic Obstructive Cardiomyopathy

Xavier Jeanrenaud, MD and Lukas Kappenberger, MD

Hypertrophic cardiomyopathy is associated in approximately 30% of cases with dynamic subaortic obstruction. This obstruction, which is caused by the systolic displacement of mitral leaflets against the hypertrophied septum, contributes to the disease-related symptoms (angina, dyspnea, syncope, arrhythmias). If first-step therapy consists of β-blockers, calcium antagonists and/or disopyramide administration, surgical resection of the septum has long been considered as the only option for patients refractory to drug therapy. In the literature, the first successful attempt of myotomy was attributed to Cleland in 1958, but this experience was published only in 1963,[1] but though there has been constant modification since that time[2] this well-established and effective method still represents the gold standard of treatment for such patients.

Since the mid-1980s, dual-chamber pacing has been proposed as an alternative therapy to surgery[3] and has demonstrated its efficacy in a number of patients. However, after an initial period of enthusiasm, this method has been subject to some criticism and is challenged by a new and promising strategy of alcohol septal ablation.[4] The aim of this review is to summarize current knowledge on pacing therapy in hypertrophic obstructive cardiomyopathy (HOCM).

Historical background

The history of pacing in HOCM begins in the 1960s with the observation that patients developing left bundle branch block (LBBB) after myotomy–myectomy had a better clinical outcome than those with normal intraventricular conduction. Soon afterwards, Hassenstein and Wolter[5] and Gilgenkrantz and colleagues[6] observed, during hemodynamic studies performed in HOCM patients with complete atrioventricular block, that a right apical stimulation, which mimics LBBB, reduced the degree of obstruction. In 1971, Rothlin and Moccetti[7] confirmed these results in six patients and underlined the importance of the pacing site, i.e. obstruction was decreased when the right ventricular (RV) apex was paced but was enhanced by pulmonary infundibulum stimulation.

In 1975, Hassenstein and colleagues[8] tested the hypothesis that RV pacing could be a primary treatment for HOCM in the absence of intrinsic conduction abnormalities. On the basis of their experience in four patients implanted with a ventricular atrial-triggered (VAT) device, they concluded that permanent atrial-triggered RV pacing improved symptoms as well as obstruction and could be therefore considered as an alternative to surgery. Synchronous (VAT) systems were chosen as they prevent the fall in stroke volume and aortic pressure which is observed when the atrial contribution to left ventricular filling is lost. Other clinical[9–10] and haemodynamic[11] reports supported this concept, but real enthusiasm for pacing began in 1985 after the first implantation of a DDD programmable pacemaker by Erwin and colleagues from Dublin.[3] Three years later, the group published the first series of patients.[12]

Guidelines for optimal efficiency

Previous hemodynamic studies have demonstrated that the key factor for the optimal efficiency of pacing is full ventricular pre-excitation from the right ventricular apex, i.e. a complete reversal of normal activation of the heart. This precondition justifies the careful positioning of the lead, as stimulation from other regions of the right ventricle, for example the basal septum or pulmonary infundibulum, is ineffective and may even be deleterious.[7,13] Once the lead is implanted, full capture of the left ventricle depends upon the programmed atrioventricular delay. The atrioventricular delay must be shorter than the native PR interval but long enough to prevent loss of atrial contribution to filling. Individual adaptation is mandatory and a compromise has to be found between pre-excitation and preload. Echo-Doppler is of aid in analyzing the repercussion of programmed atrioventricular delay adaptation on mitral flow. In order to ensure full ventricular capture during exercise, drug therapy (β-blocker/calcium antagonists) should be maintained in order to prolong PR conduction. Also, the use of DDD devices with atrioventricular delay adaptive features—sensed and paced atrioventricular delay as well as rate adaptive functions—will improve the efficiency of pacing. Treadmill testing and/or 24-hour ECG monitoring are helpful in controlling (in daily life conditions) the adequacy of programming. In patients who lose capture due to a short PR interval at rest or to excessive shortening during exercise, despite reinforcement of drug therapy, ablation of the atrioventricular node is a very effective solution.[14,15]

Mechanisms of action

How pacing exerts its beneficial effects is still poorly understood, but it is mainly attributed to pressure gradient reduction. Apical pre-excitation modifies regional wall motion as well as the global function, and both of these mechanisms can influence obstruction. By the use of contrast ventriculography, apical pre-excitation has been shown to induce early contraction of the apex, delayed contraction of the base and a reduction of septal motion.[16,17] Moreover, prolongation of the delay in mitral leaflet–septal contact has been observed during pacing by M-mode. This may allow a greater proportion of end-diastolic volume to be ejected before obstructive mechanisms occur. Pollick and colleagues[18] demonstrated that the subaortic pressure gradient is inversely proportional to the delay in the appearance of systolic anterior motion (SAM). Other data suggest that pacing could also influence obstruction by exerting a negative inotropic effect comparable to that of β-blockers. Leclercq and colleagues[19] observed a reduction of left ejection fraction and positive dp/dt during DDD pacing compared with AAI. Similar observations have been confirmed in HOCM patients by Nishimura and colleagues.[20]

Improvement by pacing could also be explained by another concept, elaborated by Pak and colleagues[21] and predicated on hemodynamic studies performed in five patients with HOCM and in six patients with hypertensive hypertrophy and cavity obliteration. Pressure–volume relations were recorded at baseline and then during pre-excitation obtained by VDD pacing and short atrioventricular interval. VDD pacing was shown to increase end-systolic volume by shifting the end-systolic pressure–volume relation rightward, to reduce intracavitary pressure gradients, and to lower the total chamber workload. They suggested that, by reducing metabolic demand, pacing can improve symptoms even in the absence of subaortic obstruction.

Other hemodynamic effects of pacing

Diastolic function

The major potential diastolic consequence of DDD pacing is on the preload, as a short atrioventricular delay may induce a severe alteration in active filling, as has been reported by Nishimura and colleagues.[2] Since the hemodynamic study of Zile and colleagues,[22] DDD pacing has also been known to alter the relaxation properties of the myocardium. This alteration can be related to asynchrony of contraction, which, as shown by Brutsaert and colleagues, is one of the determinant factors of relaxation.[23] In HOCM, prolongation of constant τ of relaxation and a delay in early peak filling rate have been demonstrated by catheterization[20] and radionuclide scintigraphy.[24] Apical stimulation also induces regional asynchrony of relaxation, particularly at the apex, which relaxes earlier than the base. This is at the origin of abnormal diastolic intraventricular flows (Fig. 17.1). The long-term clinical consequences of these electrically induced diastolic alterations are not yet known.

Mitral insufficiency

Subaortic obstruction frequently coexists with a variable degree of functional mitral insufficiency due to systolic distortion of the valve. By influencing the mechanisms of obstruction, DDD pacing decreases in parallel the degree of functional regurgitation.[25]

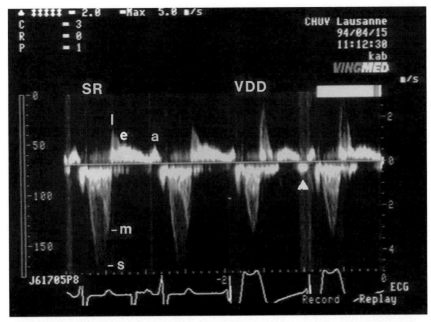

Fig 17.1 Effect of DDD pacing on intraventricular flows. Subaortic and transmitral flow velocities are recorded from a four-chamber apical view in sinus rhythm then VDD pacing mode, and an arterioventricular interval of 80 ms. During systole, a reduction of subaortic flow velocity (s) from 4.8 to 3.4 m/s is observed during pacing. A superimposed component of midventricular obstruction (m) at the level of the papillary muscle is also reduced, from 3.0 to 1.9 m/s. During diastole, the isovolumic relaxation flow (I), which is frequently present in hypertrophic and hyperdynamic left ventricle, is significantly increased during apical stimulation compared with baseline, from 1.7 to 2.8 m/s. As regards mitral flow (e and a waves, corresponding to the passive and active filling periods), the atrial contribution to left ventricular filling (a) is slightly reduced compared with sinus rhythm. Finally, during pacing only, a small negative flow (white arrow) appears in mid-diastole, indicating the presence of a small but positive intraventricular gradient between apex and base.

Coronary flow

In dogs, apical stimulation has been shown to decrease fiber strain[26] and to reduce mean and phasic flows[27] in the early activated descending coronary region. A positron emission tomography study of HOCM patients observed that pacing causes a decrease in resting left ventricular myocardial blood flow (which could reflect a lower myocardial oxygen demand) together with a redistribution of myocardial flow and a more homogeneously distributed myocardial perfusion reserve.[28] Whether these changes in myocardial perfusion explain the improvement of angina is still hypothetical.

Remodeling

The long-term effect of pacing on left ventricular parameters is still unresolved. A non-randomized study described slight dilatation of the left ventricle but no reduction of hypertrophy after a mean pacing period of 62 months.[16] With regard to septal thickness, van Oosterhout and colleagues[29] observed in dogs a localized thinning of the left ventricular wall at the site of stimulation, which was attributed to decreased mechanical work in early activated areas. In HOCM patients, a slight reduction in septal thickness has been described in a nonrandomized study.[30] Data obtained from randomized trials have not confirmed these results.[31,32]

Clinical trials: observational studies

In 1988, McDonald and colleagues[12] were the first to report, in 11 HOCM patients refractory to drug therapy, an improvement of symptoms and an increase in exercise tolerance. Soon afterwards, other independent centers reported results consistent with this.[16,33–36] Their results can be summarized as follows. Pacing induces a long-lasting reduction in subaortic obstruction together with a significant improvement of symptoms. Mean pressure gradient reduction varies from 43% to 85%, with considerable inter-individual variation. Pacing efficacy on obstruction is not immediate after implantation but increases with time.[16,33] New York Heart Association (NYHA) functional class is improved from a mean value of 3–4 to 1.5–2. Angina and especially syncopes improve to a greater extent than dyspnea.[16,35] Longer exercise duration time has been observed on a treadmill test.[33] However, no relationship between pressure gradient reduction and functional improvement could be established, suggesting that factors other than relief of obstruction may provide a beneficial effect.

Prospective and randomized trials

Three prospective, randomized, crossover trials are now available: the Pacing in Cardiomyopathy (PIC) study,[37] the M-PATHY study[31] and the Mayo Clinic study.[38]

These studies differ in terms of population size and length of follow-up but their study design is very similar, comprising a 6-month crossover period. After pacemaker implantation, patients were randomized in a blinded fashion to 3 months each of active (DDD mode with optimized atrioventricular interval) or inactive (AAI rate 30) pacing period. In the PIC study, patients were permanently paced for 22–42 months in their preferred mode after completion of the crossover period (DDD mode was chosen by 94%). In the M-PATHY study, all patients were stimulated in DDD mode during 6 additional months. The

Mayo Clinic study reports the results of the 6-month crossover period, with no further follow-up. The results obtained from these trials in HOCM patients refractory to drug therapy are as follows.

The PIC study, which collected data from 12 European centers, included 83 patients. One died during a temporary pacing study due to ventricular perforation. After a mean period of 36 months (22–46 months), 73 of 82 patients were still being stimulated in DDD mode. Ablation of the arterioventricular conduction had to be performed in eight of them in order to ensure full left ventricular capture. Of the other nine patients, five were sent for surgery, three preferred AAI mode and one was lost to follow-up. In the 73 DDD-stimulated patients, the mean maximal pressure gradient was reduced from 72 ± 35 to 28 ± 21 mm Hg ($P < 0.001$). The mean NYHA functional class significantly improved with pacing from 2.4 at baseline to 1.4 ($P < 0.01$), with 97% in class I or II and only 3% in class III. NYHA functional class and quality of life (QoL) score revealed a preference for DDD pacing but significant improvement was also observed in 28% of patients during AAI pacing mode, suggesting the existence of a placebo/study effect.[39] After a 36-month pacing period, and despite subjective improvement, objective measurements of functional capacity, including exercise duration time or peak oxygen consumption ($\dot{V}O_2$), showed no significant modifications during pacing compared with baseline (except in the most limited patients). The authors concluded that pacing should be considered as a reasonable alternative to surgery.

The M-PATHY study included 48 patients recruited from 14 centers in the USA, Canada and the UK. Only 32 of the patients completed the 1-year protocol. No significant differences between the DDD pacing and non-pacing periods were found with regard to either subjective assessment (NYHA functional class), QoL score, or more rigorous objective measurements, such as treadmill exercise time and peak $\dot{V}O_2$. At 1 year, pressure gradient decreased 40%, from 82 ± 32 mm Hg to 48 ± 32 mm Hg ($P < 0.001$) and was reduced in 57% of patients but unchanged or increased in 43%. Peak $\dot{V}O_2$ was unchanged with the exception of six patients aged more than 65 years. No significant reduction in left ventricular wall thickness was observed.

The Mayo Clinic study included 21 patients, of whom 19 completed the 6-month crossover protocol. Results were very similar to those of the M-PATHY study. The pressure gradient significantly decreased after DDD pacing compared with baseline value or AAI mode. QoL score and exercise duration were significantly improved from baseline after pacing but were not significantly different between the DDD and AAI periods. Moreover, peak $\dot{V}O_2$ was unchanged. Overall, 63% of patients improved in DDD mode and 42% in AAI. In addition, 36% felt no change or deteriorated.

Based on these results, the authors of the M-PATHY and Mayo Clinic studies concluded that pacing does not usually affect clinical outcome.

Remarks

In all three studies, various degrees of clinical improvement were observed after pacemaker implantation, part of which may have been influenced by placebo/protocol effects. The evidence of a placebo effect, which is not unexpected as one has been described for every technique, has considerably dampened the enthusiasm for this method. As a result, experts have called for caution in its use. In our view, the importance given to the placebo effect is exaggerated. As it is expected to wane with time, a placebo effect is unlikely to explain the protracted clinical benefit observed in the PIC study after more than 1 year of permanent pacing. The fact that 14 of the 41 patients, initially programmed in DDD in the PIC study then reprogrammed to AAI, deteriorated clinically provides strong support for a direct effect of pacing. The independent observation by Gadler and colleagues[40] of clinical deterioration occurring in patients suddenly unpaced after months of stimulation is also evidence of an intrinsic effect of pacing. It is, however, becoming clearer that some individual patients benefit from pacing whereas others do not. Unfortunately, there is at present no specific predictor of long-term pacing efficacy. Therefore, for individual patient management it is still useful, in our view, to proceed to a temporary pacing study prior to implantation in order to assess responsiveness in terms of relief of obstruction.

Patient selection may be one of the explanations for the differences in results observed between the three randomized studies. The M-PATHY study implanted more symptomatic patients than the PIC study, since 80% of patients were initially in NYHA class III or IV *vs* 55% in the PIC study. Moreover, and in contrast to the M-PATHY and Mayo Clinic studies, which included only patients with a resting or provocable pressure gradient at least 50 mm Hg, the PIC study included patients with values of at least 30 mm Hg and 22% of the study population had latent obstruction.

Indications for pacing in HOCM

The ACC/AHA (American College of Cardiology/American Heart Association) guidelines for the implantation of cardiac pacemakers consider pacing in HOCM to be a class IIb indication (level of evidence A) in the absence of sinus node dysfunction or complete atrioventricular block.[41] Until a consensus is found on the specific role of each method—surgical myectomy, nonsurgical septal ablation, DDD stimulation—it is our view that pacing therapy can be considered as an alternative to more invasive treatments in many patients. Candidates with HOCM for pacemaker implantation should fulfill the following criteria: (1) adults with angina and/or dyspnea of at least NYHA class II or syncope and who are refractory to drugs; and (2) the presence of a sub-

Table 17.1 Factors influencing decision for DDD pacemaker implantation. PG = subaortic maximal pressure gradient; SAM = systolic anterior motion of mitral valve; LVOT = left ventricular outflow tract

	In favor of pacing	Not in favor
Age	>50 years	<40 years
Obstruction	Latent or low to moderate PG at rest (<60 mm Hg)	High PG at rest (>60 mm Hg)
Mechanism of obstruction	SAM	Aberrant papillary muscle SAM and basal septum protruding markedly into LVOT SAM and mitral annulus calcification
Temporary pacing study	Residual PG <30 mm Hg	Residual PG >60 mm Hg
Chronotropic incompetence	Present	Absent

aortic obstruction due to SAM with a maximal pressure gradient of at least 30 mm Hg at rest or after a provocative maneuver.

Factors affecting our decision to implant a DDD pacemaker are summarized in Table 17.1. Our current strategy is to consider pacing as a first-line therapy in patients aged 50 years or older, or somewhat younger subjects with latent obstruction.[36] In the case of no response or a partial response to pacing, subsequent radiofrequency ablation/modulation of the atrioventricular node conduction, nonsurgical septal ablation and surgery are considered. In younger patients (less than 40 years) with a high pressure gradient at rest (greater than 60 mm Hg) who fail to benefit from pacing, our preferred approach is surgery or alcohol septal ablation. Pacing should be considered when medical treatment is not tolerated due to chronotropic incompetence.

Left ventricular morphology appears, in our experience, to be an important factor in the hemodynamic response to pacing. As illustrated in Fig. 17.2, dynamic subaortic obstruction not due to systolic anterior motion of the mitral valve, such as aberrant papillary muscle or severe forms of basal septal hypertrophy with excessive protrusion into the left ventricular outflow tract, respond poorly to pacing. Fixed obstruction by a fibrous membrane and aberrant mitral valve is a rare cause of dynamic obstruction and should be treated by surgery.

Significant mitral insufficiency due to organic mitral valve disease, with ruptured chordae tendinae or prolapse are contraindications for stimulation and must be excluded with the use of transesophageal echocardiography.

Experience in children is limited[42] and does not support the use of pacing in this age group.

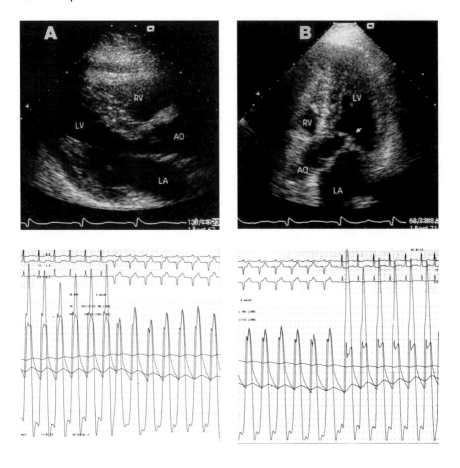

Fig. 17.2 Influence of left ventricular morphology on hemodynamic behavior observed during temporary DDD pacing. (Left-hand page) Case I, a 66-year-old woman in NYHA class III. (**A**) Two-dimensional echocardiographic stop-frames. Parasternal long-axis view. The septum is slightly hypertrophied (15 mm) and no other anomaly exists. (**B**) Apical view showing the presence of a frank systolic anterior motion of mitral valve with septal contact. (**C**) Simultaneous recording of the left ventricular and peak aortic pressure during a temporary pacing study. When changing from sinus rhythm and a PR interval of 220 ms to VDD pacing mode and an atrioventricular interval of 120 ms, the subaortic pressure gradient is abolished and the aortic pressure increases. Obstruction recurs immediately after switching off the pacemaker (right panel).

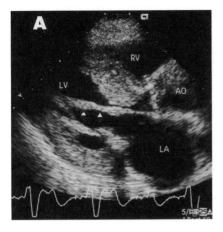

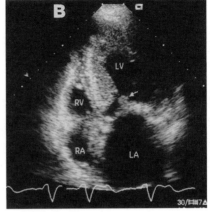

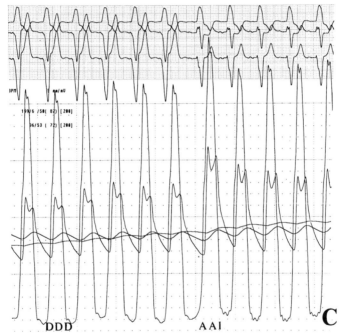

(Right-hand page) Case II, a 74-year-old woman in NYHA class III–IV. (**A**) Parasternal long-axis view. The septum is severely hypertrophied (23 mm) compared with the posterior wall (12 mm), protruding largely into the left ventricular outflow tract. The mitral annulus is sclerosed and there is a malposition of the anterolateral papillary muscle (white arrow). (**B**) Four-chamber apical view showing the presence of a systolic anterior motion of mitral valve with septal contact at rest. (**C**) Hemodynamic study. During DDD pacing mode and an atriovenous interval of 100 ms (left panel), the maximal subaortic pressure gradient of 103 mm Hg is unchanged compared with AAI mode at the same rate (right panel). LV = left ventricle; RV = right ventricle; LA = left atrium; RA = right atrium; AO = aorta.

The pacemaker should be implanted by experienced centers as pacing efficacy depends upon careful and individual adaptation of pacing characteristics and implantation is not exempt from complications.[43]

References

1 Cleland WP. The surgical management of obstructive cardiomyopathy. *J Cardiovasc Surg* 1963; **4**: 489–461.
2 Schoendube FA, Klues HG, Reith S *et al.* Long-term clinical and echocardiographic follow-up after surgical correction of hypertrophic obstructive cardiomyopathy with extended myectomy and reconstruction of the subvalvular mitral apparatus. *Circulation* 1995; **92** (Suppl. II): II-122–7.
3 Erwin J, McWilliams E, Gearty G *et al.* Hemodynamic and symptomatic improvement using dual-chamber pacing in hypertrophic cardiomyopathy [abstract]. *Br Heart J* 1985; **54**: 641.
4 Sigwart U. Non-surgical myocardial reduction for hypertrophic obstructive cardiomyopathy. *Lancet* 1995; **346**: 211–14.
5 Hassenstein P, Wolter HH. Therapeutische Beherrschung einer bedrohlichen Situation bei der idiopathischen hypertrophischen Subaortenstenose. *Verh Dtsch Ges Kreisl* 1967; **33**: 242–6.
6 Gilgenkrantz JM, Cherrier F, Petitier H *et al.* Cardiomyopathie obstructive du ventricule gauche avec bloc auriculo-ventriculaire complet. *Arch Mal Cœur* 1968; **60**: 439–53.
7 Rothlin M, Moccetti T. Influencing of the muscular subaortic stenosis by intraventricular stimulus propagation *Verhandl Dtsch Ges Kreislaufforsch* 1971; **37**: 411–15.
8 Hassenstein P, Storch HH, Schmitz W. Erfahrungen mit der Schrittmacherdauberbehandlung bei patienten mit obstruktiver Kardiomyopathie. *Thoraxchirurgie* 1975; **23**: 469–98.
9 Johnson AD, Daily PO. Hypertrophic subaortic stenosis complicated by high degree heart block: Successful treatment with atrial synchronous ventricular pacemaker. *Chest* 1975; **23**: 496–9.
10 Duport G, Valeix B, Lefebvre J *et al.* Intérêt de la stimulation droite permanente dans la cardiomyopathie obstructive. *Nouv Presse Med* 1978; **32**: 2868–9.
11 Duck HJ, Hutschenreiter W, Pankau H *et al* Vorhofsynchrone Ventrikelstimulation mit verkurzter a.v. verzogerungszeit als Therapieprinzip der hypertrophischen obstruktiven Kardiomyopathie. *Z Gesamte Inn Med* 1984; **39**: 437–47.
12 McDonald K, McWilliams E, O'Keeffe B *et al* Functional assessment of patients treated with permanent dual-chamber pacing as a primary treatment for hypertrophic cardiomyopathy. *Eur Heart J* 1988; **9**: 893–8.
13 Gadler F, Linde C, Juhlin-Dannfeldt A *et al.* Influence of right ventricular pacing site on left ventricular outflow tract obstruction in patients with hypertrophic obstructive cardiomyopathy. *J Am Coll Cardiol* 1996; **27**: 1219–24.
14 Jeanrenaud X, Schläpfer J, Fromer M *et al.* Dual chamber pacing in hypertrophic obstructive cardiomyopathy: Beneficial effect of atrioventricular junction ablation for optimal left ventricular capture and filling. *Pacing Clin Electrophysiol* 1997; **20**: 293–300.
15 Gras D, De Place C, Le Breton H *et al.* L'importance du synchronisme auriculo-ventriculaire dans la cardiomyopathie hypertrophique obstructive traitée par stimulation cardiaque. *Arch Mal Cœur* 1995; **88**: 215–23.

16 Jeanrenaud X, Goy JJ, Kappenberger L. Functional assessment of patients treated with permanent dual chamber pacing as a primary treatment for hypertrophic cardiomyopathy. *Lancet* 1992; **339**: 1318–23.

17 Jeanrenaud X, Kappenberger L. Regional wall motion during pacing for hypertrophic obstructive cardiomyopathy. *Pacing Clin Electrophysiol* 1997; **20**: 1673–81.

18 Pollick C, Rakowski H, Wigle ED. Muscular subaortic stenosis: The quantitative relationship between systolic anterior motion and the pressure gradient. *Circulation* 1984; **69**: 43–9.

19 Leclercq C, Gras D, Le Helloco A *et al*. Hemodynamic interest of preserving a normal sequence of ventricular activation in permanent cardiac pacing. *Am Heart J* 1995; **129**: 1133–1141.

20 Nishimura RA, Hayes DL, Ilstrup DM *et al*. Effect of dual-chamber pacing on systolic and diastolic function in patients with hypertrophic cardiomyopathy. *J Am Coll Cardiol* 1996; **27**: 421–30.

21 Pak PH, Maughan LW, Baughman KL *et al*. Mechanism of acute mechanical benefit from VDD pacing in hypertrophied heart. Similarity of responses in hypertrophic cardiomyopathy and hypertensive heart disease. *Circulation* 1998; **98**: 242–8.

22 Zile MR, Blaustein AS, Shimizu G *et al*. Right ventricular pacing reduces the rate of left ventricular relaxation and filling. *J Am Coll Cardiol* 1987; **10**: 702–9.

23 Brutsaert DL, Rademakers FE, Sys SU. Triple control of relaxation: Implications in cardiac disease. *Circulation* 1984; **69**: 190–6.

24 Betocchi S, Losi M-A, Piscione F *et al*. Effects of dual-chamber pacing in hypertrophic cardiomyopathy on left ventricular outflow tract obstruction and on diastolic function. *Am J Cardiol* 1996; **77**: 498–502.

25 Pavin D, de Place C, Le Breton H *et al*. Effects of permanent dual chamber pacing on mitral regurgitation in hypertrophic obstructive cardiomyopathy. *Eur Heart J* 1999; **20**: 203–10.

26 Prinzen FW, Hunter WC, Wyman BT *et al* Mapping of regional myocardial strain and work during ventricular pacing: Experimental study using magnetic resonance imaging tagging. *J Am Coll Cardiol* 1999; **33**: 1735–42.

27 Amitzur G, Manor D, Pressman A *et al*. Modulation of the arterial coronary blood flow by asynchronous activation with ventricular pacing. *Pacing Clin Electrophysiol* 1995; **18**: 697–710.

28 Posma JL, Blanksma PK, van der Wall EE *et al*. Effects of permanent dual chamber pacing on myocardial perfusion in symptomatic hypertrophic cardiomyopathy. *Heart* 1996; **76**: 358–62.

29 Van Oosterhout MF, Arts T, Muijtjens AM *et al*. Remodeling by ventricular pacing in hypertrophying dog hearts. *Cardiovasc Res* 2001; **49**: 771–8.

30 Fananapazir L, Epstein ND, Curiel RV *et al*. Long-term results of dual-chamber (DDD) pacing in obstructive hypertrophic cardiomyopathy: Evidence for progressive symptomatic and hemodynamic improvement and reduction of left ventricular hypertrophy. *Circulation* 1994; **90**: 2731–42.

31 Maron BJ, Nishimura RA, McKenna W *et al*. for the M-PATHY Study Investigators. Assessment of permanent dual-chamber pacing as a treatment for drug-refractory symptomatic patients with obstructive hypertrophic cardiomyopathy: A randomized, double-blind, crossover study (M-PATHY). *Circulation* 1999; **99**: 2927–33.

32 Jeanrenaud X, Aebischer N, Kappenberger L and the PIC Study Group. Influence of DDD pacing on LV parameters in hypertrophic obstructive cardiomyopathy: Results of the PIC Study [abstract]. *J Am Coll Cardiol* 1998; **31**: 183.

33 Fananapazir L, Cannon RO, Tripodi D *et al.* Impact of dual-chamber permanent pacing in patients with obstructive hypertrophic cardiomyopathy with symptoms refractory to verapamil and beta-adrenergic blocker therapy. *Circulation* 1992; **85**: 2149–61.

34 Sadoul N, Simon JP, de Chillou C *et al.* Intérêts de la stimulation cardiaque permanente dans les myocardiopathies hypertrophiques et obstructives rebelles au traitement médical. *Arch Mal Cœur* 1994; **87**: 1315–23.

35 Slade AKB, Sadoul N, Shapiro L *et al.* DDD pacing in hypertrophic cardiomyopathy. A multicentre clinical experience. *Heart* 1996; **75**: 44–9.

36 Gadler F, Linde C, Juhlin-Dannfelt A *et al.* Long-term effects of dual chamber pacing in patients with hypertrophic cardiomyopathy without outflow tract obstruction at rest. *Eur Heart J* 1997; **18**: 636–42.

37 Kappenberger L, Linde C, Jeanrenaud X *et al.* for the Pacing in Cardiomyopathy (PIC) Study Group. *Europace* 1999; **1**: 77–84.

38 Nishimura RA, Trusty JM, Hayes DL *et al.* Dual-chamber pacing for hypertrophic cardiomyopathy: A randomized, double-blind, crossover trial. *J Am Coll Cardiol* 1997; **29**: 435–41.

39 Linde C, Gadler F, Kappenberger L *et al.* for the PIC Study Group. Placebo effect of pacemaker implantation in obstructive hypertrophic cardiomyopathy. *Am J Cardiol* 1999; **83**: 903–7.

40 Gadler F, Linde C, Ryden L. Rapid return of left ventricular outflow tract obstruction and symptoms following cessation of long-term atrioventricular synchronous pacing for obstructive hypertrophic cardiomyopathy. *Am J Cardiol* 1999; **83**: 553–7.

41 ACC/AHA/NASPE Guideline Update for Implantation of Cardiac Pacemakers and Antiarrhythmia Devices. *Circulation* 2002; **106**: 2146–61.

42 Rishi F, Hulse EJ, Auld DO *et al.* Effects of dual-chamber pacing for pediatric patients with hypertrophic obstructive cardiomyopathy. *J Am Coll Cardiol* 1997; **29**: 734–40.

43 Kappenberger L, Linde C, Daubert C *et al.* Pacing in hypertrophic obstructive cardiomyopathy: A randomized cross-over study. *Eur Heart J* 1997; **18**: 1249–56.

CHAPTER 18

Alcohol Septal Ablation

**Hubert Seggewiss, MD Prof, Angelos Rigopoulos, MD,
Lothar Faber, MD, and Peer Ziemssen, MD**

Treatment of symptomatic patients with hypertrophic obstructive cardiomy-opathy (HOCM) aims to reduce symptoms, improve functional capacity and provide better quality of life.[1,2] This can be achieved by reducing the extent of the outflow tract gradient and improving diastolic filling. Medical therapy, with the administration of negatively inotropic drugs, e.g. β-blockers,[3–5] vera-pamil[4,6] or disopyramide,[7,8] is always the first line of treatment. Unfortunately, at least 10% of patients with marked outflow tract obstruction have severe symptoms, which are unresponsive to medical therapy.[9] In this group, surgical treatment with myectomy–myotomy has been the mainstay for decades, providing long-term symptomatic relief in a substantial proportion of patients, albeit with relatively high mortality, which is now reduced to <2% in highly experienced centers.[10–13] Dual-chamber pacing was subsequently introduced as an alternative to surgery. Although it was initially presented as a very effective treatment,[14] it has not proven to be as efficacious in randomized trials, most of the reported reduction of symptoms being due to a substantial placebo effect.[15–17] Percutaneous transluminal septal myocardial ablation (PTSMA), through alcohol-induced occlusion of a septal branch, aims directly to reduce the hypertrophied interventricular septum with associated expansion of the left ventricular outflow tract (LVOT) and reduction of the subaortic gradient.[18] This is achieved through a circumscribed infarction of the area supplied by the occluded septal branch.

Historical perspective

The idea of percutaneous septal myocardial ablation by inducing a localized therapeutic myocardial infarction due to alcohol-induced septal branch occlusion was considered in the 1980s, as a consequence of the favorable hemodynamic and clinical results of surgical myectomy and the growing experience of interventional cardiologists. The PTSMA technique was originally described in 1989 (G. Berghoefer, personal communication) after a similar chemical septal branch ablation procedure had already been described as a therapy of ventricular dysrhythmia.[19] Initial studies showed that temporary balloon occlusion of the first larger septal branch resulted in substantial resting outflow gradient reduction in a minority of patients.[20,21] Sigwart was the first to report a successful nonsurgical myocardial reduction after occlusion of the septal branch using 96% alcohol.[20]

Technique

The original technique of PTSMA has undergone several modifications with the intention of improving the identification of the target septal perforator branch, in order to achieve the optimal hemodynamic result with fewer complications.[20,22,23] The technique described below is the one currently performed by most of the active PTSMA groups.[18]

All operators agree that a temporary pacemaker should be placed in the right ventricle because of the risk of trifascicular block during PTSMA. Following exclusion of an aortic valve gradient, the left ventricular outflow tract gradient is recorded simultaneously via a PTCA (percutaneous transluminal coronary angioplasty) guiding catheter placed in the ascending aorta and a 5F specially designed pigtail catheter, with holes only in its distal part and not on the shaft (Cordis), placed in the apex of the left ventricle. The potential risk of trans-septal puncture can be avoided in this way. The LVOT gradient is then recorded both at rest and during provocative maneuvers, such as the Valsalva maneuver and after an extrasystolic beat (Fig. 18.1a). In order to avoid thromboembolic complications, weight-adjusted heparin should be administered intravenously. Furthermore, analgesic premedication is necessary to suppress pain during the alcohol injection.

After angiographic identification of the target septal branch that is presumed to be responsible for the blood supply to the hypertrophied septal area involved in obstruction (Fig. 18.2a), wiring of this vessel is performed with a 0.014-inch angioplasty guidewire. Afterwards, a short (≤1 cm in length) over-the-wire balloon catheter is advanced and inflated in the septal branch. This type of short balloon catheter, specially produced by some companies for this procedure, prevents the balloon from being positioned in the left anterior descending coronary artery (LAD) (Fig. 18.2b), which could potentially cause reduction of blood flow or dissection of the LAD. To avoid alcohol leakage in the LAD, a slightly oversized balloon (compared with septal branch diameter) is used. In addition, injection of a small amount of dye (1–2 ml) through the guidewire lumen of the inflated balloon catheter angiographically determines the supply area of the septal branch and excludes the possibility of reflux of contrast medium (and thus of alcohol) into the LAD (Fig. 18.2c). In order to identify the target septal branch and to exclude alcohol injection into wrong areas (e.g. the papillary muscle or the left ventricular free wall), echocardiographic monitoring of the procedure was introduced.[23,24] Prior to alcohol injection, 1–2 ml of echo contrast medium (Levovist®; Schering, Berlin, Germany) is administered through the central lumen of the balloon catheter under color Doppler and two-dimensional echocardiographic monitoring (Fig. 18.3). Injection into the optimal septal branch results, on the one hand, in complete coverage of the echo-contrast-marked septal area and the color

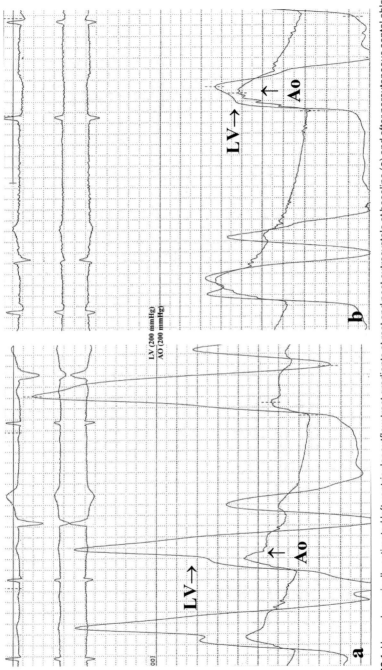

Fig. 18.1 Hemodynamically estimated left ventricular outflow tract gradients at rest and post extrasystole at baseline (**a**) and after percutaneous septal ablation (**b**). LV = left ventricular outflow tract pressure; Ao = aortic pressure.

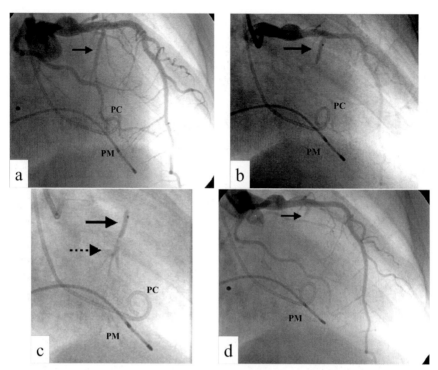

Fig. 18.2 Left coronary angiography shows the target septal branch (arrow) typically originating from the left antery descending artery (LAD) in RAO (**a**). Optimal position of the ballon catheter (arrow) in the proximal part of the septal artery without compromise of the LAD (**b**). Injection of dye through the central lumen of the inflated ballon (arrow) determines the supply area of the septal branch (dotted arrow) and excludes leakage into the LAD (**c**). Final visualization of the vessel stump (arrow) after alcohol-induced septal branch occlusion (**d**). PC = pigtail catheter; PM = pacemaker lead.

Doppler-estimated area of maximal flow acceleration, as well as the area of systolic anterior motion septal contact, without, on the other hand, opacification of any other cardiac structure (Fig. 18.4). Several echocardiographic views are examined and compared with baseline echocardiograms. Once the above criteria are fulfilled, 2 ml (to 4 ml) of 96% alcohol in 1-ml portions is injected through the central lumen of the over-the-wire balloon, irrespective of the hemodynamic result from preliminary balloon occlusion. The amount of alcohol depends on the acute hemodynamic effect and the echocardiographically estimated size of the contrasted septal area. At least 10 minutes after the last injection of alcohol, the balloon catheter is deflated and removed, thus ensuring that no alcohol can flow into the LAD.[25] A final angiographic control excludes LAD damage and verifies septal branch occlusion (Fig. 18.2d), whereas final hemodynamic measurements confirm the acute result of septal ablation (Fig. 18.1b). Finally, hemodynamic and arrhythmia monitoring at the coronary care unit is required for at least 24–48 hours.

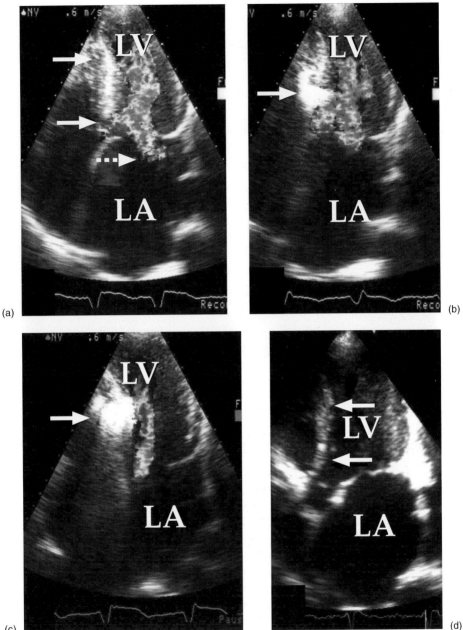

Fig. 18.3 Apical four-chamber view in a patient with subaortic and midcavitary obstruction (arrows) and gradient-associated mitral regurgitation (dotted arrow) after surgical myectomy (**a**). Myocardial contrast-echo of the first septal branch shows coverage of the subaortic area (**b**). Myocardial contrast-echo of the second septal branch after alcohol ablation of the first branch shows significant reduction of the subaortic gradient and coverage of the midcavitary gradient area of the ventricular septum (arrow) (**c**). Three months after PTSMA, thinning of the subaortic and midcavitary septum can be seen (**d**). LV = left ventricle; LA = left atrium.

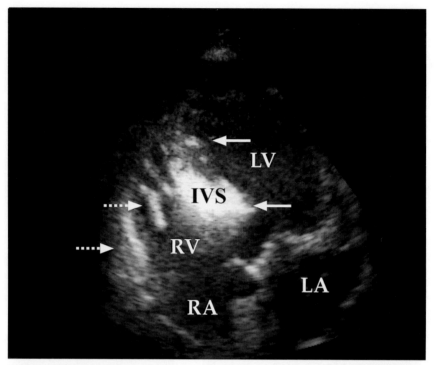

Fig. 18.4 Angulated apical four-chamber view with echo-contrast opacification of the intraventricular septum (IVS; arrows), right ventricular free wall and papillary muscle (dotted arrows). RV = right ventricle, RA = right atrium; LV = left ventricle, LA = left atrium.

Indications and contraindications

A clinical indication for PTSMA is given in symptomatic patients with a New York Heart Association (NYHA) class of at least III and/or Canadian Cardiovascular Society (CCS) class III despite optimal drug therapy, and in patients with substantial side-effects of medication in whom high outflow tract gradients (≥50 mm Hg at rest or ≥100 mm Hg under stress) can be verified.[18] Patients with less severe symptoms should only be treated if they have high gradients and additional findings, such as recurrent exercise-induced syncope, abnormal blood pressure response at exercise, paroxysmal atrial fibrillation and/or objective reduction of exercise capacity. Nevertheless, it should be taken into consideration that there are no data that suggest that gradient reduction reduces the risk for sudden death, although a resting gradient of more than 30 mm Hg has been correlated with a higher risk for HCM-related death.[26,27] A morphologic indication for echocardiographically guided septal ablation is given in patients with subaortic as well as midcavitary obstruction (Fig. 18.3).

Patients with previous, but hemodynamically unsuccessful, surgical myectomy or DDD pacemaker implantation can also be treated with alcohol ablation. Patients with concomitant cardiac diseases indicating surgery, such as extensive coronary artery disease, valvular disease, and morphologic changes of the mitral valve or papillary muscle responsible for gradient formation or mitral regurgitation, should not be treated interventionally. Furthermore, hypertrophic cardiomyopathy without significant resting or provocable outflow tract gradient is a clear contraindication for PTSMA. Alcohol should not be injected when myocardial contrast echocardiography fails to identify a target septal branch or reveals opacification of any cardiac structure other than the target septal area (Fig. 18.4), or when balloon positioning carries a risk of alcohol reflux during injection.

Symptomatic patients with both HOCM and coronary artery disease requiring revascularization are normally referred for a combined surgical treatment (myectomy and bypass grafting), which is, however, associated with an increased surgical risk. In cases with single-vessel disease amenable to dilatation and stenting, a combined percutaneous treatment (PTCA and PTSMA) can be performed.[28]

Results

Acute results

At the present time, more than 1000 patients are known to have been treated worldwide. LVOT gradient reduction can be achieved acutely in about 90% of treated patients.[20,22,23,25,29–36]

In our experience, an acute reduction of LVOT gradients, from 72 ± 36 to 20 ± 22 mm Hg ($P < 0.00001$) at rest and from 148 ± 43 to 62 ± 44 mm Hg after extrasystole ($P < 0.00001$), has been achieved.[18] Younger patients (less than 40 years of age) had less gradient reduction than elderly patients,[37] probably due to greater septal thickness and additional morphologic changes, such as abnormal papillary muscles. Nevertheless, about 50% of young patients with an insufficient acute result show improvement of gradient reduction at follow-up due to postinfarction remodeling and shrinkage of the ablated septal area. Patients with functional class IV showed acute results comparable with those in less symptomatic patients.[38]

Reasons for insignificant gradient reduction can be procedure- and patient-related. Suboptimal scar localization can be ruled out by echocardiographic monitoring of PTSMA. Before diagnosing a definitive insufficiently large PTSMA scar, completion of the remodeling process, which lasts up to 12 months, should be awaited. One possible reason for an insufficient scar is the underlying histologic change in the hypertrophied septum. If fibrosis is predominant, a sufficient scar of the myocardium may not be achieved. Additional pre-interventional noninvasive estimation of the underlying histologic change will probably be helpful in the future in excluding these patients from PTSMA. Careful pre-PTSMA echo is helpful in identifying elongation of the mitral leaflet, which can result in less pronounced hemodynamic success.

Value of echo guidance

Echo guidance with myocardial contrast echocardiography (MCE) had a crucial impact on the selection of the ablated area in about one-fourth of our patients. Echo contrast helped to identify an atypically originating septal branch as the target vessel (Fig. 18.5) or to avoid alcohol misplacement by changing the vessel if there had been echo contrast opacification of the wrong septal areas or other cardiac structures, such as the papillary muscles or ventricular free walls (Fig. 18.4). Our findings were confirmed by an autopsy study by Singh and colleagues.[39] They showed large variability in the size and distribution of the first septal perforating artery with supply of the right ventricular free wall in 20% of patients and an incomplete supply of the subaortic septum by the first septal branch in 40% of patients. Furthermore, in our hands a target septal area could not be identified in about 5% of cases; in these cases the procedure was stopped before injecting alcohol, thus avoiding possible complications due to necrotization of non-target cardiac structures.

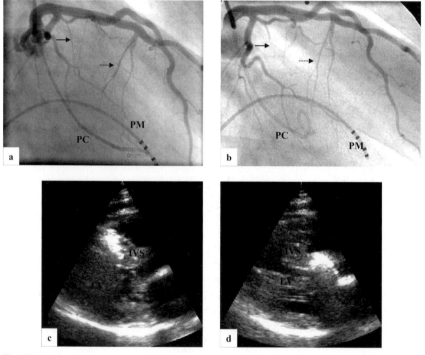

Fig. 18.5 Left coronary angiography shows the target septal branch (arrow) atypically originating from the intermediate branch in RAO (**a**). Injection of echo-contrast dye into the first typically originating septal branch (dotted arrow) determines the supply area in the midcavitary part (dotted arrow) of the ventricular septum (IVS) whereas the subaortic area (**b**, arrow) is not supplied by this branch (**c**). Change to the atypically originating septal branch (b; arrow) results in optimal opacification of the subaortic IVS (arrow) (**d**). PC = pigtail catheter; PM = pacemaker lead; LV = left ventricle; LA = left atrium.

Moreover, the induced scar can be limited to an optimally necessary size by using myocardial contrast echocardiography, thus avoiding the development of a large septal scar with all its associated potential negative consequences for left ventricular systolic and diastolic function. This has been shown by the reduced increase in creatine kinase after the introduction of echo guidance,[23] in conjunction with the higher percentage of patients with an outflow tract gradient reduction greater than 50% (in 86% of patients with MCE, compared with only 70% of patients without MCE) ($P < 0.05$). As Ruzyllo and colleagues reported, a gradient reduction of 50% compared with baseline values is required in order to achieve an improvement in objective exercise measurements.[25]

Furthermore, echocardiographic monitoring of the procedure has probably helped to avoid most of the potential complications related to acute myocardial infarction, such as the occurrence of ventricular and supraventricular dysrhythmia, infranodal trifascicular blocks depending on the course and supply of the His bundle, and iatrogenic ventricular septal defects, cerebral embolisms, and papillary muscle rupture with ensuing acute mitral insufficiency, depending on the distribution pattern of the injected alcohol. Furthermore, the need for re-interventions, with occlusion of several septal branches, was reduced, thus avoiding unnecessary enlargement of the septal scar with all its associated potential negative consequences for left ventricular systolic or diastolic function and increased risk of sudden death. Echocardiographic monitoring also permits the interventional treatment of combined subaortic and midventricular obstruction, and of a pronounced midventricular obstruction following the reduction of its afterload after successful subaortic myectomy.[40]

Complications

In-hospital death is the most significant complication observed to date, with a rate of up to 4%.[34] Our own experience with PTSMA in about 500 patients showed hospital mortality of less than 1.0%, which is at least comparable to rates at experienced surgical myectomy centers (Table 18.1). These deaths have only occurred in elderly patients and during the postinterventional period, which underlines the importance of careful hospital monitoring. Particular attention should be paid to reports of delayed occurrence of complete heart block up to 10 days after the intervention, which underlines the need for close arrhythmic monitoring for several days following the intervention.[41]

The most frequent complications are peri- and postinterventional trifascicular blocks, which occur at a rate of 60%, but in most cases these blocks are only transitory. After the introduction of MCE the number of permanent pacemaker implantations due to permanent trifascicular block was reduced to less than 5%, a nearly postoperative range.[10] Furthermore, the development of complete heart block after septal ablation can be predicted using a score that has been introduced by Faber and colleagues.[42] Besides trifascicular blocks, all groups reported on the occurrence of bundle branch block in about 50% of patients, predominantly involving the right bundle branch, in contrast to many patients after surgical myectomy, who show left bundle branch block.

Table 18.1 Published acute results of alcohol septal ablation. LAD = left anterior descending coronary artery; NR = not reported. *Six patients with pacemaker implantation before PTSMA

Author	Patients (n)	Success without complication (%)	Death (%)	Pacer (%)	Comments
Seggewiss et al.[22]	25	88	4.0	20	No echo monitoring
Faber et al.[23]	91	97	2.2	11	Improvement of results by echo monitoring
Gietzen et al.[34]	50	NR	4.0	NR	12 re-interventions; no echo monitoring
Nagueh et al.[33]	29	NR	0	34	4 patients with only provocable gradients at dobutamine infusion
Knight et al.[29]	18	89	0	5*	1 patient alcohol leakage down the LAD
Kornacewicz–Jach et al.[32]	9	100	0	22	Echo monitoring
Kuhn et al.[43]	172	NR	2.3	NR	No echo monitoring
Seggewiss[18]	290	90	1.0	5.5	DDD pacer rate with echo monitoring 4.2%
Boekstegers et al.[46]	50	NR	0	10	No echo monitoring; 2 septal branches in 6 patients
Schweinfurt (5/00 to 4/02)	150	92	0.7	1.3	Echo monitoring

Contrary to the incidence of significant ventricular dysrhythmia in patients with myocardial infarction due to coronary artery disease, the incidence of such dysrhythmia during and after ablation is rare. The reason for this may be found in the findings of pathologic examinations, which illustrate a marked distinction between the myocardial necrosis induced by the ablation and the noninfarcted myocardium, in contradiction to patients with myocardial infarction due to coronary artery disease.[43] In addition, the QT interval decreases to under the pre-interventional values during follow-up, possibly contributing to the lack of occurrence of ventricular dysrhythmia following induced infarction.[22]

A dreaded complication that has been reported is iatrogenic reflux of alcohol into the LAD with transitory vessel occlusion and anterolateral ischemia.[25,29] This can be avoided by the use of a slightly oversized balloon and angiography of the LAD after each injection of alcohol, which should be slowly administered in fractions of 1 ml, and septal branch balloon occlusion for 10 minutes after the last alcohol injection. Ruzyllo and colleagues managed to avoid alcohol leakage by prolonging septal branch balloon occlusion after having seen this dangerous phenomenon in the three of the first 12 patients in whom the balloon was deflated after only 5 minutes after the last alcohol injection.[25]

Balloon-induced dissections of the LAD can be avoided by positioning the balloon completely in the septal branch. Other reported complications included the occurrence of a peri-interventional ventricular septal defect at day 11, a cerebral embolism with persisting neurological deficit, LAD and left main coronary dissections due to the guidewire requiring emergency stent implantation or emergency bypass surgery and causing a large myocardial infarction, acute mitral regurgitation (probably due to necrosis of a papillary muscle), and large right and left ventricular free wall infarctions due to unexpected alcohol runoff into these areas. Most of these complications underline the importance of echocardiographic monitoring of the procedure, which may well have avoided many of them.

Follow-up studies

Clinical and hemodynamic follow-up studies of up to 6 years have shown no increased risk of sudden death or arrhythmic complications.[44] During a mean follow-up period of 43 months (up to 72 months), seven out of 178 (4%) patients died. Two of these patients died due to sudden cardiac death and stroke, respectively, whereas the other patients died from malignant diseases. Only two patients (one patient with additional coronary artery disease) in the series required the implantation of a cardioverter–defibrillator due to clinically relevant ventricular tachycardias. Furthermore, septal perforation has not been reported during follow-up.

The most important finding is an impressive symptomatic improvement during short- and long-term follow-up after outflow tract gradient reduction, which is reported by all groups. Mean functional class improved from

NYHA 2.8 ± 0.6 to 1.6 ± 0.7 after a mean follow-up period of more than 3 years ($P < 0.001$).

Objective measurements showed an increase in exercise capacity from 88 ± 57 to 110 ± 40 watts after 3 months ($P < 0.0001$), with an ongoing effect evident after 2 years (122 ± 43 watts).[18] Long-term follow-up studies showed that the increase of exercise capacity was a long-lasting effect (Fig. 18.6).[44] These observations are similar to reports from other groups with a follow-up period up to 3 years in the original London series.[29] Spiro-ergometry data of a subgroup of our own patients and those of other authors show a significant increase in oxygen consumption.[45,46]

From the hemodynamic standpoint, the most important finding is the continuing and increasing reduction of the LVOT gradients (Fig. 18.7).[18,44] Compared with the acute results, 56% of our patients revealed a further reduction in their resting and provocable gradients after 3 months. Compared with the 3-month follow-up, 43% of the patients had a further gradient reduction after 1 year. These changes resulted in complete reduction of gradients in 40% of the patients after 3 months and in 62% after 1 year ($P < 0.01$). After a mean follow-up of 43 months, 90% of the patients showed complete elimination of the outflow tract gradient. This should be appraised as an expression of post-interventional remodeling following an induced septal infarction, analogous to the remodeling that occurs after acute myocardial infarction. These findings also underscore the rationale of our strategy in inducing septal necrosis by alcohol ablation, which, whilst sufficiently large, should be as small as possible.

Remodeling after PTSMA results in reduction of both the ventricular septal thickness and the left ventricular posterior wall thickness[18,44,47] (Fig. 18.8). As in

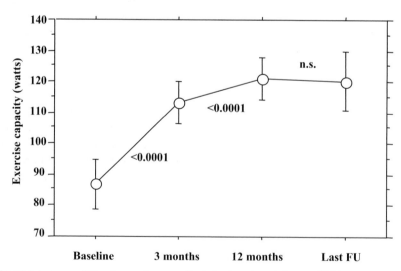

Fig. 18.6 Increase of bicycle exercise capacity during long-term follow-up (FU) in 178 patients.

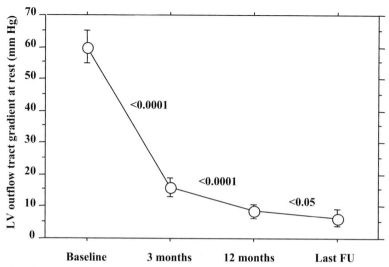

Fig. 18.7 Ongoing reduction of left ventricular outflow tract gradients at rest during long-term follow-up (FU) in 178 patients.

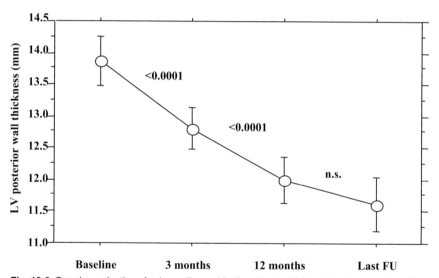

Fig. 18.8 Ongoing reduction of echocardiographically estimated left ventricular posterior wall thickness during long-term follow-up (FU) in 178 patients.

the case of surgical myectomy,[48] these findings must be interpreted as a result of the elimination (or at least reduction) of the pressure overload. Negative effects of the induced septal infarction, especially left ventricular enlargement, have not been described. Our studies found a decrease in left atrial diameter and mitral regurgitation. Furthermore, some groups report reduction of both left ventricular end-diastolic pressure and mean pulmonary arterial pressure.[9,23,29,34,46] Preliminary studies have shown a reduction in the risk factors that have been reported for sudden cardiac death, such as exertional syncope, abnormal blood pressure response, and exercise-induced ischemia, after successful PTSMA.[49]

HOCM and concomitant cardiac disease

HOCM and mitral regurgitation

In patients with subaortic obstruction, the severity of mitral regurgitation is directly related to the severity of systolic anterior motion of the mitral leaflet. The effective thinning of the septum and the resulting widening of the outflow tract after PTSMA lead to a reduction or obliteration of systolic anterior motion and mitral regurgitation. However, care should be taken during the echocardiographic assessment to exclude structural abnormalities, such as anomalous papillary muscle or mitral valve prolapse, which can cause mitral regurgitation that is not associated with systolic anterior motion and therefore cannot be expected to decrease with PTSMA. Patients with such structural abnormalities of the mitral valve should be referred for surgical treatment.

HOCM and coronary artery disease

Symptomatic patients with HOCM and concomitant coronary artery disease requiring revascularization constitute a special group that calls for individualized treatment. Our own data show that about 12% of symptomatic patients suffer from additional coronary artery disease.[50] Patients with a clear surgical indication for revascularization can be referred for a combined operation that includes myectomy, but the increased risk associated with this kind of treatment needs to be acknowledged. Patients with single-vessel coronary artery disease amenable to interventional treatment can have coronary angioplasty and PTSMA at the same time when the coronary lesion is in the left anterior descending artery.[28] This way, the PTSMA is performed first and is followed by the coronary intervention. The combined procedure does not increase the interventional risk if the patients have been selected carefully.[50] Otherwise, it should be more prudent to treat the coronary lesion, i.e. in the right or the circumflex coronary artery, and reassess the patient after 6 months. If the symptoms persist PTSMA should be performed then, provided that the result of the coronary angioplasty remains satisfactory.

HOCM and conduction disease

Any kind of arrhythmia or conduction disturbance that is considered to cause hemodynamic decompensation in patients with HOCM should be treated first, before there is any thought of PTSMA or myectomy. In particular, pacemaker implantation in patients with severe bradycardia or conduction abnormality should preferably precede any other invasive treatment. After all, DDD pacemaking has been shown to be beneficial in some patients with HOCM, leading to symptomatic improvement.[16]

Comparison of PTSMA with myectomy

Up to now, no randomized trials comparing surgical and percutaneous treatment of septal reduction in HOCM have been published. Nonrandomized trials have shown a significant reduction of LVOT obstruction and symptomatic improvement with both treatment options.[51–53] Therefore, the benefits and drawbacks of each therapeutic method must be balanced when deciding on treatment for LVOT obstruction. This decision must take into consideration several clinical, morphological, and technical aspects.

The advantages of percutaneous septal ablation comprise the avoidance of cardiopulmonary bypass with its attendant risks (especially in elderly patients with concomitant noncardiac disease), as well as shorter hospital stay and recovery time. Nevertheless, it is necessary to take into consideration that too short a period of hospitalization may carry the risk of late out-of-hospital heart block. Furthermore, the percutaneous approach is less expensive.

Potential drawbacks of PTSMA in comparison with myectomy are the risk of damage to the left coronary artery, requiring emergency bypass surgery or left main/LAD stenting, and the technical impossibility of reaching or identifying a target septal branch. In these patients elective myectomy can be performed. Mitral valve leaflet and papillary muscle abnormalities can prevent a good result after septal ablation.

Furthermore, younger patients with large septal thickness must be informed about the possibility of less frequently successful ablation. On the other hand, it has been be shown that, in contrast to previous ideas,[54] even patients with isolated midcavitary[40] or combined subaortic and midcavitary obstruction (Fig. 18.3) can be successfully treated by echo-guided percutaneous septal ablation.

The advantages of myectomy surgery are more immediate and complete relief of resting and provoked obstruction and concomitant mitral regurgitation, in addition to good long-term results (up to 30 years) in contrast to the 7-year follow-up results after percutaneous septal ablation. Although there is no risk of coronary dissection or unwanted myocardial infarction, most surgical series report a low risk of aortic regurgitation after surgery. Arrhythmogenic effects after myectomy have not been described. While there are some reports of the successful combined simultaneous or staged percutaneous treatment of HOCM and coronary artery disease[28,50] surgery can deal with HOCM and coexistent cardiac diseases, such as coronary artery disease, valve replacement, right ventricular obstruction, and constricting muscle bridges over the left anterior descending coronary artery. Extended myectomy, as introduced by Messmer and Schoendube, allows additional treatment of papillary muscle abnormalities, which are common in hypertrophic cardiomyopathy.[13] As in percutaneous septal ablation, echocardiographic monitoring of the myectomy is important for the optimization of surgical results.[55]

However, there are some reports of left ventricular deterioration resulting in heart transplantation after extended myectomy during long-term follow-up. One of the possible reasons for this may be the high incidence of left bundle branch block, with its possible negative impact in patients with impaired LV function due to the asynchronous contraction.

Overall, surgery and percutaneous septal ablation should be regarded as alternatives in HOCM. An individual decision has to be taken in each patient in order to achieve optimal results. Beside the points we have mentioned, the individual experience of the center should be taken into consideration.

Summary

Nearly one decade after its introduction, percutaneous septal ablation is a promising treatment option for symptomatic patients with HOCM that is refractory to medical treatment. The morphologic, hemodynamic, and clinical effects (Fig. 18.9) have been well described. Intra-procedure echocardiographic monitoring results in optimization of the ablated septal area with reduction of peri-interventional complications and improvement of acute and mid-term hemodynamic results. However, possible complications and limited long-term effects mandate careful patient selection. In order to avoid overuse of the technique we would underline the importance of restricting alcohol septal ablation

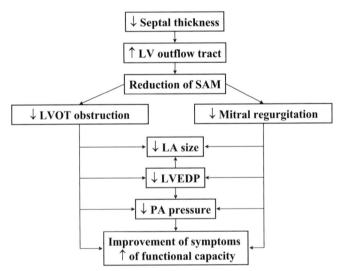

Fig. 18.9 Morphologic, hemodynamic, and clinical effects of percutaneous septal ablation (↓ = reduction; ↑ = increase; LV = left ventricle; SAM = systolic movement of the mitral valve apparatus; LVOT = left ventricular outflow tract; LA = left atrium; LVEDP = left ventricular end-diastolic pressure; PA = pulmonary artery).

to a few centers with large interventional and echocardiographic experience and knowledge of this uncommon disease.

References

1 Wigle ED, Rakowski H, Kimball BP, Williams WG. Hypertrophic cardiomyopathy: Clinical spectrum and treatment. *Circulation* 1995; **92**: 1680–92.

2 Spirito P, Seidman CE, McKenna WJ, Maron BJ. The management of hypertrophic cardiomyopathy. *N Engl J Med* 1997; **336**: 775–85.

3 Frank MJ, Abdulla AM, Canedo MI, Saylors RE. Long-term medical management of hypertrophic obstructive cardiomyopathy. *Am J Cardiol* 1978; **42**: 993–1001.

4 Haberer T, Hess OM, Jenni R, Krayenbühl HP. Hypertrophic obstructive cardiomyopathy: Spontaneous course in comparison to long-term therapy with propanolol and verapamil. *Z Kardiol* 1983; **72**: 487–93.

5 Harrison DC, Braunwald E, Glick G, Mason DT, Chidsey CA, Ross J Jr. Effects of beta adrenergic blockade on the circulation with particular reference to observations in patients with hypertrophic subaortic stenosis. *Circulation* 1964; **29**: 84–98.

6 Kaltenbach M, Hopf R, Kober G, Bussmann WD, Keller M, Petersen Y. Treatment of hypertrophic obstructive cardiomyopathy with verapamil. *Br Heart J* 1979; **42**: 35–42.

7 Pollick C. Muscular subaortic stenosis: Hemodynamic and clinical improvement after disopyramide: *N Engl J Med* 1982; **307**: 997–9.

8 Kimball BP, Bui S, Wigle ED. Acute dose–response effects of intravenous disopyramide in hypertrophic obstructive cardiomyopathy. *Am Heart J* 1993; **125**: 1691–7.

9 Maron BJ. Appraisal of dual-chamber pacing therapy in hypertrophic cardiomyopathy: Too soon for a rush to judgment? *J Am Coll Cardiol* 1996; **27**: 431–2.

10 Schulte HD, Gramsch-Zabel H, Schwartzkopff B. Hypertrophe obstruktive Kardiomyopathie: Chirurgische Behandlung. [In German.] *Schweiz Med Wochenschr* 1995; **125**: 1940–9.

11 Robbins RC, Stinson EB, Daily PO. Long-term results of left ventricular myotomy and myectomy for obstructive hypertrophic cardiomyopathy. *J Thorac Cardiovasc Surg* 1996; **111**: 586–94.

12 Heric B, Lytle BW, Miller DP *et al.* Surgical management of hypertrophic obstructive cardiomyopathy: Early and late results. *J Thorac Cardiovasc Surg* 1995; **110**: 195–208.

13 Schoendube FA, Klues HG, Reith S *et al.* Long-term clinical and echocardiographic follow-up after surgical correction of hypertrophic obstructive cardiomyopathy with extended myectomy and reconstruction of the subvalvular mitral apparatus. *Circulation* 1995; **92** (Suppl. II): 122–7.

14 Fananapazir L, Epstein ND, Curiel RV, Panza JA, Tripodi D, McAreavey D. Long-term results of dual-chamber (DDD) pacing in obstructive hypertrophic cardiomyopathy: Evidence for progressive symptomatic and hemodynamic improvement and reduction of left ventricular hypertrophy. *Circulation* 1994; **90**: 2731–42.

15 Nishimura RA, Trusty JM, Hayes DL *et al.* Dual-chamber pacing for hypertrophic cardiomyopathy: A randomized, double-blind, crossover trial. *J Am Coll Cardiol* 1997; **29**: 435–41.

16 Maron BJ, Nishimura RA, McKenna WJ, Rakowski H, Josephson ME, Kieval RS. Assessment of permanent dual-chamber pacing as a treatment for drug-refractory symptomatic patients with obstructive hypertrophic cardiomyopathy. A randomized, double-blind, crossover study (M-PATHY). *Circulation* 1999; **99**: 2927–33.

17 Linde C, Gadler F, Kappenberger L, Ryden L. Placebo effect of pacemaker implantation in obstructive hypertrophic cardiomyopathy. PIC Study Group. Pacing In Cardiomyopathy. *Am J Cardiol* 1999; **83**: 903–7.

18 Seggewiss H. Current status of alcohol septal ablation for patients with hypertrophic cardiomyopathy. *Curr Cardiol Rep* 2001; **3**: 160–6.

19 Brugada P, de Swart H, Smeets JL *et al.* Transcoronary chemical ablation of ventricular tachycardia. *Circulation* 1989; **79**: 475–82.

20 Sigwart U. Non-surgical myocardial reduction of hypertrophic obstructive cardiomyopathy. *Lancet* 1995; **346**: 211–14.

21 Kuhn H, Gietzen F, Leuner C *et al.* Induction of subaortic ischaemia to reduce obstruction in hypertrophic obstructive cardiomyopathy. *Eur Heart J* 1997; **18**: 846–51.

22 Seggewiss H, Gleichmann U, Faber L *et al.* Percutaneous transluminal septal myocardial ablation (PTSMA) in hypertrophic obstructive cardiomyopathy: Acute results and 3-month follow-up in 25 patients. *J Am Coll Cardiol* 1998; **31**: 252–8.

23 Faber L, Seggewiss H, Gleichmann U. Percutaneous transluminal septal myocardial ablation in hypertrophic obstructive cardiomyopathy: Acute and 3-months follow-up results with respect to myocardial contrast echocardiography. *Circulation* 1998; **98**: 2415–21.

24 Faber L, Seggewiss H, Fassbender D *et al.* Guiding of percutaneous transluminal septal myocardial ablation in hypertrophic obstructive cardiomyopathy by myocardial contrast echocardiography. *J Intervent Cardiol* 1998; **11**: 443–8.

25 Ruzyllo W, Chojnowska L, Demkow M *et al.* Left ventricular outflow tract gradient decrease with non-surgical myocardial reduction improves exercise capacity in patients with hypertrophic obstructive cardiomyopathy. *Eur Heart J* 2000; **21**: 770–7.

26 Maron BJ, Casey SA, Poliac LC, Gohman TE, Almquist AK, Aeppli DM. Clinical course of hypertrophic cardiomyopathy in a regional United States cohort. *JAMA* 1999; **281**: 650–5.

27 Maron MS, Olivotto I, Betocchi S *et al.* Effect of left ventricular outflow tract obstruction on clinical outcome in hypertrophic cardiomyopathy. *N Engl J Med* 2003; **348**: 295–303.

28 Seggewiss H, Faber L, Meyners W *et al.* Simultaneous percutaneous treatment in hypertrophic obstructive cardiomyopathy and coronary artery disease: A case report. *Cathet Cardiovac Diagn* 1998; **44**: 65–9.

29 Knight C, Kurbaan AS, Seggewiss H *et al.* Non-surgical septal reduction for hypertrophic obstructive cardiomyopathy: Outcome in the first series of patients. *Circulation* 1997; **95**: 2075–81.

30 Lakkis N, Kleiman N, Killip D *et al.* Hypertrophic obstructive cardiomyopathy: Alternative therapeutic options. *Clin Cardiol* 1997; **20**: 417–18.

31 Bhargava B, Agarval R, Kaul U *et al.* Transcatheter alcohol ablation of the septum in a patient of hypertrophic obstructive cardiomyopathy. *Cathet Cardiovasc Diag* 1997; **41**: 56–8.

32 Kornacewicz-Jach Z, Gil R, Wojtarowicz A *et al.* Early results of alcohol ablation of the septal branch of coronary artery in patients with hypertrophic obstructive cardiomyopathy. [In Polish.] *Kardiol Pol* 1998; **48**: 105–12.

33 Nagueh SF, Lakkis NM, He Z-X *et al.* Role of myocardial contrast echocardiography during nonsurgical reduction therapy for hypertrophic obstructive cardiomyopathy. *J Am Coll Cardiol* 1998; **32**: 225–9.

34 Gietzen FH, Leuner CJ, Raute-Kreinsen U *et al.* Acute and long-term results after transcoronary ablation of septal hypertrophy (TASH). Catheter interventional treatment for hypertrophic obstructive cardiomyopathy. *Eur Heart J* 1999; **20**: 1342–54.

35 Seggewiss H, Faber L, Gleichmann U. Percutaneous transluminal septal ablation in hypertrophic obstructive cardiomyopathy. *Thorac Cardiovasc Surg* 1999; **47**: 94–100.

36 Faber L, Meissner A, Ziemssen P, Seggewiss H. Percutaneous transluminal septal myocardial ablation for hypertrophic obstructive cardiomyopathy: Long term follow up of the first series of 25 patients. *Heart* 2000; **83**: 326–31.

37 Seggewiss H, Faber L, Ziemssen P *et al*. Age related acute results in percutaneous septal ablation in hypertrophic obstructive cardiomyopathy [abstract]. *J Am Coll Cardiol* 2000; **35** (Suppl. A): 188A.

38 Seggewiss H, Faber L, Ziemssen P, Meyners W. Non-surgical septal ablation (PTSMA) in patients with NYHA class IV and hypertrophic obstructive cardiomyopathy (HOCM) [abstract]. *Circulation* 1999; **100** (Suppl. I): 515.

39 Singh M, Edwards WD, Holmes DR Jr, Tajil AJ, Nishimura RA. Anatomy of the first septal perforating artery: A study with implications for ablation therapy for hypertrophic cardiomyopathy. *Mayo Clin Proc* 2001; **76**: 799–802.

40 Seggewiss H, Faber L. Percutaneous septal ablation for hypertrophic cardiomyopathy and mid-ventricular obstruction. *Eur J Echocardiogr* 2000; **1**: 277–80.

41 Kern MJ, Holmes DG, Simpson C, Bitar SR, Rajjoub H. Delayed occurrence of complete heart block without warning after alcohol septal ablation for hypertrophic obstructive cardiomyopathy. *Cathet Cardiovasc Intervent* 2002; **56**: 503–7.

42 Faber L, Seggewiss H, Werlemann BC, Fassbender D, Schmidt HK, Horstkotte D. Prediction of the risk of pacemaker dependency after percutaneous septal ablation for hypertrophic obstructive cardiomyopathy [abstract]. *J Am Coll Cardiol* 2002; **39** (Suppl. A): 845–3.

43 Kuhn H, Gietzen F, Leuner CH *et al*. Transcoronary ablation of septal hypertrophy: A new treatment for hypertrophic obstructive cardiomyopathy. *Z Kardiol* 2000; **89** (Suppl. 4): 41–54.

44 Welge D, Faber L, Werlemann BC *et al*. Long-term outcome after percutaneous septal ablation for hypertrophic obstructive cardiomyopathy [abstract]. *J Am Coll Cardiol* 2002; **39**: 845A.

45 Ziemssen P, Faber L, Schlichting J, Meyners W, Horstkotte D, Seggewiss H. Percutaneous septal ablation in patients with hypertrophic obstructive cardiomyopathy results in improvement of exercise capacity [abstract]. *J Am Coll Cardiol* 2000; **35**: 182A.

46 Boekstegers P, Steinbigler P, Molnar A *et al*. Pressure-guided nonsurgical myocardial reduction induced by small septal infarctions in hypertrophic obstructive cardiomyopathy. *J Am Coll Cardiol* 2001; **38**: 846–53.

47 Mazur W, Lakkis NM, Nagueh SF *et al*. Regression of left ventricular hypertrophy after nonsurgical septal reduction therapy for hypertrophic obstructive cardiomyopathy. *Circulation* 2001; **103**: 1492–6.

48 Curtius JM, Stoecker J, Loesse B, Welslau R, Scholz D. Changes of the degree of hypertrophy in hypertrophic obstructive cardiomyopathy under medical and surgical treatment. *Cardiology* 1989; **76**: 255–63.

49 Seggewiss H, Faber L, Ziemssen P, Gleichmann U. One year follow-up after echocardiographically-guided percutaneous septal ablation in hypertrophic obstructive cardiomyopathy. [In German.] *Dtsch Med Wochenschr* 2001; **126**: 424–30.

50 Seggewiss H, Faber L, Kleikamp G, Becker J, Gleichmann U. Hypertrophic obstructive cardiomyopathy and coronary artery disease: Surgical or interventional therapy [abstract]. *Eur Heart J* 1998; **19** (Suppl.): 624.

51 Qin JX, Shiota T, Lever HM *et al.* Outcome of patients with hypertrophic obstructive cardiomyopathy after percutaneous transluminal septal myocardial ablation and septal myectomy surgery. *J Am Coll Cardiol* 2001; **38**: 1994–2000.

52 Nagueh SF, Ommen SR, Lakkis NM *et al.* Comparison of ethanol septal reduction therapy with surgical myectomy for the treatment of hypertrophic obstructive cardiomyopathy. *J Am Coll Cardiol* 2001; **38**: 1701–6.

53 Firoozi S, Elliott PM, Sharma S *et al.* Septal myotomy–myectomy and transcoronary septal alcohol ablation in hypertrophic obstructive cardiomyopathy: A comparison of clinical, haemodynamic and exercise outcomes. *Eur Heart J* 2002; **23**: 1617–24.

54 Wigle ED, Schwartz L, Woo A, Rakowski H. To ablate or operate? That is the question! *J Am Coll Cardiol* 2001; **38**: 1707–10.

55 Grigg LE, Wigle ED, Williams WG, Daniel LB, Rakowski H. Transesophageal Doppler echocardiography in obstructive hypertrophic cardiomyopathy: Clarification of pathophysiology and importance in intraoperative decision making. *J Am Coll Cardiol* 1992; **20**: 53–4.

CHAPTER 19

Alcohol Septal Ablation in the Treatment of Hypertrophic Obstructive Cardiomyopathy: A Seven-Year Experience

Horst Kuhn, MD, Thorsten Lawrenz, MD, Frank Lieder, MD, Frank H. Gietzen, MD, Ludger Obergassel, MD, Claudia Strunk-Muller, MD, Berit Stolle, MD, and Christian H. Leuner, MD

From 1991 to 1993 we performed fundamental studies in the development of a catheter-based concept of interventional treatment for hypertrophic obstructive cardiomyopathy (HOCM)[1–5] (Fig. 19.1). The new concept, which included the injection of alcohol, was suggested by our group in April 1994 (Annual Meeting of the German Cardiac Society).[1,2,4] Its first therapeutic application was in June 1994 by U. Sigwart and was published in 1995.[3] We suggested the designation transcoronary ablation of septal hypertrophy (TASH).[1,2,4] Other designations are nonsurgical septal reduction therapy (NSRT), percutaneous septal myocardial ablation (PTSMA) and alcohol septal ablation (ASA).[6–9] Since 1995, an estimated 3000 patients in more than 25 countries, predominantly in Germany and in Europe, have been treated by this new catheter-based method. In our institution, 386 patients had undergone TASH up to September 2002. In October 1997, the national multicenter TASH registry of the German Cardiac Society was created.[10] The first workshop on the new catheter-based method took place in Bielefeld, Germany, in June 1997.[4]

Technique

The concept of the technique that was suggested initially has not changed in principle (Figs 19.1–19.3), i.e. the common 'over the wire' technique of percutaneous transluminal coronary angioplasty (PTCA) has been used to date, in which highly concentrated ethanol (at least 95%) is injected into a proximal septal branch of the left coronary artery to induce local subaortic damage of the septum with subsequent septal hypokinesia and shrinkage, with widening of the outflow tract area.[11] An electrode catheter is positioned in the apex of the right ventricle for back-up pacing during ethanol-induced periods of complete heart block.

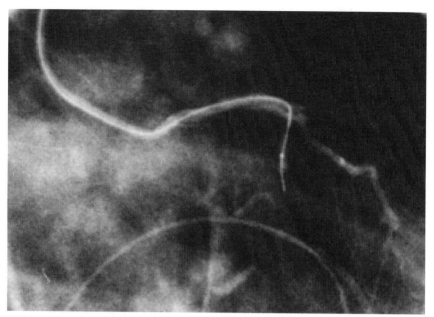

Fig. 19.1 First case with hypertrophic obstructive cardiomyopathy in which transient balloon occlusion was performed in 1991 to develop a new catheter-based concept of treatment for hypertrophic obstructive cardiomyopathy. Reprinted from Kuhn *et al.* Induction of subaortic septal ischemia to reduce obstruction in hypertrophic obstructive cardiomyopathy: studies to develop a new catheter-based concept of treatment. *Eur Heart J* 1997; **18**: 846–51, © 1997, with permission from the European Society of Cardiology.

The technique has been modified some during the last 6 years. Today, all groups performing TASH use smaller amounts of ethanol[12] (between 2 and 3 ml). Figure 19.4 shows the result of systematic alcohol reduction in our institution.[6] The nonechocardiographic gradient, angiography (fluoroscopy) and programmed electrical stimulation (GAPS; Fig. 19.3)-guided technique (compared with the echo-guided method) enabled us to use very small amounts of ethanol, to apply a more targeted approach and to identify more precisely the appropriate septal branch or side branch (see below).[6,13] Compared with results after injection of higher dose of ethanol, we achieved similar clinical and hemodynamic benefit with less myocardial damage, as indicated by reduction of peak creatine kinase activity, less frequent (mostly transient) complete heart block during the ablation and the first 2 days afterwards, and no ventricular tachycardia (see below).

Based on our experience with transient balloon occlusion of the first septal branch of the left anterior descending coronary artery,[1,2] since 1995 during therapeutic sessions we have used continuous invasive pressure gradient monitoring and programmed right ventricular electrostimulation. One extrasystolic beat every eight normal beats with a fixed coupling interval and as long a left ventricular filling period as possible was used to provoke the post-

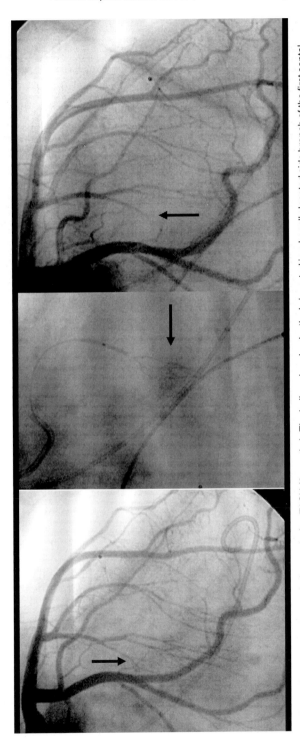

Fig. 19.2 Coronary angiogram before and after TASH (8 months). The balloon is subselectively inserted in a basally located side branch of the first septal branch of the left anterior descending coronary artery. The arrows mark the periphery (left panel) with opacification of the contrast agent (middle panel), injected through the balloon catheter. Eight months after TASH the occlusion of the side branch persisted (arrow). The corresponding transesophageal echocardiogram of the same patient is shown in Fig. 19.8. Reprinted with permission from Kuhn *et al.* Transcoronary ablation of septal hypertrophy (TASH): a new treatment option for hypertrophic obstructive cardiomyopathy. *Z Kardiol* 2000; **89**: 41–54.

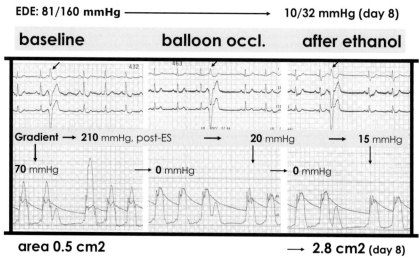

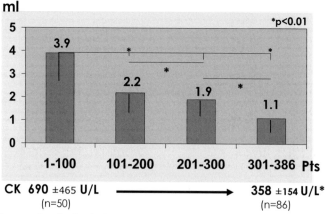

Fig. 19.3 Original recording of the TASH procedure in a 44-year-old man using the gradient angiography-programmed stimulation (GAPS)-guided method. The intraventricular gradients at baseline and after extrasystolic potentiation before TASH, during ischemia (balloon occlusion) followed by contrast injection and alcohol injection, and after the intervention are shown. Data on the increase in outflow tract area and gradient reduction, as assessed by bicycle exercise Doppler echocardiography (EDE), are also shown. The extrasystolic beat is induced after every eight normal beats by programmed electrical stimulation of the right ventricle.

Fig. 19.4 Systematic reduction in the amount of ethanol used for the TASH procedure since 1995 in patients treated in our institution up to September 2002.

extrasystolic gradient under reproducible conditions.[1,2,10,14] (Fig. 19.3). This approach is also preferred by others.[12] Compared with the resting gradient, this post-extrasystolic gradient correlates significantly with the gradient measured by Doppler echocardiography, as assessed immediately after the end of bicycle ergometry (tilt position, work load 75 W) (Figs 19.5 and 19.6).[6,15] Obviously, be-

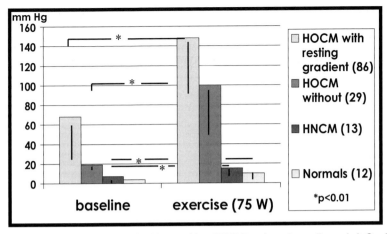

Fig. 19.5 Bicycle exercise (head-up tilting position, 75 W, Doppler echocardiography). Gradient assessment immediately after exercise in normal subjects and patients with hypertrophic obstructive cardiomyopathy (HOCM with and without resting gradient) and hypertrophic non-obstructive cardiomyopathy (HNCM). The four groups can be clearly identified by the different gradient responses.[6,14]

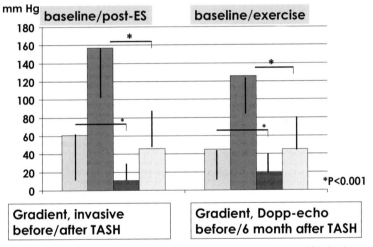

Fig. 19.6 Effect of small amounts of alcohol, defined as a maximum of 1.5 ml for the therapeutic session (1.1 ± 0.4 ml), in the last 68 consecutive patients with typical HOCM. Similar to the effect of higher amounts of ethanol,[6,10,11,14] there is a significant reduction in the pre-/post-TASH gradient, as assessed invasively in the therapeutic session at baseline and after post-extrasystolic provocation ($n = 68$), and assessed by Doppler echocardiography before and 6 months after TASH at rest and immediately after exercise [35 consecutive patients out of the 68 patients who have attended the regular 6-month control so far (September 2002)].

fore TASH in all patients careful echocardiographic evaluation of the outflow tract is performed to identify the form of HOCM and the site of obstruction, and to exclude discrete subaortic stenosis.[11,16]

With regard to the amount of alcohol, final selection of one of the proximal septal branches or their side branches, the position of the balloon within the septal branch and the appropriate injection technique, one has to consider the anatomy of the presumed culprit septal branch and predominantly the wash-out characteristics of the common anionic contrast agent injected through the balloon. The anatomy is clearly visualized under fluoroscopic guidance after the injection of the contrast agent. In our experience, septal branch angiography elucidates more precisely the capillary system, the collaterals, fistulas, and inappropriate side branches of the septal branch (e.g. leading to the apex or to the midventricular papillary muscle area) than the nonfluoroscopic myocardial echo-contrast technique. Continuous invasive gradient monitoring is most helpful. The often immediate fall in the resting or provoked gradient[1,11] after balloon occlusion or additional contrast (which enhances the ischemic effect) by at least 30% indicates the appropriateness of selective angiography and the identity of the appropriate perforator artery, allowing a more targeted approach to the obstructing area. This approach also makes it possible to identify the most appropriate branch if there are several anatomic possibilities.

Obviously, the provoked gradient is of special importance in patients without a resting gradient. The continuous simultaneous pressure recording also enables a precise, continuous evaluation of the alcohol effect on the gradient during the injection and during a 5-minute observation performed after the procedure.

The appropriate alcohol amount and injection technique depend on the flow characteristics of the contrast agent in the selected vessel. Stepwise, slow (about 0.05–0.1 ml/minute) alcohol injection is performed and higher alcohol amounts (maximum 1.5 ml) are used in case of rapid wash-out of the contrast. However, stepwise, more bolus-like (about 1.0–0.2 ml/minute) instillation of alcohol is used, and very small amounts of alcohol (minimum 0.3 ml) are injected if there is no or little wash-out of the contrast medium. The wash-out is judged under fluoroscopy about 5 seconds after the first selective injection of the contrast medium. (For further technical details see http://www.TASH-HOCM.de).

The aim should be to achieve a gradient reduction at rest and after provocation by at least 50% at the end of the procedure. This intraprocedural reduction results from the local subaortic hypokinesia, which is induced by myocardial ischemia, intravascular thrombosis, and chemical injury of the myocyte, the interstitial cells and the endothelium.[6,11] To date (September 2002), in our institution 386 patients have been treated with this GAPS-guided technique.[13]

Another technique applies a myocardial echo-contrast agent (not visible by fluoroscopy), which is injected through the occluding balloon. Echocardiographic opacification of the subaortic septum is seen.[17,18] This area may be correlated with the presumed area of obstruction, verified by color Doppler echocardiography.[18] Unlike the pressure-guided, angiographic approach, alcohol is injected into the assumed area of obstruction in the septum irrespective of whether there is gradient reduction.[18] The myocardial contrast echo-guided approach is used for the recognition of alcohol misplacement. In our experience, the angiographic approach is more helpful and sensitive in this regard.

Regarding the comparison of both techniques, the only data available can be obtained from a first 2-year analysis of the German TASH registry (1997–1999). Forty-six per cent of patients, enrolled from 10 participating centers, had been treated by the echo-guided approach and 54% by the angiographic, pressure-guided approach.[10] Both methods turned out to be effective. This is apparently due to the fact that both techniques use the identical concept of treatment and in most HOCM patients there is only one major proximal septal branch accessible for the balloon.[1,2,6] In addition, in typical HOCM the blood supply of the obstructing septal bulge always originates from a proximal septal branch[1] and the use of midventricular branches is ineffective. In the echo-monitoring group, however, a significantly greater amount of ethanol was needed (3.1 vs 2.5 ml) and the gradient reduction was less pronounced.[10]

Doppler echocardiography with bicycle ergometry (75 W) in a head-up, tilting position is a feasible, physiologic and standardized method for assessing the outflow gradient with stress and to evaluate the TASH effect during follow up[15] (Figs 19.5 and 19.6). The increase in the gradient at ergometry, which has to be assessed immediately after exercise,[6,15,19] amounts to 133% and is significantly higher than increase produced by the Valsalva maneuver (70%).[10]

Indications

The catheter interventional treatment has been performed by all groups predominantly in adult HOCM patients with typical subaortic obstruction who remain very symptomatic despite optimal medical and/or dual-chamber pacing therapy.[1–3,6,7,10,12,14–18,20–36] Regarding atypical midventricular obstruction, only a small number of patients have been treated so far. Similar to the results at surgery,[37–39] TASH has been proved to be effective not only in patients with a substantial gradient at rest but also in patients with only a provocable gradient.[6,34,36] TASH has been also shown to be effective in both the elderly and the young.[6,14] However, there is no basis upon which to perform TASH in children (i.e. in the growing heart) or in less symptomatic or even asymptomatic patients, even if they present with a substantial gradient.[6,7,9,40] In our institution we have extended the indication for TASH to patients with frequent syncope.[6,11]

Subjective outcome and objective measurements

Regarding the clinical and hemodynamic effect of TASH, original articles have been published by more than 20 centers in 15 countries so far (Internet search of Medline). All groups reported consistent beneficial results.[6,7] TASH was effective in both resting and exercise conditions, in the young and the elderly, and in patients with a resting or provocable gradient.[36] A high clinical success rate (approximately 90%) was also reported consistently. In patients who did not improve despite optimal morphologic (echocardiographic assessment) and hemodynamic results after TASH, a skeletal myopathy (predominantly mitochondriopathy) or myocardial storage disease (Fabry's disease) was identified after TASH.[41–43]

The clinical effects of TASH are seen in the first post-procedure days or they slowly evolve over months.[11,12,14,18,22,35] Only a small proportion of patients show recurrence of symptoms. In about 5% of patients, TASH has to be redone after 6–12 months to reduce the gradient in case of insufficient reduction. Partial abolition of the gradient (50%) may lead to the same clinical benefit as complete abolition of the gradient, including improvement of autonomic dysfunction, the response of blood pressure to exercise, and reduction of syncopal events.[6]

Regarding subjective assessment, there is a comprehensive improvement in quality of life,[13,44] with a significant decrease in New York Heart Association (NYHA) functional class and angina pectoris[6,7,10–12,14–18,20–32,34,35,45–47] as well as syncopal events.[6,7,14,37,38,48–50] According to questionnaires and regular control examinations, the vast majority of patients reported feeling 'much better.'[4,6,14,16,36]

With regard to objective measurements, TASH results in complete relief or significant reduction of the intraventricular gradient at rest and with stress (by at least 50%), as well as left ventricular end-diastolic pressure, mean pulmonary artery pressure at exercise and mitral insufficiency. As shown by several groups, there is also a significant increase in maximal oxygen uptake and exercise tolerance,[12,14,20,22,23,36,46,47] and the cardiac output is augmented significantly.[14] The ejection fraction, usually abnormally high in patients with HOCM, becomes normalized.[14] Echocardiographic follow-up studies revealed a small but significant increase in the subaortic left ventricular diameter, a local subaortic septal contraction disorder characterized by decreased fractional shortening of the end-diastolic diameter[11] or by strain rate imaging,[11,51] a decrease in left atrium size and an increase in outflow tract area[11,24,31] (Figs 19.7 and 19.8). Echocardiographic evidence of improved diastolic function has also been reported.[30]

Cardiac magnetic resonance imaging and transthoracic and transesophageal echocardiography demonstrated a distinct reduction in subaortic septal and global hypertrophy corresponding to pronounced septal shrinkage, observed histologically, and to regression of cell size in myocardial biopsies.[6,11,24,31,52,53] According to PET examinations, the subaortic myocardial defect volume is circumscribed, amounts to about 1–3% of left ventricular volume, and correlates significantly with the maximal increase in creatine kinase activity after TASH.[11] Decreased expression of tumor necrosis factor-α, possibly due to the regression of left ventricular hypertrophy, was also reported.[52] Autopsy studies showed an atypical, surrounding, nonpenetrating or even absent cellular reaction within the ablated area, with delayed fibrotic organization unlike that of common atherosclerotic myocardial necrosis.[6,53]

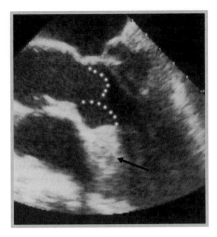 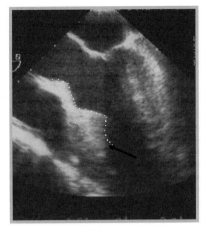

16 years after surgery   4 years after TASH

Fig. 19.7 Transesophageal echocardiogram (long-axis view) in a patient treated with surgery and a patient treated with TASH. A nearly identical subaortic notch-like deformity of the septum can be seen. Such a post-TASH septal picture was frequently seen in our patients in the past, when relatively high doses of ethanol were used (2–4 ml), but it became rare in the low-dose era. Note that the acute and chronic gradient reduction is predominantly caused by subaortic septal hypokinesia and not by septum reduction. There is also further widening of the outflow tract during exercise.

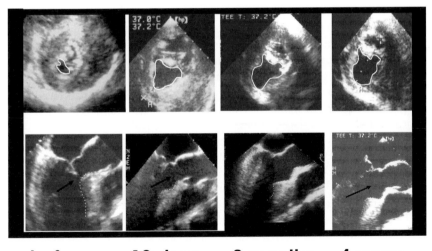

before   10 days   8 months   4 years

Fig. 19.8 Transesophageal echocardiogram before TASH and during a 4-year follow-up. The corresponding TASH procedure for the same patient is shown in Fig. 19.2.

Complications

The 2 years of in-hospital procedural outcome analysis of the national multicenter TASH Registry of the German Cardiac Society (October 1997 to September 1999) showed a TASH-related rate of major complications of 7.4% in 243 patients, including a death rate of 1.2%.[10] This total rate excludes a TASH redo rate of 5.8% and a permanent pacemaker implantation rate of 8.3%. At the beginning of the learning curve, higher in-hospital mortality rates (up to 4%) were reported.[4,14,21] In the German TASH Registry, besides death, major complications in rare cases were pericardial tamponade, pericardial effusion, ventricular fibrillation, dissection of the left anterior descending coronary artery, inguinal hematoma, abrupt coronary no-flow, *Staphylococcus aureus*-positive fever, pneumonia and cardiac decompensation under transient VVI pacing because of total atrioventricular (AV) block.[10]

The in-hospital post-TASH proportion of patients who required a permanent pacemaker was reported to be between 0% and 33%.[3,12,17,20,21,23,26] With this complication, the decision about replacing the external pacemaker by a permanent one apparently depends on the post-TASH watchful waiting interval (there is currently a 10% pacemaker implantation rate at a waiting interval of 48 hours in our institution). There is rapid recovery to normal sinus rhythm in the vast majority of patients.[6,14,17,21] Recently we analyzed the first 163 patients 7 months after TASH, thus including the early TASH cases. The pacemaker implantation rate in this early series of patients was 23% based on the '48-hour strategy'.[14] Seven months later, only a small proportion of patients (5.6%) were found who needed the pacemaker because of permanent total AV block within the first 48 hours after the TASH session.

Major complications in our patients were also analyzed recently (Table 19.1).[13] The overall TASH-related in-hospital mortality rate to date is 1.5% (6 out of 386 patients). This rate includes the early period of the learning curve 6–7 years ago (three patients died), when we performed TASH predominantly in patients with severe coexisting illness, in whom surgical treatment was at least relatively contraindicated.[6,11,50] The mortality was 0.4% in patients without severe comorbidity or NYHA functional class IV. (One out of 262 patients died. This man had no comorbidity but there were severe attacks of paroxysmal tachyarrhythmia due to atrial fibrillation. He died in hospital from ventricular fibrillation after successful TASH.) In patients with severe comorbidity and/or NYHA IV class the mortality was 7% (5 of 71 patients).

Attention should be drawn to two special complications. The first is in-hospital, sudden, unexpected, complete heart block after an uncomplicated intervention. Its frequency is 4.2%, including sudden AV block observed for at least some seconds or minutes during continuous in-hospital monitoring. This complication also occurred in the low-dose alcohol era. Therefore, in our institution continuous electrocardiographic monitoring is performed up to post-TASH day 10 (2 days in the intensive care unit and 8 days using telemetry

Table 19.1 Major in-hospital complications in all patients undergoing TASH in our institution up to January 2002.[6,13] Number of patients = 333; number of procedures = 361. + = patients who died

Death	1.8% (6)
Sudden unexpected AV III	4.2% (14)
Ventricular tachycardia/fibrillation	1.8% (6)++
Abrupt coronary no-flow	1.5% (5)+
Thrombosis (arm, leg)	0.9% (3)
Fever (*Staphylococcus aureus*-positive)	0.9% (3)
Pulmonary embolism	0.6% (2)
Pacemaker lead perforation	0.3% (1)+
Pericardial effusion	0.3% (1)
Perivascular coronary hematoma	0.3% (1)
Cardiac decompensation (VVI)	0.3% (1)
Asystole (and AV III, tachyarrhythmia)	0.3% (1)+
Stroke	0.3% (1)+
Total	13.7%

in a special rhythmologic unit). However, the risk for sudden complete heart block after day 5 is low (0.8%).

The second complication with the potential of a lethal outcome concerns the abrupt coronary no-flow phenomenon (severe multivessel peripheral spasm). In patients with HOCM, it may occur after the injection of ethanol,[54] or independently of TASH during routine coronary angiography before any alcohol is injected.[54,55] It is well known after coronary interventions, due to atherosclerotic coronary artery disease.[55,56] Intracoronary injection of urapidil (10 mg) may be very effective in resolving the spasm and restoring normal coronary flow.[9] During routine diagnostic coronary angiography, patients with hypertrophic cardiomyopathy seem more prone to this complication than patients without hypertrophic cardiomyopathy. Very stressed, anxious patients also seem to be at risk. Therefore, deep intravenous sedation before performing TASH and during any diagnostic or therapeutic procedure is recommended.[54] In addition, we now prophylactically administer verapamil (5 mg bolus) intravenously at the beginning of the procedure, followed by a body weight-adjusted infusion of verapamil (approximately 6 mg/hour).

Prognosis and limitations

TASH is a new method performed with increasing experience and technical modifications (e.g. a 75% reduction in the amount of alcohol in our institution). Consequently, as for any new method (e.g. in the early era of PTCA), the evaluation of the clinical, hemodynamic and prognostic effects of TASH is limited by the relatively short follow-up time and the obstacles to randomized prognostic studies.[6,8,57]

Recently, for patients treated in our institution up to December 2001 ($n = 329$), a nearly complete follow-up (98.8%, mean follow-up 2.1 years) was performed and Kaplan–Meier curves were calculated.[13,44] Four patients died suddenly after hospital discharge. Nineteen patients died from noncardiac, nonTASH-related reasons (e.g. carcinoma). Total annual cardiac mortality was 1.5%, the annual out-of-hospital mortality was 0.6% and total annual mortality 4.3%. The annual cardiac mortality after TASH turned out to be significantly better in patients treated with smaller amounts of ethanol (≤2.0 vs >2.0 ml; an independent predictor of mortality in Cox regression analysis). Regarding the learning curve, no significant prognostic difference was found in two large series (mortality of patient 1–165 vs patient 166–329). The results of a comprehensive quality-of-life evaluation in the two subsets (≤2.0 vs >2.0 ml; quality-of-life score +3.96 vs +3.95; clinical improvement rate 84.3 vs 90.2%) were also similar.

Serial electrophysiologic testing before and up to 6 months after TASH and serial Holter monitoring at regular control examinations did not indicate a TASH-induced risk for malignant ventricular arrhythmia.[14,48] As is the case after surgery (annual mortality 0.6%),[58,59] the annual post-TASH out-of-hospital rate of cardiac death is low (0.6%[6,13,22,34,48,44]). This indicates an improved prognosis compared with the much worse prognosis after medical treatment in historical cohorts of substantially ill patients admitted to hospital (similar to those patients selected today for TASH).[50,60,61] Naturally, longer post-TASH follow-up studies are needed for comprehensive prognostic evaluation. Regarding randomized prognostic studies, there is the major obstacle of patient recruitment, as has been shown in the Hypertrophic Obstructive Ablation Pacing Study (HOCAP) study (see chapter comparison with other interventional options).[57]

After hospital discharge, the rate of high-grade AV block (0.4–0.5% per year, mean follow-up 25 and 27 months), also is low; however, longer follow-up is necessary.[6,22,48] Regarding the theoretic potential of late malignant rhythm disorders after alcohol septal ablation, it is an open question whether chemically induced myocardial injury and infarction may lead to similar arrhythmogenic substrates as does the common atherosclerotic scar.

Unlike the common atherosclerotic myocardial infarction, TASH induces an inhomogeneous, transmural scar. The early round-cell infiltration and fibrotic process of the TASH-induced ablated septal area surround rather than penetrate the alcohol-induced myocardial center of necrosis.[6,53] The late consequences of all these changes remain to be determined with reference to arrhythmogeneity.

Comparison with surgical and dual-chamber pacing treatment

There is only one randomized study comparing different interventional treatment modalities in patients with HOCM (HOCAP study).[57] Regarding surgical treatment, there have been no randomized trials, even though this method was introduced 40 years ago.

The randomized HOCAP study (pacemaker treatment *vs* TASH) was terminated early because of lack of patient recruitment.[57] Although only 30 patients were enrolled, there was significant clinical improvement after 6 and 12 months, indicating a high grade of efficacy of both treatment options— pacemaker therapy and TASH. However, because of the lack of sustained clinical benefit, there was a high crossover rate pacemaker therapy to TASH during a 2-year follow-up of more than 50%, and ongoing beneficial changes were found in the TASH branch, including quality-of-life scores and hemodynamic measures.

Regarding the comparison of the effect of alcohol septal ablation with results of pacemaker studies for HOCM, dual-chamber pacing was reported to be effective in subgroups only and overall seemed less effective.[62–68]

Clinical success and objective measurements after TASH compare favorably with results after surgery.[6,7,14,50,60,61] In Germany, the number of patients undergoing surgery for HOCM has been reduced by approximately 90% since the introduction of the catheter-based method.[6,7,50]

The overall in-hospital mortality after surgery in selected series may be 0%. However, it was 4.4% in a review of the literature[58,59] and 3.1% (191 patients) between 1991 and 1998 at one of the most experienced centers.[59] In very severely ill patients (functional class IV and V) the mortality was between 42 and 100% compared with 7% (functional class IV) in severely ill patients treated by TASH.[6,13,50,69] These results indicate a higher risk of surgery compared with TASH for HOCM.

Based on a questionnaire study performed by us in 2001 among cardiac surgeons in Germany during the 5-year interval from 1991 to 1995, approximately 350 patients have been treated by surgery. Based on the TASH registry data and an annual questionnaire of the German Cardiac Society regarding all cardiac invasive procedures between January 1998 and December 2000, 971 patients were treated by TASH.[70]

Conclusions

Ten years after the first transient balloon occlusion of a septal branch in a study to develop a catheter-based concept of treatment for HOCM and 7 years after its therapeutic introduction, TASH has been shown to constitute a new treatment option for severely symptomatic adult patients who fail to improve adequately with medical treatment. This new catheter-based method also opens a new area of comprehensive research in a unique clinical infarct model.

TASH has become an alternative to surgical treatment, which, however, remains the gold standard of therapy.[68] Further careful follow-up studies and the enrollment of all patients into a national or international TASH registry seem to be required.[6,8,10,71]

References

1 Kuhn H, Gietzen F, Leuner C, Gerenkamp T. Induction of subaortic septal ischemia to reduce obstruction in hypertrophic obstructive cardiomyopathy: Studies to develop a new catheter-based concept of treatment. *Eur Heart J* 1997; **18**: 846–51.

2 Gietzen F, Leuner C, Gerenkamp T, Kuhn H. Abnahme der Obstruktion bei hypertrophischer Kardiomyopathie während passagerer Okklusion des ersten Septalastes der linken Koronararterie [abstract]. *Z Kardiol* 1994; **83** (Suppl. 1): 146.

3 Sigwart U. Non-surgical myocardial reduction for hypertrophic obstructive cardiomyopathy. *Lancet* 1995; **346**: 211–14.

4 Kuhn H. Transkoronare Ablation der Septum-Hypertrophie (TASH). Bericht über das 1 Bielefelder Werkstattgespräch. *Z Kardiol* 1998; **87**: 244–8.

5 Braunwald E. A new treatment for hypertrophic cardiomyopathy? *Eur Heart J* 1997; **18**: 709–10.

6 Kuhn H, Gietzen FH, Leuner CH *et al.* Transcoronary ablation of septal hypertrophy (TASH): A new treatment option for hypertrophic obstructive cardiomyopathy. *Z Kardiol* 2000; 89, **4**: 41–54.

7 Kuhn H. Transcoronary ablation of septal hypertrophy (TASH): A 5-year experience. *Z Kardiol* 2000; **89**: 559–64.

8 Maron BJ. Role of alcohol septal ablation in treatment of obstructive hypertrophic cardiomyopathy. *Lancet* 2000; **355**: 425–6.

9 Gregorini L, Marco J, Farah B *et al.* Effects of selective alpha1- and alpha2-adrenergic blockade on coronary flow reserve after coronary stenting. *Circulation* 2002; **106**: 2901–7.

10 Kuhn H, Seggewiss H, Gietzen F *et al.* Catheter interventional therapy for hypertrophic obstructive cardiomyopathy: First two year analysis of the national registry of the German Cardiac Society [abstract]. *Eur Heart J Abstr Suppl* 2000; **21**: 413.

11 Kuhn H, Gietzen F, Schäfers M *et al.* Changes of left ventricular outflow tract after transcoronary ablation of septum hypertrophy (TASH) for hypertrophic obstructive cardiomyopathy as assessed by transesophageal echocardiography and measuring of myocardial glucose utilization and perfusion. *Eur Heart J* 1999; **20**: 1808–17.

12 Boekstegers P, Steinbigler P, Molnar A *et al.* Pressure-guided nonsurgical myocardial reduction induced by small septal infarctions in hypertrophic obstructive cardiomyopathy. *J Am Coll Cardiol* 2001; **38**: 846–53.

13 Kuhn H, Lawrenz T, Gietzen F, Obergassel L, Lieder F, Leuner C. Catheter based treatment for HOCM: Technique, complications and prognosis. *J Heart Fail Abstr* 2002; **7**: 16.

14 Gietzen FH, Leuner CJ, Raute-Kreinsen U *et al.* Acute and long-term results after transcoronary ablation of septum hypertrophy (TASH). Catheter interventional treatment for hypertrophic obstructive cardiomyopathy. *Eur Heart J* 1999; **20**: 1342–54.

15 Kuhn H, Gietzen F, Lerch M, Lieder F, Meyer zu Vilsendorf D, Kruse J. The impact of exercise Doppler echocardiography in patients treated by transcoronary ablation of septal hypertrophy [abstract]. *Eur Heart J Abstr Suppl* 2000; **21**: 113.

16 Beer G, Strunk-Müller C, Gietzen FH, Kuhn H. Discrete subvalvular aortic stenosis (DSAS) – pitfall in the diagnosis of patients with hypertrophic obstructive cardiomyopathy (HOCM). *Eur Heart J Abstr Suppl* 2002; **23**: 313.

17 Lakkis NM, Nagueh SF, Kleiman NS *et al.* Echocardiography-guided ethanol septal reduction for hypertrophic obstructive cardiomyopathy. *Circulation* 1998; **98**: 1750–5.

18 Faber L, Seggewiss H, Gleichmann U. Percutaneous transluminal septal myocardial ablation in hypertrophic obstructive cardiomyopathy: Results with respect to intraprocedural myocardial contrast echocardiography. *Circulation* 1998; **98**: 2415–21.

19 Klues HG, Leuner C, Kuhn H. Left ventricular outflow tract obstruction in patients with hypertrophic cardiomyopathy: Increase in gradient after exercise. *J Am Coll Cardiol* 1992; **19**: 527–33.

20 Ruzyllo W, Chojnowska L, Demkow M *et al.* Left ventricular outflow tract decrease with non-surgical myocardial reduction improves exercise capacity in patients with hypertrophic obstructive cardiomyopathy. *Eur Heart J* 2000; **21**: 770–7.

21 Seggewiss H, Gleichmann U, Faber L, Fassebender D, Schmidt HK, Strick S. Percutaneous transluminal septal myocardial ablation in hypertrophic obstructive cardiomyopathy: Acute results and three months follow up in 25 patients. *J Am Coll Cardiol* 1998; **31**: 252–8.

22 Krater L, Seggewiss H, Meissner A, Faber L, Horstkotte B. Long-term clinical and hemodynamic outcome after percutaneous septal ablation for hypertrophic obstructive cardiomyopathy. *J Am Coll Cardiol* 2001; **37**: 203A.

23 Kim JJ, Lee CW, Park SW *et al.* Improvement in exercise capacity and exercise blood pressure responds after transcoronary alcohol ablation therapy of septal hypertrophy in hypertrophic cardiomyopathy. *Am J Cardiol* 1999; **83**: 1220–3.

24 Schulz-Menger J, Strohm O, Waigand J, Uhlich F, Dietz R, Friedrich MG. The value of magnetic resonance imaging of the left ventricular outflow tract in patients with hypertrophic obstructive cardiomyopathy after septal artery embolization. *Circulation* 2000; **18**: 1764–6.

25 Seggewiss H, Faber L, Ziemssen P. Alcohol septal ablation for hypertrophic obstructive cardiomyopathy. *Cardiol Rev* 1999; **7**: 316–23.

26 Knight C, Kurbaan AS, Seggewiss H *et al.* Non-surgical septum reduction for hypertrophic obstructive cardiomyopathy: Outcome in the first series of patients. *Circulation* 1997; **95**: 2075–81.

27 Kern MJ, Rajjoub H, Bach R. Hemodynamic round series II: Hemodynamic effects of alcohol-induced septal infarction for hypertrophic obstructive cardiomyopathy. *Cath Cardiovasc Intervent* 1999; **47**: 221–8.

28 Omman A, Ramachandran P, Subramanyan K, Kalarickal MS, Osman MN. Percutaneous transluminal septal myocardial ablation in drug-resistant hypertrophic obstructive cardiomyopathy: 18-month follow-up results. *J Invasive Cardiol* 2001; **13**: 526–30.

29 Spirito P, Rubartelli P. Alcohol septal ablation in the management of obstructive hypertrophic cardiomyopathy. *Ital Heart J* 2000; **1**: 721–5.

30 Henein MY, O'Sullivan CA, Ramzy IS, Sigwart U, Gibson DG. Electromechanical left ventricular behavior after nonsurgical septal reduction in patients with hypertrophic obstructive cardiomyopathy. *J Am Coll Cardiol* 1999; **34**: 1117–22.

31 Mazur W, Nagueh SF, Lakkis NM *et al.* Regression of left ventricular hypertrophy after non surgical septal reduction therapy for hypertrophic obstructive cardiomyopathy. *Circulation* 2001; **103**: 1492–6.

32 Sitges M, Kapadia S, Rubin DN, Thomas JD, Tuzcu ME, Lever HM. Percutaneous transluminal alcohol septal myocardial ablation after aortic valve replacement. *Catheter Cardiovasc Intervent* 2001; **53**: 524–6.

33 Cecchi F, Olivotto I, Montereggi A, Santoro G, Dolara A, Maron BJ. HCM in Tuscany: Clinical course and outcome in an unselected regional population. *J Am Coll Cardiol* 1995; **26**: 1529–36.

34 Lakkis N, Plana JC, Nagueh S, Killip D, Roberts R, Spencer WH. Efficacy of nonsurgical septal reduction therapy in symptomatic patients with obstructive hypertrophic cardiomyopathy and provocable gradients. *Am J Cardiol* 2001; **88**: 583–6.

35 Lakkis NM, Nagueh SF, Dunn JK, Killip D, Spencer WH. Non surgical septal reduction therapy for hypertrophic obstructive cardiomyopathy: One-year follow-up. *J Am Coll Cardiol* 2000; **36**: 852–5.

36 Gietzen FH, Leuner CJ, Obergassel L, Strunk-Müller C, Kuhn H. Role of transcoronary ablation of septal hypertrophy in patients with hypertrophic cardiomyopathy, NYHA functional class III or IV and outflow obstruction only under provocable conditions. *Circulation* 2002; **106**: 454–9.

37 Morrow AG, Reitz BA, Epstein SE *et al.* Operative treatment in hypertrophic subaortic stenosis. Techniques, and the results of pre and postoperative assessments in 83 patients. *Circulation* 1975; **52**: 88–102.

38 Maron BI, Merrill WH, Freier PA *et al.* Long term clinical course and symptomatic status of patients after operation for hypertrophic subaortic stenosis. *Circulation* 1978; **57**: 1205–13.

39 Robbins RC, Stinson EB. Long term results of left ventricular myotomy and myectomy for obstructive hypertrophic cardiomyopathy. *J Thorac Cardiovasc Surg* 1996; **111**: 586–94.

40 Maron BJ. Role of alcohol septal ablation in treatment of obstructive hypertrophic cardiomyopathy. *Lancet* 2000; **355**: 425–6.

41 Beer G, Gietzen F, Gabbert HE, Lieder F, Kuhn H. Incidental diagnosis of Fabry's disease in a patient with hypertrophic obstructive cardiomyopathy not responding to catheter interventional therapy [abstract]. *Eur Heart J* 2001; **22**: 407.

42 Lieder F, Gellerich F, Lawrenz T, Beer G, Holzhausen HJ, Kuhn H. Skeletal myopathy with fiber type I predominance and ultrastructural abnormalities in patients with hypertrophic obstructive cardiomyopathy. *Eur Heart J* 2003; **24** (Abstr. Suppl.): 561.

43 Beer G, Reinecke P, Gabbert HE, Hort W, Kuhn H. FABRY disease in patients with hypertrophic cardiomyopathy (HCM). *Z Kardiol* 2002; **91**: 992–1002.

44 Lawrenz T, Gietzen F, Lieder F, Obergassel L, Kuhn H. Prognosis of patients with hypertrophic obstructive cardiomyopathy after transcoronary ablation of septal hypertrophy (TASH). *Eur Heart J Abstr Suppl* 2002; **4**: 734.

45 Mogensen J, Egeblad H, Hansen PS, Jensen HK, Thysen L. Percutaneous transluminal septal myocardial ablation in hypertrophic obstructive cardiomyopathy. A new therapeutic option. *Ugeskr Laeger* 2000; **162**: 1371–5.

46 Airoldi F, Di Mario C, Catanoso A *et al.* Progressive decrease of outflow gradient and septum thickness after percutaneous alcoholization of the interventricular septum in hypertrophic obstructive cardiomyopathy. *Ital Heart J* 2000; **1**: 200–6.

47 Keren A, Nanai S. Transcatheter ablation of septal hypertrophy: A promising alternative to surgery in hypertrophic obstructive cardiomyopathy. *Isr Med Assoc J* 2002; **4**: 114–16.

48 Obergassel L, Gietzen F, Strunk-Müller C *et al.* Does transcoronary ablation of septal hypertrophy (TASH) in hypertrophic obstructive cardiomyopathy (HOCM) induce an arrhythmogenic substrate? Clinical results and Holter-ECG-data. *Pacing Clin Electrophysiol* 2001; **24** (II): 694.

49 Gietzen FH, Leuner CH, Obergassel L, Strunk-Müller C, Kuhn H. Role of transcoronary ablation of septal hypertrophy for relief of syncope in hypertrophic obstructive cardiomyopathy. *Eur Heart J Abstr Suppl* 2001; **22**: 704.

50 Kuhn H, Gietzen F. Transcoronary ablation of septal hypertrophy (TASH): Supersedes it the surgery (myectomy)? *Herz* 1999; **24**: 647–51.

51 Abraham TP, Nishimura RA, Holmes DR, Belohlavek M, Seward JB. Strain rate imaging for assessment of regional myocardial function. Results from a clinical model of septal ablation. *Circulation* 2002; **105**: 1403–6.

52 Nagueh SF, Stetson SJ, Lakkis NM *et al.* Decreased expression of tumor necrosis factor-a and regression of hypertrophy after non surgical septal reduction therapy for patients with hypertrophic obstructive cardiomyopathy. *Circulation* 2001; **103**: 1844–50.

53 Raute-Kreinsen U. Morphology of necrosis and repair after transcoronary ethanol ablation of septal hypertrophy. *Pathol Res Pract* 2003; **199**: 121–7.

54 Kuhn H, Gietzen F, Leuner C. The abrupt no-flow: A no-reflow like phenomenon in hypertrophic cardiomyopathy. *Eur Heart J* 2002; **23**: 91–3.

55 Wu DJ, Ueng KC, Lin CS *et al.* Multivessel spasm during coronary angiographic procedure in catheterization laboratory. *Acta Cardiol Sin* 1999; **15**: 45–50.

56 Eeckhout E, Kern MJ. The coronary no-reflow phenomenon: A review of mechanisms and therapies. *Eur Heart J* 2001; **22**: 729–39.

57 Kuhn H, Gietzen FH, Breithardt G *et al.* Pacemaker therapy and alcohol ablation for HOCM: A randomized study [abstract]. *Eur Heart J* 2001; **22**: 20.

58 Schulte HD, Bircks WH, Lösse B, Godehardt EAJ, Schwartzkopff B. Prognosis of patients with HOCM after transaortic myectomy. *J Thorac Cardiovasc Surg* 1993; **106**: 709–17.

59 Schulte HD, Borisov K, Gams E, Gramsch-Zabel H, Lösse B, Schwartzkopff B. Management of symptomatic hypertrophic obstructive cardiomyopathy. Long term results after surgical therapy. *Thorac Cardiovasc Surg* 1999; **47**: 213–18.

60 Kuhn H, Krelhaus W, Bircks W, Schulte HD, Loogen F. Indication for surgical treatment in patients with hypertrophic obstructive cardiomyopathy. In: Kaltenbach M, Loogen F, Olsen EGJ, eds. *Cardiomyopathy and Myocardial Biopsy*. Berlin: Springer, 1978: 308–15.

61 Loogen F, Kuhn H, Gietzen F, Lösse B, Schulte HD, Bircks W. Clinical course and prognosis of patients with typical and atypical hypertrophic obstructive and with hypertrophic non obstructive cardiomyopathy. *Eur Heart J* 1983; **4** (Suppl. F): 145–53.

62 Gadler F, Linde C, Juhlin-Dannfelt A, Ribeiro A, Ryden L. Long term effects of dual chamber pacing in patients with hypertrophic cardiomyopathy without outflow tract obstruction at rest. *Eur Heart J* 1997; **18**: 636–42.

63 Fananapazir L, Epstein ND, Curiel RV, Panza JA, Tripodi D, McAreavey D. Long-term results of dual-chamber pacing in obstructive hypertrophic cardiomyopathy. *Circulation* 1994; **90**: 2731–42.

64 Nishimura RA, Trusty JM, Hayes DL *et al.* Dual-chamber pacing for hypertrophic cardiomyopathy: A randomized, double-blind, crossover trial. *J Am Coll Cardiol* 1997; **29**: 435–41.

65 Kappenberger L, Linde C, Daubert C *et al.* Pacing in hypertrophic obstructive cardiomyopathy: A randomized crossover study. PIC Study Group. *Eur Heart J* 1997; **18**: 1249–56.

66 Maron BJ, Nishimura RA, McKenna WJ, Rakowski H, Josephson ME, Kieval RS. Assessment of permanent dual-chamber pacing as a treatment for drug-refractory symptomatic patients with obstructive hypertrophic cardiomyopathy. *Circulation* 1999; **99**: 2927–33.

67 Ommen SR, Nishimura RA, Squires RW, Shaff HV, Danielson GK, Tajik AJ. Comparison of dual-chamber pacing versus septal myectomy for the treatment of patients with hypertrophic obstructive cardiomyopathy: A comparison of objective hemodynamic and exercise end points. *J Am Coll Cardiol* 1999; **34**: 191–6.

68 Maron BJ, Danielson GK, Kappenberger LJ *et al.* ACC/ESC Expert Consensus Document on Hypertrophic Cardiomyopathy: A report of the American College of Cardiology/ American Heart Association Task Force on Clinical Expert Consensus Documents. *J Am Coll Cardiol.* (In press.)

69 Schulte HD, Gramsch-Zabel H, Schwartzkopff R. Hypertrophic obstructive cardiomy-opathy (HOCM): Surgical management. *Schweiz Med Wochenschr* 1995; **125**: 1940–9.

70 Mannebach H, Hamm C, Horstkotte D. 17 Bericht über die Leistungszahlen der Herz-katheterlabore in der Bundesrepublik Deutschland. *Z Kardiol* 2001; **90**: 665–7.

71 Spencer WH 3rd, Roberts R. Alcohol septal ablation in hypertrophic obstructive cardio-myopathy: The need for a registry. *Circulation* 2000; **102**: 600–1.

CHAPTER 20

Role of Septal Ablation in a Surgical Center

Harry M. Lever, MD

Hypertrophic cardiomyopathy (HCM) is a disease that was first described in England by Drs Donald Teare[1] and Russell Brock.[2] HCM was initially thought to be a rare disorder but recent studies suggest that it occurs in 1 in 500 people.[3] Early descriptions of HCM suggested that most patients had left ventricular outflow tract (LVOT) obstruction.[4] Since then, it has become clear that this disease has a wide spectrum of anatomic and hemodynamic subgroups, and may actually constitute more than one disease.[5] There are subgroups with obstruction under resting conditions or only after a provoking maneuver. In addition, there is another subgroup without resting or inducible obstruction. In addition, there is a wide spectrum of anatomic distribution of hypertrophy,[6] some of which is related to the age of the patient.[5] While it is recognized that the mitral valve is involved in LVOT obstruction, there is anatomic variability in mitral valve structure that may affect the treatment of this disease.[7–9]

For patients without LVOT obstruction, treatment is only medical, with β-blockers, calcium channel blockers, disopyramide and, in some cases, afterload-reducing agents. For those with LVOT obstruction, if there is failure to benefit with medical treatment there are three treatment modalities available: surgical myectomy; percutaneous transluminal myocardial septal ablation (PTMSA) [also called nonsurgical septal reduction therapy (NSRT), transcoronary ablation of septal hypertrophy (TASH) or alcohol septal ablation], and implantation of a permanent DDD pacemaker. The present chapter will compare PTMSA with surgical myectomy.

Some important questions have arisen concerning the use of PTMSA. Which patients anatomically are good candidates for the procedure? Which ones are poor candidates for it? What are the long-term effects of PTMSA? Is PTMSA now the treatment of choice for patients who have medically resistant HCM? Does surgery still have a role in these patients? What are the indications for surgery?

Mechanisms of obstruction and mitral regurgitation

Echocardiography is not only the principal diagnostic tool in HCM but helps in understanding the causes for outflow obstruction and directs the anatomic approach to the treatment of this disease. It differentiates the anatomic subgroups and defines the anatomy of the mitral valve, which is so important in the disease process and the mechanism of mitral regurgitation.

Before considering the role of each type of treatment, the mechanism of LVOT obstruction should be understood. The hypertrophied proximal septum tends to encroach and thus narrows the outflow tract of the left ventricle. With this narrowing, there is increased flow, which results in Venturi forces that suck the mitral valve anteriorly. In some patients, the papillary muscles are positioned more anteriorly, thus placing the mitral leaflets into the outflow stream and resulting in increased drag forces.[10]

Systolic anterior motion (SAM) of the mitral valve results in mitral regurgitation that can range from mild to severe. The severity of the mitral regurgitation is, in part, related to the length of the mitral leaflets. If the leaflets are of sufficient length, they can maintain coaptation and thus there will be less mitral regurgitation. However, if one or both leaflets are relatively short, then there may be severe mitral regurgitation. In general, there is a poor correlation between the outflow tract gradient and the degree of mitral regurgitation.[11]

There are other mechanisms for mitral regurgitation that must be considered when evaluating a patient with HCM, such as intrinsic mitral valve disease. Patients with HCM, particularly if they are old, can have mitral annular calcification that results in lack of contraction of the mitral annulus and mitral regurgitation. Alternatively, the mitral valve may have myxomatous changes that, over time, can result in flail segments, particularly if there is increased intraventricular pressure. There is also a subgroup of patients who have large leaflets that develop SAM associated with relatively little septal hypertrophy.

Differentiating the mechanism of mitral regurgitation is greatly aided by transthoracic echocardiography or transesophageal echocardiography, if the transthoracic echocardiography is not of sufficient quality, and by color-flow Doppler, which shows the direction of the mitral regurgitant jet. When mitral regurgitation is related to the SAM of the mitral valve, the jet direction is posterior and lateral. If the jet is directed anteriorly, intrinsic mitral valve disease should be suspected.[12] Usually, in this circumstance there is a posterior leaflet abnormality, such as partial flail. If the jet direction is central, the regurgitation is usually caused by calcification of the mitral annulus or restricted leaflet motion.

In order to decide on which invasive procedure is indicated, the mechanism of the obstruction and the mitral regurgitation must be determined. PTMSA, as will be described below, will only reduce the thickness of the septum and only alter the mitral regurgitation if it is related to the SAM. If there is intrinsic mitral valve disease, causing mitral regurgitation, PTMSA will be ineffective. An accurate septal thickness measurement is also mandatory. If the septum is in the range of 15–18 mm the mechanism for obstruction frequently involves large myxomatous mitral leaflets and PTMSA will be of no value. The advent of PTMSA has made echocardiography even more important in the management of patients with HCM.

Septal myectomy

Septal myectomy is a surgical procedure that was popularized by Dr Andrew Morrow.[13] Since 1960 there have been a number of operative series reported (Table 20.1)[14–22] (B. Lytle, pers. comm.). A portion of the proximal septum is removed to open the LVOT via a transaortic approach. There are a number of refinements that have occurred in myocardial protection during surgery to preserve the hypertrophied muscle. Transesophageal echocardiography now guides the surgeon in locating the proper site to perform the myectomy.[23] The depth of the myectomy should be based on the thickness of the proximal septal muscle. The distal extent of the myectomy is determined by the location of SAM–septal contact.

The early experience with surgery for HCM revealed an operative mortality as high as 10%.[24] Some small series have reported zero mortality.[25] In more recent operative series mortality has been reported to be between 1 and 3.5%. As would be expected with advancing age, the mortality increases and is in the range of 10–15% (Table 20.1). As HCM has been more often recognized, it is clear that there is a large group of elderly patients with this disease. The current indications for surgery are severely symptomatic New York Heart Association (NYHA) class III and IV patients who are unresponsive to medical treatment and have a gradient of at least 50 mm Hg at rest or with provocation.

Our most recent experience at the Cleveland Clinic with septal myectomy shows an operative mortality of 0.8% in a group of 459 patients from 1994 to 2003.[22] Over the same time period, in 279 consecutive patients with pure myectomy, there was no mortality. In 75 patients with myectomy and coronary artery bypass grafting there was only 1 death (1.3%). However, 3 of 105 patients with combined myectomy and valve replacement died, giving a mortality rate of 2.9%. Our present permanent pacemaker rate for pure myectomy is 7.2%.[22]

PTMSA

PTMSA was conceived by Dr Sigwart[26] after he observed a few patients who had HCM and experienced a myocardial infarction and then lost their LVOT gradient. He felt if he could produce a controlled myocardial infarction in the proximal septum in patients with HCM, he could also cause the outflow gradient to disappear or lessen. He injected ethyl alcohol down the first septal perforator, using a balloon-tipped catheter to cause the infarction. He noted that by just inflating the balloon the outflow tract gradient would immediately lessen. Subsequently, Sigwart collaborated with Hubert Seggeweiss[27] in a group of patients who had HCM and the technique rapidly developed. There was clear success in the early group, with no mortality and low mor-

Table 20.1 Surgical series. TSM = transaortic septal myectomy; CABG = coronary artery bypass graft; RBBB = right bundle branch block

Study	No. of patients (study years)	Mortality overall	Mortality with other procedures	Mortality <65 years	Mortality >65 years	Permanent pacemaker
Maron et al. (1978)[16]	120 (1960–75)	8.3%		8.3%		3.7%
Bircks (1986)[14]	160 (1963–84)	7.5% (1963–1984) 5.0% (1977–1984) 3.8% 5/130 TSM	56% 5/9			3.1%
Williams et al. (1987)[15]	61 (1971–86)	1.6% 1/61		1.6%		1.6%
Mohr et al. (1989)[17]	115 (1972–87)	5.2% 6/115 2.5% 2/80 TSM	11.4% 4/35	1.2%	15.6%	5.2%
Heric et al. (1995)[18]	178 (1975–93)	6.2% 11/178 4% 4/95 TSM	5% 2/41 TSM + CABG 8% 2/25 TSM + valve 21% 3/14 TSM + CABG + valve	1.3%	10%	10% 6%TSM
Schoendube et al. (1994)[19]	58 (1979–92)	1.7%				5.2%
Robbins and Stinson (1996)[20]	158 (1972–94)	3.2% 5/158 2.3% 3/131 TSM	7.4% 2/27	0.8%	11.4%	2.5% 3 prior RBBB
Schulte et al. (1999)[21]	519 (1963–98)	4.4% 23/519 3.5% 13/368 TSM	6.6% 10/151			
B. Lytle (pers. comm.)	459 (1994–2003)	0.8% 4/459 0% 279 TSM	1.3% 1/25 TSM + CABG 2.9% 3/105 TSM + valve	1	3	9.2% 42/459 7.2% 20/279 TSM 13.3% 10/75 TSM + CABG 11.4% 12/105 TSM + valve

bidity. Based on this early experience, other investigators began performing this procedure on larger numbers of patients with reasonably good success, although with some morbidity and mortality. One group of investigators felt that echocardiographic guidance was important in planning and carrying out the procedure,[28] while another felt that mechanical obstruction of the septal perforator with the balloon-tipped catheter with gradient drop would be sufficient to localize where the infarction should occur.[29]

To date, there have been well over 1000 patients who have had PTMSA performed. Faber and Seggewiss[30] now have follow-up of up to 2 years in 171 patients. However, in 9% of a larger series PTMSA could not be performed for technical reasons. Of the 171 patients who were followed for longer than 2 years, 88% had complete relief of the gradient, 8% had greater than 50% relief and 4% had less than 50% relief. The hospital mortality in 178 patients was 2% and the late death rate was 2.3%. Permanent pacemakers were required in 7%. However, in the subgroup who were younger (less than 40 years old) and tended to have thicker hearts there was only a 70% success rate. In the older age group (over the age of 65 years), who tended to have less left ventricular wall thickening there was greater than 90% success. It is possible that with thicker left ventricular muscle, alcohol may not cause enough necrosis to open the outflow tract sufficiently.

Gietzen and colleagues[29] studied 50 patients in whom the mean resting gradient was reduced from 45 ± 38 to 5 ± 7 mm Hg and the post-extrasystolic gradient from 135 ± 50 to $25 \pm$ mm Hg. However, the early death rate was 4% and 38% required permanent pacemakers. There was improvement by at least one functional class in 26 and by at least two classes in 18. Objective improvement in exercise performance was by an average improvement of 23% in $\dot{V}O_2$max. In a recent study by Gietzen and colleagues,[31] patients with PTMSA and provocable obstruction were compared with those with resting obstruction. They found equal success in both groups in reducing the gradient and relieving symptoms; there was 4.8% mortality in the group with resting obstruction and no mortality in the provocable group. In addition, in both groups a significant number of patients required a permanent pacemaker (27% in the provocable group and 25% in the resting group).

Lakkis and colleagues[32] reported on 50 PTMSA patients with 1 year of follow-up. The reduction in mean resting gradient was from 74 ± 23 mm Hg to 6 ± 18 mm Hg; the dobutamine-provoked gradient decreased from 84 ± 28 to 30 ± 35 mm Hg. There was significant improvement in functional class. Two patients died early after the procedure and one had cardiac arrest 22 weeks after the procedure, with successful resuscitation and implantation of a defibrillator. Eleven patients required permanent pacemakers and eight were still in complete heart block at 1 year. Seven patients required a second procedure because of symptoms and a significant residual gradient. This group, along with investigators from the Mayo Clinic,[33] compared their results of PTMSA with those of surgical myectomy in a non-randomized study. Relief of symptoms, reduction in gradient, thinning of the septum, and improvement in exercise tolerance appeared similar when the mean data were considered. In terms of complications, there was one death in the PTMSA group (related to a dissection of the left anterior descending coronary artery) and none in the surgical group. There was a higher incidence of implantation of permanent pacemakers in the patients who had the percutaneous approach compared with those who had surgical myectomy (22 and 2%, respectively). The group who underwent ablation therapy had no post-procedure atrial fibrillation, whereas the surgical group had a 20% incidence of atrial fibrillation. There was also a higher incidence of post-procedure mild aortic insufficiency after surgical myectomy.

Cleveland Clinic experience

At the Cleveland Clinic we have taken a somewhat different approach to the invasive management of these patients. We have two excellent surgeons who perform the septal myectomy operation. During the years 2000 and 2001, we performed 144 septal myectomies for pure HCM with no mortality and 32 septal ablations with one death in a patient with chronic renal failure on dialysis. We have felt that septal ablation is still investigational; for example, there is no animal model to study the long-term effects of alcohol ablation on the heart. The domestic cat has a relatively high incidence of HCM but the heart is too small to selectively catheterize a septal perforator. It is not clear yet if the infarction that is caused is homogeneous or patchy, and thus possibly predisposes to re-entrant arrhythmias. While there have been no reports of late ventricular arrhythmias, a large number of patients have not been followed systematically. Therefore, we have felt that PTMSA, while effective in many patients, should be reserved for those patients who have comorbidities that would make surgery high-risk. These higher-risk patients might include the elderly, the obese, and those with renal failure or chronic pulmonary disease. We have recently reviewed our experience with PTMSA and compared it with septal myectomy at our institution.[34] There were 25 patients who had PTMSA (63 ± 14 years, range 39–85) and 26 who underwent septal myectomy (48 ± 13 years, range 30–70) over the same time period. Both groups had a significant improvement in NYHA functional class and reduction in outflow tract gradient. However, when the individual patients were analyzed, it was clear that septal myectomy gave a much more consistent drop in the resting and provocable LVOT gradients. Five patients in our PTMSA group subsequently required septal myectomy because of persistent symptoms (two patients with resting gradients greater than 50 mm Hg and two with provocable gradients of 100 and 180 mm Hg). One patient was scheduled for repeat PTMSA for a high gradient that had not lessened, along with continued symptoms, when she developed an acute dissection of the ascending aorta. All five patients who required myectomy after PTMSA also received a permanent pacemaker in the immediate postoperative period. There were no patients who required repeat septal myectomy in our group. There was a 24% incidence of permanent pacemaker in the PTMSA patients and 8% after myectomy. There were no deaths in either group. The hospital stay in the PTMSA group was shorter than in the surgical group (5.6 ± 2.3 *vs* 8.1 ± 3.5 days).

PTMSA
Advantages
The hospital stay is relatively short and there is little postoperative discomfort. The patient can be active and back to daily activities more quickly. The elderly patient may have less mortality and morbidity associated with PTMSA than patients undergoing surgery. Compared with surgery, there is less frequent post-procedure atrial fibrillation with PTMSA.

Limitations
The success of PTMSA is limited by the size, distribution and flow through the septal perforator. If the vessel is particularly small, it may not be possible to pass a catheter into the lumen. Also, there may not be a perforator large enough to supply the area of the proximal septum where SAM–septal contact occurs, especially in patients with severe hypertrophy. The flow through the perforators may be so swift that the alcohol could be carried to a portion of the heart distant from the location intended, and thus an infarction will occur. It is also clear that not all patients are candidates for PTMSA. In our surgical series of 459 patients noted above, only 60.8% could have been considered as potential candidates for PTMSA.[22]

Surgery
Advantages
Surgery achieves a more consistent and permanent relief of the gradient, and allows possible mitral valve repair or replacement if necessary. LVOT obstruction and mitral regurgitation can be eliminated upon completion of surgery, which can be documented by transesophageal echocardiography before the patient leaves the operating room.

Disadvantages
Septal myectomy requires a surgeon experienced with this procedure. The risk of surgery tends to be increased in the elderly patient. The recovery time from surgery is longer than for PTMSA and there is a higher incidence of atrial fibrillation in the immediate postoperative period compared with the immediate post-PTMSA period.

Summary

PTMSA and septal myectomy should be considered effective techniques for the management of drug-refractory patients with HCM. However, a careful assessment of the patient's cardiac anatomy by echocardiography and angiography is required to properly select the patient for the most appropriate procedure. In addition, since long-term follow-up is not available for PTMSA, it should not be considered the first invasive treatment of choice in young patients. PTMSA should be considered in the elderly or in patients with other comorbid conditions that might increase the risk of surgery. Surgical myectomy is a safe and predictable procedure when performed by an experienced surgeon. At this time there is not sufficient information to abandon surgical myectomy in favor of PTMSA. In a center with qualified surgeons, septal myectomy is still the treatment of choice, particularly in young patients.

References

1 Teare D. Asymmetrical hypertrophy of the heart in young adults. *Br Heart J* 1958; **20**: 1–8.

2 Brock R. Functional obstruction of the left ventricle. *Guys Hosp Rep* 1957; **106**: 221–38.

3 Maron BJ, Gardin JM, Flack JM *et al.* Prevalence of hypertrophic cardiomyopathy in a general population of young adults. Echocardiographic analysis of 4111 subjects in the CARDIA Study. Coronary Artery Risk Development in (Young) Adults. *Circulation* 1995; **92**: 785–9.

4 Frank S, Braunwald E. Idiopathic hypertrophic subaortic stenosis: Clinical analysis of 126 patients with emphasis on the natural history. *Circulation* 1968; **37**: 759–88.

5 Lever HM, Karam RF, Currie PJ, Healy BP. Hypertrophic cardiomyopathy in the elderly. Distinctions from the young based on cardiac shape. *Circulation* 1989; **79**: 580–9.

6 Wigle ED, Sasson Z, Henderson MA *et al.* Hypertrophic cardiomyopathy. The importance of the site and the extent of hypertrophy. A review. *Prog Cardiovasc Dis* 1985; **28**: 1–83.

7 Klues HG, Proschan MA, Dollar AL *et al.* Echocardiographic assessment of mitral valve size in obstructive hypertrophic cardiomyopathy. Anatomic validation from mitral valve specimen. *Circulation* 1993; **88**: 548–55.

8 Klues HG, Roberts WC, Maron BJ. Morphological determinants of echocardiographic patterns of mitral valve systolic anterior motion in obstructive hypertrophic cardiomyopathy. *Circulation* 1993; **87**: 1570–9.

9 Klues HG, Maron BJ, Dollar AL, Roberts WC. Diversity of structural mitral valve alterations in hypertrophic cardiomyopathy. *Circulation* 1992; **85**: 1651–60.

10 Nakatani S, Schwammenthal E, Lever HM *et al.* New insights into the reduction of mitral valve systolic anterior motion after ventricular septal myectomy in hypertrophic obstructive cardiomyopathy. *Am Heart J* 1996; **131**: 294–300.

11 Schwammenthal E, Nakatani S, He S *et al.* Mechanism of mitral regurgitation in hypertrophic cardiomyopathy: Mismatch of posterior to anterior leaflet length and mobility. *Circulation* 1998; **98**: 856–65.

12 Grigg LE, Wigle ED, Williams WG *et al.* Transesophageal doppler echocardiography in obstructive hypertrophic cardiomyopathy: Clarification of pathophysiology and importance in intraoperative decision making. *J Am Coll Cardiol* 1992; **20**: 42–52.

13 Morrow AG, Koch JP, Maron BJ *et al.* Left ventricular myotomy and myectomy in patients with obstructive hypertrophic cardiomyopathy and previous cardiac arrest. *Am J Cardiol* 1980; **46**: 313–16.

14 Bircks W. Surgical treatment of hypertrophic cardiomyopathy (Dusseldorf experience). *Postgrad Med J* 1986; **62**: 571–4.

15 Williams WG, Wigle ED, Rakowski H *et al.* Results of surgery for hypertrophic obstructive cardiomyopathy. *Circulation* 1987; **76**: V104–8.

16 Maron BJ, Merrill WH, Freier PA *et al.* Long-term clinical course and symptomatic status of patients after operation for hypertrophic subaortic stenosis. *Circulation* 1978; **57**: 1205–13.

17 Mohr R, Schaff HV, Danielson GK *et al.* The outcome of surgical treatment of hypertrophic obstructive cardiomyopathy. Experience over 15 years. *J Thorac Cardiovasc Surg* 1989; **97**: 666–74.

18 Heric B, Lytle BW, Miller DP *et al.* Surgical management of hypertrophic obstructive cardiomyopathy: Early and late results. *J Thorac Cardiovasc Surg* 1995; **110**: 195–208.

19 Schoendube FA, Klues HG, Reith S, Messmer BJ. Surgical correction of hypertrophic obstructive cardiomyopathy with combined myectomy, mobilisation and partial excision of the papillary muscles. *Eur J Cardiothorac Surg* 1994; **8**: 603–8.

20 Robbins RC, Stinson EB. Long-term results of left ventricular myotomy and myectomy for obstructive hypertrophic cardiomyopathy. *J Thorac Cardiovasc Surg* 1996; **111**: 586–94.

21 Schulte HD, Borisov K, Gams E *et al.* Management of symptomatic hypertrophic obstructive cardiomyopathy – long-term results after surgical therapy. *J Thorac Cardiovasc Surg* 1999; **47**: 213–18.

22 Lytle B. Personal communication, 2001.

23 Marwick TH, Stewart WJ, Lever HM *et al.* Benefits of intraoperative echocardiography in the surgical management of hypertrophic cardiomyopathy. *J Am Coll Cardiol* 1992; **20**: 1066–72.

24 Beahrs MM, Tajik AJ, Seward JB *et al.* Hypertrophic obstructive cardiomyopathy: Ten- to 21-year follow-up after partial septal myectomy. *Am J Cardiol* 1983; **51**: 1160–6.

25 Cohn LH, Trehan H, Collins JJ Jr. Long-term follow-up of patients undergoing myotomy/myectomy for obstructive hypertrophic cardiomyopathy. *Am J Cardiol* 1992; **70**: 657–60.

26 Sigwart U. Non-surgical myocardial reduction for hypertrophic obstructive cardiomyopathy. *Lancet* 1995; **346**: 211–14.

27 Knight C, Kurbaan AS, Seggewiss H *et al.* Nonsurgical septal reduction for hypertrophic obstructive cardiomyopathy: Outcome in the first series of patients. *Circulation* 1997; **95**: 2075–81.

28 Seggewiss H, Faber L, Gleichmann U. Percutaneous transluminal septal ablation in hypertrophic obstructive cardiomyopathy. *J Thorac Cardiovasc Surg* 1999; **47**: 94–100.

29 Gietzen FH, Leuner CJ, Raute-Kreinsen U *et al.* Acute and long-term results after transcoronary ablation of septal hypertrophy (TASH). Catheter interventional treatment for hypertrophic obstructive cardiomyopathy. *Eur Heart J* 1999; **20**: 1342–54.

30 Faber L, Werlemann B, Krater L *et al.* Septal ablation for hypertrophic obstructive cardiomyopathy: An analysis of the patients with dissatisfactory reduction of the outflow gradient. *J Am Coll Cardiol* 2001; **37** (Suppl. A): 200A.

31 Gietzen FH, Leuner CJ, Obergassel L *et al.* Role of transcoronary ablation of septal hypertrophy in patients with hypertrophic cardiomyopathy, New York Heart Association functional class III or IV, and outflow obstruction only under provocable conditions. *Circulation* 2002; **106**: 454–9.

32 Lakkis NM, Nagueh SF, Dunn JK *et al.* Nonsurgical septal reduction therapy for hypertrophic obstructive cardiomyopathy: One-year follow-up. *J Am Coll Cardiol* 2000; **36**: 852–5.

33 Nagueh SF, Ommen SR, Lakkis NM *et al.* Comparison of ethanol septal reduction therapy with surgical myectomy for the treatment of hypertrophic obstructive cardiomyopathy. *J Am Coll Cardiol* 2001; **38**: 1701–6.

34 Qin JX, Shiota T, Lever HM *et al.* Outcome of patients with hypertrophic obstructive cardiomyopathy after percutaneous transluminal septal myocardial ablation and septal myectomy surgery. *J Am Coll Cardiol* 2001; **38**: 1994–2000.

CHAPTER 21

Molecular and Clinical Tools for Sudden Death Risk Assessment in Hypertrophic Cardiomyopathy

Asifa Quraishi, MB, MRCP, Mohammad S. Hamid, MB, MRCP, and William J. McKenna, MD, FRCP

Hypertrophic cardiomyopathy (HCM) is a familial heart muscle disorder caused by mutations in genes encoding sarcomeric proteins.[1,2] In most patients the natural history of HCM is benign. However, the incidence of sudden death may be as high as 2–4% in referral center populations and 1% in the community.[3] Sudden death may occur at any age but is most commonly seen in the young; that is, people less than 30 years of age.

Sudden death may be the result of several potential mechanisms including ventricular and supraventricular arrhythmia, atrioventricular block, myocardial ischemia, hemodynamic alterations (including inappropriate vasodilatation), or other factors, such as vigorous physical exercise.[1,3]

Role of risk stratification for sudden death in HCM

Given the incidence of sudden death, it is important to identify patients at high risk, especially as most sudden deaths occur in young, asymptomatic individuals.[4] Identification of patients who are at risk of sudden death represents an increasingly important aspect of management, in view of the improvements in the availability and delivery of effective treatment with implantable cardioverter–defibrillators (ICDs).[5]

Molecular tools for risk stratification

Genetic abnormalities

More than 150 mutations in eight sarcomeric disease-causing genes have been identified to date.[1,6,8–11] Between them they are responsible for 50–60% of cases of HCM.[1] The proteins involved are β-myosin heavy chain (β-MHC),[1,8] essential and regulatory myosin light chains (MLC-1, MLC-2), cardiac troponin T (cTnT),[1,9] cardiac troponin I (cTnI), α-tropomyosin (α-TM),[1,9] myosin-binding protein C (MyBP-C), and cardiac actin.[6] Three other contractile protein gene abnormalities (titin, α-myosin heavy chain, troponin C) have been identified, but whether they cause disease remains to be established.

Preliminary studies suggest that certain genetic abnormalities may carry a higher risk of sudden death; for example, cTnT and certain β-MHC mutations (Arg403Gln, Arg453Cys, and Arg719Trp).[1,2,8–10] Implementation of DNA diagnosis in prognostic management is, however, hindered by a number of factors. The majority of families appear to have their own 'private' mutations; the number of families with the same individual mutations is relatively small and additional characterization of genetic abnormalities and their phenotypes is required before definitive clinical correlations can be made.[1] There also remains a significant proportion of familial HCM for which the gene involved remains to be isolated. Studies to date have selection bias because most genotyped patients are from tertiary referral centres, where overt disease may be more prevalent. The same mutations, which are classified as high-risk in such a population, may have a more benign prognosis in patients seen within the community.[10]

There is a wide spectrum of phenotypic expression seen in HCM, even within families carrying the same mutation, with up to a quarter of genetically affected individuals showing no disease expression.[1,11] The environmental and genetic determinants of this clinical heterogeneity are largely unknown. For example, a family with troponin T disease experienced eight sudden deaths under the age of 25 but also had eight members who carried the same genetic mutation but survived into the seventh decade. This suggests that mutation analysis in isolation is unlikely to be highly predictive of the risk of sudden death and that genetic information will need to be integrated into clinical risk assessment.

In summary, though there is potential for mutation analysis to aid in the identification of high-risk individuals, preliminary data will require confirmation and DNA diagnosis will need to become more readily available to clinicians.

Clinical tools for risk stratification

Family history of sudden death

Of HCM probands, 10–20% have a family history of premature sudden death, approximately 5% displaying a 'malignant' family history with two or more sudden deaths.[3,12] However, there are problems in identifying an adverse family history of sudden death and in its use as a risk factor for sudden death. Reliance is placed on the family history, as direct pedigree analysis with cardiovascular evaluation of relatives or genetic testing is not usually feasible. By history, it is often not possible to determine the precise number of affected relatives or the precise cause of death. These factors may contribute to the low positive predictive accuracy of a family history of sudden death.[3]

An adverse family history of sudden death has been arbitrarily defined by one group of investigators[13] as two or more sudden deaths from HCM in family members aged less than 40. This definition has been formulated on the basis that the likelihood of identifying a prognostically useful adverse family history increases when a greater number of affected individuals who have died suddenly are correctly identified. A cutoff of 40 years has been used to aid differentiation of sudden death due to HCM versus coronary artery disease and other cardiac conditions, which are more prevalent in the older population. A detailed family history may be a 'poor man's' gene test and efforts to ascertain the status of relatives (e.g. medical records, ECG and echo evaluation) may increase the predictive power of a family history of sudden death as a risk marker for sudden death.

Syncope

Approximately 30% of patients with HCM suffer syncope or presyncope. In a retrospective review of 254 patients with HCM, McKenna and colleagues[14] found that, amongst the 32 patients who died suddenly, syncope was the only symptom associated with death. The findings were influenced by the children included in the study, who had a greater incidence of syncope compared with older patients, and they concluded that syncope carried a worse prognosis if the patient was young, syncope in patients less than 45 years of age being associated with sudden death ($P < 0.01$).[14] This has been substantiated by other investigators.[15] In adults, the predictive power of syncope rises when episodes occur with an adverse family history.[16] In this circumstance it carries a relative risk from sudden death of about 5.[15,16]

In some patients, syncope occurs during or immediately after exercise, in which case this may be associated with an abnormal blood pressure response, atrial and ventricular arrhythmias or increasing left ventricular outflow obstruction. Nienaber and colleagues[15] suggested that the risk of syncope in HCM was higher in patients with lower left ventricular filling volumes, but this observation has not been reproduced in a larger series.[14] However, no systematic studies in large cohorts looking at predictors of syncope are available in the literature. This may in part reflect the fact that extensive investigations into the cause of syncope in patients with HCM identified a probable mechanism in only 20–30%. At the present time it is not possible to predict syncope in HCM.

Echocardiographic risk factors

A recent cross-sectional study[17] reported an association between a maximal left ventricular wall thickness of at least 30 mm, and an increased risk of sudden death in HCM. Recent studies have confirmed this finding. Spirito and colleagues[18] demonstrated an increased risk of sudden death with extreme hypertrophy and concluded that the magnitude of left ventricular hypertrophy is an independent predictor of prognosis. However, the analysis was confined to data from the clinical history and echocardiographic features and assessment in relation to other major recognized risk factors was not performed.

In prospective studies of the prognostic significance and relation of multiple risk factors for sudden death, Elliott and colleagues confirmed that extreme hypertrophy is associated with an increased risk of sudden death, and univariate analysis demonstrated a sudden death risk ratio of 4.1 for maximal left ventricular wall thickness (95% confidence interval 0.8–4.5, $P = 0.001$).[13,16] However, the positive predictive accuracy for a wall thickness of 30 mm of greater was less than 20% in both studies (13 and 16% respectively),[16,18] confirming the fact that most patients with extreme hypertrophy do not die suddenly.[19]

Spirito and colleagues[18] also suggested that young patients with extreme left ventricular hypertrophy were at greatest risk and in these cases an ICD was warranted. This was concluded in light of the observation that five of the seven patients with extreme hypertrophy in whom sudden death occurred were less than 18 years old, but again assessment in relation to other recognized risk factors was not performed.

In the prospective prognostic study of Elliott and colleagues, extreme left ventricular hypertrophy was strongly associated with the presence of other risk factors, and those patients with extreme left ventricular hypertrophy, young or old, who had other risk factors had a significantly increased risk of sudden death (Fig. 21.1).[13] In contrast, young patients with extreme left ventricular hypertrophy and no other risk factors did not die suddenly.[13] In addition, there was no continuous relationship between age and sudden death alone ($P = 0.13$).[13] Hence, extreme hypertrophy in a young patient with no other risk factors for sudden death cannot be said to be a mandatory indication for ICD implantation. Wall thickness may be a useful marker for the risk of sudden death but its interpretation requires broader assessment of the phenotype and of other risk factors.[13]

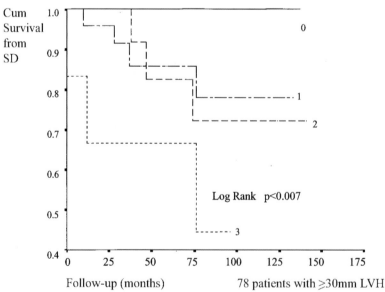

Fig. 21.1 Survival from sudden death in relation to extreme left ventricular hypertrophy and the number of risk factors. Kaplan–Meier survival curves for different numbers of risk factors in the group of patients with ≥30 mm left ventricular hypertrophy (LVH). From Elliott *et al.*[13]

Other echocardiographic features that have been assessed as risk markers for sudden death in HCM include left ventricular outflow obstruction. However, the presence or absence of outflow obstruction is not related to the incidence of sudden death ($P = 0.76$).[18] Data in relation to severe left ventricular outflow gradients (>100 mm Hg), however, are limited. Existing data do not suggest a relation between the pattern of hypertrophy (asymmetric, concentric, apical or eccentric) and sudden death ($P = 1.0$).[16]

Abnormal vascular responses

Frenneaux and colleagues first demonstrated that 33% of HCM patients out of a series of 129 had exercise-induced hypotension (a failure to increase blood pressure by 20 mm Hg or more during upright exercise).[20] Subsequent studies have supported these observations.[21,22]

Invasive hemodynamic monitoring during the course of the study by Frenneaux and colleagues also revealed that abnormal blood pressure responses occurred despite an adequate increase in cardiac output. The features were consistent with an exaggerated fall in systemic vascular resistance secondary to inappropriate vasodilatation in nonexercising muscles.[3,20] This is particularly significant as exercise is associated with sudden death in HCM.[19,23]

Abnormal blood pressure responses are seen more commonly in the young and are associated with a family history of sudden death and an increased risk of sudden death (Fig 21.2).[24] A normal blood pressure response has been

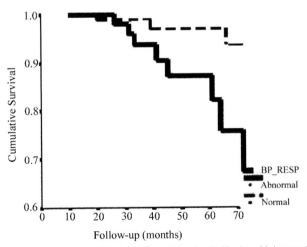

Fig. 21.2 Blood pressure response in relation to sudden death. Kaplan–Meier survival curve for normal blood pressure response and abnormal normal blood pressure response. Solid line denotes the normal blood pressure response group; dotted line represents the abnormal blood pressure response group. BP RESP = blood pressure response. Reproduced with permission from Sadoul N, Prasad K, Elliott PM *et al.* Prospective prognostic assessment of blood pressure response during exercise in patients with hypertrophic cardiomyopathy. *Circulation* 1997; **96**: 2987–91.

shown to be an accurate marker of the low risk cohort with a high negative predictive accuracy (97%), allowing this subset to be reassured.[3,24] Conversely, in isolation an abnormal blood pressure response has a low positive predictive value (15%) for the risk of sudden death.[3,16,24] However, it is a sensitive marker of the patient at high risk of sudden death (under 40 years of age), which then allows further risk stratification and monitoring of this subset.

The most likely mechanism by which abnormal blood pressure responses could cause sudden death is by provoking hemodynamic collapse in an HCM patient in conjunction with another factor, such as sinus tachycardia, ischemia and atrial or ventricular arrhythmia.[24]

Nonsustained ventricular tachycardia

Nonsustained ventricular tachycardia (NSVT) is seen in approximately 20% of adults with HCM on 24-hour ambulatory Holter monitoring. It is uncommon in adolescents and children.[3] Clinically analogous to a normal blood pressure response, the absence of NSVT on 24-hour Holter monitoring in adults is a sensitive marker of the low-risk patient, allowing these patients to be reassured with regard to prognosis.

Historically, there have been conflicting views regarding the implications for the management of patients with NSVT. Two contemporary studies reported that NSVT was associated with a high risk of sudden death.[25,26] Combined data in 169 patients showed that NSVT was a sensitive and specific marker of sudden death within 3 years, with a high negative (97%) and low positive (22%) predictive accuracy.[25-27] Patients with NSVT had an annual mortality rate of approximately 8%.[25,26] NSVT was defined as at least three beats at a rate of at least 120 beats per minute. Data were insufficient to permit analysis in relation to the frequency, rate or duration of episodes. Subsequently, improved survival was noted in HCM patients with NSVT who received amiodarone.[7] Some investigators, however, concluded that sudden death mortality associated with infrequent bursts of NSVT was low and that this cohort should not be treated with amiodarone,[28,29] particularly in view of amiodarone's potential side-effects. Do all patients with NSVT warrant prophylactic treatment? Spirito and colleagues studied a selected low-risk population that excluded patients with symptoms, recurrent syncope and those on antiarrhythmic drugs.[28] The relative risk of NSVT was approximately 2. In contrast, data from preliminary analysis of the prognostic significance of NSVT in the young reveals a relative risk of at least 5-fold in the young compared with 2- to 3-fold in older cohorts.

NSVT seen on Holter monitoring is reflective of arrhythmogenic potential.[27] The prevalence and significance of NSVT differs with age. When seen in the young it warrants serious consideration for prophylactic treatment, whereas in isolation in older patients it may not.

Previous cardiac arrest and sustained ventricular tachycardia

Previous cardiac arrest, especially where sustained ventricular tachycardia (VT) or ventricular fibrillation (VF) has been documented, is a powerful predictor of the risk of sudden death.[3,4] Prior to the availability of ICD implants, the subsequent annual mortality rate was 4% in these patients,[3] while the ICD discharge rate in high-risk patients is 5%. These data strongly support the recommendation of an ICD in this subgroup.

Role of electrophysiologic studies in determining risk factors for sudden death

Electrophysiologic studies have an established role in the diagnosis and management of survivors of sudden cardiac arrest, syncope and arrhythmias in patients with various cardiac conditions, other than HCM. Several studies have investigated the role of electrophysiological studies in determining the risk of sudden death in HCM.[30,31]

Fananapazir and colleagues studied 155 consecutive patients with HCM using standard invasive electrophysiologic techniques and identified numerous electrophysiological abnormalities, including inducible NSVT in 14%, sustained monomorphic VT in 10% and polymorphic VT and VF in 32%.[31] The authors concluded that the induction of sustained ventricular arrhythmias in these patients was an important prognostic marker of sudden death. Of these 155 patients, 145 were at high risk of sudden death by conventional noninvasive criteria. Seventy-three per cent of the sustained ventricular arrhythmias induced were polymorphic VT/VF, both of which are regarded as nonspecific findings of limited clinical importance when induced in electrophysiologic studies carried out for other cardiac conditions. In addition, this study provided limited data on the low risk cohort. Interpretation of the data set is problematic, especially as it is known that a significant number of low-risk patients would also demonstrate polymorphic VT/VF at the levels of stimulation used by Fananapazir and colleagues.[31]

Electrophysiologic studies may have a role in HCM in the assessment of patients with accessory pathways and in the management of clinical arrhythmias. However, the use of electrophysiologic studies routinely as a means for risk stratification for sudden death in HCM is not advocated, as analogous information to identify patients at high risk of sudden death, with similar positive predictive accuracy, can be gained by noninvasive means (Table 21.1).

Other risk factors

Other noninvasive electrophysiological markers, such as QT interval dispersion,[32] signal-averaged electrocardiography, heart rate variability and T-wave alternans reveal abnormalities in HCM patients but their role as markers of increased risk of sudden death in HCM patients remains to be demonstrated.[3]

Myocardial ischemia is known to occur in hypertrophic cardiomyopathy.[33–35] The mechanism of the ischemia in an individual patient is often difficult to establish. Postulated causes include small vessel disease, increased extravascular compression, systolic compression of epicardial and septal perforator arteries, obstruction of left ventricular outflow and reduced capillary density.[35]

Table 21.1 Sensitivity, specificity and predictive accuracy of risk factors for sudden death. PPA = positive predictive accuracy; NPA = negative predictive accuracy; BP = blood pressure; NSVT = nonsustained ventricular tachycardia; VT = ventricular tachycardia; VF = ventricular fibrillation; FHSD = family history of premature (<40 years) sudden death. Data generated from Sadoul et al.,[24] McKenna et al.,[14] Fananapazir et al.,[31] and Elliott et al.[13,16]

Risk factor	Sensitivity (%)	Specificity (%)	PPA (%)	NPA (%)
Abnormal exercise BP response	75	66	15	97
NSVT	69	80	22	97
Inducible VT/VF	82	68	17	98
Syncope				
Overall	29	83	25	86
<45 years	42	82	29	89
FHSD	42	79	28	88

Myocardial ischemia in HCM may be a significant trigger for sudden death but its identification and significance in HCM patients is inherently difficult.[5] It is not possible to advocate a specific marker of ischemia as predictive of sudden death, though assessment of the individual patient should include evaluation of anginal symptoms, ST segment change on exercise as well as risk of coexistent coronary artery disease.

Development of an individual patient's risk factor profile

Experience of risk factor stratification at our institution (St George's Hospital Medical School, London) reveals that approximately 50% of patients have none of the risk factors evaluated in Table 21.2, 25% have one risk factor while the remainder will have at least 2. An increasing number of risk factors confers an increased risk of sudden death (Fig. 21.3).[13,16] The presence of two or more of the above risk factors is associated with annual sudden death rates of 2–4% and warrants consideration of prophylactic treatment. For patients with a single risk factor, with annual sudden death rates of approximately 1%, decisions about prophylactic treatment need to be individualized in relation to the intensity of the risk factor and particularly the age of the patient, *viz.* NSVT in adults

Table 21.2 List of risk factors for sudden death and estimated 6-year survival rates from sudden death. Risk factors: family history of sudden death, syncope; NSVT on Holter; abnormal blood pressure response; extreme left ventricular hypertrophy (≥30 mm). NSVT = nonsustained ventricular tachycardia. Data generated from Elliott et al.[13,16]

Number of risk factors	Six-year survival rate (%)	95% confidence interval (%)
0	95	91–99
1	93	87–99
2	82	67–96
3	36	0–75

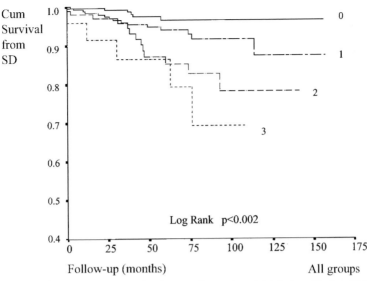

Fig. 21.3 Survival from sudden death in relation to the number of risk factors. Kaplan–Meier survival curves for different number of risk factors in the whole group. Reproduced with permission from McKenna W. Hypertrophic cardiomyopathy. In: Topol EJ, Califf RM, Isner J *et al.* (eds). *Textbook of Cardiovascular Medicine*. Lippincott Williams & Wilkins, Copyright 2002, p. 697.

vs young patients. Ideally, the absence of risk factors would be associated with 100% survival. In our prospective analysis a small proportion of patients without risk factors died suddenly. Retrospective review revealed evidence of significant ischemia with coexistent coronary artery disease, the prognostic significance of which was not fully appreciated. The absence of risk factors and evidence of ischemia at low workloads provides sufficient predictive accuracy to permit confident reassurance.

Recommendations

The prevalence of HCM in the adult population is approximately 1:500, making HCM a relatively common cardiac condition.[36] It is estimated that only 10–15% of affected patients are recognized clinically, and of these between 1 and 4%, depending on the population, die suddenly. The identification of these high-risk patients remains an ongoing concern, particularly as this subset includes young, often asymptomatic patients in whom sudden death is a devastating event.

The availability of effective treatments for the prevention of sudden death in HCM also underscores the importance of identifying the high-risk cohort who will benefit most. Patients with previous cardiac arrest, documented sustained ventricular arrhythmias, multiple premature sudden deaths in affected relatives, and young patients with severe and diffuse left ventricular hypertrophy or recurrent arrhythmic syncope related to exercise are at obvious risk and warrant treatment. Many patients who die suddenly, however, do not exhibit clinical markers that are particularly obvious. The greatest challenge in preventing premature sudden death in HCM may well be ensuring systematic stratification of risk factors for those patients who do not exhibit severe disease markers. All patients should undergo risk stratification with history, two-dimensional echocardiogram/Doppler, 24- to 48-hour Holter and maximal upright exercise testing with continuous assessment of blood pressure.

Experience suggests that risk stratification for sudden death using the above-mentioned risk factors is sufficiently accurate to provide a useful guide to prophylactic treatment, which can be individualized in relation to the level of acceptable risk for the patient.

References

1 Bonne G, Carrier L, Richard P *et al.* Familial hypertrophic cardiomyopathy: From mutation to functional defects. *Circ Res* 1998; **83**: 580–93.

2 McKenna WJ. The future in hypertrophic cardiomyopathy: Important clues and potential advances from an understanding of the genotype phenotype relationship. *Ital Heart J* 2000; **1**: 17–20.

3 Priori SG, Aliot E, Blomstrom-Lundqvist C *et al.* Task force on sudden cardiac death of the European Society of Cardiology. *Eur Heart J* 2001; **22**: 1374–450.

4 Spirito P, Seidman CE, McKenna WJ, Maron BJ. The management of hypertrophic cardiomyopathy. *N Engl J Med* 1997; **336**: 775–85.

5 Maron BJ, Shen W-K, Link MS *et al.* Efficacy of the implantable cardioverter–defibrillators for the prevention of deaths in patients with hypertrophic cardiomyopathy. *N Engl J Med* 2000; **342**: 365–73.

6 Mogensen J, Klausen IC, Pedersen AK *et al.* Alpha-cardiac actin is a novel disease gene in familial hypertrophic cardiomyopathy. *J Clin Invest* 1999; **103**: R39–43.

7 McKenna WJ, Oakley C, Krikler DM, Goodwin JF. Improved survival with amiodarone in patients with hypertrophic cardiomyopathy and ventricular tachycardia. *Br Heart J* 1895; **53**: 412–6.

8 Watkins H, Rosenzweig A, Hwang D *et al.* Characteristics and prognostic implications of myosin missense mutations in familial hypertrophic cardiomyopathy. *N Engl J Med* 1992; **326**: 1108–14.

9 Watkins H, McKenna WJ, Thierfelder L *et al.* Mutations in the genes for cardiac troponin T and α-tropomyosin in hypertrophic cardiomyopathy. *N Engl J Med* 1995; **332**: 1058–64.

10 Burn J, Camm J, Davies MJ *et al.* The phenotype/genotype relation and the current status of genetic screening in hypertrophic cardiomyopathy, Marfan syndrome, and the long QT syndrome. *Heart* 1997; **78**: 110–16.

11 Watkins H. Multiple disease genes cause hypertrophic cardiomyopathy. *Br Heart J* 1994; **72** (Suppl.): S4–9.

12 Maron BJ, Lipson LC, Roberts WC *et al.* 'Malignant' hypertrophic cardiomyopathy: Identification of a subgroup of families with unusually frequent premature death. *Am J Cardiol* 1978; **41**: 1133–40.

13 Elliott PE, Gimeno Blanes JR, Mahon NG *et al.* Relation between the severity of left ventricular hypertrophy and prognosis in patients with hypertrophic cardiomyopathy. *Lancet* 2001; **357**: 420–4.

14 McKenna WJ, Deanfield J, Faruqui A *et al*. Prognosis in hypertrophic cardiomyopathy: Role of age, clinical, electrocardiographic and haemodynamic features. *Am J Cardiol* 1981; **47**: 532–8.

15 Nienaber CA, Hiller S, Spielmann R *et al*. Syncope in hypertrophic cardiomyopathy: Multivariate analysis of prognostic determinants. *J Am Coll Cardiol* 1990; **15**: 948–55.

16 Elliott PE, Poloniecki J, Dickie S *et al*. Sudden death in hypertrophic cardiomyopathy: Identification of high risk patients. *J Am Coll Cardiol* 2000; **36**: 2212–18.

17 Spirito P, Maron BJ. Relation between extent of left ventricular hypertrophy and occurrence of sudden cardiac death in hypertrophic cardiomyopathy. *J Am Coll Cardiol* 1990; **15**: 1521–6.

18 Spirito P, Bellone P, Harris KM *et al*. Magnitude of left ventricular hypertrophy and risk of sudden death in hypertrophic cardiomyopathy. *N Engl J Med* 2000; **342**: 1778–85.

19 Maron BJ, Roberts WC, Epstein SE. Sudden death in hypertrophic cardiomyopathy: A profile of 78 patients. *Circulation* 1982; **65**: 1388–94.

20 Frenneaux MP, Counihan PJ, Alida LP *et al*. Abnormal blood pressure response during exercise in hypertrophic cardiomyopathy. *Circulation* 1990; **82**: 1995–2000.

21 Olivotto I, Maron BJ, Montereggi A *et al*. Prognostic value of systemic blood pressure response in a community-based patient population with hypertrophic cardiomyopathy. *J Am Coll Cardiol* 1999; **33**: 2044–51.

22 Yoshida N, Ikeda H, Wada T *et al*. Exercise-induced abnormal blood pressure responses are related to subendocardial ischaemia in hypertrophic cardiomyopathy. *J Am Coll Cardiol* 1998; **32**: 1938–42.

23 Maron BJ, Roberts WC, McAllister HA *et al*. Sudden death in young athletes. *Circulation* 1980; **62**: 218–29.

24 Sadoul N, Prasad K, Elliott PM *et al*. Prospective prognostic assessment of blood pressure response during exercise in patients with hypertrophic cardiomyopathy. *Circulation* 1997; **96**: 2987–91.

25 McKenna WJ, England D, Doi YL *et al*. Arrhythmia in hypertrophic cardiomyopathy. I: Influence on prognosis. *Br Heart J* 1981; **46**: 168–72.

26 Maron BJ, Savage DD, Wolfson JK, Epstein SE. Prognostic significance of 24 hour ambulatory electrocardiographic monitoring in patients with hypertrophic cardiomyopathy: A prospective study. *Am J Cardiol* 1981; **48**: 252–7.

27 McKenna WJ, Sadoul N, Slade AKB *et al*. The prognostic significance of non-sustained ventricular tachycardia in hypertrophic cardiomyopathy. *Circulation* 1994; **90**: 3115–17.

28 Spirito P, Rapezzi C, Autore MD *et al*. Prognosis of asymptomatic patients with hypertrophic cardiomyopathy and nonsustained ventricular tachycardia. *Circulation* 1994; **90**: 2743–7.

29 Cecchi F, Olivotto I, Montereggi A *et al*. Prognostic value of nonsustained ventricular tachycardia and the potential role of amiodarone treatment in hypertrophic cardiomyopathy: Assessment in an unselected non-referral based patient population. *Heart* 1998; **79**: 331–6.

30 Fananapazir L, Tracy CM, Leon MB *et al*. Electrophysiologic abnormalities in patients with hypertrophic cardiomyopathy: A consecutive analysis of 155 patients. *Circulation* 1989; **80**: 1259–68.

31 Fananapazir L, Chang AC, Epstein SE *et al*. Prognostic determinants in hypertrophic cardiomyopathy: Prospective evaluation of a therapeutic strategy based on clinical, Holter, hemodynamic, and electrophysiological findings. *Circulation* 1992; **86**: 730–40.

32 Yi G, Poloniecki J, Dickie S et al. Can the assessment of dynamic QT interval dispersion on exercise electrocardiogram predict sudden cardiac death in hypertrophic cardiomyopathy? *Pacing Clin Electrophysiol* 2000; **23**: 1953–6.

33 Cannon RO III, Dilsizian V, O'Gara PT et al. Myocardial metabolic, haemodynamic, and electrocardiographic significance of reversible thallium-201 abnormalities in hypertrophic cardiomyopathy. *Circulation* 1991; **83**: 1660–7.

34 Elliott PM, Rosano GM, Gill JS et al. Changes in coronary sinus pH during dipyridamole stress in patient with hypertrophic cardiomyopathy. *Heart* 1996; **75**: 179–83.

35 Wigle ED, Rakowski H, Kimball BP et al. Hypertrophic cardiomyopathy: Clinical spectrum and treatment. *Circulation* 1995; **92**: 1680–92.

36 Maron BJ, Gardin JM, Flack JM, Gidding SS, Kurosaki TT, Bird DE. Prevalence of hypertrophic cardiomyopathy in a general population of young adults. Echocardiographic analysis of 4111 subjects in the CARDIA Study. Coronary artery risk development in (young) adults. *Circulation* 1995; **92**: 785–9.

IN MEMORIAM ASIFA QURAISHI, 1973–2002

Asifa Quraishi was a promising cardiologist who encompassed curiosity with grace and humor. She commenced her career in cardiology in October 2000 at the Royal Brompton Hospital, where she initially attended a course on cardiac magnetic resonance imaging. She subsequently applied for, and was granted, a British Heart Foundation Junior Research Fellowship Grant under the supervision of Professors W.J. McKenna and Dudley Pennell. This enabled her to start working on establishing the right and left ventricular phenotypic characteristics of patients with arrhythmogenic right ventricular cardiomyopathy, and to subsequently screen family members for the disease. It was only a few months later that she was diagnosed with cancer. In spite of drug therapy, she was full of determination to complete the job in hand, and worked until the end.

Despite her illness, she achieved a great deal in a short time. Her patients will remember her for her patience and care, and her colleagues for her bravery, energy, enthusiasm for her work and her infectious sense of humor.

She made a difference to those who knew her because of who she was, and what she did.

CHAPTER 22

Risk Stratification for Sudden Death in Hypertrophic Cardiomyopathy: Extreme Left Ventricular Hypertrophy as a New Indicator of Risk

Paolo Spirito, MD and Barry J. Maron, MD

Since Teare's modern description of hypertrophic cardiomyopathy (HCM) in 1958, sudden death has remained the most visible and devastating feature in the natural history of this disease.[1-6] The fact that sudden death frequently occurs in young patients in the absence of previous symptoms makes this event particularly dramatic. However, despite several decades of research, the complex pathophysiology and diverse clinical course of HCM continue to represent a major obstacle to the identification of patients who are at high risk of sudden death. These difficulties in risk stratification have acquired even greater relevance since the implantable cardioverter–defibrillator (ICD) has proved highly effective in preventing sudden death in HCM, thereby further increasing the need for accurate indicators of risk.[7]

Risk stratification

The spectrum of HCM is particularly heterogeneous in its morphologic, functional and clinical presentation.[2-5] During the last decade, a number of investigations performed in relatively unselected cohorts have shown that the natural history of the overall HCM population is more benign than previously reported, and that only a small minority of HCM patients die suddenly.[8-12] Therefore, the great challenge is to identify, within the broad clinical spectrum of the disease, those few high risk patients who require aggressive management for prevention of sudden cardiac death.

At present, patients who survive a cardiac arrest or have one or more episodes of sustained ventricular tachycardia are judged to be at the highest risk and are regarded as definite candidates for aggressive treatment with the ICD for secondary prevention of sudden death.[3-5] Greater uncertainty persists regarding ICD indications for the prophylactic primary prevention of sudden death. While several disease features are generally considered markers of increased risk, each has important limitations in terms of risk stratification. Therefore, aggressive management decisions must usually be based on a careful evaluation of the weight of each of these risk factors within the overall risk profile of the individual patient.

Family history of sudden death

A history of premature sudden and unexpected death in family members is regarded as an indicator of risk.[3–5] However, several studies have not proved in statistical terms that a family history of single or multiple sudden deaths is associated with a significant increase in risk, possibly because the study populations did not include a sufficient number of events.[12–14]

Because of these uncertainties, the clinical management of HCM families in which a sudden cardiac death has occurred remains particularly challenging, and these difficulties are increased by the understandable concerns of surviving affected relatives. Should a single catastrophic event in a large HCM family lead to implantation of an ICD in all young affected relatives? In a pedigree with only two young patients with HCM, should the sudden death of one lead to implantation of a device in the other? At present, there are no definitive answers to these compelling questions. Nevertheless, because of the limitations of risk stratification and despite the absence of definitive statistical support, it would be unethical to withhold information regarding the option of the ICD from patients with sudden cardiac death in first-degree relatives. The patient's attitude toward their disease and its inherent risks should also be considered, and the presence of additional risk factors may contribute to the final management decision.

Nonsustained ventricular tachycardia during Holter ECG monitoring

In the early 1980s, two studies suggested that short bursts (even a single three-beat run) of nonsustained ventricular tachycardia on ambulatory Holter monitoring was a marker of risk for sudden death and an indication for long-term anti-arrhythmic therapy.[15,16] A subsequent investigation did not confirm a significant association between nonsustained ventricular tachycardia and the risk of sudden death, although the presence of this arryhthmia conveyed a relative risk of about 2.[17] Recently, a study performed in a larger HCM population confirmed that the presence of nonsustained ventricular tachycardia carried a relative risk of about 2, without achieving statistical significance.[14] Therefore, at present, it remains unresolved whether brief, sporadic runs of ventricular tachycardia on Holter are associated with increased risk in HCM. No data are available regarding the predictive power of recurrent and/or prolonged runs of nonsustained ventricular tachycardia (about 10 or more beats). Nevertheless, it would appear reasonable to attribute greater weight to such arrhythmias in the general assessment of prognosis.

Abnormal blood pressure response during exercise

Two investigations have identified a hypotensive or attenuated blood pressure response during exercise in a large proportion of HCM patients (20–40%) and found a significant association between this vascular abnormality and the risk of sudden death.[18,19] More recently, in a larger patient population, an abnormal blood pressure response during exercise was associated with a relative risk of about 2 and reached statistical significance in univariate, but not multivariate, analysis.[14] Therefore, as in the case of nonsustained ventricular tachycardia, a certain level of uncertainty persists as to whether this functional abnormality conveys a definite increase in the level of risk. Nevertheless, because nonsustained ventricular tachycardia and an abnormal blood pressure response during exercise were both associated with a 2-fold increase in risk in several of the studies, it seems plausible that the inclusion of these parameters in the overall patient risk profile may improve the ability to stratify risk.

Syncope

Syncope has often been regarded as a surrogate for aborted sudden death in HCM and thus an indication for intervention. However, the diversity of mechanisms potentially responsible for syncopal episodes in HCM and the transient character of these events have been a major obstacle in defining their prognostic significance.[3–5,20,21] Several observations suggest that syncopal episodes in HCM can be due to autonomic dysfunction and hemodynamic instability rather than arrhythmias, and thus have less serious prognostic implications.[20,21] Also, the possible differences in the risk of sudden death associated with syncope during exercise, at rest, or with postural changes have not been systematically investigated. When considered as a clinical event, independently of its precise mechanism, syncope has not proved to be a significant risk marker in HCM patient populations.[12,14] Nevertheless, based on clinical intuition and experience in individual clinical cases, syncope related to exercise (or repetitive episodes of syncope) in young patients appears to have ominous clinical implications associated with a high risk of sudden death. Therefore, syncopal event(s) with such presentation may be considered *per se* sufficient justification for an ICD.

Electrophysiologic testing

Electrophysiologic testing does not appear to have an important role in identifying HCM patients at high risk. Stimulation protocols with two ventricular premature depolarizations seldom induce monomorphic ventricular tachycardia even in high-risk patients (such as those with a previous cardiac arrest). On the other hand, aggressive protocols with triple ventricular premature depolarizations or ventricular bursts frequently trigger a response judged to be nonspecific, such as polymorphic ventricular tachycardia or ventricular fibrillation, even in many patients known to be at low risk.[22–24] Therefore, the available data do not provide convincing evidence that programmed electrical stimulation has a major impact on identifying those high-risk patients with HCM who require aggressive management for the prevention of sudden death.

Genetic markers of risk

In the early 1990s, a novel approach to risk stratification evolved that focused on certain HCM-causing gene mutations which appeared to convey either a favorable or an adverse prognosis.[25-28] However, over the subsequent years, the number of genes known to cause HCM has gradually increased to ten.[29,30] This intergenic heterogeneity is further augmented by high intragenic heterogeneity, since disease-causing mutations usually differ in unrelated families or patients (more than 150 individual mutations have been reported to date).[25-30] At present, genetic characterization remains complex, time-consuming, particularly expensive and not widely available. Furthermore, the chances that a given patient carries one of the molecular defects designated either as 'benign' or 'malignant' are exceptionally low and the notion that certain mutations are tightly linked to specific clinical outcomes has been challenged.[30] Therefore, genetic screening cannot at present be regarded as an effective, clinically applicable approach for stratifying risk in HCM.

Extreme left ventricular hypertrophy: a new risk factor for sudden death

In the present context of HCM risk stratification, and in an effort to improve the assessment of prognosis, attention has recently focused on the magnitude of left ventricular hypertrophy (LVH) as a potential predictor of increased risk for sudden death. Indeed, a large body of data indicates that this morphologic feature, particularly when interpreted in the context of the overall clinical profile, is important for the stratification of risk in HCM.

Observations in the late 1980s suggested that patients at the extreme end of the HCM morphologic spectrum have reduced survival.[31] More recently, echocardiographic cross-sectional data in more than 800 patients with HCM identified an inverse relation between left ventricular wall thickness and age. Extreme LVH (30 mm or thicker) was relatively frequent in young patients but uncommon in older patients. In particular, fewer than 0.5% of the patients older than 50 years had wall thickness of 35 mm or more (Fig. 22.1).[32] Consistent with these observations is the reported association between greater magnitude of LVH and the occurrence of nonsustained ventricular tachycardia, itself considered a risk factor for sudden death.[33,34] Finally, a relation between extreme hypertrophy (30 mm or more) and sudden death in HCM had been identified in a retrospective study.[35]

More recently, the incremental risk associated with greater degrees of LVH has been quantified in two investigations of large and consecutively enrolled HCM populations.[13,36] One of these studies, performed in about 500 HCM patients, showed that the risk of sudden death increased progressively in direct relation to maximal left ventricular wall thickness measured by echocardiography (Fig 22.2).[13] At the extremes of the morphologic spectrum, patients with mild forms of hypertrophy (wall thickness less than 20 mm) appeared to be at low risk in the absence of other generally accepted risk factors, while those

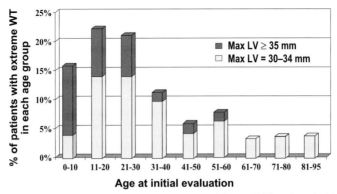

Fig. 22.1 Relation between extreme left ventricular wall thickness (WT) and age in 807 patients with hypertrophic cardiomyopathy. Extreme hypertrophy was relatively common in young patients but rare after middle age.

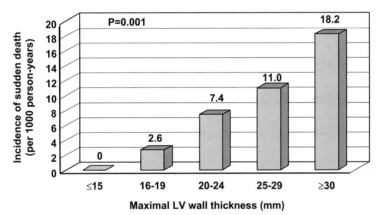

Fig. 22.2 Relation between incidence of sudden death and maximal left ventricular wall thickness in 480 patients with hypertrophic cardiomyopathy. Risk of sudden death increases progressively in direct relation to maximal wall thickness ($P = 0.001$). Reproduced from Spirito *et al.* Magnitude of left ventricular hypertrophy and risk of sudden death in hypertrophic cardiomyopathy. *N Engl J Med* 2000; **342**: 1778–85, © 2000 Massachusetts Medical Society. All rights reserved.

with wall thickness 30 mm or more were predominantly adolescents or young adults with no or only mild symptoms and had a substantial long-term risk of sudden death (about 20% at 10 years and 40% at 20 years) (Fig. 22.3). Based on these data, the magnitude of hypertrophy has become the first continuous indicator of risk reported in HCM, since all previously proposed predictors of sudden death are categorical-binary variables.

The second study, in more than 600 patients, confirmed the results of the first investigation. The risk of sudden death was highest in patients with extreme hypertrophy (30 mm or thicker) and increased continuously and significantly with each 5 mm increment in wall thickness.[36] Also, in both studies,

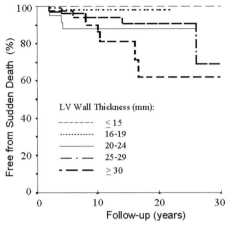

Fig. 22.3 Kaplan–Meier estimates of survival free from sudden cardiac death in 480 patients with hypertrophic cardiomyopathy and different magnitudes of left ventricular hypertrophy. Reproduced from Spirito, *et al*. Magnitude of left ventricular hypertrophy and risk of sudden death in hypertrophic cardiomyopathy. *N Engl J Med* 2000; **342**: 1778–85. © 2000 Massachusetts Medical Society. All rights reserved.

patients with extreme hypertrophy represented about 10% of the overall HCM population but accounted for more than 25% of the sudden deaths.[13, 36] In both studies, the patient subgroup at the extreme of the morphologic spectrum had an estimated long-term risk of sudden death of about 20% at 10 years.

This large body of evidence has important implications for patient management.[13, 31–36] In the absence of any of the other generally accepted risk factors, patients with mild HCM phenotypes appear to be at low risk and deserve reassurance. These patients at the low end of the morphologic spectrum constitute an important proportion of the overall HCM population and are more frequently encountered at nonreferral centers.[8–12] On the other hand, patients with extreme hypertrophy are mostly young and have high long-term risk for sudden death. Since these young patients with massive LVH usually do not have symptoms of heart failure and/or systolic dysfunction, prevention of sudden death with the ICD could offer a normal or near-normal life expectancy.

Therefore, independently of whether other potential risk indicators are present, young patients with extreme LVH and their families should be fully informed regarding the life-saving capabilities of the ICD (and its possible complications), as well as the present uncertainties in HCM risk stratification. Patient (and family) attitudes toward both the disease and the ICD will contribute importantly to final therapeutic decisions.

References

1 Teare D. Asymmetrical hypertrophy of the heart in young adults. *Br Heart J* 1958; **20**: 1–8.

2 Wigle ED, Rakowski H, Kimball BP *et al*. Hypertrophic cardiomyopathy. Clinical spectrum and treatment. *Circulation* 1995; **92**: 1680–92.

3 Spirito P, Seidman CE, McKenna WJ *et al*. The management of hypertrophic cardiomyopathy. *N Engl J Med* 1997; **336**: 775–85.

4 Maron BJ. Hypertrophic cardiomyopathy. *Lancet* 1997; **350**: 127–33.

5 Maron BJ. Hypertrophic cardiomyopathy. A systematic review. *JAMA* 2002; **287**: 1308–20.

6 Maron BJ, Olivotto I, Spirito P *et al*. Epidemiology of hypertrophic cardiomyopathy-related death revisited in a large non-referral-based patient population. *Circulation* 2000; **102**: 858–64.

7 Maron BJ, Shen WK, Link MS *et al*. Efficacy of the implantable cardioverter–defibrillator for the prevention of sudden death in hypertrophic cardiomyopathy. *N Engl J Med* 2000; **342**: 365–73.

8 Spirito P, Chiarella F, Carratino L *et al*. Clinical course and prognosis of hypertrophic cardiomyopathy in an outpatient population. *N Engl J Med* 1989; **320**: 749–55.

9 Kofflard MJ, Waldstein DJ, Vos J, ten Cate FJ. Prognosis in hypertrophic cardiomyopathy: A retrospective study. *Am J Cardiol* 1993; **72**: 939–43.

10 Cecchi F, Olivotto I, Montereggi A *et al*. Hypertrophic cardiomyopathy in Tuscany: Clinical course and outcome in an unselected regional population. *J Am Coll Cardiol* 1995; **26**: 1529–36.

11 Cannan CR, Reeder GS, Bailey KR *et al*. Natural history of hypertrophic cardiomyopathy. A population-based study, 1976 through 1990. *Circulation* 1995; **92**: 2488–95.

12 Maron BJ, Casey SA, Poliac LC *et al*. Clinical course of hypertrophic cardiomyopathy in a regional United States cohort. *JAMA* 1999; **281**: 650–5.

13 Spirito P, Bellone P, Harris KM *et al*. Magnitude of left ventricular hypertrophy and risk of sudden death in hypertrophic cardiomyopathy. *N Engl J Med* 2000; **342**: 1778–85.

14 Elliott PM, Poloniecki J, Dickie S *et al*. Sudden death in hypertrophic cardiomyopathy: Identification of high risk patients. *J Am Coll Cardiol* 2000; **36**: 2212–18.

15 McKenna WJ, England D, Doi YL *et al*. Arrhythmia in hypertrophic cardiomyopathy. I. Influence on prognosis. *Br Heart J* 1981; **46**: 168–72.

16 Maron BJ, Savage DD, Wolfson JK *et al*. Prognostic significance of 24-hour ambulatory electrocardiographic monitoring in patients with hypertrophic cardiomyopathy: A prospective study. *Am J Cardiol* 1981; **48**: 252–7.

17 Spirito P, Rapezzi C, Autore C *et al*. Prognosis in asymptomatic patients with hypertrophic cardiomyopathy and nonsustained ventricular tachycardia. *Circulation* 1994; **90**: 2743–7.

18 Sadoul N, Prasad K, Elliott PM *et al*. Prospective prognostic assessment of blood pressure response during exercise in patients with hypertrophic cardiomyopathy. *Circulation* 1997; **96**: 2987–91.

19 Olivotto I, Maron BJ, Montereggi A *et al*. Prognostic value of systemic blood pressure response during exercise in a community-based patient population with hypertrophic cardiomyopathy. *J Am Coll Cardiol* 1999; **33**: 2044–55.

20 McKenna W, Harris L, Deanfield J. Syncope in hypertrophic cardiomyopathy. *Br Heart J* 1982; **47**: 177–9.

21 Gilligan DM, Nihoyannopoulos P, Chan WL *et al*. Investigation of a hemodynamic basis for syncope in hypertrophic cardiomyopathy. *Circulation* 1992; **85**: 2140–8.

22 Kuck K-H, Kunze KP, Schluter M *et al*. Programmed electrical stimulation in hypertrophic cardiomyopathy: Results in patients with and without cardiac arrest and syncope. *Eur Heart J* 1988; **9**: 177–85.

23 Fananapazir L, Chang AC, Epstein SE *et al*. Prognostic determinants in hypertrophic cardiomyopathy: Prospective evaluation of a therapeutic strategy based on clinical, Holter, hemodynamic, and electrophysiological findings. *Circulation* 1992; **86**: 730–40.

24 Wellens H, Brugada P, Stevenson WG. Programmed electrical stimulation of the heart in patients with life-threatening arrhythmias: What is the significance of induced arrhythmias and what is the correct stimulation protocol? *Circulation* 1985; **72**: 1–7.

25 Watkins H, Rosenzweig A, Hwang DS *et al*. Characteristics and prognostic implications of myosin missense mutations in familial hypertrophic cardiomyopathy. *N Engl J Med* 1992; **326**: 1108–14.

26 Schwartz K, Carrier L, Guicheney P *et al*. Molecular basis of familial cardiomyopathies. *Circulation* 1995; **91**: 532–40.

27 Marian AJ, Roberts R. Recent advances in the molecular genetics of hypertrophic cardiomyopathy. *Circulation* 1995; **92**: 1336–47.

28 Watkins H, McKenna WJ, Thierfelder L *et al*. The role of cardiac troponin T and alfa-tropomyosin mutations in hypertrophic cardiomyopathy. *N Engl J Med* 1995; **332**: 1058–64.

29 Seidman JG, Seidman C. The genetic basis for cardiomyopathy: From mutation identification to mechanistic paradigms. *Cell* 2001; **104**: 557–67.

30 Ackerman MJ, VanDriest SL, Ommen SR *et al*. Prevalence and age-dependence of malignant mutations in the beta-myosin heavy chain and troponin T genes in hypertrophic cardiomyopathy. *J Am Coll Cardiol* 2002; **39**: 2042–8.

31 Spirito P, Maron BJ. Relation between extent of left ventricular hypertrophy and age in hypertrophic cardiomyopathy. *J Am Coll Cardiol* 1989; **13**: 820–3.

32 Maron BJ, Piccininno M, Bernabò P *et al*. Relation of extreme left ventricular hypertrophy to age in hypertrophic cardiomyopathy. *Am J Cardiol* 2003; **91**: 626–8.

33 Ruddy TD, Henderson MA, Downar E *et al*. Ventricular tachycardia and degree of left ventricular hypertrophy in hypertrophic cardiomyopathy [abstract]. *Circulation* 1982; **66** (Suppl. 2): 343.

34 Spirito P, Watson RM, Maron BJ. Relation between extent of left ventricular hypertrophy and occurrence of ventricular tachycardia in hypertrophic cardiomyopathy. *Am J Cardiol* 1987; **60**: 1137–42.

35 Spirito P, Maron BJ. Relation between extent of left ventricular hypertrophy and occurrence of sudden cardiac death in hypertrophic cardiomyopathy. *J Am Coll Cardiol* 1990; **15**: 1521–6.

36 Elliot PM, Gimeno Blanes JR, Mahon NG *et al*. Relation between severity of left ventricular hypertrophy and prognosis in patients with hypertrophic cardiomyopathy. *Lancet* 2001; **357**: 420–4.

CHAPTER 23

Implantable Defibrillator for Prevention of Sudden Death in Hypertrophic Cardiomyopathy

Barry J. Maron, MD, Win-Kuang Shen, MD, and Paolo Spirito, MD

Sudden and unexpected death has been recognized as the most devastating consequence of hypertrophic cardiomyopathy (HCM) since the initial description of this disease over 40 years ago.[1] Over this period of time, considerable investigative interest has been generated regarding risk stratification, definition of the mechanisms responsible for sudden death, and treatment strategies to prevent these unexpected catastrophes.[2–24] This review focuses on observations linking ventricular tachyarrhythmias with sudden death in HCM and the future potential role of preventive interventions such as the implantable cardioverter–defibrillator (ICD).

Historical context

Since Teare's original pathologic report of this disease,[1] recognition that a small but important subgroup of patients with HCM are at increased risk for sudden cardiac death has for many years generated considerable interest in the role of arrhythmias and the process of risk stratification,[2–5,8–14,20–23] as well as stimulating a continuing debate regarding the most appropriate measures for effective prevention of these unexpected events.[13,24] Over the years, many authors have emphasized that sudden death in HCM occurs not uncommonly in young asymptomatic patients,[1–24] with annual mortality rates reported as high as 4–6% in tertiary referral center populations disproportionately comprising high-risk patients.[2,3,11,12,25,26]

Pharmacologic treatment

Historically, the management of high-risk HCM patients had been confined to prophylactic pharmacologic treatment with β-blockers, verapamil, and antiarrhythmic agents such as procainamide and quinidine, and more recently with amiodarone.[2,3,5,15] However, there are limited data in HCM supporting the efficacy of prophylactic drug treatment for sudden death.[2,3,5,15] For example, no controlled studies have addressed the effects of β-blockers or verapamil on sudden death. Type IA anti-arrhythmic agents have been largely abandoned as prophylactic treatment for those HCM patients with isolated or infrequent runs of nonsustained ventricular tachycardia on ambulatory (Holter) ECG, due to the acknowledged potential pro-arrhythmic effects of these drugs.[5,8,16] Since the sole report 15 years ago proposing the protective effects of amiodarone against sudden death primarily in symptomatic or mildly symptomatic HCM patients with nonsustained ventricular tachycardia (i.e. using a retrospective and non-randomized study design with historical controls),[15] there have been no further reports regarding the long-term protective efficacy of this drug in high-risk patients. Also, the not infrequent adverse side-effects associated with the chronic administration of amiodarone severely limits its application to sudden death prevention for young patients with HCM, who characteristically have extended periods of risk.[7,13] Therefore, due to the paucity of efficacy data and the concern for patient compliance with drugs over many years of potential risk, pharmacologic treatment for the prevention of sudden death in HCM has been largely abandoned.

Ventricular arrhythmias and mechanisms of sudden death

Although supraventricular arrhythmias (particularly atrial fibrillation) are of great clinical importance for a substantial proportion of HCM patients by virtue of their association with heart failure, acute hemodynamic decompensation, and the risk for embolic stroke,[7,19,27,28] ventricular arrhythmias have been most devastating in HCM due to a clear linkage with the risk for sudden unexpected death.[2,3,5,7,10,11,13,18,23] Ventricular tachyarrhythmias, as recorded by ambulatory Holter ECG, are particularly common in HCM, and include premature ventricular depolarizations and complex forms such as couplets and nonsustained ventricular tachycardia.[8,10,11,29] Short bursts of nonsustained ventricular tachycardia (usually three to six beats), initially identified in the early 1980s as a marker for sudden death in two studies from tertiary HCM centers,[10,11] focused attention on clinically occult ventricular tachycardia as a rhythm premonitory to major cardiac events in this disease.[10–12,16,17]

More recently, arrhythmia sequences in HCM have been documented with stored electrocardiographic recordings in patients with ICDs experiencing appropriate device interventions.[13,30] These observations offer a unique window for understanding the mechanisms responsible for sudden death in HCM. In this regard, a multicenter ICD study in high-risk HCM patients showed that ventricular tachycardia or fibrillation triggered appropriate device activations,[13] supporting the long-standing hypothesis that primary ventricular tachyarrhythmias are most commonly responsible for unexpected catastrophes in this disease.[2–5,17,18] It was not possible, however, to conclusively exclude bradycardia-mediated events in that analysis because of the back-up pacing capability operative in many of the devices; indeed, other, more diverse arrhythmia mechanisms may ultimately prove to be involved in device interventions.[19,30,31] Expanded memory and greater use of dual-chamber devices will likely provide significant insights into any atrial arrhythmia-triggered ventricular event in this patient population.

In HCM, ventricular tachyarrhythmias probably emanate from an electrically unstable myocardial substrate with distorted electrophysiologic propagation and repolarization created by disorganized cellular architecture in the left ventricle, or from bursts of myocardial ischemia (probably due to structurally abnormal, narrowed intramural arterioles leading to myocyte necrosis and repair in the form of replacement scarring).[1–5,32–37] This arrhythmogenic myocardial substrate may be vulnerable to a variety of incompletely defined triggers, either intrinsic to the HCM disease process (e.g. vascular instability), or extrinsic environmental factors such as intense physical exertion.[38,39] Also, there is undoubtedly substantial individual patient susceptibility which plays a role in determining which individual HCM patients experience clinical events.

Risk stratification

Sudden cardiac death is a well-recognized and devastating anticipated complication of HCM, which occurs in a small but important minority of patients.[1–8,11–19,22–24,31,38–40] A major clinical challenge has been the identification of this high-risk subset among all portions of the broad HCM disease spectrum, which in fact includes many more patients judged to be in low-risk categories. Certainly, a measure of uncertainty and lack of precision persist regarding the stratification of sudden death risk for individual HCM patients, and it is generally accepted that no single test is capable of reliably stratifying all patients in a HCM population.

Nevertheless, at present, based on the available evidence it is reasonable to conclude that the highest levels of risk are associated with the following noninvasive clinical markers (Fig. 23.1):[2,3,5,9,10,12,14,21–23,41] (1) prior cardiac arrest or sustained (spontaneous) episodes of ventricular tachycardia; (2) a family history of premature HCM-related death, particularly if sudden, in close relatives and multiple; (3) syncope, when exertional or recurrent and particularly in the young; (4) bursts of nonsustained ventricular tachycardia on serial ambulatory (Holter) ECGs, particularly if multiple repetitive or prolonged; (5) extreme phenotypic disease expression with massive degrees of left ventricular hypertrophy (maximum wall thickness ≥30 mm); and (6) hypotensive (or attenuated) blood pressure response to exercise. However, in clinical practice it is rare for an HCM patient to be judged to be at high risk solely or largely based on an abnormal blood pressure response to exercise or the presence of asymptomatic ventricular tachycardia on Holter.

While there is no definitive evidence that the presence or magnitude of left ventricular outflow obstruction,[40,42,43] the occurrence of atrial fibrillation[27] and that of myocardial ischemia (possibly due to tunneled coronary artery)[44] constitute independent risk factors for sudden death in groups of HCM patients,

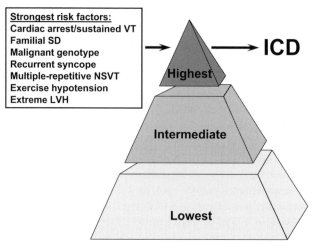

Strongest risk factors:
Cardiac arrest/sustained VT
Familial SD
Malignant genotype
Recurrent syncope
Multiple-repetitive NSVT
Exercise hypotension
Extreme LVH

ICD

Highest

Intermediate

Lowest

Fig. 23.1 Assessment of risk for sudden cardiac death in the overall hypertrophic cardiomyopathy population. At present, treatment for prevention of sudden death is focused on the small subset of patients perceived to be at the highest risk. ICD = implantable cardioverter–defibrillator; NSVT = nonsustained ventricular tachycardia; LVH = left ventricular hypertrophy; SD = sudden death; VT = ventricular tachycardia.

a role for these mechanisms in determining events in individual selected patients cannot be excluded.

Implementing interventions

Sudden death prevention (i.e. with the ICD) is strongly warranted for those patients with prior cardiac arrest or sustained and spontaneously occurring ventricular tachycardia.[13,45,46] While the presence of multiple clinical risk factors confers increasing risk for sudden death, it is also clear that in selected patients a single risk factor may be sufficient to justify aggressive treatment with the ICD for primary prevention of sudden death. Indeed, some investigators, particularly in the USA, favor strong consideration for a primary prevention ICD, even in the presence of one risk factor regarded as major in the clinical profile of that patient (e.g. a family history of sudden death in close relatives),[47] while other (largely European) investigators are much more conservative and restrictive, requiring two or more risk factors before recommending prophylactic treatment.[22,23] It is possible, however, that the HCM spectrum may be too heterogeneous and sudden death too unpredictable to allow sole reliance on arbitrarily defined risk factors to identify definitively each individual patient predisposed to cardiac arrest.[48] Therefore, such management decisions must often be based on individual judgment for the particular patient by taking into account the overall clinical profile, including age, the strength of the risk factor identified, the known strengths and limitations of the risk stratification process, the level of uncertainty acceptable to the patient and family, and the not inconsequential frequency of complications largely related to the lead systems (particularly inappropriate device discharges). It is also worth noting that physician and patient attitudes to ICDs (and the access to such devices within the respective health-care system) can vary considerably among countries and cultures, and thereby impact importantly on clinical decision-making and the threshold for implantation in HCM.[49,50] The ACC/AHA/NASPE 2002 guidelines have designated the ICD for primary prevention of sudden death as a class IIb indication and for secondary prevention (after cardiac arrest) as a class I indication.[45]

There is, at present, an understandable reluctance on the part of pediatric cardiologists to implant such devices chronically in children (particularly for primary prevention), in view of the necessary and ongoing commitment to maintenance and the likelihood of lead or other (ICD-related) complications occurring over very long time periods. However, while adolescence may represent a psychologically difficult age to be encumbered by an ICD, it should also be emphasized that this is coincidentally the period of life which has consistently shown the greatest predilection for sudden death in HCM. One alternative, but empiric, strategy proposed for some very young high-risk children is the administration of amiodarone as a bridge to later ICD placement after sufficient growth and maturation has occurred.

The strategy of electrophysiologic testing with the programmed electrical stimulation of ventricular tachyarrhythmias, for independently detecting the substrate of sudden death risk in individual HCM patients,[20] has been largely abandoned in clinical practice.[2,3] Acknowledged limitations to this technique include the infrequency with which monomorphic ventricular tachycardia is inducible in HCM (only about 10% of patients) and the fact that the electrical response of the HCM substrate to ventricular stimulation appears to be highly dependent on the precise laboratory protocol employed. For example, aggressive electrophysiologic testing using three premature ventricular extrastimuli can be expected to trigger sustained polymorphic ventricular tachycardia or ventricular fibrillation in a substantial proportion of patients; consequently, these inducible arrhythmias have been regarded largely as nonspecific responses in patients with the more common cardiac conditions, including coronary artery disease.[5] The precise clinical significance that should be attached to ventricular tachyarrhythmias induced with two extrastimuli is unresolved in HCM. Therefore, given the inherent risks and inconvenience of the procedure, the considerable uncertainty which surrounds the significance of induced arrhythmias, and the fact that most high-risk patients can be identified using noninvasive clinical markers independent of programmed ventricular stimulation,[2,22,23,47,50] the routine use of such laboratory-based testing to replicate clinical arrhythmias now appears to have little practical value in predicting outcome in HCM.

Due to the complex, time-consuming and expensive techniques necessary for genotyping, DNA analysis in HCM is at present largely confined to research-oriented investigations of highly selected pedigrees.[2] Also, caution is warranted before drawing strong conclusions regarding prognosis based only on the available genetic data, which is skewed toward high-risk families and reflects biases in patient selection.

Prevention of sudden death with the ICD

Since its introduction by Michel Mirowski[51] 20 years ago, the ICD has achieved widespread acceptance as a preventive treatment for sudden death, by virtue of indisputable evidence of its efficacy in terminating life-threatening ventricular tachyarrhythmias and prolonging life, principally in high-risk patients with ischemic heart disease.[52,53] In such patients, the superiority of the ICD to anti-arrhythmic drug treatment has recently been documented in several prospective, randomized trials, either for primary or secondary prevention.[52–54] Of particular importance in this regard was the evolution of the ICD from a thoracotomy-based procedure with epicardial leads to a transvenous endocardial electrode system with pectoral implantation of the pulse generator. This greatly facilitated its clinical employment, particularly as a prophylactic measure. However, despite the widespread and increasing use of the ICD in subsets of patients with coronary artery disease over two decades, there had been relatively little systematic application of the device to less common genetic cardiovascular conditions which are also associated with sudden death risk, such as the long QT and Brugada syndromes,[55] arrhythmogenic right ventricular cardiomyopathy,[56] as well as HCM.[30,57]

Sudden death prevention trial with the ICD in HCM

When the risk level for sudden death is judged by contemporary criteria to be unacceptably high and deserving of intervention, the ICD appears to be the most effective and reliable treatment option available, having the potential for absolute protection and altering the natural history of this disease in some patients.[58] Efficacy of the ICD was investigated in a large group of HCM patients judged to be at high risk for sudden death as part of a retrospective, multicenter study in the USA and Italy (Figs 23.2–23.4).[13] The study group of 128 HCM patients, all of whom had ICDs implanted for sudden death prevention due to the perception of high-risk status, were followed for an average period of about 3 years. Appropriate device discharges (either defibrillation shocks or antitachycardia pacing), triggered by ventricular tachycardia/fibrillation, occurred in almost 25% of patients, with an average overall annual discharge rate of

Fig. 23.2 Primary prevention of sudden cardiac death in hypertrophic cardiomyopathy. Stored ventricular electrogram from an asymptomatic 35-year-old man who received an ICD prophylactically because of a family history of hypertrophic cardiomyopathy-related sudden death and marked ventricular septal hypertrophy (wall thickness 31 mm). Intracardiac electrogram was triggered almost 5 years after the defibrillator implant (at 1:20 a.m. during sleep). Continuous recording at 25 mm/s, shown in four contiguous panels with the tracing recorded left-to-right in each segment. (a) Begins with four beats of sinus rhythm, and thereafter ventricular tachycardia begins abruptly (at 200 beats/min). (b) Device senses ventricular tachycardia and charges.

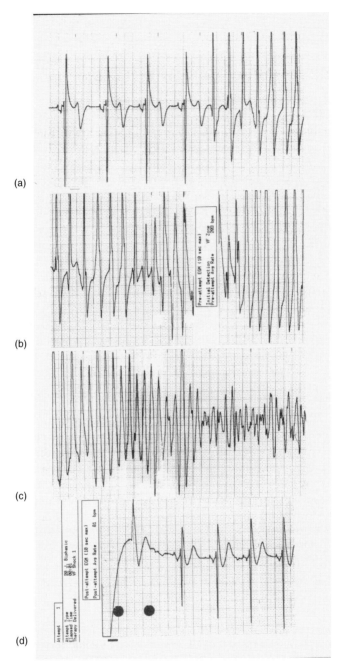

(a)

(b)

(c)

(d)

(**c**) Ventricular tachycardia deteriorates into ventricular fibrillation. (**d**) Defibrillator discharges appropriately (20-J shock) during ventricular fibrillation and restores the sinus rhythm. In the 5 years since this event the patient has remained asymptomatic without device activity. From Maron *et al.* Aborted sudden cardiac death in hypertrophic cardiomyopathy. *J Cardiovasc Electrophysiol* 1999; **10**: 263, with permission from Blackwell Publishing.

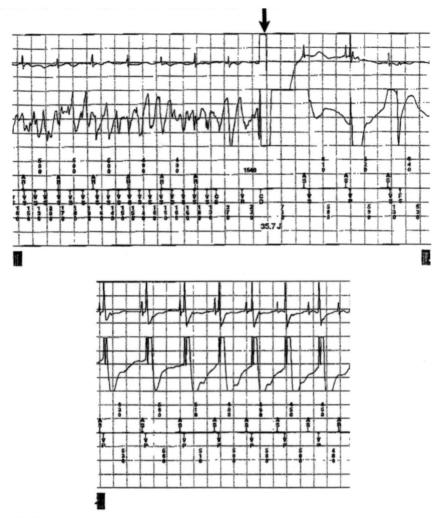

Fig. 23.3 Primary prevention of sudden death in an asymptomatic 14-year-old boy with hypertrophic cardiomyopathy and only one risk factor (massive left ventricular hypertrophy, 35 mm in thickness). Continuous recording of a stored intracardiac ventricular electrogram in which the ICD senses ventricular fibrillation and automatically delivers a defibrillation shock (arrow), which restores normal rhythm.

7–11% for secondary prevention and about 5% per year for primary prevention (Figs 23.2–23.5). Furthermore, about 60% of those patients who received appropriate defibrillator therapy had experienced multiple interventions. Of note, the ICD proved effective in HCM despite the substantially increased cardiac mass characteristic of this disease.[58,59] There was only a 4:1 ratio of devices implanted to lives saved, a favorable excess compared with that in primary prevention trials in coronary artery disease following myocardial infarction, in which this

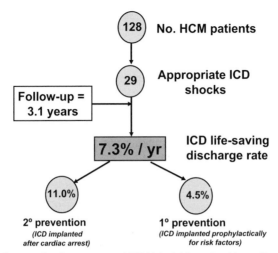

Fig. 23.4 Flow diagram showing outcome of 128 high-risk hypertrophic cardiomyopathy patients with implantable defibrillators for primary prevention (ICD for at least one risk factor) or secondary prevention (ICD following ventricular fibrillation or sustained ventricular tachycardia). Two patients (not shown here) died of hypertrophic cardiomyopathy with refractory end-stage heart failure and systolic dysfunction (despite the ICD).

ratio may be as high as 11:11.[53] Similar data from a European registry, limited largely to ICD therapy following cardiac arrest,[60] have been reported in preliminary form. There are also reports of ICD application in high-risk children.[61,62]

Furthermore, at the time of appropriate defibrillator interventions more than one-half of the patients were taking amiodarone or other anti-arrhythmic drugs. This observation, while ancillary to the main end-points of the trial, substantiates the superiority of the ICD over pharmacologic strategies in preventing sudden death as well as in disputing previous claims that amiodarone is absolutely protective against sudden death in HCM patients.[15]

Secondary prevention

Not unexpectedly, life-saving defibrillator interventions were most frequent in those patients implanted specifically for secondary prevention; i.e., following fortuitous resuscitation from cardiac arrest (with documented ventricular fibrillation) or after an episode of spontaneous and sustained ventricular tachycardia (Figs 23.4 and 23.5).[63] Over 40% of these patients received defibrillator therapy for secondary prevention during the relatively brief follow-up period. Such frequent recurrences of potentially lethal ventricular tachyarrhythmias following cardiac arrest are consistent with a previously reported experience involving similar HCM patients in the pre-ICD era.[62]

Primary prevention

Of particular note, those patients receiving ICDs solely for primary prevention also showed a substantial appropriate device intervention rate of about 5%

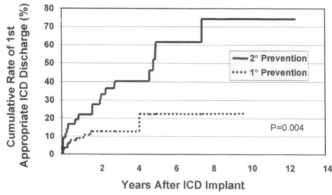

Fig. 23.5 Estimated cumulative rates of first appropriate ICD discharges in 128 patients with hypertrophic cardiomyopathy. Calculated separately for 85 patients with defibrillators placed for primary prevention and 43 patients with defibrillators for secondary prevention. Reproduced from Maron *et al.* Efficacy of implantable cardioverter–defibrillators for the prevention of sudden death in patients with hypertrophic cardiomyopathy. *N Engl J Med* 2000; **342**: 365–73, © 2000 Massachusetts Medical Society. All rights reserved.

per year (Figs 23.1, 23.2, 23.4 and 23.5). These primary prevention strategies represent prophylactic implants based on a clinical profile with one or more identifiable risk factors for sudden death.

By extrapolating the reported primary prevention discharge rate, it can be estimated that within 10 years about 50% of the defibrillators implanted prophylactically in young patients will intervene and abort a sudden death event. Indeed, the 5% annual discharge rate achieved in this subset of patients represents a figure reminiscent of that reported for sudden death in the selected high-risk HCM patient cohorts evaluated at tertiary referral centers.[2,3,11,25] It should be emphasized that prophylactic ICD employment for sudden death, as practiced in HCM, represents a novel and particularly pure form of primary prevention, given that it is based solely on the assessment of noninvasive risk factors in asymptomatic (or only mildly symptomatic) patients and typically in the absence of a major cardiovascular event or evidence of spontaneous arrhythmias.

Extended sudden death risk period

Crucial to understanding the role of the ICD within the broad HCM disease spectrum is an appreciation of certain demographic distinctions from ICD therapy in patients with coronary artery disease and heart failure.[47,58] The latter patients are of relatively advanced age at the time of implant (average, about 65 years), often with severe, progressive heart failure as a consequence of prior myocardial infarction. In sharp contrast, ICDs in HCM often involve young asymptomatic patients with an extended period of risk for sudden death.[7,13,22,23,40] In the multicenter ICD in HCM trial,[13] mean age at implant and the age at the time of first appropriate device intervention was only 40 years; furthermore, almost 25% of the patients were under 30 years old when they received an ICD.

Annual appropriate intervention rates for HCM are lower than those reported in coronary artery disease[52–54] but are nevertheless significant, given the important distinction that the experience with ICDs in HCM must be considered in the context of a much younger patient population that is usually free of significant heart failure (and with preserved systolic function). Protected by the ICD, these patients could survive many decades of productive life, even with normal or near-normal life expectancy. Therefore, ICD therapy can be regarded as potentially life-saving in HCM. However, annual ICD primary prevention intervention rates in HCM should not be compared directly in absolute terms with those in coronary artery disease,[53] for that would skew and underestimate the clinical value of the ICD in young HCM patients.

Of particular note, the time interval between implant and first appropriate ICD intervention may be quite variable, and particularly long time delays—of up to almost 10 years for the initial life-saving intervention—are not uncommon (Fig 23.6).[13,47] This observation underlines the unpredictable timing of sudden death in HCM, in which the ICD may remain dormant for substantial periods before it is ultimately required to intervene appropriately.

The decision to prophylactically implant an ICD in an HCM patient is often fortuitously based on the precise time at which risk stratification is undertaken and high-risk status identified.[46] Once there is recognition of risk in a patient, temporizing or delaying potentially preventive treatment is not appropriate. Therefore, a patient identified as high-risk at age 20 (and implanted with a device prophylactically) will still be young and at increased risk for an event at age 35, even if the ICD has not been triggered appropriately during that 15-year period. Consequently, once the decision to implant an ICD in a high-risk HCM patient is made, it is also likely to represent a lifelong preventive measure.

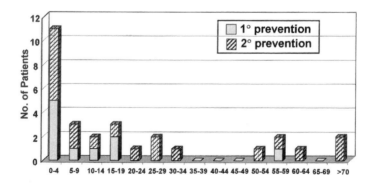

Implant to First Appropriate ICD Intervention (months)

Fig. 23.6 Time elapsed from implantation of the cardioverter–defibrillator (ICD) to first appropriate shock.

Strategic limitations

Risk stratification

Although there is now little reason to doubt the efficacy of the ICD in preventing sudden death in HCM, several important issues regarding prophylactic treatment remain incompletely resolved.[58] For example, precisely which clinical markers most definitively identify high-risk status and which patients within the broad HCM disease spectrum should receive implantable devices for primary prevention are constrained by imperfections in available risk stratification profiles, which ultimately emanate from the relatively low prevalence in cardiologic practice and heterogeneous clinical expression of HCM.[2–4,26,58,64] Indeed, almost 50% of patients in a clinically identified HCM cohort have some evidence of increased risk and almost 5% of those without any risk factors nevertheless experience sudden death (Fig. 23.7).

Given that definitive risk stratification data are not available to govern all possible at-risk clinical circumstances, decisions regarding ICD implantation may unavoidably reside with the best clinical judgment of the treating cardiologist in some cases.[47] Equally important, however, are patient motivation and compliance, since an ICD implanted over many years requires regular maintenance and carries the distinct possibility of complications. Specific examples of potential risk stratification ambiguity relative to consideration for ICD therapy concern a family history of HCM-related sudden death, generally regarded as a justification for a primary prevention implant. However, should 'only' one sudden death in a close relative of a surviving affected individual

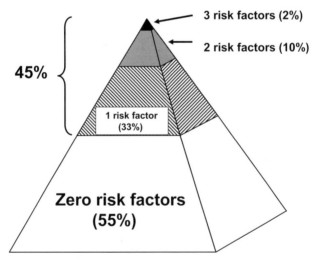

Fig. 23.7 Percentages of clinically identified, hospital-based hypertrophic cardiomyopathy patients with known risk factors for sudden death. It is evident that a substantial proportion of hypertrophic cardiomyopathy patients (45%) have some evidence of increased risk. Adapted from the data of Elliott *et al.*[23]

be sufficient to trigger a prophylactic ICD in that individual? Alternatively, should two or more such deaths be required for this treatment strategy?[50,65] Also, should *all* affected members in a large HCM family be offered an ICD because of a familial occurrence of one (or two) sudden deaths? Data governing such critical questions are sparse, and definitive answers are not always available. Therefore, it is reasonable to conclude, at present, that the power and sophistication of the ICD to effectively abort sudden cardiac death exceeds that of available risk stratification profiles to reliably discriminate all appropriate candidates with HCM for an ICD.

Further studies with much larger numbers of HCM patients are under way (completion scheduled for 2004), with the expectation of defining with greater precision those patients who should be targeted for (and would benefit most from) prophylactic defibrillator therapy. Such investigations will necessarily be retrospective and prospective in design, but uncontrolled and nonrandomized due to the relatively uncommon and heterogeneous nature of the disease[2,58] and the particularly long risk period characteristic of young HCM patients, which would make any such study prolonged in design and impractical,[7,13,14] as well as certain obvious ethical considerations that would necessarily arise by virtue of denying the ICD option to some at-risk patients.

Complications and other considerations

It is important to recognize the potential complications of ICD therapy that may impact on implant decisions, including inappropriate and spurious device discharges,[13] fractured or disrupted leads, and infection. The substantial cost of the ICD may be another important obstacle (particularly over the long time periods required), as is the limited access to ICDs and restrictions on its acceptability as a legitimate treatment modality in certain countries (Fig. 23.8).[49,50] Of course, all these issues must be weighed against the ultimate potential benefit of the ICD for individual high-risk patients; i.e. the preservation of life.

Implications

Primary ventricular tachyarrhythmias arising from an unstable myocardial substrate appear to be the basis of sudden and unexpected death in HCM. While the precise identification of the HCM patient subset at high risk for a catastrophic event continues to present challenges and some uncertainty, prevention of sudden death is now an achievable aspiration for high-risk patients with HCM, due to recent application of the ICD to this genetic disease. It is evident that the ICD is efficacious and can be life-saving in HCM, with an important role in both secondary and primary prevention of sudden cardiac death.

It is also possible that the ICD could afford some HCM patients normal or near-normal longevity. Most HCM patients will not develop atrial fibrillation or severely limiting heart failure-related symptoms. Therefore, in those patients for whom the consequences of this disease are largely or completely confined to sudden electrically based events with ventricular fibrillation, the

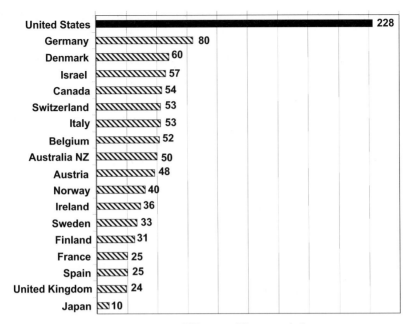

ICDs per million population

Fig. 23.8 Defibrillator implants worldwide in the year 2001, shown by country (per 1 000 000). The rates shown are for all ICD indications, but largely represent implants in high-risk patients with coronary artery disease.

ICD could potentially treat successfully (and repetitively) their only disease complication, which, in fact, may arise only very infrequently during a lifetime. However, the defibrillator should not be regarded as a treatment strategy for all (or even most) patients with HCM, and should be confined to that relatively small subset of patients judged to be at high risk for sudden death in accord with current risk stratification profiles.

References

1 Teare D. Asymmetrical hypertrophy of the heart in young patients. *Br Heart J* 1958; **20**: 1–8.
2 Maron BJ. Hypertrophic cardiomyopathy: A systematic review. *JAMA* 2002; **287**: 1308–20.
3 Maron BJ. Hypertrophic cardiomyopathy. *Lancet* 1997; **350**: 127–33.
4 Wigle ED, Rakowski H, Kimball BP *et al.* Hypertrophic cardiomyopathy. Clinical spectrum and treatment. *Circulation* 1995; **92**: 1680–92.
5 Spirito P, Seidman CE, McKenna WJ, Maron BJ. The management of hypertrophic cardiomyopathy. *N Engl J Med* 1997; **336**: 775–85.
6 Maron BJ, Roberts WC, Epstein SE. Sudden death in hypertrophic cardiomyopathy: Profile of 78 patients. *Circulation* 1982; **65**: 1388–94.

7 Maron BJ, Olivotto I, Spirito P *et al.* Epidemiology of hypertrophic cardiomyopathy-related death: Revisited in a large non-referral based patient population. *Circulation* 2000; **102**: 858–64.

8 Spirito P, Rapezzi C, Autore C *et al.* Prognosis of asymptomatic patients with hypertrophic cardiomyopathy and nonsustained ventricular tachycardia. *Circulation* 1994; **90**: 2743–7.

9 Olivotto I, Maron BJ, Montereggi A *et al.* Prognostic value of systemic blood pressure response during exercise in a community-based patient population with hypertrophic cardiomyopathy. *J Am Coll Cardiol* 1999; **33**: 2044–51.

10 Maron BJ, Savage DD, Wolfson JK *et al.* Prognostic significance of 24-hour ambulatory electrocardiographic monitoring in patients with hypertrophic cardiomyopathy: a prospective study. *Am J Cardiol* 1981; **48**: 252–7.

11 McKenna WJ, Camm AJ. Sudden death in hypertrophic cardiomyopathy: Assessment of patients at high risk. *Circulation* 1989; **80**: 1489–92.

12 Maron BJ, Cecchi F, McKenna WJ. Risk factors and stratification for sudden cardiac death in patients with hypertrophic cardiomyopathy. *Br Heart J* 1994; **72** (Suppl.): S13–18.

13 Maron BJ, Shen W-K, Link MS *et al.* Efficacy of implantable cardioverter–defibrillators for the prevention of sudden death in patients with hypertrophic cardiomyopathy. *N Engl J Med* 2000; **342**: 365–73.

14 Spirito P, Bellone P, Harris KM *et al.* Magnitude of left ventricular hypertrophy predicts the risk of sudden death in hypertrophic cardiomyopathy. *N Engl J Med* 2000; **324**: 1778–85.

15 McKenna WJ, Oakley CM, Krikler DM *et al.* Improved survival with amiodarone in patients with hypertrophic cardiomyopathy and ventricular tachycardia. *Br Heart J* 1985; **53**: 412–16.

16 Cecchi F, Olivotto I, Montereggi A *et al.* Prognostic value of non-sustained ventricular tachycardia and the potential role of amiodarone treatment in hypertrophic cardiomyopathy: Assessment in an unselected non-referral based patient population. *Heart* 1998; **79**: 331–6.

17 Maron BJ, Bonow RO, Cannon RO *et al.* Hypertrophic cardiomyopathy: Interrelation of clinical manifestations, pathophysiology, and therapy (Parts I and II). *N Engl J Med* 1987; **316**: 780–789 and 844–852.

18 Nicod P, Polikar R, Peterson KL. Hypertrophic cardiomyopathy and sudden death. *N Engl J Med* 1988; **318**: 1255–6.

19 Stafford WJ, Trohman RG, Bilsker M *et al.* Cardiac arrest in an adolescent with atrial fibrillation and hypertrophic cardiomyopathy. *J Am Coll Cardiol* 1986; **7**: 701–4.

20 Fannapazir L, Chang AC, Epstein SE *et al.* Prognostic determinants in hypertrophic cardiomyopathy: Prospective evaluation of a therapeutic strategy based on clinical, Holter, hemodynamic and electrophysiologic findings. *Circulation* 1992; **86**: 730–40.

21 Sadoul N, Prasad L, Elliott PM *et al.* Prospective diagnostic assessment of blood pressure response during exercise in patients with hypertrophic cardiomyopathy. *Circulation* 1997; **96**: 2987–91.

22 Elliott PM, Gimeno JR, Mahon NG *et al.* Relation between severity of left-ventricular hypertrophy and prognosis in patients with hypertrophic cardiomyopathy. *Lancet* 2001; **357**: 420–4.

23 Elliott PM, Poloniecki J, Dickie S *et al.* Sudden death in hypertrophic cardiomyopathy: Identification of high risk patients. *J Am Coll Cardiol* 2000; **36**: 2212–18.

24 Watkins H. Sudden death in hypertrophic cardiomyopathy [editorial]. *N Engl J Med* 2000; **342**: 422–4.

25 Maron BJ, Spirito P. Impact of patient selection biases on the perception of hypertrophic cardiomyopathy and its natural history. *Am J Cardiol* 1993; **72**: 970–2.

26 Spirito P, Chiarella F, Carratino L *et al.* Clinical course and prognosis of hypertrophic cardiomyopathy in an outpatient population. *N Engl J Med* 1989; **320**: 749–55.

27 Olivotto I, Cecchi F, Casey SA *et al.* Impact of atrial fibrillation on the clinical course of hypertrophic cardiomyopathy. *Circulation* 2001; **104**: 2517–24.

28 Maron BJ, Olivotto I, Bellone P *et al.* Clinical profile of stroke in 900 patients with hypertrophic cardiomyopathy. *J Am Coll Cardiol* 2002; **39**: 301–7.

29 Adabag AS, Casey SA, Maron BJ. Sudden death in hypertrophic cardiomyopathy: Patterns and prognostic significance of tachyarrhythmias on ambulatory Holter ECG [abstract]. *Circulation* 2002; **106** (Suppl. II): II-710.

30 Elliott PM, Sharma S, Varnava A *et al.* Survival after cardiac arrest in patients with hypertrophic cardiomyopathy. *J Am Coll Cardiol* 1999; **33**: 1596–601.

31 Boriani G, Rapezzi C, Biffi M, Branzi A, Spirito P. Atrial fibrillation precipitating sustained ventricular tachycardia in hypertrophic cardiomyopathy. *J Cardiovasc Electrophysiol* 2002; **13**: 954.

32 Maron BJ, Roberts WC. Quantitative analysis of cardiac muscle cell disorganization in the ventricular septum of patients with hypertrophic cardiomyopathy. *Circulation* 1979; **59**: 689–706.

33 Maron BJ, Anan TJ, Roberts WC. Quantitative analysis of the distribution of cardiac muscle cell disorganization in the left ventricular wall of patients with hypertrophic cardiomyopathy. *Circulation* 1981; **63**: 882–94.

34 Maron BJ, Wolfson JK, Epstein SE *et al.* Intramural ('small vessel') coronary artery disease in hypertrophic cardiomyopathy. *J Am Coll Cardiol* 1986; **8**: 545–57.

35 Tanaka M, Fujiwara H, Onodera T *et al.* Quantitative analysis of myocardial fibrosis in normal, hypertensive hearts, and hypertrophic cardiomyopathy. *Br Heart J* 1986; **55**: 575–81.

36 Tanaka M, Fujiwara H, Onodera T *et al.* Quantitative analysis of narrowings of intramyocardial small arteries in normal hearts, hypertensive hearts, and hearts with hypertrophic cardiomyopathy. *Circulation* 1987; **75**: 1130–9.

37 Cannon RO, Rosing DR, Maron BJ *et al.* Myocardial ischemia in hypertrophic cardiomyopathy: Contribution of inadequate vasodilator reserve and elevated left ventricular filling pressures. *Circulation* 1985; **71**: 234–43.

38 Maron BJ, Shirani J, Poliac LC *et al.* Sudden death in young competitive athletes: Clinical, demographic and pathological profiles. *JAMA* 1996; **276**: 199–204.

39 Maron BJ, Carney KP, Lever HM *et al.* Relationship of race to sudden cardiac death in competitive athletes with hypertrophic cardiomyopathy. *J Am Coll Cardiol* 2003; **41**: 974–80.

40 Maron BJ, Casey SA, Poliac LC *et al.* Clinical consequences of hypertrophic cardiomyopathy in an unselected regional United States cohort. *JAMA* 1999; **281**: 650–5.

41 Monserrat L, Elliott PM, Gimeno JR, Sharma S, Penas-Lado M, McKenna WJ. Nonsustained ventricular tachycardia in hypertrophic cardiomyopathy: an independent marker of sudden death risk in young patients. *J Am Coll Cardiol* 2003; **42**: 873–9.

43 Maron MS, Olivotto I, Betocchi S *et al.* Effect of left ventricular outflow tract obstruction on clinical outcome in hypertrophic cardiomyopathy. *N Engl J Med* 2003; **348**: 295–303.

43 Maki S, Ikeda H, Muro A *et al.* Predictors of sudden cardiac death in hypertrophic cardiomyopathy. *Am J Cardiol* 1998; **82**: 774–8.

44 Yetman AT, McCrindle BW, MacDonald C, Freedom RM, Gow R. Myocardial bridging in children with hypertrophic cardiomyopathy – a risk factor for sudden death. *N Engl J Med* 1998; **339**: 1201–9.

45 Gregoratos G, Abrams J, Epstein AE *et al.* ACC/AHA/NASPE 2002 Guideline Update for Implantation of Cardiac Pacemakers and Antiarrhythmia Devices: Summary article: A report of the American College of Cardiology/American Heart Association Task Force on Practice Guidelines. *Circulation* 2002; **106**: 2145–61.

46 Silka MJ, Kron J, Dunnigan A, Dick M. Sudden cardiac death and the use of implantable cardioverter–defibrillators in pediatric patients. The Pediatric Electrophysiology Society. *Circulation* 1993; **87**: 800–7.

47 Maron BJ, Estes NAM III, Maron MS, Almquist AK, Link MS, Udelson J. Primary prevention of sudden death as a novel treatment strategy in hypertrophic cardiomyopathy. *Circulation* 2003; **107**: 2872–5.

48 Spirito P, Maron BJ. Sudden death and hypertrophic cardiomyopathy [correspondence]. *Lancet* 2001; **357**: 1975–6.

49 Camm AJ, Nisam S. The utilization of the implantable defibrillator – a European enigma. *Eur Heart J* 2000; **21**: 1998–2004.

50 Maron BJ. Contemporary considerations for risk stratification, sudden death and prevention in hypertrophic cardiomyopathy [editorial]. *Heart* 2003; **89**: 1–2.

51 Mirowski M, Reid PR, Mower MM *et al.* Termination of malignant ventricular arrhythmias with an implanted automatic defibrillator in human beings. *N Engl J Med* 1980; **303**: 322–4.

52 The Antiarrhythmics Versus Implantable Defibrillators (AVID) Investigators: A comparison of antiarrhythmic-drug therapy with implantable defibrillators in patients resuscitated from near-fatal ventricular arrhythmias. *N Engl J Med* 1997; **337**: 1576–83.

53 Moss AJ, Zareba W, Hall WJ *et al.* Prophylactic implantation of a defibrillator in patients with myocardial infarction and reduced ejection fraction. *N Engl J Med* 2002; **346**: 877–83.

54 Buxton AE, Lee KL, Fisher JD *et al.* A randomized study of the prevention of sudden death in patients with coronary artery disease. *N Engl J Med* 1999; **341**: 1882–90.

55 Moss AJ, Daubert JP. Internal ventricular defibrillation. *N Engl J Med* 2000; **342**: 398.

56 Link MS, Wang PJ, Haugh CJ *et al.* Arrhythmogenic right ventricular dysplasia: Clinical results with implantable cardioverter defibrillator. *J Intervent Card Electrophysiol* 1997; **1**: 41–8.

57 Primo J, Geelen P, Brugada J *et al.* Hypertrophic cardiomyopathy: Role of the implantable cardioverter–defibrillator. *J Am Coll Cardiol* 1998; **31**: 1081–5.

58 Maron BJ, Danielson GK, Kappenberger LJ *et al.* American College of Cardiology/European Society of Cardiology Clinical Expert Consensus Document on Hypertrophic Cardiomyopathy. A report of the American College of Cardiology Task Force on Clinical Expert Consensus Documents and the European Society of Cardiology Committee for Practice Guidelines and Policy Conferences. *J Am Coll Cardiol* 2003; **42**: 1687–713.

59 Klues HG, Schiffers A, Maron BJ. Phenotypic spectrum and patterns of left ventricular hypertrophy in hypertrophic cardiomyopathy: Morphologic observations and significance as assessed by two-dimensional echocardiography in 600 patients. *J Am Coll Cardiol* 1995; **26**: 1699–708.

60 Maron BJ, Gross BW, Stark SI. Extreme left ventricular hypertrophy. *Circulation* 1995; **92**: 2748.

61 Borggrefe MM, McKenna WJ. Primary and secondary prevention of sudden death with the ICD in hypertrophic cardiomyopathy. Results of the European Registry on ICD in HCM [abstract]. *Circulation* 2002; **106**: II-710.

62 Stefanelli CB, LeRoy S, Bradley DJ *et al.* Implantable cardioverter–defibrillator therapy for life-threatening arrhythmias in young patients [abstract]. *Pacing Clin Electrophysiol* 2001; **24**: 571.

63 Shah MJ, Rhodes LA, Sehra R *et al.* Efficacy of implantable cardioverter-defibrillator in prevention of sudden death in children with hypertrophic cardiomyopathy [abstract]. *Pacing Clin Electrophysiol* 2001; **24**: 571.

64 Cecchi F, Maron BJ, Epstein SE. Long-term outcome of patients with hypertrophic cardiomyopathy successfully resuscitated after cardiac arrest. *J Am Coll Cardiol* 1989; **13**: 1283–8.

65 Maron BJ, Gardin JM, Flack JM *et al.* Assessment of the prevalence of hypertrophic cardiomyopathy in a general population of young adults: Echocardiographic analysis of 4111 subjects in the CARDIA Study. *Circulation* 1995; **92**: 785–9.

66 Maron BJ, Lipson LC, Roberts WC *et al.* 'Malignant' hypertrophic cardiomyopathy: Identification of a subgroup of families with unusually frequent premature deaths. *Am J Cardiol* 1978; **41**: 1133–40.

CHAPTER 24

Hypertrophic Cardiomyopathy and Other Causes of Sudden Death in the Trained Athlete: An Electrophysiologist Perspective on the Management of Benign and Not So Benign Arrhythmias

N. A. Mark Estes III, MD, Paul J. Wang, MD, Munther K. Homoud, MD, and Mark S. Link, MD

The evaluation and management of athletes with a documented cardiac arrhythmia or symptoms attributable to an arrhythmia represents a challenge for the clinician. Arrhythmias in the athlete can range over a full spectrum of risk from benign and asymptomatic to highly symptomatic and life-threatening. There is a risk of not diagnosing an important cardiovascular condition which may predispose to a serious or life-threatening arrhythmia. At the same time there is the risk of unnecessarily restricting the athlete with a more benign condition. Furthermore, the evaluation of the athlete is confounded by many complex, psychological, social and, in some instances, economic implications. Benign arrhythmias, such as many bradyarrhythmias and atrial and ventricular premature contractions, are common in the young and older athlete. Supraventricular arrhythmias, such as atrial fibrillation, atrioventricular (AV) nodal re-entrant tachycardia, and Wolff–Parkinson–White (WPW) syndrome, are less common. The least common, but clearly the most important for diagnosis and appropriate treatment, are life-threatening ventricular arrhythmias, which may predispose patients to a clinical syndrome of sudden cardiac death. Although the annual risk of sudden death in the athlete appears to be low (5–10 athletes for one million participants per year), selected athletes, such as those with hypertrophic cardiomyopathy, may be at particularly high risk. In this chapter, the perspectives of the electrophysiologist on the management of benign and not so benign arrhythmias in the young and older athlete will be reviewed. In this regard, we will provide the current recommendations for the evaluation and management of bradyarrhythmias, supraventricular arrhythmias, and ventricular arrhythmias in the athlete and review the current status of the automatic external defibrillator. In addition, we will provide recommendations for participation in athletics based on the 26th Bethesda Conference recommendations for determining the eligibility for competition of athletes with cardiovascular abnormalities[1] and the NASPE (North American Society of Pacing and Electrophysiology) Consensus Statement on Arrhythmias in the Athlete.[2]

Evaluation and management

The evaluation and management of the athlete with a cardiac arrhythmia begins with a detailed history. The physician should always ask the individual whether they have any symptoms of an arrhythmia. These might include palpitations, lightheadedness, 'skipped beats', 'extra beats', chest pressure, shortness of breath, presyncope or syncope. When any symptoms are present, the physician should determine whether these are associated with exertion, post-exertion or rest. In general, any symptoms of an arrhythmia which occur with exertion are more likely to be serious than those occurring at rest.[3,4] Rarely a neurocardiogenic reflex can be the cause of syncope during exertion.[5-8] The duration and frequency of the symptoms are important. In this respect, symptoms that are frequent and sustained (lasting longer than 30 seconds) are probably less likely to be serious or life-threatening compared with those that are short-lived and shorter in duration. The decision to further evaluate the athlete with symptoms possibly due to an arrhythmia needs to be made in the context of the patient's family history of any significant cardiovascular condition or premature sudden death and the presence or absence of any structural heart disease in the athlete. In general, when an athlete presents with symptoms consistent with a more serious arrhythmia with sudden onset, syncope, and exertionally related symptoms, a full evaluation is warranted. By contrast, for the athlete with symptoms which suggest a less serious condition, such as post-exertional lightheadedness or orthostatic symptoms, it may be appropriate to undertake a more limited evaluation.

When evaluating symptoms in the athlete, the physician needs to be mindful of the family medical history and the presence or absence of structural heart disease as determined by the physical examination, supplemented selectively by an ECG and echocardiogram.[9-15] Symptoms in association with many types of structural heart disease, including hypertrophic cardiomyopathy, may be associated with an increased risk of sudden death. Premature ventricular contractions and nonsustained ventricular tachycardia in the absence of structural heart disease generally have no prognostic significance and need to be treated only if the symptoms are moderate or severe.[2] However, in the presence of structural heart disease, symptoms such as presyncope or syncope, nonsustained ventricular tachycardia, and sustained ventricular tachycardia could be markers of risk for sudden cardiac death.[2,16]

In the younger athlete (less than 35 years of age), hypertrophic cardiomyopathy is the most common underlying structural heart disease predisposing to sudden cardiac death.[17-22] Hypertrophic cardiomyopathy accounts for about 35% of the sudden deaths in athletes in North America. Anomalous origin

Table 24.1 Cardiovascular conditions associated with sudden cardiac death in athletes

Hypertrophic cardiomyopathy
Coronary artery disease
Arrhythmogenic right ventricular dysplasia
Left ventricular hypertrophy
Myocarditis
Conduction system abnormalities
Mitral valve prolapse
Congenital heart disease
Valvular heart disease
Aortic dissection
Cerebral embolus
Pulmonary embolus
Arteriovenous malformation
Berry aneurysm
Wolff–Parkinson–White syndrome
Myocardial bridge
Coronary aneurysm
Subvalvular aortic stenosis
Long QT syndrome
Idiopathic ventricular fibrillation
Dilated cardiomyopathy

of the coronary arteries, arrhythmogenic right ventricular dysplasia, as well as a number of less common conditions causing sudden death in the athlete are listed in Table 24.1. Coronary artery disease is the underlying condition that predisposes to sudden cardiac death in most patients over the age of 35 years.[17–22] By contrast, the experience outside of North America in Italy is that arrhythmogenic right ventricular dysplasia more commonly predisposes to sudden cardiac death in the young athlete compared with hypertrophic cardiomyopathy.[4]

Electrocardiographic changes in the athlete

The evaluation of the athlete is confounded by changes in surface electrocardiogram which are commonly based on the physiologic adaptations that occur in myocardial conduction, repolarization, impulse formation and the response to athletic conditioning and changes in autonomic tone.[9–15,23] Many of these electrocardiographic changes (Table 24.2) are subject to misinterpretation as representing underlying cardiac disease. It is not uncommon for athletes to undergo diagnostic evaluations based on ECG abnormalities, including ventricular hypertrophy, bradyarrhythmias, and repolarization abnormalities, which are physiologic rather than pathologic. Such diagnostic tests might include stress testing, ambulatory monitoring, echocardiogram or even invasive tests such as electrophysiologic evaluation or cardiac catheterization.[9–15,23] Occasionally unnecessary restriction from exercise or unwarranted therapy may be instituted based on ECG changes. An ECG may also manifest changes

Table 24.2 Common electrocardiographic findings in athletes

Sinus bradycardia
Sinus arrhythmia
First-degree atrioventricular block
Second-degree Wenckebach atrioventricular block
Incomplete right bundle branch block
Notched P waves
Right ventricular hypertrophy by voltage criteria
Left ventricular hypertrophy by voltage criteria
Repolarization abnormalities including J point and ST-segment evaluation and depression
Corrected QT interval at the upper limit of normal
Tall, peaked, and inverted T wave

which indicate the potential for life-threatening arrhythmia which should be recognized by the physician.[9–15] These include the pseudo-infarct pattern seen in hypertrophic cardiomyopathy with septal Q waves, the epsilon wave and T-wave inversions across the precordium with arrhythmogenic right ventricular dysplasia, the ST-segment elevation in lead V1 with Brugada syndrome, and the delta waves which are present in patients with WPW syndrome.[9–15,24–26] In addition, individuals with long QT syndrome have a spectrum of repolarization abnormalities recognizable on the surface ECG.[9–15,27]

Spontaneous arrhythmias may be detected by monitoring the patient by Holter, loop or event monitoring as part of the evaluation for symptoms. In addition to the abnormalities on ECGs, there is a spectrum of cardiac arrhythmias which occur more commonly in the athlete.[2,12–14] These include sinus bradycardia, first- and second-degree AV block and occasionally third-degree AV block. In addition, atrial premature contractions and short runs of supraventricular tachycardia, ventricular premature contractions and short runs of nonsustained ventricular tachycardia are also found in the absence of symptoms and in the absence of structural heart disease.[2,12–14] The sinus bradycardia and AV conduction abnormalities are generally felt to be due to withdrawal of sympathetic tone and an increase in vagal tone. As such, they are reversible with atropine and exercise, and in the absence of symptoms do not need further evaluation or therapy. Any spontaneous arrhythmias need to be evaluated and treated based on the patient's symptoms and underlying structural heart disease, as determined by the history, physical examination and ECG, and an echocardiogram. Evaluation of symptoms such as palpitations, presyncope, and syncope is most frequently effectively evaluated with event monitors and loop monitors, which can be activated at the time of the patient's symptoms. For individuals having exercise-related symptoms, selected use of stress testing would be appropriate.[28]

Electrophysiologic observations

In individuals with documented sustained arrhythmias or symptoms suggestive of a sustained arrhythmia (or structural heart disease), selective use of invasive electrophysiologic evaluation for further analysis and guiding therapy of the arrhythmia may be appropriate. The invasive techniques of electrophysiologic evaluation are identical in the athlete and nonathlete; however, the spectrum of normal sinus node and AV node function may be altered considerably as a result of the heightened vagal tone in athletes.[12] With the usual diagnostic electrophysiologic evaluation, catheters are placed through the femoral vein, to the high right atrium, AV junction to record from the bundle of His and the right ventricular apex. The initial comprehensive evaluation and diagnostic portion includes the evaluation of sinus node function with sinus node recovery times, sinoatrial conduction times, assessment of AV nodal conduction with onset of Wenckebach, onset of 2:1 and AV node curves antegrade and retrograde. In addition, the His–Purkinje system is assessed by recording the His potential and assessing the HV interval as well as assessing its response to antegrade and retrograde premature stimuli. This portion of the test would identify the electrophysiologic substrate for arrhythmias such as atrioventricular bypass tracts (WPW) or dual AV nodal physiology. When present, programmed atrial and ventricular stimulation can be used to induce sustained arrhythmias. This evaluation is performed in the drug-free state. When appropriate, programmed ventricular stimulation is performed at the right ventricular apex and outflow tract. In selected individuals who do not have underlying coronary disease, programmed atrial or ventricular stimulation may be supplemented by isoproterenol administration. The predictive value of electrophysiologic studies, sensitivity and specificity are very dependent upon the type of underlying structural heart disease and clinical presentation. It is widely appreciated, for example, that programmed ventricular stimulation has high sensitivity and specificity in individuals with underlying coronary artery disease but has considerably lower sensitivity and specificity in patients with dilated cardiomyopathies or other types of primary electrical diseases, such as long QT syndrome or Brugada syndrome.[12]

The use of electrophysiologic studies in patients with hypertrophic cardiomyopathy remains controversial.[30–32] In the largest series of patients with hypertrophic cardiomyopathy reported with programmed stimulation, 230 patients underwent electrophysiologic evaluation.[30] These patients all had clinically and echocardiographically hypertrophic cardiomyopathy but were not selected based on the occurrence of spontaneous clinical arrhythmias. In these individuals, sustained ventricular arrhythmias were induced in 36%, polymorphic ventricular tachycardia being three times more common than monomorphic ventricular tachycardia. In the group of individuals who had previously been resuscitated from sudden cardiac death, 66% had an induced arrhythmia.[30] Thirty per cent of individuals with asymptomatic hypertrophic cardiomyopathy had inducible ventricular arrhythmia.[30] In the subset of individuals with inducible ventricular arrhythmias, there was a higher incidence of subsequent cardiac arrest in prospective follow-up, particularly in those who had had prior episodes of presyncope or syncope. However, three of

17 patients with a subsequent cardiac arrest did not have any inducible ventricular arrhythmias. All three of these individuals previously had syncope or resuscitated sudden death. Based on this data, it would seem that electrophysiologic evaluation in patients with hypertrophic cardiomyopathy has the greatest utility in patients with prior episodes of syncope or cardiac arrest. However, even in the subset segment of individuals who are not inducible the risk of sudden death remains high, particularly if they had previous syncope or resuscitated sudden death. Therefore, there appears no clinical utility for using invasive electrophysiologic evaluation for the screening of patients with asymptomatic hypertrophic cardiomyopathy.

The sensitivity and specificity of electrophysiologic evaluations in individuals with arrhythmogenic right ventricular dysplasia is in the clinically acceptable range of 70–80%.[12,33–35] In patients with inducible sustained arrhythmia at electrophysiologic evaluation in arrhythmogenic right ventricular dysplasia, there is an increased risk of subsequent sudden death.[12,33–35] There are very limited data on the use of electrophysiologic evaluation for evaluation of patients with other types of congenital heart disease.[36] Recurrence of sudden death presumptively due to ventricular arrhythmias or bradyarrhythmias in patients with surgically repaired tetralogy of Fallot has been reported to be up to 7%. Unfortunately, there are also limited data regarding the prognostic utility of electrophysiologic studies for risk stratification.[36] It is widely appreciated that in patients with primary electrical disease, such as the long QT syndrome, programmed ventricular stimulation has no prognostic use.[37] However, it appears that catecholamine infusion, including isoproterenol and epinephrine, and exercise testing have some clinical utility in evaluating those patients with suspected long QT syndrome.[12,37] Paradoxically, in individuals with long QT syndrome, catecholamine infusions and exercise increase the QTc interval.[37] In the Brugada syndrome, manifested by ST segment elevation in the right precordial leads with a pattern of atypical right bundle branch block,[38] programmed ventricular stimulation serves as a risk stratifier for this condition.[38]

Bradyarrhythmias

Due to increase in vagal tone, a broad spectrum of bradyarrhythmias and other electrophysiologic alterations is commonly observed in conditioned athletes. Multiple studies have documented that vagal tone is increased in athletes with withdrawal of sympathetic tone relative to the level of fitness.[9–13,15,23] In the absence of symptoms, evaluation is not usually warranted.[9–13] However, extreme bradycardia with resting rates less than 30 b.p.m. or sinus pauses longer than 3 seconds can result in symptoms. This is most commonly seen in endurance athletes, such as long-distance runners, bicyclists, and long-distance swimmers. Symptomatic or extreme bradyarrhythmias can be evaluated with a history, physical examination, electrocardiogram supplemented with a 24-hour ambulatory monitoring and exercise tolerance testing. If there is any indication from the history, physical examination, and ECG of structural heart disease, an echocardiogram should be performed. In individuals with either symptoms or structural heart disease, there is no need to restrict athletic activity.[1,2,39] By contrast, in the presence of structural heart disease, restriction should be based on particular heart disease.[1,2] It rarely will become necessary to restrict training and competition in well-conditioned athletes because of symptomatic resting bradycardias. In such athletes without structural heart disease (including coronary artery disease), all training and competitive athletics are allowed if the heart rate increases appropriately with exercise and the patient is asymptomatic at rest.[1,2] An exercise stress test or Holter monitor with exercise can be useful for evaluation of athletes with resting sinus bradycardia.[1,2,28] It is generally accepted that in athletes with symptoms such as presyncope or syncope, participation in athletics should be restricted for a period of 3–6 months.[1,2] When permanent pacemaker therapy is necessary, restriction from contact sports is recommended.[1,2] Indications for permanent pacing in athletes with sinus bradycardia are based on symptoms and exercise limitation due to chronotropic incompetence as opposed to the absolute heart rate.[1,2,39] Unfortunately, electrophysiologic studies are neither sensitive nor specific for evaluation of sinus node dysfunction and sinus bradycardia in athletes and nonathletes; consequently, there is a very limited role for invasive electrophysiologic evaluation in the evaluation of sinus bradycardia.[12]

First-degree AV block and Wenckebach (Mobitz I heart block) are also common in athletes due to the heightened vagal tone.[9–12,15,23,40] Most commonly, first-degree AV block and Wenckebach are manifestations of heightened vagal tone which is withdrawn with exercise and resolves with atropine. It is not uncommon to find Wenckebach-type block at rest or particularly during sleep in an athlete who has no symptoms of bradyarrhythmia. However, if symptoms of presyncope, syncope, or fatigue are present, further evaluation and occasionally therapy is warranted.[1,2] Uncommonly, Mobitz type II block or complete heart block (third-degree AV block) are present in an athlete.[9–12,15] Occasionally, an athlete will present with 2:1 atrial:ventricular conduction. It can be difficult, based on the surface ECG, to determine whether the level of block is at the AV node or the His–Purkinje system. Noninvasive maneuvers such as administration of atropine can be helpful. This typically results in improvement in the conduction ratio if it is at the level of the AV node and worsening if it is below the AV node (infra-Hisian). In this setting, invasive electrophysiologic evaluation with recording of the His bundle potential also can provide insights into the level of block. Mobitz type II block occurs below the bundle of His and is readily diagnosed with intracardiac recordings. If the QRS complex is of normal duration without an intraventricular conduction delay, it would be unusual for 2:1 AV block to be at the level of the His–Purkinje system. If it is determined that the patient had symptoms related to any level of AV block (Wenckebach, Mobitz type II, or complete heart block), consideration of permanent pacing is warranted (Table 24.3). In the absence of symptoms of worsening of AV block with exercise or underlying structural heart dis-

Table 24.3 Algorithm for bradyarrhythmias. Note should be made of the recommendations for prophylactic pacemaker insertion for patients with Mobitz II heart block or higher. Note should also be made of the recommendations for avoiding sports with bodily contact after a pacemaker is inserted (based on the 26th Bethesda Conference). HB = heart block; ECG = electrocardiogram; LH = lightheadedness; PPM = permanent pacemaker; CHB = complete heart block. Modified from Link *et al.* Cardiac arrhythmias and electrophysiologic observations in the athletes. In: Williams RA, ed. *The Athlete and Heart Disease: Diagnosis, Evaluation & Management.* Philadelphia, PA: Lippincott Williams & Wilkins, 1999: 197–216

Condition	Symptoms	Diagnosis	Treatment options	Competitive athletics
Sinus bradycardia	None	ECG	None	No restrictions
Sinus arrhythmia	None	ECG	None	No restrictions
1st-degree HB	None	ECG	None	No restrictions
Wenckebach	None	Monitor, ECG	None	No restrictions
Wenckebach	LH, syncope	Monitor, ECG	PPM	No bodily collision if PPM
Mobitz II or CHB	None	Monitor, ECG	PPM	No bodily collision if PPM
Mobitz II or CHB	Dizziness, syncope	Monitor, ECG	PPM	No bodily collision if PPM

ease, there is generally no need for therapy or restriction from athletic activity.[1,2,9–12,15,23] For athletes without structural heart disease, congenital complete heart block, and no symptoms with a resting rate greater than 40 b.p.m. (and without ventricular arrhythmias during exercise), no restrictions in exercise are recommended.[1,2]

Supraventricular arrhythmias

Supraventricular arrhythmias in the athlete may be benign, asymptomatic and not require therapy. Occasionally, however, they may be associated with more severe symptoms or cause hemodynamic collapse and require definitive treatment. Atrial fibrillation in the presence of hypertrophic cardiomyopathy can result in loss of atrial contraction, lowering of cardiac output and hemodynamic collapse.[42] In general, a careful history, physical examination, and 12-lead ECG is recommended.[1,2,12] Premature atrial contractions may be symptomatic and detected by the athlete or the physician. Without evidence of structural heart disease with clinically important symptoms, evaluation beyond a 12-lead ECG is unwarranted.[1,2] By contrast, in athletes with clinically important symptoms such as palpitations, presyncope, or longer runs of atrial tachycardia, therapy might be warranted, most commonly with β-blockers. There is no need to bar athletes with premature atrial contractions from competitive athletics.[1,2,11,12]

Atrial fibrillation or flutter is more common in the athlete than in an aged-match population of nonathletes.[40–42] Vagally mediated atrial fibrillation may also be more common in athletes.[12,41] Additionally, it is felt that focal atrial tachycardias if as rapid as focal atrial fibrillation (more than 250 b.p.m.) may be more common in the younger age group.[43] Athletes presenting with atrial fibrillation or flutter should undergo a comprehensive history and physical examination, including a detailed history with regard to alcohol, caffeine or illicit drug use, ECG, echocardiogram, as well as thyroid-stimulating hormone to screen for thyroid abnormalities. Atrial fibrillation represents the most common sustained arrhythmia in hypertrophic cardiomyopathy.[41] Approximately 20–25% of patients with hypertrophic cardiomyopathy will develop atrial fibrillation. Increasing left atrium size and age are associated with an increased risk of atrial fibrillation. Atrial fibrillation is not associated with an increased risk of sudden death and is reasonably well tolerated by approximately one-third of hypertrophic cardiomyopathy patients. It is, however, associated with an increased risk for stroke and progression of heart failure. Amiodarone is considered relatively effective in maintaining normal sinus rhythm in patients with hypertrophic cardiomyopathy. However, when paroxysms of atrial fibrillation or persistent atrial fibrillation develop, rate control with β-blockers, verapamil, or atrioventricular junction and pacing and anticoagulation is warranted.[41]

If the patient experiences sustained atrial fibrillation or flutter, the maximal ventricular response should be assessed with an exercise stress test and ambulatory monitoring while the patient is exercising. Strategies for treatment of atrial fibrillation include rhythm control (by re-establishing and maintaining normal sinus rhythm) and rate control during atrial fibrillation.[2,12,41] The rhythm control strategy has the advantage of avoiding anticoagulation but the limitation of side-effects and costs of anti-arrhythmic drug therapy or β-blockers needed to increase the probability of maintaining NSR.[2,12,41] Control of the ventricular response with β-blockers or calcium channel blockers can be difficult in athletes as their ventricular response may accelerate rapidly with exercise. The physician managing the athlete with atrial fibrillation should be mindful that β-blockers are prohibited in some competitive athletics.[12] In addition, β-blockers are generally tolerated poorly by the athlete. When anticoagulation is required for reducing the risk of stroke, athletes should be restricted from sports in which there is a danger of bodily collision.[1,2] For individuals with (and without) structural heart disease in whom atrial fibrillation results in a ventricular response during physical activity comparable to the appropriate sinus tachycardia, while receiving no therapy with rate-slowing agents, participation in competitive athletics is restricted according to the type of structural heart disease present.[1,2] Based on the high cure rates of focal atrial fibrillation and atrial flutter with radiofrequency ablation techniques, it is preferable to undertake a curative approach with radiofrequency ablation.[12,43,44] When athletes are cured definitively of their focal atrial fibrillation or flutter, resumption of athletic activity within a period of approximately 3 months[1,2] is appropriate.

Sustained supraventricular tachycardia most commonly has its mechanistic basis in re-entry within the AV node in the athlete (Table 24.4). Based on a low complication rate and a high cure rate when an athlete presents with symptomatic supraventricular, invasive electrophysiologic evaluation is justi-

Table 24.4 Supraventricular arrhythmias in the athlete. APC = atrial premature contractions; AVNRT = atrioventricular nodal re-entrant tachycardia within normal limits; ECG = electrocardiogram; EPS = electrophysiology study; RFA = radiofrequency ablation; WNL = within normal limits; WPW = Wolf–Parkinson–White syndrome. Modified from Link et al. Cardiac arrhythmias and electrophysiologic observations in the athletes. In: Williams RA, ed. *The Athlete and Heart Disease: Diagnosis, Evaluation & Management*. Philadelphia, PA: Lippincott Williams & Wilkins, 1999: 197–216

Arrhythmia	Baseline ECG	Symptoms	Diagnosis	Treatment options	Guidelines for athletic participation[1,2]
APCs	Often WNL	Palpitations	Monitor	Reassurance	No restrictions β-Blocker if highly symptomatic
Atrial fibrillation	Often WNL	Palpitations	Monitor	Anti-arrhythmics, anticoagulation, and with warfarin rate control	Body contact prohibited
Atrial flutter	Often WNL	Palpitations	Monitor	RFA Anti-arrhythmics Rate control and anticoagulation	Body contract prohibited with warfarin
Ventricular pre-excitation (WPW)	Short PR Delta waves	Asymptomatic	Monitor ECG	No therapy RFA if high risk	Consider EPS to risk stratify
Ventricular pre-excitation (WPW)	Short PR Delta waves	Palpitations	Monitor ECG	RFA Anti-arrhythmics	No restrictions after 3–6 months without symptoms
AVNRT	Normal	Palpitations	Monitor EPS	RFA Anti-arrhythmics	No restrictions after 3–6 months without symptoms

fied to define the mechanism and cure the arrhythmia.[2,12,44] With success rates approaching 98% and complication rates less than 1%, radiofrequency ablation of patients with supraventricular tachycardia due to AV nodal re-entry is considered to be the appropriate first-line therapy.[1,2,12,44] For individuals who elect for radiofrequency ablation therapy, therapy should be proven to be effective for a period of 3 months before resumption of competitive athletics.[1,2] In individuals who have less severe symptoms without presyncope or syncope, or for selected individuals at extremely low risk for arrhythmia recurrence, consideration should be given to allowing resumption of athletic activities on pharmacological therapy earlier than 6 months. In such individuals, the performance of a stress test on pharmacologic therapy to assess for arrhythmia recurrence is reasonable. However, no prospective data are available regarding the predictive accuracy of this approach. Although the guidelines of the 26th Bethesda Conference allow the resumption of all competitive athletics 3 months after radiofrequency ablation[1] for individuals at low risk for arrhythmia recurrence or severe symptoms, many experts will allow resumption of athletic activity at a time earlier than 3 months.[2] Currently, follow-up electrophysiologic evaluation after institution of medical therapy or successful radiofrequency ablation is not warranted. However, in athletes selected on the basis of the severity of symptoms (syncope or presyncope) and participation in high-risk sports, where arrhythmia recurrence may put them at particularly high risk (automobile racing, swimming, biking, horseback riding, downhill skiing), repeat electrophysiologic evaluation to ensure continued success of the definitive therapy prior to participation is reasonable.[1,2,12]

WPW syndrome, manifested by ventricular pre-excitation in the form of a delta wave, is another cause of supraventricular arrhythmias in the athlete. A delta wave is found in approximately 3 out of 1000 individuals.[24–26] The evaluation of the athlete, or any individual with asymptomatic ventricular pre-excitation or a WPW pattern on the surface ECG, remains controversial. Some electrophysiologists recommend observation without restriction of athletic participation since the risk of sudden death appears to be extremely low.[1,2,12] Because WPW syndrome is associated with some congenital abnormalities, such as Ebstein anomaly, a history, physical examination, 12-lead ECG, 24-hour ambulatory monitoring, stress test, and echocardiography should be performed to exclude associated cardiovascular abnormalities.[1,2] Some experts recommend electrophysiological evaluation in the asymptomatic athlete with WPW to define the properties and location of the bypass tract.[1,2,24–26] If conduction to the ventricle is present through the bypass tract at a rate greater than 240 b.p.m., consideration should be given to radiofrequency ablation to eliminate the risk of future life-threatening arrhythmias.[1,2,12,24–26]

Occasionally in an individual presenting with supraventricular tachycardia without delta wave or manifest pre-excitation on the surface ECG, a bypass tract is found conducting from the ventricle to the atrium. This 'concealed' bypass tract allows retrograde conduction from the ventricle to the atrium during the tachycardia with antegrade conduction through the AV node. In individuals with any symptoms of an arrhythmia, including palpitations, lightheadedness, presyncope, syncope, shortness of breath, or chest pressure, catheter ablation is the preferred therapeutic option.[1,2,11,24–26,44] In addition, catheter ablation is the recommended approach in those with structural heart disease with a manifest or concealed bypass tract participating in the circuit during supraventricular tachycardia. This is based on high success rates (greater than 98%) and low complication rates (less than 1%). In addition, it is widely agreed that, in athletes undergoing successful ablation of concealed or manifest bypass tracts without inducible arrhythmias or spontaneous arrhythmia recurrence, participation in competitive athletics for a period of approximately 3 months is reasonable.[1,2]

Ventricular arrhythmias

In evaluating the athlete with ventricular arrhythmias, the nature of the ventricular arrhythmia, the presence or absence of symptoms and the presence or absence of structural heart disease are critical factors in determining the need for therapy or restriction from athletic activity (Table 24.5).[1,2,12,14,16] Most commonly, individuals at risk for sudden cardiac death have underlying structural heart disease, hypertrophic cardiomyopathy being the most common.[17–22,45–50] Only 3 of 134 athletes with a cardiac cause of death had no structural heart disease in a recent review of the topic.[20] Of the remaining 131 patients, 48

Table 24.5 Diagnosis and management of ventricular arrhythmias in athletes. Recommendations for competitive athletics are based on the 26th Bethesda Conference. ECG = electrocardiogram; VPC = ventricular premature contractions; NL = normal; SHD = structural heart disease; BB = β-blockers; NSVT = nonsustained ventricular tachycardia; VT = ventricular tachycardia; VF = ventricular fibrillation; RFA = radiofrequency ablation; ICD = implantable cardioverter–defibrillator; AAD = anti-arrhythmic drugs. Modified from Link *et al.* Cardiac arrhythmias and electrophysiologic observations in the athletes. In: Williams RA, ed. *The Athlete and Heart Disease: Diagnosis, Evaluation & Management.* Philadelphia, PA: Lippincott Williams & Wilkins, 1999: 197–216

Condition	Symptoms	ECG	Diagnosis	Treatment options	Competitive athletics
VPCs	Palpitations	NL	Monitor	Reassurance	No restrictions
NSVT	Palpitations	Often NL	Monitor	Assess for SHD If no SHD, reassure. If SHD, further evaluation needed	No restrictions if no SHD. If SHD, see Table 24.6
VT/VF	Palpitations	Can be NL	Monitor	RFA if no SHD ICD or AAD if SHD present	No restrictions if no SHD and cure by RFA. Restricted to low-intensity sports for all others

had hypertrophic cardiomyopathy, 14 patients having possible hypertrophic cardiomyopathy. Anomalous coronary arteries were found in 17 individuals. In the young athlete, hypertrophic cardiomyopathy and anomalous coronary arteries most commonly account for sudden cardiac death in North America.[17-22,46-50] Over 35 years of age, up to 80% of individuals have underlying coronary artery disease as the anatomic substrate for their sudden death. By contrast, arrhythmogenic right ventricular dysplasia is the most common type of structural heart disease found in young athletes with sudden cardiac death in Italy.[4,48] It is possible that rigorous screening techniques used in Italy for athletes undergoing competition identify individuals at risk with hypertrophic cardiomyopathy and that disproportionate elimination of such individuals from competitive athletics decreases the frequency of sudden death with this condition in competitive athletics.[4,48]

Among patients with hypertrophic cardiomyopathy there is a small subset for whom the risk for sudden death is approximately 5% per year.[41] Noninvasive markers of risk for sudden cardiac death include prior cardiac arrest or spontaneous sustained ventricular tachycardia. Other markers of risk include a family history of sudden death, syncope or near-syncope, spontaneous nonsustained ventricular tachycardia, a hypotensive blood pressure response to exercise, and extreme left ventricular hypertrophy with maximal wall thickness 30 mm or more, particularly in adolescents and young adults.[41] Outflow tract obstruction is not independently associated with an increased risk of sudden death. A novel method for risk stratification has been proposed based on analysis of the fractionation of patterns of right ventricular electrograms in response to programmed ventricular stimulation. However, there are no prospective follow-up data with this technique.[50]

Most patients with hypertrophic cardiomyopathy should undergo a risk stratification assessment, including a thorough history and physical examination, echocardiography, Holter monitoring for 24–48 hours, and treadmill testing. Patients older than 60 years might reasonably be excluded from this evaluation. Unfortunately, there are no data showing that medical therapy (with amiodarone, β-blockers, or verapamil) prevents sudden death in patients with hypertrophic cardiomyopathy. The implantable cardioverter–defibrillator (ICD) currently is the only modality with proven efficacy in sudden death prevention. In a large multicenter study of ICDs in patients with hypertrophic cardiomyopathy, appropriate device interventions occurred in 11% of patients annually for secondary prevention (implant following cardiac arrest) and about 5% annually for primary prevention based on risk factors.[41,42] Based on the observations from this study, the ICD is warranted in hypertrophic cardiomyopathy patients with prior cardiac arrest or spontaneous sustained ventricular tachycardia.[41,42] Furthermore, a single risk factor for sudden cardiac death may be sufficient to justify serious consideration of ICD implantation for primary prevention. Unfortunately, none of the nonpharmacologic therapies for outflow tract obstruction, including DDD pacing, surgical myotomy–myectomy and alcohol septal ablation, have been shown to reduce the risk of sudden death in patients with hypertrophic cardiomyopathy.[41]

Ventricular arrhythmias in the setting of common types of congenital heart disease, such as Ebstein anomaly, tetralogy of Fallot, and other valvular heart diseases, are also markers for higher risk of sudden cardiac death.[1,2,36] Additionally, idiopathic dilated cardiomyopathy and acute myocarditis are accepted as conditions associated with a higher risk of life-threatening arrhythmic events.[1,2,16,18] Premature ventricular contractions in the athlete are felt to be common and they rarely cause symptoms severe enough to warrant therapy. For athletes, in the absence of any congenital or acquired structural heart disease, there is no increased risk due to arrhythmias.[1,2,12,16] In a recent study of 355 competitive athletes with ventricular tachyarrhythmias assessed by 24-hour ambulatory monitors, frequent and complex ventricular arrhythmias were common in trained athletes and were usually unassociated with cardiovascular abnormalities.[33] These ventricular arrhythmias, when unassociated with cardiovascular abnormalities, did not have any prognostic significance. The authors suggest that ventricular arrhythmias may be a manifestation of 'athlete's heart syndrome' and probably do not *per se* justify disqualification from competitive athletics.[33]

The routine evaluation of athletes with premature ventricular contractions includes history, physical examination, ECG and echocardiogram (Table 24.6). In the presence of hypertrophic cardiomyopathy, arrhythmogenic right ventricular dysplasia, anomalous origin of the coronary arteries, coronary artery disease, dilated cardiomyopathy or myocarditis as well as long QT syndrome, therapy is warranted.[1,2,12] When there is no underlying structural heart disease, therapy with β-blockers may decrease symptoms with or without reduction in the frequency of premature ventricular contractions. Drug therapy with other anti-arrhythmic agents generally is not required unless the symptoms are sufficiently severe and persistent on β-blocker therapy.[2,12] In the absence of symptoms, and in the absence of structural heart disease, no therapy is needed.[2,12]

In athletes without structural heart disease, nonsustained ventricular tachycardia that is monomorphic does not indicate any additional risk for sudden cardiac death.[1,2,12,16,33] The evaluation and management of athletes with nonsustained ventricular tachycardia, in general, is similar to that for premature ventricular contractions. A notable exception, however, is in those athletes with nonsustained polymorphic ventricular tachycardia, in whom there may be a higher risk for life-threatening ventricular arrhythmias.[2,12,16,37,51,52] β-Blocker therapy is considered to be the first approach in these individuals and barring them from athletic activity should be considered.[2,51,52]

When an athlete has had a prior episode of sustained ventricular tachycardia or prior episodes of ventricular fibrillation, thorough evaluation of cardiac status with history, physical, ECG, echocardiogram and selected use of stress test, cardiac MRI, cardiac catheterization, and electrophysiologic evaluation is warranted.[1,2,12] Sustained ventricular tachycardia originating from the right ventricular outflow tract or other regions of the right or left ventricle (idio-

Table 24.6 Ventricular arrhythmias in different forms of structural heart disease. ECG = electrocardiogram; VT = ventricular tachycardia; LV = left ventricle; LH = lightheadedness; NL = normal; RB = right bundle; RFA = radiofrequency ablation; RVOT = right ventricle outflow tract; VT = ventricular tachycardia; LB = left bound; HCM = hypertrophic cardiomyopathy; SCD = sudden cardiac death; BB = β-blockers; AAD = anti-arrhythmic drugs; ICD = implantable cardioverter defibrillator; inv ant = inverted anteriorly; ARVD = arrhythmogenic right ventricular dysplasia; RBBB = right bundle-branch block; sot = sotalol; amio = amiodarone; PPM = permanent pacemaker; CABG = coronary artery bypass surgery. Modified from Link *et al. Cardiac arrhythmias and electrophysiologic observations in the athletes.* In: Williams RA, ed. *The Athlete and Heart Disease: Diagnosis, Evaluation & Management.* Philadelphia, PA: Lippincott Williams & Wilkins, 1999: 197–216

Condition	Symptoms	ECG	VT morph	Treatment options	Competitive athletics
Idiopathic	Palpitations LH, syncope	NL	RB, left axis	RFA	No restrictions 3 months after RFA
Idiopathic RVOT, VT	Palpitations LH, syncope	NL	LB, inf axis	RFA	No restrictions 3 months after RFA
HCM	Palpitations Syncope SCD	Q's-ant		BB AAD Myomectomy ICD	Only low intensity
ARVD	Palpitations Syncope SCD	T = inv ant RBBB Epsilon wave	LB, inf axis	Sot or amio ICD RFA	Only low intensity
CAD	Palpitations Syncope SCD	Infarcts Ischemic ST	RB or LB	AAD ICD	Only low intensity
LQTS	Palpitations Syncope SCD	Long QTc	Torsades de pointes	BB PPM ICD	Only low intensity
Anomalous CAD	SCD	NL	VF	CABG	No restrictions after CABG

pathic ventricular tachycardia) typically occur in the absence of any identifiable structural heart disease. In this setting, there is extremely low risk for sudden cardiac death.[2,12,13,16] Programmed ventricular stimulation, sometimes supplemented by isoproterenol infusion, generally can induce the sustained arrhythmia. Mapping the site of origin and obliteration with radiofrequency ablation is generally possible. As with athletes who undergo ablative therapy for supraventricular arrhythmias, these athletes can return to athletic competition after a period of approximately 3 months if free of arrhythmias.[1,2,12]

In athletes presenting with sustained ventricular tachycardia or prior episodes of resuscitated ventricular fibrillation there is usually some type of underlying structural heart disease. In the athlete under age 35, hypertrophic cardiomyopathy, anomalous origin of a coronary artery, arrhythmogenic right ventricular dysplasia, or other congenital abnormalities typically serve as a substrate for these arrhythmias.[1,2,18,19,20] By contrast, over 80% of athletes older than 35 years have underlying coronary disease with an ischemic basis for their arrhythmias.[1,2,17–22,36,46–49] In these athletes, the ICD has been shown to provide superior protection from sudden death compared with anti-arrhythmic therapy,[1,2,12] particularly in the setting of underlying coronary artery disease.[12] Once an athlete with underlying structural heart disease has had episodes of sustained ventricular tachycardia or fibrillation and receives a defibrillator, competitive sports are prohibited by current guidelines.[1,2] A physician may give consideration to allowing the athlete to return to competitive athletic activity in the setting of anomalous coronary which has definitively been treated with surgery with documentation of absence of ischemia with stress testing.[1,2,12]

Exercise may exacerbate arrhythmias in many types of structural heart disease predisposed to sudden cardiac death.[2,3,12,28,53] In particular, with the sustained monomorphic ventricular tachycardia associated with arrhythmogenic right ventricular dysplasia and ventricular tachycardia of right ventricular outflow tract origin, exercise frequently accentuates the arrhythmia.[4,12,33–35] In patients with anomalous origin of the coronary arteries and long QT syndrome, life-threatening ventricular arrhythmias frequently occur with exertion or immediately after exertion.[2,12,27,28,37] With the most common form of underlying structural heart disease, hypertrophic cardiomyopathy, arrhythmias are induced by exertion in approximately one-half of individuals.[12,17,21,41] In patients with idiopathic ventricular fibrillation, approximately 15% of individuals have their cardiac arrest in the setting of intense physical exertion.[12,51,52] Finally, in the setting of underlying coronary artery disease, there is a multifold increase in the frequency of sudden death related to exertion.[53]

Automatic external defibrillators

Automatic external defibrillators (AEDs), first introduced for clinical use in 1979, have revolutionized the approach to out-of-hospital cardiac arrest, with clear implications for their use at athletic events.[54–72] An AED is a lightweight portable device containing a battery, capacitors, and circuitry designed to analyze cardiac rhythm and prompt the operator when a shock is indicated for a life-threatening ventricular arrhythmia. Manufacturers were challenged by the American Heart Association to develop a device so reliable in sensitivity and specificity for life-threatening heart rhythms and with ease of use so that fear of misuse and inappropriate shocks would be unfounded. Reductions in size, weight, cost and maintenance by manufacturers have allowed these devices to be incorporated into the American Heart Association's Public Access to Defibrillation programs.

The concept of public access to defibrillation promotes expansion of the role of the defibrillation to both minimally trained first responders (such as trainers, coaches, police officers, firefighters, security guards and flight attendants) and trained lay persons who are present at the time of arrest. It also promotes the placement of the AED in such venues as sports arenas, athletic fields, airports, convention centers, casinos, shopping malls, large office buildings and airlines. It is possible that the AED will become as commonplace as a fire extinguisher in the future. There is a growing body of evidence to suggest that public access to defibrillation using the AED has resulted in greatly improved survival for sudden cardiac arrest (Table 24.7).

Cardiac arrest in athletics may occur in a variety of settings that should be considered in designing a response system for these emergencies. Most of the reported episodes of cardiac arrest in athletes occur in football or basketball.[67] Accordingly, a logical focus of AED use as a response system would be in these two sports. In addition, it is known that more than one-half of the emergencies occur during training sessions as opposed to actual competition.[67] It is widely accepted that team athletic trainers, rather than team physicians, are most likely to be present during these sessions.[67] Approximately one-third of the episodes of sudden cardiac arrest occur in athletes during or immediately after competition, when a physician is most likely to be present.[67] Importantly, cardiac emergencies also frequently develop amongst spectators attending the athletic event. In fact, the probability of AED use during such emergencies is likely to be greater in the spectators and other attendees than in the athletic participants. The AED needs to be incorporated into a formal response system that adheres to the principles of the chain of survival promoted by the Ameri-

Table 24.7 Public-access defibrillation programs using nontraditional first responders

Author	First responder	Survival from ventricular fibrillation (%)
O'Rourke et al.[63]	Flight attendant	26
Page et al.[64]	Flight attendant	40
Valenzuela et al.[66]	Casino security personnel	53
Becker et al.[68]	Medical/dental practice staff	56
Myerburg et al.[69]	Police vs EMT	17
Capucci et al.[70]	Police, lay volunteers	44

can Heart Association. This concept is straightforward, with early activation of emergency medical care, early cardiopulmonary resuscitation, early defibrillation (using the AED) and early advanced life support.[55,56]

It has been demonstrated that emergency medical technicians (EMTs) and paramedics can effectively and safely use manual defibrillators.[54] A small number of studies[55,57] have shown that use of the AED is safe and effective. Multiple studies have documented improved survival with addition of EMT defibrillation using the AED.[56–73] These studies also showed that use by emergency personal such as police officers, firefighters and trained first responders dramatically reduces the time to defibrillation and enhances survival in selected communities (Table 24.7). Early experience with the AEDs was with Qantas Airlines, beginning in 1991.[63] Over a 64-month period they documented 46 cardiac arrests with long-term survival of 26%, which was comparable to the most effective prehospital emergency services.[63] Subsequently, American Airways documented 200 AED uses over a 2-year period.[64] From 15 documented episodes of ventricular fibrillation, six passengers (40%) ultimately survived because of AED therapy. Sensitivity and specificity for ventricular fibrillation was 100%. Based on these experiences, several US and international airlines have implemented AED programs.[64,65] Also, AEDs used by security personnel at casinos[66] resulted in survival in 53% of patients in whom the initial rhythm was ventricular fibrillation. Importantly, in this public access defibrillation program, the mean time to response was 4.4 ± 2.9 minutes while the paramedic response time was 9.8 ± 4.3 minutes.

Conclusion

The evaluation and management of athletes with documented cardiac arrhythmia or symptoms attributable to an arrhythmia represents a clinical challenge. Multiple clinical, social, psychological, and economic factors may confound the decisions regarding testing, therapy, and restriction from athletics. The overlap of normal and abnormal electrocardiographic changes, the lack of sensitivity and specificity of screening techniques, and the imperfect risk stratification techniques and therapies further complicate clinical decision-making. Based on these considerations, the available guidelines for evaluation and management, as well as restrictions from competition, should be used by all physicians involved in the assessment of trained athletes.[1–2]

References

1 Zipes DP, Garson A Jr. Task Force 6. In: Maron BJ, Mitchell J, eds. 26th Bethesda Conference. Recommendations for determining eligibility for competition in athletes with cardiovascular abnormalities. *J Am Coll Cardiol* 1994; **24**: 892–9.
2 Estes NAM III, Link MS, Cannom D *et al.* NASPE consensus statement report of the NASPE policy conference on arrhythmias and the athlete. *J Cardiovasc Electrophysiol* 2001; **12**: 1208–19.

3 McGovern BA, Liberthson R. Arrhythmias induced by exercise in athletes and others. *S Afr Med J* 1996; **89**: 588–96.

4 Corrado D, Thiene G, Nava A, Rossi L, Pennelli N. Sudden death in young competitive athletes: Clinicopathologic correlations in 22 cases. *Am J Med* 1990; **89**: 588–96.

5 Sneddon JF, Scalia G, Ward DE, McKenna WJ, Camm AJ, Frenneaux MP. Exercise induced vasodepressor syncope. *Br Heart J* 1994; **71**: 554–7.

6 Sakaguchi S, Shultz JJ, Remole SC, Adler SW, Lurie KG, Benditt DG. Syncope associated with exercise, a manifestation of neurally mediated syncope. *Am J Cardiol* 1995; **75**: 476–81.

7 Calkins H, Siefert M, Morady F. Clinical presentation and long-term follow up of athletes with exercise induced vasodepressor syncope. *Am Heart J* 1995; **129**: 1159–64.

8 Kosinski D, Grubb BP, Kip K, Hahn H. Exercise induced neurocardiogenic syncope. *Am Heart J* 1996; **132**: 451–2.

9 Foote CB, Michaud G. The athletes electrogram: Distinguishing normal from abnormal. In: Estes NAM, Salem DN, Wang PJ, eds. *Sudden Cardiac Death in the Athlete*. Armonk, NY: Futura Publishing, 1998: 110–14.

10 Zehender M, Meinertz T, Keul J *et al.* ECG variants and cardiac arrhythmias in athletes: Clinical relevance and prognostic importance. *Am Heart J* 1990; **119**: 1378–91.

11 Estes NAM, Thompson PJ. EKG changes in the athlete. In: Topol EJ, ed. *A Textbook of Cardiovascular Medicine*, 2002.

12 Link MS, Wang PJ, Estes NAM III. Cardiac arrhythmias and electrophysiologic observations in the athletes. In: Williams RA, ed. *The Athlete and Heart Disease: Diagnosis, Evaluation & Management*. Philadelphia, PA: Lippincott Williams & Wilkins, 1999: 197–216.

13 Link MS, Olshansky B, Estes NAM III. Cardiac arrhythmias in the athlete. *Curr Opin Cardiol* 1999; **14**: 24–9.

14 Link MS, Estes III NAM. Ventricular arrhythmias. In: Estes NAM, Salem DN, Wang PJ, eds. *Sudden Cardiac Death in the Athlete*. Armonk, NY: Futura Publishing, 1998: 253–75.

15 Balady GJ, Cadigan JB, Ryan TJ. Electrocardiogram of the athlete: An analysis of 289 profession football players. *Am J Cardiol* 1985; **53**: 1339–43.

16 Kinder C, Tamburro P, Kopp D, Kall J, Olshansky B, Wilber D. The clinical significance of nonsustained ventricular tachycardia: Current perspectives. *Pacing Clin Electrophysiol* 1994; **17**: 637–64.

17 Maron BJ, Epstein SE, Roberts WC. Cause of sudden death in competitive athletes. *J Am Coll Cardiol* 1986; **7**: 204–14.

18 Liberthson RR. Sudden death from cardiac causes in children and young adults. *N Engl J Med* 1996; **334**: 1039–44.

19 Katcher M, Maron BJ, Homoud M. Risk profiling and screening strategies. In: Estes NAM, Salem DN, Wang PJ, eds. *Sudden Cardiac Death in the Athlete*. Armonk, NY: Futura Publishing, 1998: 57–87.

20 Maron BJ, Shirani J, Poliac LC, Mathenge R, Roberts WC, Mueller FO. Sudden death in young competitive athletes: Clinical, demographic, and pathologic profiles. *JAMA* 1996; **276**: 199–204.

21 Van Camp SP, Bloor CM, Mueller FO, Cantu RC, Olsen HG. Nontraumatic sports death in high school and college athletes. *Med Sci Sports Exerc* 1995; **27**: 641–7.

22 Burke AP, Farb A, Virmani R. Causes of sudden death in athletes. *Cardiol Clin* 1992; **10**: 303–17.

23 Smith ML, Hudson DL, Graitzer HM *et al.* Exercise training bradycardia: The role of the autonomic balance. *Med Sci Sports Exerc* 1989; **21**: 40–4.

24 Wellens HJ, Rodriguez L, Timmermanns C, Smeets JL. The asymptomatic patient with Wolff–Parkinson–White electrocardiogram. *Pacing Clin Electrophysiol* 1997; **20**: 2082–6.

25 Leitch JW, Klein GJ, Yee R, Murdock C. Prognostic value of electrophysiologic testing in asymptomatic patients with Wolff–Parkinson–White pattern. *Circulation* 1990; **82**: 1718–23.

26 Krahn AD, Klein GJ, Yee R. The approach to the athlete with Wolff–Parkinson–White Syndrome: In: Estes NAM, Salem DN, Wang PJ, eds. *Sudden Cardiac Death in the Athlete*. Armonk, NY: Futura Publishing, 1998: 237–52.

27 Roden DM, Lazzara R, Rosen M, Schwartz PJ, Towbin J, Vincent GM. Multiple mechanisms in the long QT syndrome: Current knowledge, gaps, and future directions. *Circulation* 1996; **94**: 1996–2012.

28 Sloan S, Wang PJ. The role of exercise testing in the evaluation of the athlete. In: Estes NAM, Salem DN, Wang PJ, eds. *Sudden Cardiac Death in the Athlete*. Armonk, NY: Futura Publishing, 1998: 123–55.

29 Fananapazir, McAreavey D. Hypertrophic cardiomyopathy: Evaluation and treatment of patients at high risk for sudden cardiac death. *Pacing Clin Electrophysiol* 1997; **20**: 478–500.

30 Fananapazir L, Chang AC, Epstein SE, McAreavey D. Prognostic determinants in hypertrophic cardiomyopathy. *Circulation* 1992; **86**: 730–40.

31 Fananapazir L, Tracy CM, Leon MB et al. Electrophysiologic abnormalities in patients with hypertrophic cardiomyopathy. *Circulation* 1989; **80**: 1259–68.

32 Saumerez RC, Slade AK, Grace AA et al. The significance of paced electrograms fractionation in hypertrophic cardiomyopathy. *Circulation* 1995; **91**: 2762–8.

33 Biffi A, Pelliccia A, Verdile L et al. Long-term clinical significance of frequent and complex ventricular tachyarrhythmias in trained athletes. *J Am Coll Cardiol* 2002; **40**: 446–52.

34 Corrado D, Fontaine G, Marcus FI et al. Arrhythmogenic right ventricular dysplasia/cardiomyopathy: Need for an international registry. Study Group on Arrhythmogenic Right Ventricular Dysplasia/Cardiomyopathy of the Working Groups on Myocardial and Pericardial Disease and Arrhythmias of the European Society of Cardiology and of the Scientific Council on Cardiomyopathies of the World Heart Federation. *Circulation* 2000; **101**: E101–6.

35 Link MS, Wang PJ, Haugh CJ et al. Arrhythmogenic right ventricular dysplasia: Clinical results with implantable cardioverter defibrillators. *J Interv Cardiovasc Electrophysiol* 1997; **1**: 41–8.

36 Gillette P. Sudden cardiac death in athletes with congenital heart disease. In: Estes NAM, Salem DN, Wang PJ, eds. *Sudden Cardiac Death in the Athlete*. Armonk, NY: Futura Publishing, 1998: 373–8.

37 Jackman WM, Friday KJ, Anderson JL, Aliot EM, Clark M, Lazzara R. The long QT syndromes: A critical review, new clinical observations and a unifying hypothesis. *Progr Cardiovasc Dis* 1988; **31**: 115–72.

38 Brugada P, Brugada J. Right bundle branch block, persistent ST segment evaluation and sudden cardiac death. A distinct clinical and electrophysiologic syndrome. *J Am Coll Cardiol* 1992; **20**: 1391–6.

39 Gregoratos G, Cheitlin MD, Conill A et al. ACC/AHA guidelines for implantation of cardiac pacemakers and antiarrhythmic devices. *J Am Coll Cardiol* 1998; **31**: 1175–209.

40 Coumel P. Autonomic influence in atrial tachyarrhythmias. *J Cardiovasc Electrophysiol* 1997; **8**: 1175–89.

41 Maron BJ. Hypertrophic cardiomyopathy: A systematic review. *JAMA* 2002; **237**: 1308–20.

42 Maron BJ, Shen W-K, Link MS *et al.* Efficacy of implantable cardioverter-defibrillator for the prevention of sudden death in patients with hypertrophic cardiomyopathy. *N Engl J Med* 2000; **342**: 365–73.

43 Haissaguerre M, Jais P, Shah DC *et al.* Spontaneous initiation of atrial fibrillation by ectopic beats originating in the pulmonary veins. *N Engl J Med.* 1998; **339**: 659–66.

44 Manolis AS, Wang PJ, Estes NAM III. Radiofrequency catheter ablation for cardiac tachyarrhythmias. *Ann Intern Med* 1994; **121**: 452–61.

45 Priori SG, Aliot E, Blomstrom-Lundqvist C *et al.* Task force on sudden cardiac death of the European Society of Cardiology. *Eur Heart J* 2001; **22**: 1374–450.

46 Topaz B, Edwards JE. Pathologic features of sudden cardiac death in children, adolescents, and young adults. *Chest* 1985; **87**: 476–82.

47 McCaffery FM, Bruden DS, Strong WB. Sudden cardiac death in young athletes. *Am J Dis Child* 1991; **145**: 177–83.

48 Corrado D, Basso C, Schiavon M, Thiene G. Screening for hypertrophic cardiomyopathy in young athletes. *N Engl J Med* 1998; **339**: 364–9.

49 Rowland TW. Sudden unexpected death in sports. *Pediatric Ann* 1992; **21**: 193–5.

50 McKenna W, Firoozi S, Sharma S. Arrhythmias and sudden death in hypertrophic cardiomyopathy. *Card Electrophysiol Rev* 2002; **6**: 26–31.

51 Eisenberg SJ, Scheinman MM, Dullett NK *et al.* Sudden cardiac death and polymorphous ventricular tachycardia in patients with normal QT interval and normal systolic cardiac function. *Am J Cardiol* 1995; **75**: 687–92.

52 Viskin S, Belhassen B. Idiopathic ventricular fibrillation. *Am Heart J* 1990; **120**: 661–7.

53 Thompson PD, Funk EJ, Carleton RA, Sturner WQ. Incidence of death during jogging in Rhode Island from 1975 through 1980. *JAMA* 1982; **247**: 2635–8.

54 Stults KR, Brown DD, Kerber RE. Efficacy of an automated external defibrillator in the management of out of hospital cardiac arrest: Validation of the diagnostic algorithm and the clinical experience in a rural environment. *Circulation* 1986; **73**: 701–9.

55 Cummings RO, Eisenberg MS, Litwin PE. Automatic external defibrillators used by emergency medical technicians: A controlled clinical trial. *JAMA* 1987; **27**: 1605–10.

56 Marenco JP, Wang PJ, Link MS, Homoud MK, Estes NAM III. Improving survival from sudden cardiac arrest: The role of the automated exertional defibrillator. *JAMA* 2001; **285**: 1193–200.

57 Weaver WD, Hill D, Fahrenbuch CE *et al.* Use of automated external defibrillators in the management of out of hospital cardiac arrest. *N Engl J Med* 1988; **319**: 661–6.

58 Gray AJ, Redmond AD, Martin MA. Use of the automatic external defibrillator–pacemaker by ambulance personnel: The Stockport experience. *BMJ* 1987; **294**: 1133–5.

59 Eisenberg MS, Hallstrom AP, Copass MK. Treatment of ventricular fibrillation: Emergency medical technician defibrillation and paramedic services. *JAMA* 1984; **251**: 1723–6.

60 Vukov IF, White RD, Backman JW. New perspectives on rural EMT defibrillation. *Ann Emerg Med* 1988; **17**: 318–21.

61 Watts DD. Defibrillation by basic emergency medical technicians: Effect on survival. *Ann Emerg Med* 1995; **26**: 635–9.

62 Auble TE, Menegazzi JL, Paris PM. Effect of out-of-hospital defibrillation by basic life support providers on cardiac arrest mortality: A meta-analysis. *Ann Emerg Med* 1995; **25**: 642–8.

63 O'Rourke MF, Donaldson EE, Geddes JS. An airline cardiac arrest program. *Circulation* 1997; **96**: 2849–53.

64 Page RL, Joglar JA, Kowal RC *et al.* Use of automated external defibrillators by a US airline. *N Engl J Med* 2000; **343**: 1210–16.

65 Zimmermann PG, Campbell L. Automatic defibrillators on commercial airplanes. *J Emerg Nurs* 1997; **23**: 340–2.

66 Valenzuela TD, Roe DJ, Nichol G, Clark LL, Spaite DW, Hardman RG. Outcomes of rapid defibrillation by security officers after cardiac arrest in casinos. *N Engl J Med* 2000; **343**: 1206–9.

67 Cummings RO, Hazinski MF. Public access to defibrillation: Response to emergencies at athletic events—economic training and cost implications. In: Estes NAM, Salem D, Wang P, eds. *Sudden Cardiac Death in the Athlete.* Armonk, NY: Futura Publishing, 1998: 189–204.

68 Becker L, Eisenberg M, Fahrenbruch C, Cohen L. Cardiac arrest in medical and dental practices. *Arch Intern Med* 2001; **161**: 1509–12.

69 Myerburg R, Fenster J, Velez M *et al.* Impact of community-wide police care deployment of automatic external defibrillators on survival from out-of-hospital cardiac arrest. *Circulation* 2002; **106**: 1058–64.

70 Capucci A, Daniela A, Piepoli M, Bardy G, Konumu E, Arvedi M. Tripling survival from sudden cardiac arrest via early defibrillation without traditional education in cardiopulmonary resuscitation. *Circulation* 2002; **106**: 1065–70.

71 Hoffman C, Marenco J, Wang P, Link, M, Homoud M, Estes NAM III. Public access defibrillation programs: The role of the automated external defibrillator. *Cardiovasc Rev Rep* 2002; **23**: 286–91.

72 Balady GJ, Chaitman B, Foster C, Froelicher E, Gordon N, Van Camp S. American Heart Association. American College of Sports Medicine. Automated external defibrillators in health/fitness facilities: Supplement to the AHA/ACSM recommendations for cardiovascular screening, staffing and emergency policies at health/fitness facilities. *Circulation* 2002; **105**: 1147–50.

73 Caffrey SL, Willoughby PJ, Pepe PE, Becker LB. Public use of automated external defibrillators. *N Engl J Med* 2002; **347**: 1242–7.

CHAPTER 25

The Athlete's Heart, ECG, and Differential Diagnosis with Hypertrophic Cardiomyopathy and Other Cardiomyopathies

Antonio Pelliccia, MD and Barry J. Maron, MD

The athlete's heart

Historical context

The 'athlete's heart' was introduced as a distinct nosologic entity at the end of the 19th century by Henschen, who described enlarged cardiac area in cross-country skiers by carefully performed percussion of the chest.[1] For many years, heart enlargement in athletes was identified by physical examination and chest radiography, or inferred by electrocardiogram (ECG) alterations.[2] Subsequently, echocardiography allowed direct assessment of the morphologic and functional cardiac changes induced by athletic conditioning.[3] Since the original study by Morganroth and colleagues in 1975,[4] several investigators have explored cardiac morphologic changes in a variety of athlete populations, including elite competitors, providing extensive surveys of the adaptive cardiac alterations induced by chronic athletic training.[3-11]

Mechanisms of left ventricular remodeling
Type of sport

Morphologic left ventricular (LV) changes in athletes have been primarily attributed to type of hemodynamic overload induced by different conditioning programs.[11-13] Specifically, endurance types of sports (e.g. cycling, cross-country skiing, rowing) are associated with large volume overload, and power disciplines (e.g. weight and power lifting, shot-put, discus) are associated with pressure overload. In our experience, elite athletes engaged in endurance sport demonstrate the largest alterations in LV cavity size, wall thickness and mass[9] (Fig. 25.1). Absolute LV cavity dimensions in these athletes are usually well above the accepted normal limits (i.e. end-diastolic diameter ≥55 mm)[14,15] and not infrequently may be markedly increased (i.e. ≥60 mm). LV wall thicknesses are also increased, and in a small but important subset of elite endurance athletes exceed the upper limits of normal (i.e. ≥13 mm).[14,15]

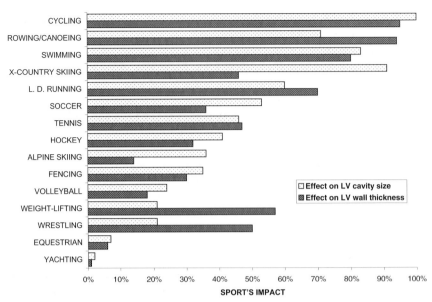

Fig. 25.1 Representation of the impact of different sport disciplines on left ventricular (LV) cavity dimension (gray bars) and maximum wall thickness (dark bars) assessed in a large population of 947 elite competitive athletes. Most disciplines have a parallel impact on LV cavity size and wall thickness; however, power sports (such as weight-lifting and wrestling) show a disproportionately greater effect on LV wall thickness. Adapted and modified from Pelliccia and Maron. Cardiovascular adaptation to exercise training. In: Harries *et al.*, eds. *Oxford Textbook of Sports Medicine*, 2nd edn. Oxford: Oxford University Press, 1998: 301–320, by permission of Oxford University Press.

Athletes engaged in power disciplines show a disproportionately larger impact on LV wall thickness than cavity size; while LV cavity dimensions remain within normal limits, the relative wall thickness is increased (Fig. 25.1). However, although increased in comparison with matched untrained controls, absolute LV wall thicknesses rarely exceed upper normal limits (i.e. they usually remain less than 13 mm).[9,16]

Other disciplines, such as soccer, rugby, and hockey, which are based on mixed (aerobic and anaerobic) metabolism, show a moderate impact on LV cavity dimensions and have absolute values that may exceed upper normal limits, but wall thicknesses usually remain within normal values.[9] Finally, technical disciplines (such as equestrian and yachting) have only a minimal effect, if any, on LV morphology.[9]

Body size and composition

Cardiac dimensions are closely related to body size and composition.[14,15] In our experience, based on a large population of elite athletes, body surface area proved to be the strongest determinant of cardiac dimensions, independently accounting for about 50% of the variability in LV cavity dimension and wall thicknesses.[9] Indeed, athletes with the greatest body surface area, such as those engaged in rowing, rugby, basketball, and water-polo, have usually the greatest absolute LV cavity dimensions.[10]

Gender

Women athletes have larger LV cavity dimension (average, +6%) and maximal wall thickness (average, +14%) compared with sedentary controls.[17] Nevertheless, and not unexpectedly, women show smaller absolute LV cavity dimensions (average, –10%) and wall thicknesses (average, –20%) in comparison with male athletes of the same age, ethnic origin and sporting disciplines.[8,17] These differences are likely to be the consequence of several determinants, including the smaller body size (and lean body mass), and the lesser absolute cardiac output and systolic blood pressure attained during exercise in women compared with men.

Genetic determinants

At present, evidence for a genetic influence in the cardiac remodeling of athletes has been demonstrated for the renin–angiotensin system.[18,19] Montgomery and colleagues[18] examined military recruits undergoing 10-week exercise training and observed that individuals with the angiotensin-converting enzyme genotype ACE-DD had LV mass increased by 42%, compared with 2% ($P < 0.001$) in individuals with the ACE-II genotype. Karjalainen and colleagues[19] have demonstrated that angiotensinogen (AGT) M235T polymorphism may regulate the rate of transcription and secretion of AGT and the extent of cardiac morphologic remodeling; elite endurance athletes with AGT-TT expression had larger LV mass than those with the AGT-MM genotype (+10%; $P < 0.004$), independently of gender and intensity of training.

Outer limits of LV remodeling

The extent to which LV dimensions are altered in trained athletes is usually mild—absolute dimensions are increased by an average of 10% for cavity size and 15% for wall thicknesses compared with matched untrained controls.[3] Therefore, in the vast majority of athletes increased cardiac dimensions remain within the accepted normal limits and differ considerably from those found in patients with structural cardiac diseases, such as cardiomyopathies.[20] Elite athletes, however, represent a unique subset of the athlete population, not only because of their more strenuous and prolonged exercise training and level of achievement, but also due to a measure of self-selection with respect to body composition and, possibly, genetic constitution. Therefore, in elite athletes LV remodeling may be more substantial, and absolute LV dimensions (particularly cavity dimension) are often increased well above the generally accepted upper normal limits. In our experience, marked LV cavity dilatation (i.e. end-diastolic dimension ≥60 mm), compatible with the clinical diagnosis of idiopathic dilated cardiomyopathy (DCM), occurs in about 15%,[10] while substantial wall thickening (≥13 mm), suggestive of hypertrophic cardiomy-opathy (HCM), occurs in about 2%.[8]

These morphologic findings raise the differential diagnosis between an extreme cardiac adaptation to intensive exercise training and a pathologic cardiac condition with the potential for adverse clinical consequences. Resolu-tion of this problem may be difficult in the individual athlete, but a number of morphologic and clinical criteria have been suggested that may aid in this often compelling diagnostic dilemma.[20]

Differential diagnosis between athlete's heart and HCM

The most common clinical occasion in which the differential diagnosis be-tween athlete's heart and structural cardiac disease arises is with respect to HCM.[20] HCM is a primary cardiac disease, with the characteristic morpho-logic pattern of a hypertrophied and nondilated left ventricle, in the absence of cardiac or systemic disease itself capable of producing LV hypertrophy of that magnitude.[21] The clinical distinction of HCM from physiologic LV hyper-trophy in trained athletes is of crucial importance, and has ethical, economic and legal implications, since sudden death may be the initial clinical event in young individuals with HCM, often related to physical exertion.[21,22] Therefore, the diagnosis of HCM is the basis for disqualification of the young athlete from competition in an effort to minimize the risk of sudden cardiac death.[23]

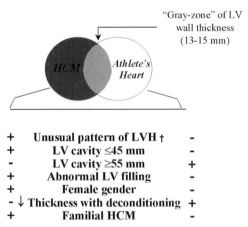

Fig. 25.2 Flow chart showing clinical criteria used to distinguish hypertrophic cardiomyopathy from athlete's heart when left ventricle wall thickness is in the gray zone of overlap consistent with both diagnoses. †Unusual pattern of left ventricular hypertrophy, including heterogeneous distribution of the hypertrophy, in which asymmetry is prominent and adjacent regions may be of greatly different thicknesses, with sharp transition evident between segments; also, patterns in which the anterior ventricular septum is spared from the hypertrophic process and the predomi-nant thickening may be in the posterior portion of the septum, or anterolateral or posterior free wall, or the apex. LV = left ventricle; LA = left atrium; ↓ = decreased. Reproduced with permis-sion from Maron *et al. Circulation* 1995; **91**: 1596–601, © Lippincott Williams & Wilkins.

On the other hand, the correct identification of a physiologic LV hypertrophy may avoid an unnecessary withdrawal of the athlete from competitions, and the unjustified loss of the varied (including economic) benefits derived from sport.

The protocol shown in Fig. 25.2 encompasses morphologic and clinical criteria that may offer a measure of clarification for this differential diagnosis.

LV wall thickness

The maximum LV wall thickness found in highly trained young athletes is 15–16 mm, which likely represents the upper limit of physiologic wall thickening.[8] Instead, in patients with HCM, including those who are asymptomatic and regularly involved in active lifestyles, maximum LV wall thickness averages 21–22 mm, and in about 10% of patients it is at least 30 mm.[21,24] However, an important minority of patients with HCM show only mild LV hypertrophy, with wall thickness in a gray zone of 13–15 mm,[25] which overlaps that found in elite athletes;[8] therefore, the single criterion of LV wall thickening may not differentiate physiologic from pathologic hypertrophy.

In the physiologic hypertrophy of trained athletes, different segments of LV walls have similar thickness (2 mm or less between contiguous segments) and the overall pattern of LV hypertrophy is symmetric and substantially homogeneous.[8] In patients with HCM, the distribution of LV hypertrophy is, in contrast, usually asymmetric.[21,24] Although the anterior ventricular septum is generally the most thickened segment, not uncommonly other areas (such as the posterior ventricular septum, anterior free wall or the apex) may show the most marked degree of thickening. In addition, contiguous portions of the LV walls often show strikingly different thicknesses, with abrupt transition between adjacent segments.[24]

LV cavity dimension

Enlarged LV cavity (end-diastolic diameter at least 55 mm) is commonly present in highly trained athletes.[8,10] Conversely, in patients with HCM, LV cavity size is characteristically normal or reduced (i.e. end-diastolic diameter is 45 mm or less),[21,24] and may be enlarged (i.e. larger than 55 mm) only in the end-stage HCM patients with progressive LV failure and systolic dysfunction.[26] Therefore, in most instances it is possible to resolve the diagnostic ambiguity of borderline LV wall thickening in athletes based solely on cavity dimension, when either small (up to 45 mm), or enlarged (55 mm or more). Indeed, the enlarged LV cavity in athletes maintains the normal ellipsoid shape, with mitral valve normally positioned,[27] while in patients with HCM the LV geometry is usually greatly distorted.[24]

Diastolic LV filling

Most patients with HCM, including those with mild hypertrophy that could possibly be confused with athlete's heart, show abnormal Doppler diastolic indexes of LV filling, independently of whether symptoms or outflow obstruction are present. Typically, the early peak of transmitral flow velocity (E) is decreased, the deceleration time of the early peak is prolonged, the late (atrial, A) peak is increased, and the E/A ratio is inverted.[28]

In contrast, trained athletes with LV hypertrophy consistently show a normal LV filling pattern.[29] Consequently, in an athlete suspected to have HCM, a distinctly abnormal LV filling pattern strongly suggests this diagnosis. A normal diastolic LV filling pattern, however, is not particularly useful for differential diagnosis because it is compatible with either athlete's heart or HCM.

Regression of hypertrophy with deconditioning

It is possible to demonstrate, by serial echocardiography, that LV hypertrophy is a physiologic consequence of athletic training, by virtue of a decrease in wall thicknesses after a relatively brief period of complete deconditioning. In our experience, highly trained athletes examined at peak conditioning (when maximum LV wall thicknesses was 13–15 mm) showed a significant reduction (by 2–5 mm) after a 3-month deconditioning period.[30] This potential for normalization of physiologic LV wall thickening is supported by a recent longitudinal study in which we prospectively evaluated the extent of LV remodeling in athletes with LV hypertrophy over a 6-year period after cessation of their athletic careers.[31] We observed complete normalization of LV wall thickness in each, and no occurrence of adverse cardiovascular events.[31] Conversely, no substantial alteration in wall thickness would be expected to occur in patients with HCM in response to changes in habitual physical activity. However, it should be emphasized that identification of changes in wall thickness with deconditioning requires high-quality serial echocardiographic studies, as well as compliance of the athlete for a temporary complete interruption of the training program.

Other criteria useful for differential diagnosis are knowledge of the type of sport in which the athlete participates and peak oxygen consumption. Marked physiologic LV wall thickening (in the range of 13–15 mm) is virtually limited to elite, highly trained athletes engaged in endurance disciplines (primarily rowing, canoeing and cycling).[8] Consequently, such marked LV wall thickening in an athlete training in other sporting disciplines is unlikely to represent the physiologic effect of exercise conditioning. Indeed, elite athletes engaged in endurance disciplines have superior exercise performance and attain high peak oxygen consumption (i.e. VO_2max greater than 50 ml/kg per minute, and often greater than 70 ml/kg per minute). On the other hand, asymptomatic patients with HCM and only mild LV hypertrophy (13–16 mm) show a reduced aerobic power (i.e. $VO_2max < 50$ ml/kg per minute).

Gender

Gender may be another criterion for differential diagnosis between physiologic LV hypertrophy and HCM. While LV absolute maximum wall thickness may exceed 13 mm in 2% of male athletes,[8] LV wall thicknesses do not usually exceed 12 mm in female athletes.[17] These observations suggest that intense athletic conditioning represents an insufficient stimulus to place women within the morphologic gray zone of LV wall thickness (13–15 mm). Therefore, such a finding in a female athlete is more likely to represent HCM than the physiologic consequence of cardiac adaptation to training.

Genetic defects

Recent advances in molecular biology have enhanced our understanding of genetic alterations associated with HCM and have raised the possibility of DNA diagnosis in individuals suspected of having this disease.[32] At present, a variety of mutations in 10 genes encoding proteins of the cardiac sarcomere have been reported to be associated with familial HCM:[32] β-myosin heavy-chain, cardiac troponin T, troponin-I, α-tropomyosin, myosin-binding protein C, essential and regulatory myosin light chains, titin, actin and α-myosin heavy chain. At present, more than 150 individual disease-causing mutations have been reported for these genes and in most cases different families show different mutations; some of them are associated with an unfavorable clinical course.[32]

Recognition of genetic alterations responsible for HCM has also raised the expectation for widespread DNA testing as the definitive method to resolve the uncertainty of a clinical HCM diagnosis in the individual athlete with borderline LV wall thickening. However, due to the substantial genetic heterogeneity of the disease and the complex, time-consuming and expensive techniques needed for genetic screening, DNA analysis is at the moment restricted to research-oriented genotyping of selected pedigrees and is not yet routinely available for clinical practice.

The athlete's electrocardiogram

ECG changes in trained athletes

It has long been known that trained athletes present a wide spectrum of 12-lead ECG alterations, and several observational studies in the past 30 years have exhaustively described these ECG changes (Table 25.1).[2,33–38] Sinus bradycardia is most common, particularly in athletes engaged in endurance disciplines (in up to 85%),[2,34,38] with resting heart rates as low as 35 b.p.m., often

Table 25.1 The most common 12-lead ECG abnormalities reported in athletes. The data are derived from prior studies[2,34,38,44]

Early repolarization	*22–100%*
Increased QRS voltages, suggestive of left ventricular hypertrophy	14–85%
Prolonged PR interval	10–35%
Negative T waves	3–30%
Prolonged QTc interval	≤10%
Left/right atrial enlargement	≤7%
Abnormal precordial R-wave progression	≤5%
Left or right bundle branch block	≤2%

associated with sinus dysrhythmia, and/or sinus pauses of 2 seconds or longer (in about 30%).[2,34,38] Indeed, endurance athletes present a higher prevalence of first-degree (37 *vs* 14%) and second-degree Mobitz type 1 atrioventricular (AV) block (23 *vs* 6%) in comparison with the general population.[2,34,38] The degrees of sinus bradycardia and AV block appear to be related to the extent of athletic conditioning, and cessation of regular exercise training may reduce or even abolish these alterations.[2,34,38]

Trained athletes also demonstrate striking alterations in the ECG pattern, including a marked increase in R- and/or S-wave voltages, ST-segment elevation, T-wave changes (tall, flattened or markedly inverted), and deep Q waves.[2,33–38] Increased R- and/or S-wave voltages in precordial leads, suggesting LV hypertrophy, are present in up to 80% of athletes (depending on the precise diagnostic criteria used), particularly in subjects engaged in endurance disciplines.[2,33–38] Marked repolarization abnormalities (mostly abnormal T-wave patterns) have been documented in up to 30% of trained athletes and deep Q waves have been reported to occur in about 10%.[2,33–38]

Many of these ECG alterations, however, may closely resemble those found in patients with structural cardiac disease, such as HCM[39] or, less commonly, DCM[40] or arrhythmogenic right ventricular cardiomyopathy (ARVC),[41] which are the cardiac lesions most commonly responsible for sudden and unexpected death in young athletes.[22,42,43]

Clinical significance of abnormal ECG patterns in athletes

The clinical significance of these ECG abnormalities in trained athletes (i.e. whether they are an innocent consequence of athletic conditioning or are the first expression of structural cardiac disease with potential adverse consequences) has remained largely unresolved for many years. We recently have addressed this question by comparing in the same athletes the 12-lead ECG patterns with cardiac morphology and function (as assessed by echocardiography). The subjects were a large population of 1005 trained individuals engaged in a variety of sporting disciplines.[44] A substantial proportion of these athletes (40%) showed abnormal ECGs, and in particular about 15% of these showed distinctly abnormal ECG patterns. However, structural cardiovascular abnormalities were rarely detected and only in a minority of cases (5% of the athletes) were they responsible for ECG abnormalities.[44] Of particular clinical interest was a small subset of 5% of athletes who showed the most marked and sometimes bizarre ECG patterns, strongly suggestive of either HCM (with diffuse, symmetric and marked T-wave inversion, associated with greatly increased R- and/or S-wave voltages or with deep Q waves) (Figs 25.3 and 25.4) or ARVC (with T-wave inversion in the precordial leads V_1 to V_3), in each case without a family history or clinical or echocardiographic evidence for these diseases.[44]

Several determinants were found to be responsible for these abnormal ECG patterns in trained athletes, including the extent of morphologic LV remodel-

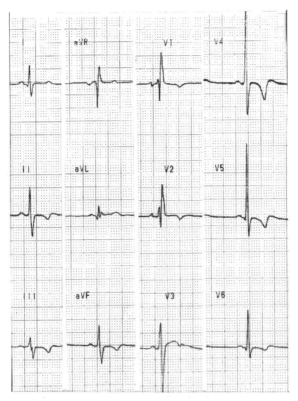

Fig. 25.3 Distinctly abnormal 12-lead ECG from an asymptomatic 19-year-old male soccer player highly suggestive of cardiac disease (such as hypertrophic cardiomyopathy). Marked and diffuse T-wave inversion is present in lateral precordial leads V_4 to V_6 and inferior leads II, III and aVF, associated with increased R-wave voltage (>30 mm in V_4 and V_5) and incomplete right bundle branch block. Reproduced with permission from Pelliccia *et al. Circulation* 2000; **102**: 278–84, © Lippincott Williams & Wilkins.

ing (athletes with the most marked ECG abnormalities showed the greatest increase in LV dimensions), participation in endurance sports (e.g. cycling, rowing, canoeing, and cross-country skiing), gender (male athletes had a higher prevalence of abnormal ECGs), and young age (less than 20 years).[44]

Therefore, it would appear that chronic conditioning may itself preferentially alter the ECG pattern in some athletes, and an abnormal ECG itself may represent another component of the 'athlete's heart syndrome'. This interpretation is also supported by our preliminary observations in a group of 50 athletes with distinctly abnormal ECG patterns (but in the absence of demonstrable cardiovascular disease) observed over a follow-up period of 8 years.[45] We have observed partial resolution (or complete normalization) of these pathologic-appearing ECGs in about 50% of athletes after cessation of their athletic career, with no adverse cardiovascular events in most of these athletes.[45]

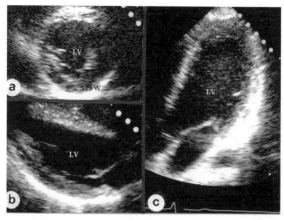

Fig. 25.4 Parasternal short- and long-axis (**a**, **b**) and apical long-axis (**c**) views in the same athlete as shown in Fig. 25.3. The echocardiogram shows no evidence of structural disease or physiologic adaptation to training (left ventricular end-diastolic cavity dimension 50 mm; ventricular septal thickness 11 mm; posterior free wall thickness 10 mm). LV = left ventricle; VS = ventricular septum; PFW = posterior free wall. Reproduced with permission of the American Heart Association from Pelliccia *et al. Circulation* 2000; **102**: 278–84, © Lippincott Williams & Wilkins.

Differential diagnosis of athlete's heart and DCM

The differential diagnosis between athlete's heart and DCM arises not uncommonly in the clinical evaluation of athletes, based on the recognition of a markedly enlarged LV cavity size (i.e. end-diastolic diameter at least 60 mm), which is present in about 15% of highly trained, elite athletes[10] and is compatible with either a marked physiologic LV enlargement or DCM. Idiopathic DCM is a primary cardiac disease, defined by the presence of LV chamber dilatation, normal wall thickness and depressed systolic function.[40,46,47] Patients with DCM usually present with symptoms related to reduced cardiac output; however, life-threatening ventricular and/or supraventricular tachyarrhythmias are not uncommonly part of the initial clinical presentation of this disorder, which may be responsible for sudden cardiac death.[22,46–48]

The protocol shown in Fig. 25.5 encompasses morphologic and clinical criteria that may offer a measure of clarification for the differential diagnosis between DCM and physiologic LV cavity dilatation consistent with the athlete's heart.

Left ventricular morphology

In patients with DCM, the LV cavity is disproportionately dilated and LV chamber morphology is modified to a more spherical shape.[46] In trained athletes, LV cavity enlargement may be substantial (and in the same range of values as DCM), but is associated with enlargement of the right ventricle and atrial cavities, as a consequence of global cardiac remodeling induced by chronic exercise training.[49] The dilated LV cavity in athletes maintains the

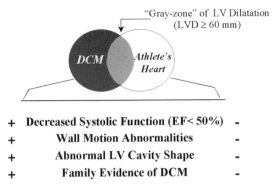

Fig. 25.5 Flow chart showing criteria to distinguish idiopathic dilated cardiomyopathy from athlete's heart when left ventricular cavity dimension is enlarged and in the gray zone of overlap consistent with both diagnoses. LV = left ventricle; EF = ejection fraction.

normal ellipsoid shape, with the mitral valve normally positioned and without mitral regurgitation.[27] Wall thicknesses are usually (mildly) increased in athletes with physiologic cavity enlargement.

Left ventricular function

The most definitive evidence for a pathologic LV dilatation such as DCM is the presence of global systolic dysfunction (i.e. ejection fraction less than 50%), and/or segmental wall motion abnormalities. Instead, athletes with physiologic LV cavity enlargement do not show global systolic dysfunction, segmental wall motion abnormalities, or abnormalities of diastolic filling pattern.[10]

Also, knowledge of the type of sport and training profile of an athlete suspected to have preclinical DCM may be relevant to the diagnosis. For example, substantial LV cavity enlargement is common in athletes training in largely aerobic disciplines, such as cycling, cross-country skiing, rowing, and long-distance running, but virtually absent in other disciplines, such as yachting, shooting, equestrian, and alpine skiing.[10] Furthermore, patients with idiopathic DCM usually present with reduced exercise tolerance, and often atrial or ventricular tachyarrhythmias are present in association with exercise.[47,48]

Differential diagnosis of athlete's heart and arrhythmogenic right ventricular cardiomyopathy

ARVC is a primary heart disease characterized by fatty or fibro-fatty replacement and functional abnormalities primarily affecting the right ventricle, and clinically by life-threatening ventricular arrhythmias at risk for sudden death in young people, especially in association with physical exercise.[41,50–52] The differential diagnosis between athlete's heart and ARVC may arise not uncommonly in the clinical evaluation of an athlete, based on the recognition of an enlargement of the right ventricular cavity, and/or ECG changes such as inverted T waves in the anterior precordial leads V_1 to V_3, or ventricular arrhythmias with LBBB (left bundle branch block) configuration.

While the recognition of ARVC is of crucial importance for the prevention of sudden death in athletes, early diagnosis may be particularly difficult. Standardized diagnostic criteria have been previously proposed, based on the presence of major and minor signs, encompassing clinical, morphologic, ECG, and genetic features of ARVC,[50] which still represent the accepted guidelines for diagnosis.

Morphologic right ventricular features

Noninvasive identification of ARVC may be difficult due to the often subtle morphologic changes. Generally, the structural abnormalities in most cases of ARVC are moderate and easily overlooked unless looked for specifically. The right ventricular morphology and function should be assessed at several levels, including the right ventricle (RV) inflow tract, apex and outflow tract because of the focal nature of the disease.

Certain features may aid in differentiating ARVC from the right ventricular changes associated with athlete's heart. In patients with ARVC, the right ventricle is more substantially enlarged than in trained athletes and shows impaired systolic function; in most ARVC patients, however, morphologic alterations are only mild and the right ventricular cavity may not be dilated, but segmental RV morphologic abnormalities are evident, and wall motion abnormalities are usually present.[52] On the other hand, trained athletes (especially those engaged in endurance disciplines) show an enlarged right ventricular cavity (associated with an enlarged LV cavity) and normal wall thickness; global right ventricular function is normal and no wall motion abnormalities are present.

The electrocardiogram

The most common abnormalities in ARVC patients include inverted T waves in the right precordial leads (V_1 to V_3), associated with increased QRS duration (monger than 110 ms) and incomplete RBBB pattern.[41,51,52] Repolarization abnormalities manifested by T-wave inversion in leads V_1 to V_3 in the absence of a complete right bundle branch block (RBBB) are considered a minor diagnostic criterion, but are extremely useful in raising the suspicion of ARVC and are present in over 50% of patients dying suddenly. However, these ECG abnormalities should be considered with caution because many children and young subjects have T-wave inversions in the right precordial leads, and this criterion may be useful only in individuals older than 12 years.[44] Furthermore, young trained athletes may occasionally show (in the absence of pathologic cardiac conditions) inverted T waves in the anterior precordial leads and right ventricular conduction delays that mimic those observed in patients with ARVC.[44]

Other ECG abnormalities that are usually found in ARVC patients (but are unusual in trained athletes) are either complete RBBB (in approximately 15%

of patients with ARVC) and selective prolongation of the QRS in leads V_1 to V_3 compared with lead V_6. The QRS precordial dispersion of 50 ms or longer generally characterizes patients with massive RV dilatation and recurrent episodes of ventricular tachycardia. A small proportion of ARVC patients (5–10%) shows a small discrete potential (an epsilon wave) just after the QRS complex in the right precordial leads, thought to be a consequence of delayed activation within the abnormal right ventricle.[51] A not minor subset of young ARVC patients show ventricular arrhythmias with LBBB configuration, particularly in association with exercise.

References

1 Rost R, Hollmann W. Athlete's heart. Review of its historical assessment and new aspects. *Int J Sports Med* 1983; **4**: 147–65.
2 Huston P, Puffer JC, MacMillan Rodney W. The athletic heart syndrome. *N Engl J Med* 1985; **315**: 24–32.
3 Maron BJ. Structural features of the athlete heart as defined by echocardiography. *J Am Coll Cardiol* 1986; **7**: 190–203.
4 Morganroth J, Maron BJ, Henry WL *et al.* Comparative left ventricular dimensions in trained athletes. *Ann Intern Med* 1975; **82**: 521–4.
5 Ikaheimo MJ, Palatsi IJ, Takkunen JT. Noninvasive evaluation of the athletic heart: Sprinters versus endurance runners. *Am J Cardiol* 1979; **44**: 24–30.
6 Nishimura T, Yamada Y, Kawai C. Echocardiographic evaluation of long-term effects of exercise on left ventricular hypertrophy and function in professional bicyclists. *Circulation* 1980; **61**: 832–40.
7 Fagard R, Aubert A, Lysens R, Staessen J, Vanhees L, Amery A. Noninvasive assessment of seasonal variations in cardiac structure and function in cyclists. *Circulation* 1983; **67**: 896–901.
8 Pelliccia A, Maron BJ, Spataro A, Proschan MA, Spirito P. The upper limit of physiologic cardiac hypertrophy in highly trained elite athletes. *N Engl J Med* 1991; **324**: 295–301.
9 Spirito P, Pelliccia A, Proschan M *et al.* Morphology of the 'athlete's heart' assessed by echocardiography in 947 elite athletes representing 27 sports. *Am J Cardiol* 1994; **74**: 802–6.
10 Pelliccia A, Culasso F, Di Paolo FM, Maron BJ. Physiologic left ventricular cavity dilatation in elite athletes. *Ann Intern Med* 1999; **130**: 23–31.
11 Pelliccia A, Maron BJ. Cardiac adaptations to exercise training. In: Harries M, Williams C, Stanish WD, Micheli LJ, eds. *Oxford Textbook of Sports Medicine*, 2nd edn. Oxford University Press, 1998: 301–20.
12 Longhurst JC, Kelly AR, Gonyea WJ *et al.* Chronic training with static and dynamic exercise: Cardiovascular adaptation and response to exercise. *Circ Res* 1981; **48** (Suppl. I): I171–8.
13 Keul J, Dickuth HH, Simon G *et al.* Effect of static and dynamic exercise on heart volume, contractility, and left ventricular dimensions. *Circ Res* 1981; **48** (Suppl. I): I162–70.
14 Henry WL, Gardin JM, Ware JH. Echocardiographic measurements in normal subjects from infancy to old age. *Circulation* 1980; **62**: 1054–61.
15 Gardin JM, Savage DD, Ware JH *et al.* Effect of age, sex, body surface area on echocardiographic left ventricular wall mass in normal subjects. *Hypertension* 1987; **9** (Suppl. II): II36–9.

16 Pelliccia A, Spataro A, Caselli G, Maron BJ. Absence of left ventricular wall thickening in athletes engaged in intense power training. *Am J Cardiol* 1993; **72**: 1048–54.

17 Pelliccia A, Maron BJ, Culasso F, Spataro A, Caselli G. The athlete's heart in women: Echocardiographic characterization of 600 highly trained and elite female athletes. *JAMA* 1996; **276**: 211–15.

18 Montgomery HE, Clarkson P, Dollery CM *et al.* Association of angiotensin-converting enzyme gene I/D polymorphism with change in left ventricular mass in response to physical training. *Circulation* 1997; **96**: 741–7.

19 Karjalainen J, Kujala HM, Stolt A *et al.* Angiotensinogen gene M235T polymorphism predicts left ventricular hypertrophy in endurance athletes. *J Am Coll Cardiol* 1999; **34**: 494–9.

20 Maron BJ, Pelliccia A, Spirito P. Cardiac disease in young trained athletes: Insights into methods for distinguishing athlete's heart from structural heart disease, with particular emphasis on hypertrophic cardiomyopathy. *Circulation* 1995; **91**: 1596–601.

21 Maron BJ. Hypertrophic cardiomyopathy: a systematic review. *JAMA* 2002; **287**: 1308–20.

22 Maron BJ. Sudden death in young athletes. *New Engl J Med* 2003; **349**: 1064–75.

23 Maron BJ, Mitchell JH. 26th Bethesda Conference: Recommendations for determining eligibility for competition in athletes with cardiovascular abnormalities. *J Am Coll Cardiol* 1994; **24**: 845–99.

24 Klues HG, Schiffers A, Maron BJ. Phenotypic spectrum and patterns of left ventricular hypertrophy in hypertrophic cardiomyopathy: Morphologic observations and significance as assessed by two-dimensional echocardiography in 600 patients. *J Am Coll Cardiol* 1995; **26**: 1699–708.

25 Maron BJ, Kragel AH, Roberts WC. Sudden death due to hypertrophic cardiomyopathy in the absence of increased left ventricular mass. *Br Heart J* 1990; **63**: 308–10.

26 Spirito P, Maron BJ, Bonow RO *et al.* Occurrence and significance of progressive left ventricular wall thinning and relative cavity dilatation in patients with hypertrophic cardiomyopathy. *Am J Cardiol* 1987; **60**: 123–9.

27 Pelliccia A, Avelar E, De Castro S, Pandian N. Global left ventricular shape is not altered as a consequence of physiologic remodeling in highly trained athletes. *Am J Cardiol* 2000; **86**: 700–2.

28 Spirito P, Maron BJ, Chiarella F *et al.* Diastolic abnormalities in hypertrophic cardiomyopathy: Relation to magnitude of left ventricular hypertrophy. *Circulation* 1985; **72**: 310–16.

29 Lewis JF, Spirito P, Pelliccia A *et al.* Usefulness of Doppler echocardiographic assessment of diastolic filling in distinguishing 'athlete's heart' from hypertrophic cardiomyopathy. *Am J Cardiol* 1992; **68**: 296–300.

30 Maron BJ, Pelliccia A, Spataro A *et al.* Reduction in left ventricular wall thickness after deconditioning in highly trained Olympic athletes. *Br Heart J* 1993; **69**: 125–8.

31 Pelliccia A, Maron BJ, De Luca R, Di Paolo FM, Spataro A, Culasso F. Remodeling of left ventricular hypertrophy in elite athletes after long-term deconditioning. *Circulation* 2002; **105**: 944–9.

32 Maron BJ, Moller JH, Seidman CE *et al.* Impact of laboratory molecular diagnosis on contemporary diagnostic criteria for genetically transmitted cardiovascular diseases: Hypertrophic cardiomyopathy, long-QT syndrome, and Marfan syndrome. *Circulation* 1998; **98**: 1460–71.

33 Venerando A, Rulli V. Frequency, morphology and meaning of the electrocardiographic anomalies found in Olympic marathon runners. *J Sports Med* 1964; **3**: 135–41.

34 Lichtman J, O'Rourke RA, Klein A, Karliner JS. Electrocardiogram of the athlete: Alterations simulating those of organic heart disease. *Arch Intern Med* 1973; **132**: 763–70.

35 Zeppilli P, Pirrami MM, Sassara M, Fenici R. T wave abnormalities in top ranking athletes: Effects of isoproterenol, atropine, and physical exercise. *Am Heart J* 1980; **100**: 213–22.

36 Nishimura T, Kambara H, Chen CH *et al*. Noninvasive assessment of T-wave abnormalities on precordial electrocardiograms in middle-aged professional bicyclists. *J Electrocardiol* 1981; **14**: 357–64.

37 Oakley DG, Oakley CM. Significance of abnormal electrocardiograms in highly trained athletes. *Am J Cardiol* 1982; **50**: 985–9.

38 Zehender M, Meinertz T, Keul J, Just H. ECG variants and cardiac arrhythmias in athletes: Clinical relevance and prognostic importance. *Am Heart J* 1990; **119**: 1378–91.

39 Maron BJ, Wolfson JK, Cirò E *et al*. Relation of electrocardiographic abnormalities and patterns of left ventricular hypertrophy identified by 2-dimensional echocardiography in patients with hypertrophic cardiomyopathy. *Am J Cardiol* 1983; **51**: 189–94.

40 Manolio TA, Baughman KL, Rodeheffer R *et al*. Prevalence and etiology of idiopathic dilated cardiomyopathy. *Am J Cardiol* 1992; **69**: 1458–66.

41 Thiene G, Nava A, Corrado D *et al*. Right ventricular cardiomyopathy and sudden death in young people. *N Engl J Med* 1988; **318**: 129–33.

42 Corrado D, Thiene G, Nava A *et al*. Sudden death in young competitive athletes: Clinicopathologic correlation in 22 cases. *Am J Med* 1990; **89**: 588–96.

43 Corrado D, Basso C, Schiavon M *et al*. Screening for hypertrophic cardiomyopathy in young athletes. *N Engl J Med* 1998; **339**: 364–9.

44 Pelliccia A, Maron BJ, Culasso F *et al*. Clinical significance of abnormal electrocardiographic patterns in trained athletes. *Circulation* 2000; **102**: 278–84.

45 Pelliccia A, DeLuca R, Di Paolo FM, Spataro A, Maron BJ. The long-term clinical significance of distinctly abnormal 12-lead ECG patterns highly suggestive of hypertrophic cardiomyopathy in trained athletes [abstract]. *Circulation* 2000; **18** (Suppl. II): II-420.

46 Gavazzi A, De Maria R, Renosto G *et al*. The spectrum of left ventricular size in dilated cardiomyopathy: Clinical correlates and prognostic implications. *Am Heart J* 1993; **125**: 410–22.

47 Lauer MS, Evans CE, Levy D. Prognostic implications of subclinical left ventricular dilatation and systolic dysfunction in men free of overt cardiovascular disease (the Framingham heart study). *Am J Cardiol* 1992; **70**: 1180–4.

48 Redfield MM, Gersh BJ, Bailey KR, Rodeheffer RJ. Natural history of incidentally discovered, asymptomatic idiopathic dilated cardiomyopathy. *Am J Cardiol* 1994; **74**: 737–9.

49 Hauser AM, Dressendorfer RH, Vos M, Hashimoto Y, Gordon S, Timmis G. Symmetric cardiac enlargement in highly trained endurance athletes: A two-dimensional echocardiographic study. *Am Heart J* 1985; **109**: 1038–44.

50 McKenna WJ, Thiene G, Nava A *et al*. Diagnosis of arrhythmogenic right ventricular dysplasia/cardiomyopathy. *Br Heart J* 1994; **71**: 215–18.

51 Marcus FI. Right ventricular dysplasia: Evaluation and management in relation to sports activities. In: Estes NAM, Salem DN, Wang PJ, eds. *Sudden Cardiac Death in the Athlete*. Armonk, NY: Futura Publishing, 1998: 277–84.

52 Nava A, Bauce B, Basso C *et al*. Clinical profile and long-term follow-up of 37 families with arrhythmogenic right ventricular cardiomyopathy. *J Am Coll Cardiol* 2000; **36**: 2226–33.

CHAPTER 26

Importance of Congenital Coronary Artery Anomalies

Cristina Basso, MD, PhD, Domenico Corrado, MD, PhD, and Gaetano Thiene, MD

Despite the low prevalence in the overall population, congenital coronary artery (CA) anomalies are frequently found to be the cause of sudden death in the young, particularly on the athletic field.[1-11] Previous studies identified hypertrophic cardiomyopathy as the most common cause of sudden death in US autopsy series,[5,6] whereas arrhythmogenic right ventricular cardiomyopathy is the leading cause in young Italian athletes.[11] All studies agree that congenital CA anomalies represent the second most frequent disease at risk for exercise-related sudden death. Table 26.1 reports previous pathologic studies on sudden death in the young, and CA anomalies account for 4–24% of the cases.[6,12-17] These anomalies consist of a wide range of structural abnormalities, which include anomalous origin, anomalous course or both.[1,7,8] These anomalies are observed both in pediatric patients and in adults, with an equal prevalence of sudden death. Why patients with coronary anomalies may survive without symptoms until adulthood and then die suddenly (without superimposition of coronary atherosclerosis) remains intriguing.

Prevalence of coronary artery anomalies

Anomalous CA origin, either the left main from the right sinus of Valsalva or the right coronary from the left sinus, represents an uncommon congenital defect, found in 0.17% of patients at autopsy[18] and in 1.2% of all patients undergoing coronary angiography.[19] Recently, Davis and colleagues[20] confirmed these figures, reporting a prevalence of 0.17% derived from a population of 2388 children and adolescents prospectively evaluated by transthoracic echocardiography. However, their population cannot be considered truly normal since it comprises asymptomatic children and adolescents preferentially referred for cardiovascular investigation. Thus, the prevalence of these coronary anomalies in a large and unselected population should likely be lower. Of note, Pelliccia and colleagues[21] did not find any CA anomalies in a population of 1360 asymptomatic competitive athletes routinely examined by echocardiography, findings which are consistent with a prevalence of less than 0.1%.

Table 26.1 Cardiovascular causes of sudden death in the young. ARVC = arrhythmogenic right ventricular cardiomyopathy; CAA = coronary artery anomaly; CAD = coronary artery disease; DCM = dilated cardiomyopathy, HCM = hypertrophic cardiomyopathy; MVP = mitral valve prolapse. *Including both acquired nonatherosclerotic and congenital CAD

Authors, time interval	Population	Age range (years)	Total no.	Causes (%)
Drory et al., 1976–85[12]	Israel	9–39	118	Atherosclerotic CAD (58) Myocarditis (25) HCM (13) Conduction system (4)
Neuspiel and Kuller, 1972–80[13]	Allegheny County, USA	1–21	51	Myocarditis (27) DCM (24) Conduction system (12) Aortic dissection (6) CAA (6) Atherosclerotic CAD (4)
Topaz and Edwards, 1960–83[14]	St Paul, Minnesota, USA	7–35	50	MVP (24) Myocarditis (25) HCM (12) CAA (4) Aortic stenosis (4)
Phillips et al., 1965–85[15]	American Forces, USA	17–28	20	Myocarditis (42) CAA (15) HCM (10) MVP (5) Atherosclerotic CAD (5) Aortic stenosis (5)
Kramer et al., 1974–86[16]	Soldiers, Israel	17–30	24	Myocarditis (29) HCM (25) MVP (13) Atherosclerotic CAD (13) Aortic dissection (8) CAA (4) DCM (4) Conduction system (4)
Maron et al., 1985[6]	Trained athletes, USA	12–40	134	HCM (36) CAA (24) Aortic rupture (5) Aortic stenosis (4) Myocarditis (3) ARVC (3)
Basso et al., 1979–99[17]	Veneto region, Italy	1–35	273	Atherosclerotic CAD (21) ARVC (14) Valve disease (12) Nonatherosclerotic CAD* (11) Myocarditis (10) Conduction system disease (9) HCM (7)

Coronary artery anomalies at risk of sudden death

Aside from anomalous origin of a CA from the pulmonary trunk, which is highly symptomatic in infancy, due to coronary blood steal from the aorta to the pulmonary artery (thus accounting for extensive myocardial infarction with either sudden death or congestive heart failure),[22] congenital CA anomalies at risk for sudden death in apparently healthy individuals comprise a wide range of clinically 'silent' lesions.[1,7,8]

Coronary ostia malformations

These consist of severe lumen stenosis, either of the right or of the left, by plication of the aortic wall leading to a valve-like ridge which may obstruct the inflow during diastolic filling, with consequent myocardial ischemia leading to life-threatening arrhythmias.[1,23,24] This anomaly may account for sudden death if the surface area of the ridge exceeds 50% of the coronary ostial luminal area.[23] Severe obstruction to the coronary ostia (and of the proximal coronary segment) may also be observed in the setting of hyperelastosis of the aortic wall, i.e. 'macaroni disease', which is a not uncommon observation in infants who have died suddenly;[25] a similar picture is described in Williams syndrome, with supravalvular aortic stenosis, in which the coronary ostia may be totally or partially insulated from the aortic lumen, due to fusion of the aortic leaflets with the wall.

High take-off of the coronary artery from the aortic wall

This anomaly has been considered a normal variant without consequences.[24] However, recently it has been described in otherwise unexplained cases of sudden death.[2] A take-off higher than 2.5 mm above the sinotubular junction may account for a vertical intramural aortic course of the CA, before reaching the aortic root and atrioventricular sulcus. Moreover, a funnel-like ostium with a slit-like lumen along the intramural aortic course might account for myocardial ischemia.[2]

Anomalous coronary artery origin from the wrong aortic sinus

Either the right CA origin from the left coronary sinus or the left CA origin from the right coronary sinus is an anomaly at highest risk of sudden death. In this setting, the proximal segment of the anomalous CA may run anterior to the pulmonary trunk, posterior to the aorta, or between the pulmonary artery and the aorta itself. The latter condition is considered to cause myocardial ischemia (particularly during exercise) by CA squeezing due to the increased cardiac output with diastolic expansion of the great vessels.[1–3,26,29]

Although both right and left CA anomalous origin from the wrong aortic sinus present an impending risk of sudden death, the anomalous left CA from the right sinus is considered more malignant because of the large amount of left ventricular myocardium at ischemic risk (Fig. 26.1). In the review by Rob-

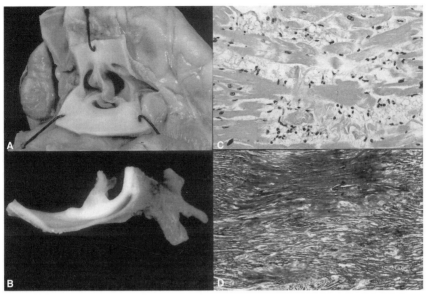

Fig 26.1 Anomalous origin of left coronary artery from the right aortic sinus in a 15-year-old asymptomatic boy who died suddenly during a soccer game. (**A**) View of the aortic root showing the anomalous left coronary artery arising with an acute angle take-off from the right sinus. (**B**) Intramural aortic course of the proximal tract of the anomalous left coronary artery just behind the commissure between the two coronary cusps. (**C**) Extensive myocardial necrosis with neutrophilic infiltrate in the myocardium supplied by the anomalous coronary artery (hematoxylin–eosin stain; magnification ×240). (**D**) Spotty area of post-necrotic replacement-type fibrosis (Heidenhain trichrome stain; magnification ×30). Reproduced from Basso *et al.* Clinical profile of congenital coronary artery anomalies with origin from the wrong aortic sinus leading to sudden death in young competitive athletes. *J Am Coll Cardiol* 2000; **35**: 1493–501, with permission from the American College of Cardiology Foundation.

erts[3] of 43 necropsy patients, 80% died due to the CA anomaly; of these, 75% died suddenly in the first two decades of life and all but one during or shortly after vigorous exertion. On the contrary, anomalous right CA origin from the left sinus may be an incidental angiographic or autopsy observation and until recently has been considered a minor congenital anomaly of no clinical significance. Of note, in a recent paper we reported that all of our cases with anomalous left CA died suddenly, compared with 43% of cases with an anomalous right CA.[2] With regard to anomalous origin of the left CA from the posterior aortic sinus, this coronary malformation is quite uncommon and even more rarely associated with sudden death.[30]

The anomalous origin of the left circumflex branch from the right CA or sinus with a separate ostium is considered the most frequent CA anomaly,[3,24] with an angiographic incidence of up to 0.7%.[31,32] Although it is frequently an incidental autopsy or angiographic finding, it has been also described in victims of unexpected arrhythmic sudden death.[1,2,33,34] After the anomalous take-off, the left circumflex branch shows an abnormal retroaortic course to reach the left atrioventricular groove crossing the mitroaortic fibrous continuity. This anomaly will be considered a benign condition until cases have been reported with evidence of myocardial infarction or sudden death in the absence of any other cause.

Myocardial bridge (tunneled epicardial coronary artery)

A coronary epicardial stem, usually the left anterior descending branch, may be embedded within the left ventricular myocardium, thus presenting with an intramural course.[35–37] Thin loops of myocardium surrounding a CA have been reported in up to 70% of patients dying from different causes, and thus should be considered as a variant of normal.[37] However, myocardial ischemia has been reported in patients in whom coronary angiography detected only systolic vessel constriction (the so-called milking effect) and in whom surgical debridging was effective in relieving both signs and symptoms of ischemia.[38–40] Moreover, sudden death has been described in patients with myocardial bridge as the only plausible substrate accounting for sudden death.[5–7,41] For example, tunneled coronary arteries have been reported in approximately 5% of athletic field deaths by Maron and colleagues[5,6] in the absence of any other structural anomaly. Effort-induced ischemia has been attributed to tachycardia, which increases the myocardial oxygen requirement and reduces coronary flow during diastole. Histopathologic analysis has established that this anomaly has pathophysiologic significance when it has a long (2–3 cm) and deep (2–3 mm) intramural course.[42] Moreover, we found that the myocardium encircling the intramural coronary segment acts as a sheath and sphincter and shows disarray and fibrosis, further hindering diastolic filling of the artery.[7] All these features are in keeping not only with systolic lumen obliteration but also with persistent occlusion during diastole, when the coronary blood flow occurs, predominantly due to relaxation of the myocardium surrounding the anomalous coronary segment. This hypothesis has been recently confirmed by intravascular ultrasound investigations.[43] The occurrence of myocardial ischemia at rest, however, could be also due to vasospasm of the intramural coronary segment[44] and transient platelet aggregation and thrombosis provoked by mechanical trauma to the vessel wall.[38,39] Surgical debridging and also interventional therapy with stent implantation have been successfully carried out in patients with this anomaly.[45]

Anomalous coronary artery origin from the wrong aortic sinus: pathophysiology, *in vivo* diagnosis and clinical management

Timely clinical identification during life of wrong aortic sinus CA origin is crucial for two reasons. First, it should result in the exclusion of affected individuals from participation in competitive sports in order to prevent sudden death that is clearly related to effort.[3,5,6,10,11] Secondly, and more importantly, these anomalies, once identified, are amenable to surgical correction.

Mechanisms precipitating sudden death.

CA anomalies produce sudden death or syncope by triggering myocardial ischemia. Our findings, paradoxically showing normal ECG patterns associated with pathologic evidence of acute myocardial ischemic damage and/or chronic ischemic injury with replacement-type fibrosis,[29] suggest that myocardial ischemia is episodic in nature, probably occurring in infrequent bursts, which may be cumulative with time.

Myocardial ischemia is the consequence of the abnormal anatomy of the anomalously arising CA, which limits coronary blood flow, including: the acute angle take-off from the aorta; narrowed slit-like lumen with a potential for a flap-like closure of the orifice; the proximal intramural course of the anomalous vessel within the aortic tunica media, which may further aggravate the obstruction; and the squeezing of the vessel along its course between the aorta and the pulmonary artery, particularly during exercise, when there is increased cardiac output with expansion of the great vessels. However, Taylor and colleagues[9] found that neither the size of the CA ostium, the degree of acute angle take-off nor the length of intramural aortic course was predictive for sudden death by comparing at post-mortem a series of 12 patients who died due to these anomalies and 18 subjects who died due to unrelated causes.

Spasm of the anomalous coronary segment, possibly as a result of endothelial injury, has also been suggested.[46] In a recent study, by comparing the various cardiovascular diseases accounting for sudden death in athletes, we found that only congenital anomalies of the CA and arrhythmogenic right ventricular cardiomyopathy occurred more frequently in athletes than in nonathletes (12.2 vs 0.5% and 22.4 vs 8.2%, respectively), supporting the idea that these diseases are particularly prone to cardiac arrest during effort.[11]

Previous symptoms and signs

Coronary artery anomalies are rarely suspected or identified during life and are usually first recognized at autopsy, largely because there is insufficient clinical suspicion and because of the difficulties implicit in routine examination or clinical testing. Although sudden death is frequently the first manifestation of the disease, by studying a series of young competitive athletes who died suddenly due to these malformations, we demonstrated that premonitory cardiac symptoms not uncommonly occurred shortly before sudden death, particularly in the setting of anomalous left main CA origin, suggesting that a history of exertional syncope or chest pain requires exclusion of this anomaly.[29] The observation that the conventional 12-lead ECG and maximal exercise stress test are usually normal suggests that myocardial ischemia is only periodically present in this disease. These findings have important implications for preventive strategies and *in vivo* identification.

Diagnostic testing

In a recent investigation describing the anatomical and clinical profile of young athletes with wrong sinus CA origin, we reported that all the resting 12-lead and exercise ECGs available during life were normal. Moreover, by reviewing the literature concerning exercise ECG findings in young patients with documented CA anomalies, only about 20% showed ischemic changes on ECG. Therefore, ECG stress testing and myocardial perfusion scintigraphy may provide little or no diagnostic information in athletes or other patients suspected of having anomalous CA.

If the index of suspicion is sufficiently high because of the presence of potential clinical markers, such as exertional syncope or chest pain, even in the setting of normal 12-lead and effort ECGs, the origin and proximal course of the coronary arteries should be defined noninvasively by transthoracic or transesophageal echocardiography. Indeed, in young individuals presenting with symptoms and/or ECG changes, echocardiography can provide correct identification of wrong aortic sinus origin, which was subsequently confirmed by coronary angiography.[47,48]

Echocardiography has the potential to address the correct diagnosis, because it potentially provides anatomic definition of the ostium and proximal epicardial course of the CA. Pelliccia and colleagues,[21] in a series of 1360 young athletes prospectively evaluated by echocardiography, were able to visualize the ostium and proximal course of the left CA in 97% and right CA in 80% of subjects. As a consequence, the failure to demonstrate that the CA actually originate from their usual location in a young person with impaired consciousness or angina suggests the need for further anatomic investigation by angiography or possibly magnetic resonance imaging or computed tomography.[49–51]

However, false negatives may occur with transthoracic echocardiography, as demonstrated by Davis and colleagues,[20] either by misinterpretation or the inability to fully identify CA origin because of a poor acoustic window. The specificity and sensitivity of echocardiography for identifying CA anomalies in a large unselected population remain to be defined.

Clinical management

Timely diagnosis of CA anomalies raises the question of clinical management. It is clear that not all patients with such anomalies are at risk of sudden death, since many have lived a full life and died of unrelated causes. The major challenge is the identification of high-risk subsets in order to determine which patients should undergo surgical therapy.

If such an anomaly, either of right or left CA anomalous origin, is found in a symptomatic patient (or in an asymptomatic patient with clinical evidence of myocardial ischemia), surgery is mandatory. Since it has been clearly demonstrated that sudden death is precipitated by exercise, competitive sports as well as strenuous effort should be strongly discouraged.[52] Surgical correction may be accomplished either by CA bypass grafting or newer techniques, such as reimplantation of the anomalous vessel in the proper coronary sinus or by 'unroofing' the common wall between the aorta and the anomalous CA, resulting in a new orifice with a more natural take-off.[53,54]

It is less clear what is the most appropriate therapeutic strategy for the asymptomatic young patient in whom diagnosis of a coronary anomaly is incidental and there is no demonstration of ischemia in the corresponding myocardial region. In this setting, the type of anomaly, whether right or left anomalous CA origin, would make the difference. We would recommend surgery in the setting of an anomalous left CA since cardiac arrest remains unpredictable, whereas right CA anomalous origin appears to have a more benign clinical course.

Acknowledgments

This study was supported by Veneto Region, Venice; MURST and the Ministry of Health, Rome; and Fondazione Cassa di Risparmio, Padova e Rovigo, Italy.

References

1 Roberts WC. Major anomalies of coronary arterial origin seen in adulthood. *Am Heart J* 1986; **111**: 941–63.

2 Frescura C, Basso C, Thiene G *et al.* Anomalous origin of coronary arteries and risk of sudden death: A study based on an autopsy population of congenital heart disease. *Hum Pathol* 1998; **29**: 689–95.

3 Roberts WC. Congenital coronary arterial anomalies unassociated with major anomalies of the heart and great vessels. In: Roberts WC, ed. *Adult Congenital Heart Diseases*. Philadelphia: FA Davis Company, 1987: 583–630.

4 Liberthson RR. Sudden death from cardiac causes in children and young adults. *N Engl J Med* 1996; **334**: 1039–44.

5 Maron BJ, Roberts WC, McAllister HA *et al.* Sudden death in young athletes. *Circulation* 1980; **62**: 218–29.

6 Maron BJ, Shirani J, Poliac LC *et al.* Sudden death in young competitive athletes: Clinical, demographic, and pathological profiles. *JAMA* 1996; **276**: 199–204.

7 Corrado D, Thiene G, Cocco P, Frescura C. Non-atherosclerotic coronary artery disease and sudden death in the young. *Br Heart J* 1992; **68**: 601–7.

8 Basso C, Frescura C, Corrado D *et al.* Congenital heart disease and sudden death in the young. *Hum Pathol* 1995; **26**: 1065–72.

9 Taylor AJ, Rogan KM, Virmani R. Sudden cardiac death associated with isolated congenital coronary artery anomalies. *J Am Coll Cardiol* 1992; **20**: 640–7.

10 Burke AP, Farb A, Virmani R *et al.* Sports-related and non-sports-related sudden cardiac death in young adults. *Am Heart J* 1991; **121**: 568–75.

11 Corrado D, Basso C, Schiavon M, Thiene G. Screening for hypertrophic cardiomyopathy in young athletes. *N Engl J Med* 1998; **339**: 364–9.

12 Drory Y, Turetz Y, Hiss Y *et al.* Sudden unexpected death in persons less than 40 years of age. *Am J Cardiol* 1991; **68**: 1388–92.

13 Neuspiel DR, Kuller LH. Sudden and unexpected natural death in childhood and adolescence. *JAMA* 1985; **254**: 1321–5.

14 Topaz O, Edwards JE. Pathologic features of sudden death in children, adolescents, and young adults. *Chest* 1985; **87**: 476–82.

15 Philips M, Robinowitz M, Higgins JR *et al.* Sudden cardiac death in Air Force recruits: A 20-year review. *JAMA* 1986; **256**: 2696–9.

16 Kramer MR, Drory Y, Lev B. Sudden death in young Israeli soldiers: Analysis of 83 cases. *Isr J Med Sci* 1989; **25**: 620–4.

17 Basso C, Calabrese F, Corrado D, Thiene G. Postmortem diagnosis in sudden cardiac death victims: Macroscopic, microscopic and molecular findings. *Cardiovasc Res* 2001; **50**: 290–330.

18 Alexander RW, Griffith GC. Anomalies of the coronary arteries and their clinical significance. *Circulation* 1956; **14**: 800–5.

19 Engel HJ, Torres C, Page HL. Major variations in anatomical origin of the coronary arteries: Angiographic observations in 4250 patients without associated congenital heart disease. *Cathet Cardiovasc Diagn* 1975; **1**: 157–69.

20 Davis JA, Cecchin F, Jones TK, Portman MA. Major coronary artery anomalies in a pediatric population: Incidence and clinical importance. *J Am Coll Cardiol* 2001; **37**: 593–7.

21 Pelliccia A, Spataro A, Maron BJ. Prospective echocardiographic screening for coronary artery anomalies in 1,360 elite competitive athletes. *Am J Cardiol* 1993; **72**: 978–9.

22 Moodie DS, Fyfe D, Gill CC *et al.* Anomalous origin of the left coronary artery from the pulmonary artery (Bland–White–Garland syndrome) in adult patients: Long-term follow-up after surgery. *Am Heart J* 1983; **106**: 381–8.

23 Virmani R, Chun PKC, Goldstein RE, Rabinovitz M, McAllister HA. Acute takeoffs of the coronary arteries along the aortic wall and congenital coronary ostial valve-like ridges: Association with sudden death. *J Am Coll Cardiol* 1984; **3**: 766–71.

24 Virmani R, Rogan K, Cheitlin MD. Congenital coronary artery anomalies: Pathologic aspects. In: Virmani R, Forman MB, eds. *Nonatherosclerotic Ischemic Heart Disease.* New York: Raven Press, 1989: 153–83.

25 Thiene G, Ho SY. Aortic root pathology and sudden death in youth: Review of anatomical varieties. *Appl Pathol* 1986; **14**: 237–45.

26 Cheitlin MD, De Castro CM, McAllister HA. Sudden death as a complication of anomalous left coronary origin from the anterior sinus of Valsalva. A not-so-minor congenital anomaly. *Circulation* 1974; **50**: 780–7.

27 Barth CW III, Roberts WC. Left main coronary artery originating from the right sinus of Valsalva and coursing between the aorta and pulmonary trunk. *J Am Coll Cardiol* 1986; **7**: 366–73.

28 Liberthson RR, Dinsmore RE, Fallon JT. Aberrant coronary artery origin from the aorta: Report of 18 patients, review of the literature and delineation of natural history and management. *Circulation* 1979; **59**: 748–54.

29 Basso C, Maron BJ, Corrado D, Thiene G. Clinical profile of congenital coronary artery anomalies with origin from the wrong aortic sinus leading to sudden death in young competitive athletes. *J Am Coll Cardiol* 2000; **35**: 1493–501.

30 Lipsett J, Byard RW, Carpenter BF, Jimenez CL, Bourne AJ. Anomalous coronary arteries arising from the aorta associated with sudden death in infancy and early childhood. *Arch Pathol Lab Med* 1991; **115**: 770–3.

31 Page HL, Engel HJ, Campbell WB, Thomas CS. Anomalous origin of the left circumflex coronary artery: Recognition, angiographic demonstration and clinical significance. *Circulation* 1974; **50**: 768–73.

32 Chaitman BR, Lespérence J, Saltiel J, Bourasse MG. Clinical, angiographic and hemody-namic findings in patients with anomalous origin of the coronary arteries. *Circulation* 1976; **53**: 122–31.

33 Corrado D, Pennelli T, Piovesana P, Thiene G. Anomalous origin of the left circumflex coronary artery from the right aortic sinus of Valsalva and sudden death. *Cardiovasc Pathol* 1994; **3**: 269–71.

34 Piovesana P, Corrado D, Contessotto F *et al.* Echocardiographic identification of anoma-lous origin of the left circumflex coronary artery from the right aortic sinus of Valsalva. *Am Heart J* 1990; **119**: 205–7.

35 Geiringer E. The mural coronary. *Am Heart J* 1951; **41**: 359–68.

36 Angelini P, Trivellato M, Donis J, Leachman RD. Myocardial bridges: A review. *Prog Car-diovasc Dis* 1983; **26**: 75–88.

37 Polacek P. Relation of myocardial bridges and loops on the coronary arteries to coronary occlusions. *Am Heart J* 1961; **61**: 44–52.

38 Feldman AM, Baughman KL. Myocardial infarction associated with a myocardial bridge. *Am Heart J* 1986; **111**: 784–7.

39 Vasan RS, Bahl VK, Rajani M. Myocardial infarction associated with a myocardial bridge. *Int J Cardiol* 1989; **25**: 240–1.

40 Faruqui AM, Maloy WC, Felner JM *et al.* Symptomatic myocardial bridging of coronary artery. *Am J Cardiol* 1978; **41**: 1305–9.

41 Morales AR, Romanelli R, Boucek RJ. The mural left anterior descending coronary artery, strenuous exercise and sudden death. *Circulation* 1980; **62**: 230–7.

42 Ferreira AG, Trotter SE, Konig B *et al.* Myocardial bridges: Morphological and functional aspects. *Br Heart J* 1991; **66**: 364–7.

43 Ge J, Erbel R, Rupprecht HJ *et al.* Comparison of intravascular ultrasound and angiogra-phy in the assessment of myocardial bridging. *Circulation* 1994; **89**: 1725–32.

44 Ciampricotti R, El Gamal M. Vasospastic coronary occlusion associated with a myocar-dial bridge. *Cathet Cardiovasc Diagn* 1988; **14**: 118–20.

45 Haager PK, Schwarz ER, vom Dahl J, Klues HG, Reffelmann T, Hanrath P. Long term angiographic and clinical follow up in patients with stent implantation for symptomatic myocardial bridging. *Heart* 2000; **84**: 403–8.

46 Cheitlin MD. Coronary anomalies as a cause of sudden death in the athlete. In: Estes NAM, Salem DN, Wang PJ, eds. *Sudden Cardiac Death in the Athlete.* Armonk, NY: Futura, 1998: 379–91.

47 Maron BJ, Leon MB, Swain JA *et al.* Prospective identification by two dimensional echo-cardiography of anomalous origin of the left main coronary artery from the right sinus of Valsalva. *Am J Cardiol* 1991; **68**: 140–2.

48 Zeppilli P, Dello Russo A, Santini C *et al.* In vivo detection of coronary artery anomalies in asymptomatic athletes by echocardiographic screening. *Chest* 1998; **114**: 89–93.

49 Serota H, Barth CW III, Seuc CA *et al.* Rapid identification of course of anomalous coro-nary arteries in adults: The 'dot and eye' method. *Am J Cardiol* 1990; **65**: 891–8.

50 McConnell MV, Ganz P, Selwyn AP *et al.* Identification of anomalous coronary arteries and their anatomic course by magnetic resonance coronary angiography. *Circulation* 1995; **92**: 3158–62.

51 Mousseaux E, Hernigou A, Sapoval M *et al.* Coronary arteries arising from the contra-lateral aortic sinus: Electron beam computed tomographic demonstration of the initial course of the artery with respect to the aorta and right ventricular outflow tract. *J Thorac Cardiovasc Surg* 1996; **112**: 836–40.

52 Maron BJ, Mitchell JE. 26th Bethesda Conference: Recommendations for determining eligibility for competition in athletes with cardiovascular abnormalities. *J Am Coll Cardiol* 1994; **24**: 845–99.

53 Cohen AJ, Grishkin BA, Helsel RA, Head HD. Surgical therapy in the management of coronary anomalies: Emphasis on utility of internal mammary artery grafts. *Ann Thorac Surg* 1989; **47**: 630–7.

54 Van Son JAM, Haas GS. Anomalous origin of left main coronary artery from right sinus of Valsalva: Modified surgical treatment to avoid neo-coronary ostial stenosis. *Eur J Cardiothorac Surg* 1996; **10**: 467–9.

Arrhythmogenic Right Ventricular Cardiomyopathy and Hypertrophic Cardiomyopathy: Identification with the Italian Preparticipation Athlete Screening Program

Domenico Corrado, MD, PhD, Cristina Basso, MD, PhD, Maurizio Schiavon, MD, and Gaetano Thiene, MD

The vast majority of sudden deaths in athletes are due to cardiovascular diseases.[1–10] In athletes over 35 years of age atherosclerotic coronary artery disease is by far the most common cause of fatal events.[2,4,5] In younger competitive athletes, hypertrophic cardiomyopathy has been implicated as the principal cause of sport-related cardiac arrest, accounting for about one-third of sudden deaths in the USA;[3,7–9] the next most frequent cause is anomalous origin of the coronary arteries from the wrong coronary sinus. Other, less common, pathologic substrates include arrhythmogenic right ventricular cardiomyopathy, myocarditis, conduction system abnormalities, and Marfan syndrome.[3–10] There is a considerable interest in the role of preparticipation athletic screening for the early identification of these cardiovascular diseases and disqualification of affected athletes at risk of sudden death, with the expectation that such a strategy makes prevention a possibility.[11,12] However, controversy remains over the cost-effectiveness of this population-based evaluation. In fact, the practicality and utility of the screening process is limited by the large size of the athletic population and the uncommon occurrence of these conditions within the general population (less than 0.1%), as well as the silent clinical course of most implicated cardiovascular diseases.

Systematic preparticipation screening by history, physical examination and electrocardiography of all young subjects embarking on competitive athletic activity has been the practice in Italy for more than 20 years.[13–15] This chapter addresses the impact of such a population-based screening strategy in detecting athletes affected by cardiovascular diseases who are at risk of life-threatening arrhythmias during sport performance and, ultimately, the efficacy of the strategy in preventing sport-related sudden death.

Screening protocols in the USA and Italy

USA

As presently employed in the USA, preparticipation athletic screening seems to be severely limited in its power to detect potentially lethal cardiovascular abnormalities. Athletic evaluation has traditionally been performed by means of only history (personal and family) and physical examination (without 12-lead ECG) and occurs largely at the discretion of the examining physician.[12] One retrospective study of 134 high school and collegiate athletes who died suddenly showed that cardiovascular abnormalities were suspected by standard history and physical examination screening only in 3%, and that less than 1% received an accurate cardiac diagnosis.[16]

The addition of 12-lead ECGs to the screening process has the potential to enhance the detection of some cardiovascular diseases. ECGs are abnormal in about 95% of patients with hypertrophic cardiomyopathy, which is the leading cause of sudden death in the athlete.[17] Moreover, ECG abnormalities are often observed in other conditions presenting a risk of sudden death in athletes, such as coronary artery anomaly, Wolff–Parkinson–White syndrome, arrhythmogenic right ventricular cardiomyopathy, and long QT and Brugada syndromes.

Italy

Systematic preparticipation screening, predominantly based on 12-lead ECG associated with a history and physical examination of all competitive athletes, has been the practice in Italy for more than 20 years.[13–15] Italian law mandates that every subject engaged in competitive sport activity must undergo an annual clinical evaluation to obtain a license to participate in competitive sports. Screening for cardiovascular disease is part of a more comprehensive medical evaluation that includes a general clinical history and a physical examination (including orthopedic evaluation, spirometry, and urinalysis). The initial cardiovascular protocol includes personal and familial histories, physical examination with blood pressure determination, basal 12-lead ECG, and a limited exercise test (Montoye step test). Additional tests, such as echocardiography, 24-hour ambulatory Holter monitoring, and exercise testing, are requested for those subjects who have positive cardiac findings at the initial evaluation. The family history is considered positive when close relative(s) have experienced a premature (before 50 years of age) cardiovascular event or sudden death or in the presence of a family history of coronary artery disease, cardiomyopathy, Marfan or long QT syndrome, clinically important arrhythmias, or other disabling conditions. The personal history is considered positive if there is prior occurrence of exertional chest pain or discomfort, syncope or near-syncope, irregular heartbeat or palpitations, or shortness of breath or fatigue out of proportion to the degree of exertion. Positive physical findings include musculoskeletal and ocular features suggestive of Marfan syndrome, diminished

Table 27.1 Criteria for a positive 12-lead electrocardiogram. *Increasing by less than 100 beats/minute during limited exercise test; †not shortening with hyperventilation or limited exercise test. Reproduced from Corrado *et al. Screening for hypertrophic cardiomyopathy in young athletes. N Engl J Med* 1998; **339**: 364–9. © 1998 Massachusetts Medical Society. All rights reserved

P wave	Left atrial enlargement: negative portion of the P wave in lead V1 ≥0.1 mV in depth and ≥0.04 s in duration Right atrial enlargement: peaked P wave in leads II and III or V1 ≥0.25 mV in amplitude
QRS complex	Frontal plane axis deviation: right ≥+120° or left −30° to −90°; increased voltage:amplitude of R or S wave in a standard lead ≥2 mV, S wave in lead V1 or V2 ≥3 mV, or R wave in lead V5 or V6 ≥3 mV Abnormal Q waves ≥0.04 s in duration or ≥25% of height of ensuing R wave or QS pattern in two or more leads Right or left bundle branch block with QRS duration ≥0.12 s R or R′ wave in lead V1 ≥0.5 mV in amplitude and R/S ratio ≥1
ST segment, T waves, and QT interval	ST-segment depression or T-wave flattening or inversion in two or more leads Prolongation of heart rate-corrected QT interval >0.44 s
Rhythm and conduction abnormalities	Premature ventricular beats or more severe ventricular arrhythmias Supraventricular tachycardias, atrial flutter, or atrial fibrillation Short PR interval (<0.12 s) with or without delta wave Sinus bradycardia with resting heart rate ≤40 beats/min* First (PR ≥0.21 s†), second- or third-degree atrioventricular block

and delayed femoral artery pulses, mid- or end-systolic clicks, a second heart sound single or widely split and fixed with respiration, pathologic heart murmurs (any diastolic or systolic murmur grade ≥2/6), irregular heart rhythm, and brachial blood pressure >145/90 mmHg (on more than one reading). Twelve-lead ECG is considered positive, according to accepted criteria,[18–20] in the presence of one or more of the findings reported in Table 27.1.

Subjects recognized as affected by clinically relevant cardiovascular abnormalities are disqualified from competitive athletic activity. Italian guidelines for assessing athletic risk are similar to those of the 16th[21] and 26th[22] Bethesda Conferences, although criteria for sports eligibility are more restrictive.[23]

Results of the Italian preparticipation screening

The Italian preparticipation screening involves nearly 6 million athletes of all ages annually (which represents about 10% of the overall Italian population), who are regularly engaged in competitive sports activities.[14] Therefore, a precise overall report on a national basis of the extent and nature of disqualification from sports over a period of more than two decades is not available. However, information on more limited athletic populations over shorter time intervals is available. Zeppilli reported a 2.5% prevalence of disqualification among 125 408 athletes who were examined in eight different sports medical centers in Italy. Cardiovascular diseases accounted for 51% of the causes of disqualification.[24] Pelliccia and Maron reported on 22 000 elite athletes (selected because of their high competitive levels) who had already been exposed to previous screening and were undergoing evaluation at the Institute of Sport Science.[14] There were 480 (2.2%) athletes disqualified for cardiovascular reasons; of interest, three of them (affected by Wolff–Parkinson–White syndrome, arrhythmogenic right ventricular cardiomyopathy, and Marfan syndrome, respectively) died during the follow-up after disregarding medical advice to cease athletic activity.

We recently reported the 17-year experience of the Center for Sport Medicine of Padova.[15] During the period from 1979 to 1996, a consecutive series of 33 735 consecutive young (under 35 years), athletes underwent preparticipation cardiovascular evaluations at the Center for Sport Medicine of Padova. Of these, 1058 were disqualified for medical reasons. Six hundred and twenty-one (2%) have been disqualified because of the recognition of clinically relevant cardiovascular abnormalities (Table 27.2). The most frequent disqualifying conditions consisted of rhythm and conduction abnormalities (38%), which included arrhythmogenic right ventricular cardiomyopathy (2%); hypertension (27%); valvular diseases including mitral valve prolapse complicated by significant ventricular arrhythmias or mitral valve regurgitation (21%); and hypertrophic cardiomyopathy (4%). Less frequent reasons for noneligibility included dilated cardiomyopathy, congenital and rheumatic heart diseases, and pericarditis.

Four of 621 athletes disqualified for cardiovascular causes died during a follow-up period of 8.2 ± 4.5 years. One athlete affected by mild mitral valve prolapse complicated by complex ventricular arrhythmias experienced sudden death, while three athletes, each disqualified because of atrial septal defect, ventricular septal defect, or bicuspid aortic valve with regurgitation, died from nonnatural causes (drug abuse, car accident, and suicide, respectively).

Table 27.2 Cardiovascular conditions causing disqualification from competitive sports in 621 athletes in Padua, 1979–96. Reproduced from Corrado *et al.* Screening for hypertrophic cardiomyopathy in young athletes. *N Engl J Med* 1998; **339**: 364–9. © 1998 Massachusetts Medical Society. All rights reserved

Conditions	No. (%)
Rhythm and conduction abnormalities	238 (38)
Systemic hypertension	168 (27)
Valvular diseases (including mitral valve prolapse)	133 (21)
Hypertrophic cardiomyopathy	22 (4)
Others	60 (10)

Identification of young competitive athletes with hypertrophic cardiomyopathy

Hypertrophic cardiomyopathy has been reported as the leading cause of sudden death in young competitive athletes, accounting for up to 30% of athletic field deaths.[3,7,8,9,12,14] Clinical diagnosis of hypertrophic cardiomyopathy relies on the demonstration, usually by echocardiography, of a hypertrophied (wall thickness at least 13 mm), nondilated left ventricle in the absence of another cardiac or systemic disease that could itself cause hypertrophy of the magnitude present in that individual.[25] Left ventricular hypertrophy in athletes is common as a response to athletic training (athlete's heart) and, in the presence of a marked response, needs careful distinction from hypertrophic cardiomyopathy.[26] Differential diagnosis is based on several echocardiographic and clinical features, such as the magnitude and extent of wall thickness and cavity dimension of the left ventricle, electrocardiographic abnormalities, the type of sport, and the results of detraining.[27-31] Criteria in favor of hypertrophic cardiomyopathy include markedly increased wall thickness (greater than 16 mm) and an unusual distribution (e.g. sparing the anterior septum) of left ventricular hypertrophy; normal left ventricular cavity (less than 45 mm); striking electrocardiographic abnormalities (marked increase of voltages, prominent Q waves, and deep, negative T waves); training in athletic disciplines other than endurance sports such as rowing and canoeing; and persistence of hypertrophy after 3–6 months of deconditioning.[27-31]

Although echocardiography is the main diagnostic tool for the clinical recognition of hypertrophic cardiomyopathy, it is prohibitively expensive and impractical for screening large athletic populations. The 12-lead ECG has been proposed as an alternative, more cost-effective test for population-based screening. It is noteworthy that the 12-lead ECG is abnormal in the majority of patients with hypertrophic cardiomyopathy.[17] Accordingly, the data of the Center for Sport Medicine of Padova shows that the Italian screening program, primarily based on ECG, has good sensitivity in detecting otherwise concealed hypertrophic cardiomyopathy in young competitive athletes.[15] Among 33 735 athletes undergoing preparticipation screening, 22 (0.07%) showed definitive echocardiographic evidence of hypertrophic cardiomyopathy. The athletes with a diagnosis of hypertrophic cardiomyopathy were 12 males and two females, aged 20 ± 4 years. Reasons for echocardiographic study were one or more of the following findings: a positive family history in three (14%); cardiac murmur in two (9%); ECG changes in 16 (80%) consisting of repolarization abnormalities in 14 (87.5%), elevated voltages in 11 (69%) and abnormal Q waves in five (31%); and premature ventricular beats in five (23%). The maximal thickness of the left ventricular wall was 19 ± 3 mm (range, 16–24 mm) and the diastolic diameter of the left ventricular cavity was 43 ± 2 mm (range, 39–46 mm). Left ventricular hypertrophy did not show a significant difference before and after deconditioning.

The 0.07% prevalence of hypertrophic cardiomyopathy in the homogeneously white, athletic population of the Veneto region of Italy, primarily screened by ECG, is very similar to the 0.1% reported in white young individuals in the USA, who were evaluated by echocardiography.[32] This shows that systematic screening by 12-lead ECG is as sensitive as echocardiography in detecting hypertrophic cardiomyopathy in the young athletic population. That adding the echocardiographic examination to the screening protocol does not result in significant improvement in its efficacy for identifying athletes with hypertrophic cardiomyopathy has been recently confirmed by Pelliccia and colleagues.[33] These authors did not diagnose hypertrophic cardiomyopathy by echocardiographic examination in 4469 elite athletes previously cleared by ECG at preparticipation evaluation.

In our experience, a protocol using ECG together with history and physical examination is successful and cost-effective for screening athletes to proceed to diagnostic echocardiography.[15] Of the 33 735 athletes initially screened, 3016 (9%) were referred for echocardiographic evaluation because of a positive history, abnormal physical findings, or electrocardiographic abnormalities, and 22 (0.7%) ultimately showed evidence of hypertrophic cardiomyopathy and were disqualified from sports. Therefore, the proportion of young athletes with normal hearts but abnormal ECGs (false positives) and thus requiring further expensive evaluation by echocardiography was 9%. This partial limitation was offset by the relatively low cost of the screening ECG and its ability to detect young athletes with hypertrophic cardiomyopathy. We recently performed a cost-effective analysis of three recommended preparticipation screening strategies and demonstrated that the identification of young competitive athletes with hypertrophic cardiomyopathy at risk of sudden death was best accomplished with a history, physical examination and ECG; this approach was twice as cost-effective as a history, physical examination, and ECG plus echocardiography.[34] Of note, history and physical examination was the least cost-effective screening strategy.

Prevention of sport-related sudden death due to hypertrophic cardiomyopathy

Two lines of evidence suggest the efficacy of Italian preparticipation screening in preventing sudden death by hypertrophic cardiomyopathy. The first comes from analysis of the follow-up of the young athletes with hypertrophic cardiomyopathy who were identified and disqualified at preparticipation athletic screening in the Padova area. None of these 22 athletes died during the follow-up.[15] In two patients who had paroxysmal atrial fibrillation, medical treatment with β-blockers and amiodarone, respectively, was effective in restoring and maintaining sinus rhythm; another asymptomatic patient with a family history of sudden death was treated with amiodarone after documentation of nonsustained ventricular tachycardia during 24-hour Holter monitoring. This supports the conclusion that preparticipation screening strategy results in the detection and elimination of such patients from competitive athletics and probably reduces mortality by such disqualification.

The second line of evidence is based on the results of systematic monitoring of sudden death in young people (up to 35 years of age) which has been carried out in the Veneto region of Italy.[15] From January 1979 to December 1996, 269 consecutive cases of juvenile sudden death were prospectively studied. Forty-nine (18%) young sudden death victims were young competitive athletes (44 males and five females, aged 23 years), who underwent preparticipation cardiovascular screening for competitive sport. These 49 athletes had participated in a variety of sports: soccer ($n = 22$), basketball ($n = 5$), swimming ($n = 4$), cycling ($n = 3$), rugby, running, gymnastics, tennis, skiing, judo, and volleyball ($n = 2$ each), and weight-lifting ($n = 1$). Fourteen athletes had previously experienced effort-dependent palpitations, syncopal episodes, or both; 16 had ECG abnormalities and/or atrioventricular conduction and rhythm disturbances. Causes of sudden death in these athletes are reported in Table 27.3. The most common causes were arrhythmogenic right ventricular cardiomyopathy ($n = 11$, 22%), atherosclerotic coronary artery disease ($n = 9$, 18%), and congenital anomalies of the coronary arteries with wrong sinus origin ($n = 8$, 16%). Hypertrophic cardiomyopathy caused only one sports-related sudden death (3%), whereas it accounted for 9% of sudden deaths in the general young population unrelated to sports. Comparison between the above findings from Italy and those of the study of Burke and colleagues in the USA[7] shows a similar occurrence (8 and 3%, respectively) of hypertrophic cardiomyopathy in sudden death unrelated to sports, but a strong difference (24 *vs* 2.5%, respectively) in sports-related deaths. These data in the nonathletic youthful population in Italy and the USA

Table 27.3 Causes of sudden deaths in athletes and nonathletes up to 35 years of age in the Veneto region of Italy, 1979–96. Data are number (%). Reproduced from Corrado *et al.* Screening for hypertrophic cardiomyopathy in young athletes. *N Engl J Med* 1998; **339**: 364–9. © 1998 Massachusetts Medical Society. All rights reserved

	Athletes (n = 49)	Nonathletes (n = 220)	Total (n = 269)
Arrhythmogenic right ventricular cardiomyopathy	11 (22.4)	18 (8.2)*	29 (10.8)
Atherosclerotic coronary artery disease	9 (18.5)	36 (16.4)	45 (16.7)
Anomalous origin of coronary artery	6 (12.2)	1 (0.4)†	7 (2.6)
Conduction system pathology	4 (8.2)	20 (9)	24 (8.9)
Mitral valve prolapse	5 (10.2)	21 (9.5)	26 (9.7)
Hypertrophic cardiomyopathy	1 (2)	16 (7.3)	17 (6.3)
Myocarditis	3 (6.1)	19 (8.6)	22 (8.2)
Myocardial bridge	2 (4)	5 (2.3)	7 (2.6)
Pulmonary thromboembolism	1 (2)	3 (1.4)	4 (1.5)
Dissecting aortic aneurysm	1 (2)	11 (5)	12 (4.5)
Dilated cardiomyopathy	1 (2)	9 (4.1)	10 (3.7)
Other	5 (10.2)	61 (27.7)	66 (24.5)

*$P = 0.008$ *vs* athletes; †$P < 0.001$ *vs* athletes.

provide strong but circumstantial evidence for a selective reduction of sudden death from hypertrophic cardiomyopathy in competitive athletes undergoing systematic preparticipation screening.

Identification of other cardiovascular diseases with a risk of sudden death in athletes

In the setting of the prospective clinicopathologic study on sudden death in athletes, we correlated pathologic findings with the athlete's clinical history and ECG in order to understand why the underlying disease was not identified or suspected during life with preparticipation athletic screening.[15] As summarized in Table 27.4, there was a statistically significant difference between athletes with arrhythmogenic right ventricular cardiomyopathy and athletes with both acquired and congenital coronary artery abnormalities with regard to prodromal symptoms and ECG abnormalities at screening. Eighty-two per cent of athletes who died from arrhythmogenic right ventricular cardiomyopathy had a history of syncope, ECG abnormalities, and ventricular arrhythmias at the cardiovascular screening evaluation, whereas 78% of athletes with atherosclerotic coronary artery disease and 75% of those with congenital coronary artery anomalies did not show any clinical prodrome ($P < 0.05$).[15]

These findings confirm that early identification of young athletes with coronary artery disease at athletic screening is limited by the scarcity of warning signs and the low sensitivity of both baseline and exercise ECG in detecting signs of myocardial ischemia in athletes with coronary atherosclerosis or anomalous coronary artery. In screening large populations of apparently healthy individuals, the use of exercise ECG to induce myocardial ischemia is limited by its low predictive value and pretest probability.[35,36] Athletes who

Table 27.4 Clinical findings at preparticipation screening of athletes who died suddenly of one of the leading three cardiovascular causes. *Includes those with anomalous origin of coronary artery and those with myocardial bridges. Reproduced from Corrado *et al.* Screening for hypertrophic cardiomyopathy in young athletes. *New Engl J Med* 1998; **339**: 364–9. © 1998 Massachusetts Medical Society. All rights reserved

	Cause of death		
Clinical finding	Arrhythmogenic right ventricular cardiomyopathy (n = 11)	Atherosclerotic coronary artery disease (n = 9)	Congenital coronary artery anomalies* (n = 8)
Familial history of sudden death from heart disease	2	0	0
Effort-induced palpitations	6	1	0
Syncope	5	1	1
Chest pain	0	0	0
ST–T abnormalities	9	0	1
Ventricular arrhythmias	6	0	2
One or more of the above	9 (82%)	2 (22%)	2 (25%)

†$P = 0.02$ *vs* those with arrhythmogenic right ventricular cardiomyopathy.

died from atherosclerotic coronary artery disease had not experienced chest pain or previous myocardial infarction and had isolated involvement of the left anterior descending coronary artery.[26]

Athletes who died from congenital anomalies of the coronary arteries were either asymptomatic or had atypical symptoms and exercise testing failed to demonstrate ischemic ST–T changes. The pathophysiological determinants of myocardial ischemia from congenital anomalies of the coronary arteries are not readily reproducible in the clinical setting.[37,38] This hinders the recognition of these potentially fatal cardiovascular malformations at athletic preparticipation screening.

Unlike athletes with coronary artery abnormalities, more than 80% of athletes who died from arrhythmogenic right ventricular cardiomyopathy had a history of syncopal episodes, ECG abnormalities with inverted T waves in the right precordial leads, and ventricular arrhythmias with the left bundle branch block pattern.[15] Nevertheless, these patients had not been identified during life. The most plausible explanation is that arrhythmogenic right ventricular cardiomyopathy was described only two decades ago and for a considerable period of time it was either underdiagnosed or regarded with skepticism by cardiologists.[39,40] We recently compared two decades of screening at the Center for Sport Medicine in Padua and found that the prevalence of disqualification due to arrhythmogenic right ventricular cardiomyopathy was significantly greater in the interval 1992–2001 than in the previous decade.[41] This indicates that, with increased awareness of clinical findings suggestive of arrhythmogenic right ventricular cardiomyopathy, more affected athletes are now being identified and this can be expected to save lives.

Conclusions

The Italian preparticipation athlete screening program, based largely on the ECG, is an efficient and cost-effective means of detecting cardiomyopathies (mostly hypertrophic cardiomyopathy and arrhythmogenic right ventricular cardiomyopathy), rhythm and conduction abnormalities, and valvular disease with the risk of sport-related sudden death. Identification of coronary artery abnormalities is limited by the low sensitivity of both baseline and exercise ECG in detecting signs of myocardial ischemia in young athletes with either coronary atherosclerosis or congenital coronary artery anomaly.

Acknowledgments

This study was supported by the Veneto Region, Venice, and the Ministry of Health, Rome, Italy.

References

1 Buddington RS, Stahl CJI, McAllister HA *et al.* Sports, death and unusual heart disease. *Am J Cardiol* 1974; **33**: 129–36.

2 Thompson PD, Stern MP, Williams P *et al.* Death during jogging or running; a study of 18 cases. *JAMA* 1979; **242**: 1265–7.

3 Maron BJ, Roberts WC, McAllister MA *et al.* Sudden death in young athletes. Circulation 1980; **62**: 218–19.

4 Waller BF, Roberts WC. Sudden death while running in conditioned runners aged 40 years or over. *Am J Cardiol* 1980; **45**: 1292–300.

5 Virmani R, Robinowitz M, McAllister HA. Nontraumatic death in joggers. *Am J Med* 1982; **72**: 874–82.

6 Corrado D, Thiene G, Nava A, Pennelli N, Rossi L. Sudden death in young competitive athletes: Clinico-pathologic correlations in 22 cases. *Am J Med* 1990; **89**: 588–96.

7 Burke AP, Farb A, Virmani R *et al.* Sports-related and non-sports-related sudden cardiac death in young adults. *Am Heart J* 1991; **121**: 568–75.

8 Van Camp SP, Bloor CM, Mueller FO, Cantu RC, Olson HG. Non-traumatic sports death in high school and college athletes. *Med Sci Sports Exerc* 1995; **27**: 641–7.

9 Maron BJ, Shirani J, Poliac LC, Mathenge R, Boberts WC, Mueller FO. Sudden death in young competitive athletes. Clinical, demographics, and pathological profiles. *JAMA* 1996; **276**: 199–204.

10 Thiene G, Pennelli N, Rossi L. Cardiac conduction system abnormalities as a possible cause of sudden death in young athletes. *Hum Pathol* 1983; **14**: 70–4.

11 Maron BJ, Bodison SA, Wesley YE, Tucker E, Green KJ. Results of screening a large group of intercollegiate competitive athletes for cardiovascular disease. *J Am Coll Cardiol* 1987; **10**: 1214–21.

12 Maron BJ, Thompson PD, Puffer JC *et al.* Cardiovascular preparticipation screening of competitive athletes. A statement for health professionals from the sudden death committee (clinical cardiology) and congenital cardiac defects committee (cardiovascular disease in the young), American Heart Association. *Circulation* 1996; **94**: 850–6.

13 Decree of the Italian Ministry of Health, February 18, 1982. Norme per la tutela sanitaria dell'attività sportiva agonistica (rules concerning the medical protection of athletic activity). *Gazzetta Ufficiale* March 5, 1982: 63.

14 Pelliccia A, Maron BJ. Preparticipation cardiovascular evaluation of the competitive athlete: Perspectives from the 30-year Italian experience. *Am J Cardiol* 1995; **75**: 827–9.

15 Corrado D, Basso C, Schiavon M, Thiene G. Screening for hypertrophic cardiomyopathy in young athletes. *N Engl J Med* 1998; **339**: 364–9.

16 Maron BJ, Shirani J, Poliac LC, Mathenge R, Boberts WC, Mueller FO. Sudden death in young competitive athletes. Clinical, demographic, and pathological profiles. *JAMA* 1996; **276**: 199–204.

17 Savage DD, Seides SF, Clark CE *et al.* Electrocardiographic findings in patients with obstructive and nonobstructive hypertrophic cardiomyopathy. *Circulation* 1978; **58**: 402–8.

18 Friedman HH. *Diagnostic Electrocardiography and Vectocardiography.* New York: McGraw-Hill, 1971.

19 Romhlit DW, Estes EH. A point score system for the ECG diagnosis of left ventricular hypertrophy. *Am Heart J* 1968; **75**: 752–9.

20 Morris JJ, Estes EH, Whalen RE, Thompson HK, McIntosh HD. P-wave analysis in valvular heart disease. *Circulation* 1964; **29**: 242–51.

21 Mitchell JE, Maron BJ, Epstein SE. 16th Bethesda Conference: cardiovascular abnormalities in the athlete: recommendations regarding eligibility for competition. *J Am Coll Cardiol*; 1985; **6**: 1186–232.

22 Maron BJ, Mitchell JH. 26th Bethesda Conference: recommendations for detecting eligibility for competition in athletes with cardiovascular abnormalities. *J Am Coll Cardiol* 1994; **24**: 845–99.

23 Comitato organizzativo cardiologico per l'idoneità allo sport (FMSI, SIC-Sport, CIC, ANCE, ANMCO). Protocolli cardiologici per il giudizio di idoneità allo sport agonistico. *G Ital Cardiol* 1989; **19**: 250–72.

24 Zeppilli P. Il concetto di idoneità e non idoneità cardiovascolare allo sport sotto il profilo clinico e medico-legale. In: Zeppilli P, ed. *Cardiologia dello Sport*. Rome: CESI Publications, 1990: 269–74.

25 Maron BJ, Epstein SE. Hypertrophic cardiomyopathy: A discussion of nomenclature. *Am J Cardiol* 1979; **43**: 1242–4.

26 Pelliccia A, Maron BJ, Spataro A, Proschan MA, Spirito P. The upper limit of physiologic cardiac hypertrophy in highly trained elite athletes. *N Engl J Med* 1991; **324**: 295–301.

27 Pelliccia A, Maron BJ, Spataro A, Caselli G. Absence of left ventricular hypertrophy in athletes engaged in intense power training. *Am J Cardiol* 1993; **72**: 1048–54.

28 Maron BJ, Gottdiener JS, Epstein SE. Pattern of significance of the distribution of left ventricular hypertrophy in hypertrophic cardiomyopathy: A wide-angle, two dimensional echocardiographic study in 125 patients. *Am J Cardiol* 1981; **48**: 418–28.

29 Wigle ED, Sasson Z, Henderson MA *et al.* Hypertrophic cardiomyopathy: The importance of the site and extent of hypertrophy: a review. *Prog Cardiovasc Dis* 1985; **28**: 1–83.

30 Shapiro LM, Smith RG. Effect of training on left ventricular structure and function: an echocardiographic study. *Br Heart J* 1983; **50**: 534–9.

31 Maron BJ, Pelliccia A, Spirito P. Cardiac disease in young trained athletes. Insights into methods for distinguishing athlete's heart from structural heart disease, with particular emphasis on hypertrophic cardiomyopathy. *Circulation* 1995; **91**: 1596–601.

32 Maron BJ, Gardin JM, Flack JM, Gidding SS, Kurosaki TT, Bild DE. Prevalence of hypertrophic cardiomyopathy in a general population of young adults: Echocardiographic analysis of 4111 subjects in CARDIA study. *Circulation* 1995; **92**: 785–9.

33 Pelliccia A, Di Paolo F, De Luca R, Buccolieri C, Maron BJ. Efficacy of preparticipation screening for the detection of cardiovascular abnormalities at risk of sudden death in competitive athletes: The Italian experience [abstract]. *J Am Coll Cardiol* 2001; **37**: 151A.

34 Corrado D, Basso C, Schiavon M, Thiene G. Cost-effectiveness analysis of screening strategies for identification of athletes with hypertrophic cardiomyopathy at risk for sudden death [abstract]. *Eur Heart J* 2002; **23**: 149.

35 Diamond GA, Forrester JS. Analysis of probability as an aid in the clinical diagnosis of coronary artery disease. *N Engl J Med* 1979; **300**: 1350–8.

36 Schlant RC, Blomqvist CG, Brandenburg RO *et al.* Guidelines for exercise testing. *J Am Coll Cardiol* 1986; **8**: 725–49.

37 Corrado D, Thiene G, Cocco P, Frescura C. Non-atherosclerotic coronary artery disease and sudden death in the young. *Br Heart J* 1992; **68**: 601–7.

38 Basso C, Maron BJ, Corrado D, Thiene G. Clinical profile of congenital coronary artery anomalies with origin from the wrong aortic sinus leading to sudden death in young competitive athletes. *J Am Coll Cardiol* 2000; **35**: 1493–501.

39 Marcus FI, Fontaine GH, Guiraudon G *et al.* Right ventricular dysplasia: A report of 24 cases. *Circulation* 1982; **65**: 384–98.

40 Thiene G, Nava A, Corrado D, Rossi L, Pennelli N. Right ventricular cardiomyopathy and sudden death in young people. *N Engl J Med* 1988; **318**: 129–33.

41 Corrado D, Basso C, Schiavon M, Thiene G. Identification of young competitive athletes with arrhythmogenic right ventricular cardiomyopathy at risk of sudden death by systematic preparticipation screening [abstract]. *Circulation* 2002; **106**: II–170.

CHAPTER 28

Cardiovascular Causes of Sudden Death, Preparticipation Screening, and Criteria for Disqualification in Young Athletes

Barry J. Maron, MD

The time you won your town the race
We chaired you through the market-place;
Man and boy stood cheering by,
And home we brought you shoulder high.

To-day, the road all runners come,
Shoulder-high we bring you home,
And set you at your threshold down,
Townsman of a stiller town.

To An Athlete Dying Young. Alfred Edward Housman, 1895

Sudden deaths of competitive athletes are personal tragedies which have a devastating impact on the lay and medical communities.[1] Such events in young people are always unexpected, and while relatively uncommon they often assume a high public profile and visibility due to the widely held perception that trained athletes constitute the healthiest segment of our society. The occasional deaths of well-known elite athletes exaggerate this visibility (Fig. 28.1).[1–14]

Over the past few years interest and concern have heightened considerably regarding the causes of the sudden and unexpected catastrophes in young trained athletes.[1] As a consequence, the underlying cardiovascular diseases responsible for sudden death in trained athletes and others participating in sporting activities have been the subject of several reports, and a large measure of clarification has resulted.[1–14]

The risks associated with participation in organized competitive sports are diverse and range from sudden collapse due to underlying (and usually unsuspected) cardiovascular disease[1–14] to nonpenetrating chest impact-related catastrophes.[15,16] Recognition that many athletic field deaths may be due to a variety of detectable cardiovascular lesions has also stimulated intense inter-

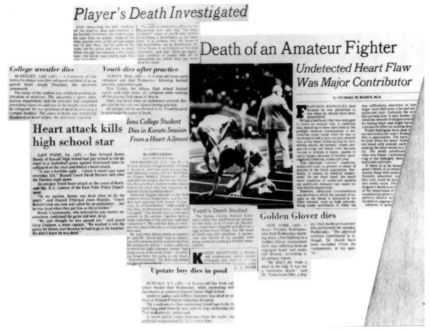

Fig. 28.1 News media accounts of sudden deaths in young athletes. Reproduced with permission from Maron BJ. Heart disease and other cardiovascular risks in competitive athletes. In: *Cardiology: Physiology, Pharmacology, Diagnosis.* Philadelphia: Lippincott-Raven, 1997.

est in preparticipation screening in high school and college-aged athletes,[11] as well as issues related to the criteria for disqualification from competitive sports.[12] Therefore, the present discussion will assess: (1) the benefits and limitations of preparticipation screening for early detection of cardiovascular abnormalities in competitive athletes; (2) cost–efficiency and feasibility issues as well as medicolegal implications of screening; (3) consensus panel recommendations and guidelines for the most prudent, practical and effective screening strategies, based on a recent American Heart Association (AHA) consensus panel;[11] and (4) consensus guidelines governing disqualification of athletes with underlying cardiovascular disease from organized competitive sports. Given the large number of competitive athletes in this country[4,17] and recent public health initiatives on physical activity and exercise, these issues, which are the subject of the present chapter, have become particularly relevant.

Definitions and background

The present considerations focus on the *competitive athlete*, previously described as one who participates in an organized team or individual sport requiring systematic training and regular competition against others, while placing a high premium on athletic excellence and achievement.[12] This definition is necessarily arbitrary, and it should be underscored that many individuals participate in 'recreational' sports in a truly competitive fashion. The purpose of *preparticipation screening*, as described here, is to provide medical clearance for participation in competitive sports through routine and systematic evaluations directed toward the identification of clinically relevant and pre-existing cardiovascular abnormalities, thereby to reduce the risks associated with organized sports. It should, however, be emphasized that raising the possibility of a cardiovascular abnormality on a standard screening examination is only the first tier of recognition, after which referral to a specialist for further diagnostic investigation will be required. When a definitive cardiovascular diagnosis is made, the consensus panel guidelines of the 26th Bethesda Conference[12] should be used to formulate recommendations for continued participation or disqualification from competitive sports.

The AHA guidelines[11] reproduced here (see Appendix) focus on the potential of large population-based screening of high school and collegiate student athletes rather than on individual clinical assessments of athletes, and are designed to apply to competitors of all ages and both genders in the USA. These recommendations may also be extrapolated to athletes in youth, middle-school, masters or professional sports, and in some instances to participants in intense recreational sporting activities. It is also recognized that the overall preparticipation screening process extends well beyond the considerations described here (which are limited to the cardiovascular system), involving many other organ systems and medical issues.

Also, the AHA screening recommendations are predicated on the probability that intense athletic training is likely to increase the risk for sudden cardiac death (or disease progression) in trained athletes with clinically important underlying structural heart disease, although presently it is not possible to quantify that risk.[3] Certainly, the vast majority of young athletes who die suddenly do so while engaged in athletic training or competition.[3–5,14] These observations support the proposition that physical exertion is an important trigger for sudden death, given the presence of certain underlying cardiovascular diseases.[3,18] Finally, the early detection of clinically significant cardiovascular disease through preparticipation screening can, in many instances, permit timely therapeutic interventions that prolong life.[19]

Causes of sudden death in athletes

Several autopsy-based studies have documented the variety of cardiovascular diseases responsible for sudden death in young competitive athletes or youthful asymptomatic individuals with active lifestyles.[2–10,13,14] These structural abnormalities are independent of the normal physiologic adaptations in cardiac dimensions and left ventricular (LV) mass evident in many trained athletes, usually consisting of increased LV end-diastolic cavity dimension or occasionally wall thickness.[20–28]

In youthful athletes (under 35 years of age) the vast majority of deaths are due to a variety of largely congenital cardiac malformations (Figs 28.2 and

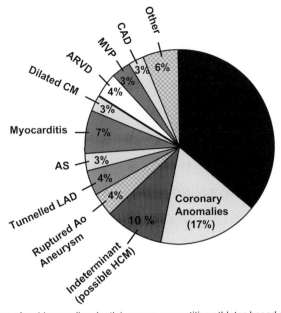

Fig. 28.2 Causes of sudden cardiac death in young competitive athletes based on systematic tracking in the USA. Adapted with permission of the American Heart Association from Maron *et al.* (1996).[11]

28.3). Indeed, virtually any disease capable of causing sudden death in young people may potentially do so in young competitive athletes. While these cardiovascular diseases may be relatively common among young athletes who die suddenly, each is uncommon within the general population.

It is also important to be cautious in assigning strict prevalence figures for the relative occurrence of various cardiovascular diseases in studies of sudden death in athletes. Patient selection biases and other limitations unavoidably influence the acquisition of such data in the absence of a systematic national registry. Indeed, the available published studies differ with regard to the methods used for documenting cardiovascular diagnosis and are derived from a variety of data bases.

Hypertrophic cardiomyopathy

In several surveys from the USA,[2–5,8,13,14] the single most common cardiovascular abnormality among the causes of sudden death in young athletes is hypertrophic cardiomyopathy (HCM), usually in the nonobstructive form,[29–32] which accounts for about 35% of these events[3] (Figs 28.2 and 28.3). However, a small proportion of all HCM patients experience sudden death with physical exertion and only some of the reported HCM-related sudden deaths occur during or just after vigorous physical activity.[3,33,34]

HCM is a primary and familial cardiac disease with heterogeneous expression, complex pathophysiology and diverse clinical course for which 10 dis-

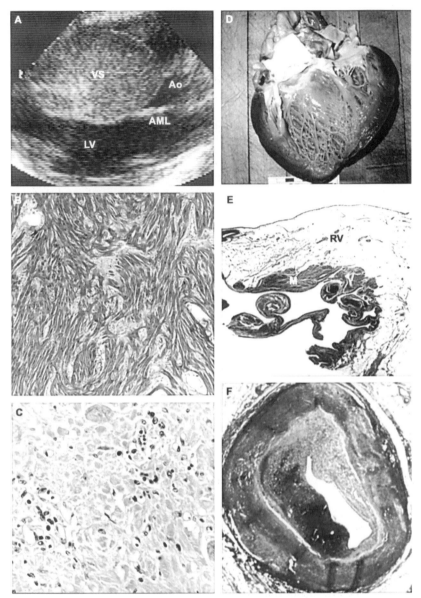

Fig. 28.3 Causes of sudden cardiac death in young competitive athletes. (**A**) Hypertrophic cardiomyopathy. Two-dimensional echocardiogram in parasternal long-axis view showing extreme
asymmetric thickening of the ventricular septum (VS) (53 mm). (**B**) Hypertrophic cardiomyopathy. Histopathology showing the substrate of disorganized cardiac muscle cells and chaotic
architectural pattern. Hematoxylin and eosin stain. (**C**) Myocarditis. Area of left ventricular
myocardium with clusters of inflammatory mononuclear cells. Hematoxylin and eosin stain; magnification ×400. (**D**) Idiopathic dilated cardiomyopathy, showing greatly enlarged left ventricular
cavity. (**E**) Arrhythmogenic right ventricular cardiomyopathy. Histologic section of right ventricular wall showing extensive fatty replacement adjacent to a small area of residual myocytes (M).
Hematoxylin and eosin stain. (**F**) Premature atherosclerotic coronary artery disease. Portion of
right coronary artery with atherosclerotic narrowing and ruptured plaque. From Maron (2003);[13]
reproduced with permission of the Massachusetts Medical Society.

ease-causing mutations in genes encoding proteins of the cardiac sarcomere have been reported,[35–38] including β-myosin heavy chain, cardiac troponin T and I, cardiac myosin-binding protein C, α-tropomyosin, α-actin, titin, essential and regulatory light chains and α-myosin heavy chain. Within the general population, HCM is a relatively uncommon malformation, occurring in about 0.2% (1:500).[39] Sudden death in HCM is most common in children and young adults, usually in individuals who have previously been asymptomatic (or only mildly symptomatic);[29,30,32] therefore, such catastrophes are often the initial clinical manifestation of the disease.[46] Because HCM is the most common cause of sudden death in young trained athletes[2–5,13,14] and these events in athletes with HCM usually occur during training or competition,[3,4,5,8] it appears likely that intense physical activity represents a trigger for sudden death[13,14,18,40] and that it is prudent to recommend the disqualification of athletes with HCM from intense competitive sports.[12,13]

The clinical diagnosis of HCM has been based on the definition (by two-dimensional echocardiography) of the most characteristic morphologic feature of the disease—asymmetric thickening of the LV wall associated with a nondilated cavity, in the absence of another cardiac or systemic disease capable of producing the magnitude of hypertrophy present (Fig. 28.3).[31,32,42] Because the nonobstructive form of HCM is predominant under resting conditions, the well-described clinical features of dynamic obstruction to LV outflow, such as a loud systolic ejection murmur, systolic anterior motion of the mitral valve or partial premature closure of the aortic valve, are not required for diagnosis.[29,30,32]

Based on both echocardiographic and necropsy analyses in large numbers of patients, it is apparent that the HCM disease spectrum is characterized by vast structural diversity with regard to the patterns and extent of LV hypertrophy (Fig. 28.3).[31,42] Indeed, virtually all possible patterns of LV hypertrophy occur in HCM, and no single phenotypic expression can be considered characteristic or typical of this disease. While many patients show diffusely distributed hypertrophy, fully 30% demonstrate localized wall thickening confined to only one segment of the left ventricle. The absolute thickness of the LV wall varies greatly, although the average reported value in tertiary center patient populations is usually 21–22 mm.[31] Wall thickness is profoundly increased in many patients, including the most severe degree of hypertrophy observed in any cardiac disease, 60 mm being the greatest wall thickness dimension reported to date.[44] On the other hand, the HCM phenotype is not invariably expressed as a greatly thickened left ventricle, and some patients show only mild increases of 13–15 mm and some genetically affected individuals have normal thicknesses (up to 12 mm).[30,32,35–38,45,46]

Some young athletes with segmental hypertrophy of the anterior ventricular septum (wall thickness 13–15 mm), consistent with a relatively mild morphologic expression of HCM, may be difficult to distinguish from those with extreme expression of physiologic LV hypertrophy, which represents an adaptation to athletic training (i.e. athlete's heart).[27] In asymptomatic, trained

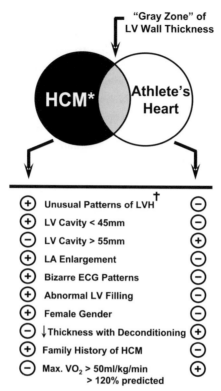

"Gray Zone" of
LV Wall Thickness

HCM*   Athlete's
           Heart

(+)	Unusual Patterns of LVH[†]	(−)
(+)	LV Cavity < 45mm	(−)
(−)	LV Cavity > 55mm	(+)
(+)	LA Enlargement	(−)
(+)	Bizarre ECG Patterns	(−)
(+)	Abnormal LV Filling	(−)
(+)	Female Gender	(−)
(−)	↓Thickness with Deconditioning	(+)
(+)	Family History of HCM	(−)
(−)	Max. VO$_2$ > 50ml/kg/min > 120% predicted	(+)

Fig. 28.4 Chart showing criteria used to distinguish HCM from athlete's heart when the left ventricular (LV) wall thickness is within the shaded gray zone of overlap (13–15 mm), consistent with both diagnoses. *Assumed to be the nonobstructive form of HCM in this discussion, since the presence of substantial mitral valve systolic anterior motion would, *per se*, confirm the diagnosis of HCM in an athlete. †May involve a variety of abnormalities, including heterogeneous distribution of left ventricular hypertrophy (LVH), in which asymmetry is prominent, and adjacent regions may be of greatly different thicknesses, with sharp transitions evident between segments. Also, patterns in which the anterior ventricular septum is spared from the hypertrophic process and the region of predominant thickening may be in the posterior portion of the septum or anterolateral or posterior free wall. ↓ = decreased; LA = left atrial. From Maron *et al.* (1995);[27] reproduced with permission of the American Heart Association.

athletes within this morphologic gray zone, the differential diagnosis between physiologic athlete's heart and HCM can often be resolved by clinical assessment and noninvasive testing (Fig. 28.4).[27]

Congenital coronary anomalies

Second in importance and frequency to HCM as a cause of sudden death in young athletes is a spectrum of congenital coronary anomalies of wrong sinus origin (occurring in about 20% of young athletic field deaths), the most common of which is anomalous origin of the left main coronary artery from the right (anterior) sinus of Valsalva (Fig. 28.5).[47–49] Coronary artery anomalies are difficult to identify since they may not be readily identifiable by conventional noninvasive imaging, and are not usually associated with cardiac symptoms or abnormalities on 12-lead or exercise ECG, or simply because the clinical index of suspicion is often not sufficiently high;[48] the vast majority of sudden deaths are associated with physical exertion. The occurrence of one or more episodes of exertional syncope in a young athlete should trigger the clinical exclusion of a coronary anomaly.[50] Also, in youthful athletes it may be possible to identify (or raise a strong suspicion of) anomalous left main coronary artery using transthoracic two-dimensional or transesophageal echocardiography,[49] which can subsequently lead to definitive confirmation with coronary arteriography. These considerations are particularly important for the echocardiographic screening of athletes[11] because, while the coronary anomalies are

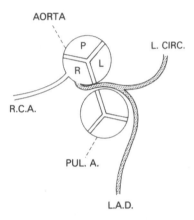

Fig. 28.5 Congenital coronary artery anomalies capable of causing sudden death in young athletes. (Top) Anomalous origin of the left main coronary artery from the right (anterior) sinus of Valsalva. The left coronary artery may have a separate or common ostium with the right coronary artery, which also arises from the right (R) sinus of Valsalva. Note the acute leftward bend of the left main coronary artery at its origin and its posterior course between the aorta and pulmonary artery (PUL. A.). (Bottom) Normal anatomy is shown for comparison. L.A.D. = left anterior descending coronary artery; L. CIRC. = left circumflex coronary artery; L = left coronary cusp; P = posterior (noncoronary) cusp; R.C.A. = right coronary artery. Reproduced with permission of the *Journal of the American College of Cardiology*, from Maron *et al.* (1986).[8]

rarely identified during life, these lesions are nevertheless amenable to corrective surgery.[48]

The mechanism by which this coronary anomaly produces syncope or sudden death remains undefined. Indeed, the episodic nature of these events contributes substantially to this uncertainty. It is possible that the acute take-off angle of the left main coronary artery from the right sinus results in narrowing of the coronary ostium. Presumably, during the basal state or with routine daily activities, the left coronary ostium remains open but oval-shaped. With the increased stroke volume and myocardial oxygen requirements associated with exercise, the ascending aorta expands and the ostium of the left main coronary artery is compressed in a slit-like fashion. This mechanical impediment to the ostial orifice may suddenly result in diminished coronary blood flow and acute myocardial ischemia.

Other unusual variants of coronary arterial anatomy may be rare causes of exercise-related sudden deaths in young athletic individuals.[3,5,8,9,51,52] These include hypoplasia of the right coronary and left circumflex arteries, the left anterior descending or right coronary artery emanating from the pulmonary trunk, virtual absence of the left coronary artery, or coronary arterial intersusception producing occlusion of the coronary lumen.

Arrhythmogenic right ventricular cardiomyopathy (ARVC)

ARVC is an unusual, often familial condition, that may be associated with important ventricular or supraventricular arrhythmias, and has been emphasized as a cause of sudden death in the young in Italy.[6,7,53,54] It is characterized morphologically by cell death in the right ventricle with myocytes replaced by fibrous or adipose tissue (Fig. 28.3). This disease process may be segmental or, alternatively, involve the right ventricle diffusely.

Of note is the investigation of Corrado and colleagues,[6] which reported ARVC to be the most common cause of sudden death in athletes in the Veneto region in northeastern Italy. While this disease is also a component of our own experience with athletic field deaths, its frequency is clearly in the range of less than 5% in reports from North America.[2,3–5,8,9] The explanation for such discrepancies is uncertain, although it is possible that the relatively frequent occurrence of ARVC in this particular region of Italy reflects a unique genetic substrate.[6,7,53–56] Furthermore, the relatively low frequency with which HCM is apparently responsible for sudden death in Italian athletes is an interesting but also a largely unresolved issue. It is possible, however, that the long-standing systematic Italian national program for cardiovascular assessment of competitive athletes[57] has had the effect of identifying and disqualifying disproportionate numbers of trained athletes with HCM (but significantly fewer with ARVC), due to the fact that HCM is more easily identifiable clinically than ARVC.[19,32,53]

Other diseases

Less common causes of sudden death include myocarditis (Fig. 28.3), dilated cardiomyopathy, Marfan syndrome with aortic rupture, sarcoidosis, mitral valve prolapse, aortic valve stenosis, atherosclerotic coronary artery disease (Fig. 28.3), and long QT syndrome.[58,59] Also, acute or chronic ingestion of agents such as cocaine may have important adverse cardiovascular consequences that can produce clinicopathologic profiles of acute myocardial infarction, myocardial fibrosis, and myocarditis.[60]

It has also been suggested periodically that major coronary arteries tunneled within the LV myocardium (i.e. myocardial 'bridges') constitute a potentially lethal anatomic variant that may cause sudden death in otherwise healthy young individuals during exertion or stress.[61,62] Such tunneled coronary arteries (usually the left anterior descending) are completely surrounded by myocardium for at least a portion of their course (about 1–3 cm). Indeed, in about 5% of our athletic field deaths a tunneled left anterior descending coronary artery was present in the absence of any other structural anomaly.[3]

Mechanisms and resuscitation

Although the precise mechanism ultimately responsible for sudden death in young athletes depends on the particular disease state involved, in the vast majority of instances (including athletes with HCM), cardiac arrest results from electrical instability due to ventricular tachyarrhythmias. There are a number of exceptions, the most common being Marfan syndrome, in which death often occurs due to a ruptured aorta.[63] However, regardless of the mechanism, very few athletes with cardiovascular disease who collapse on the athletic field are successfully resuscitated. It is possible that routine access to automatic external defibrillators at athletic events would result in the survival of greater numbers of such athletes. However, the great infrequency with which these events occur ultimately represents an obstacle to efficient resuscitation practice in the rare event of a catastrophe.

Absence of structural disease

Occasionally, athletes dying suddenly demonstrate no evidence of structural cardiovascular disease, even after careful gross and microscopic examination of the heart. In such instances (about 2% of one series),[3] it may not be possible to exclude with certainty noncardiac factors, such as drug abuse,[64] or to know whether careful inspection of the specialized conducting system and associated vasculature with serial sectioning (which is not part of the standard medical examiners' protocol) would have revealed occult but clinically relevant abnormalities.[65] Although one can only speculate on the possible etiologies in many such deaths, it is likely that some are due to either previously unidentified Wolff–Parkinson–White syndrome, rare diseases in which structural abnormalities of the heart are characteristically lacking at necropsy, such as long QT and Brugada syndromes,[58,59,66] catecholaminergic polymorphic or right ventricular outflow tachycardia,[67] exercise-induced coronary vasospasm, or undetected segmental right ventricular cardiomyopathy.[56]

Screening and preparticipation detection of cardiovascular abnormalities

Demographics

Based primarily on data assembled from broad-based US populations,[2–5,8,13,14] a profile of young competitive athletes who die suddenly has emerged. Such athletes participated in a large number and variety of sports, the most frequent being basketball and football (about 70%), probably reflecting the high participation level in these popular team sports, but also their intensity (Fig. 28.6). The vast majority of athletic field deaths occur in men (about 90%); their relative infrequency in women probably reflects lower participation rates, sometimes less intense training demands, less pronounced cardiac adaptation, and the fact that some diseases most commonly accounting for sudden death in athletes are less frequently diagnosed clinically in women (for example, HCM).[32] Most athletes are of high school age at the time of their death (about 60%); however, sudden deaths occur not uncommonly in young athletes who have achieved collegiate or even professional levels of competition.

The vast majority of athletes who incurred sudden death, regardless of their particular underlying disease, had been free of cardiovascular symptoms during their lives and were not suspected of harboring cardiovascular disease. Sudden collapse usually occurs associated with exercise, predominantly in the late afternoon and early evening hours, corresponding to peak periods of competition and training, particularly in organized team sports such as football and basketball (Fig. 28.7).[3] These observations substantiate that, in the

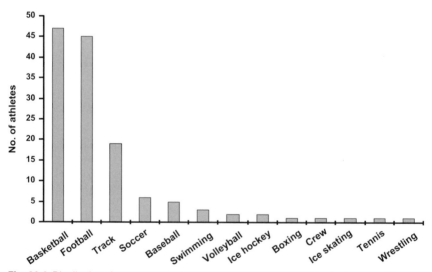

Fig. 28.6 Distribution of sports engaged in at the time of sudden death in young competitive athletes. Those competing in track events included distance runners and sprinter. From Maron *et al.* (1996);[3] reproduced with permission of the American Medical Association.

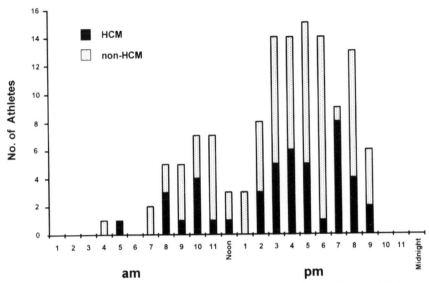

Fig. 28.7 Hourly distribution of sudden cardiac deaths. Histogram showing the time of death for 127 competitive athletes either with HCM (bold portion of bars) or a variety of other pre-dominantly congenital cardiovascular malformations (lighter portions of bars). Time of death was predominantly in the late afternoon and early evening, corresponding largely to the time of training and competition. From Maron *et al.* (1996);[3] reproduced with permission of the American Medical Association.

presence of certain underlying structural cardiovascular diseases, physical activity represents a trigger and an important precipitating factor for sudden collapse on the athletic field in susceptible individuals. The predilection for sudden death late in the day is similar in athletes with HCM and in athletes with other lesions. This observation for athletes with HCM contrasts strik-ingly with prior findings in patients with HCM (who were not competitive athletes), for whom a bimodal pattern of circadian variability over the 24-hour day was evident, including a prominent early to mid-morning peak (7 a.m. to 1 p.m.), similar to that described in patients with coronary artery disease (i.e. for sudden death, acute myocardial infarction or angina).[40]

Although the majority of reported sudden deaths in competitive athletes are in white males, a substantial proportion (over 40%) are African-American,[14] including the majority of those with HCM (55%) (Fig. 28.8). The substantial oc-currence of HCM-related sudden death in young black male athletes contrasts sharply with the infrequent identification of black patients with HCM in hos-pital and clinic-based populations from tertiary referral centers (Fig. 28.8).[14] Therefore, HCM in African-Americans is most frequently encountered when it results in sudden cardiac death on the athletic field (Fig. 28.8). These data prob-ably reflect the disproportionate access to subspecialty health-care between the African-American and white communities in the USA that makes it less likely for young black males to receive the diagnosis of HCM with echocardiography

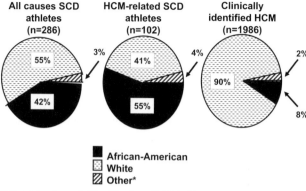

Fig. 28.8 Relationship of race to identification of HCM. Shown separately for an overall autopsy-based study population of 286 trained competitive athletes who died suddenly from a variety of cardiovascular diseases (left panel), for those athletes who died of HCM (center panel), and a clinically identified, multicenter, hospital-based cohort of 1986 HCM patients (right panel). SCD = sudden cardiac death. From Maron *et al.* (2003);[14] reproduced with permission of the American College of Cardiology.

compared with their white counterparts. Consequently, African-American athletes with HCM are also less likely to be disqualified from competition in accordance with the recommendations of the 26th Bethesda Conference[12] to reduce their risk for sudden death.

Scope of the problem

Definition of screening

In the USA, athletic screening has customarily been performed in the context of a personal and family history and physical examination.[11] Relevant to the design of any screening strategy is the fact that sudden cardiac death in young athletes is a devastating but rather infrequent event, and only a small proportion of participants in organized sports in the USA are at risk at any time. Therefore, obstacles to screening strategies for competitive athletes in the USA include the rarity of the lesions responsible for sudden death in the general population (i.e. small numerator), ranging from the relatively common (i.e. HCM)[39] to the apparently rare (e.g. coronary artery anomalies, arrhythmogenic right ventricular dysplasia, and the long QT, Brugada and Marfan syndromes). It is reasonable to estimate that all congenital malformations relevant to athletic screening may account for a combined prevalence of less than 0.5% in general athletic populations.

Also, the large reservoir of competitive athletes in the USA (i.e. large denominator) constitutes a major obstacle to screening strategies.[11,17] At present, there are approximately 7–8 million competitive athletes at the high school level (grades 9–12), in addition to lesser numbers of collegiate (500 000) and professional (10 000) athletes. These figures do not include an unspecified number of youth, middle-school, and masters level competitors, for whom reliable estimates for participation are not presently available. Therefore, the total number of trained athletes in the USA every year is probably as many as 10 million.

While the prevalence of athletic field deaths due to cardiovascular disease is not known with certainty, one report from the state of Minnesota documented one death in about 200 000 high school student athletes participating in organized interscholastic sports per year (1:70 000 over a 3-year high school career), although the rate was disproportionately higher in males than in females.[17] However, such data are limited, and the magnitude of this public health problem throughout the USA may well have been significantly underestimated. Furthermore, regardless of prevalence, the sudden death of an athlete (often fueled by the news media) has substantial impact on the community due to the youth, apparent good health, and lost potential of that person.

Regardless of precise prevalence, the emotional and social impact of athletic field catastrophes remains high. To most of the lay public and physician community (and the news media) the competitive athlete symbolizes the healthiest segment of our society and the unexpected collapse of such young people is a powerful event that inevitably strikes to the core of our sensibilities.[1,68] For these reasons, and despite its relatively low event rate, sudden death in young athletes will continue to represent an important medical issue. Indeed, it is an important responsibility of the medical community to create a fully informed public and also, where prudent and practical, to pursue the early detection of the causes of catastrophic events in young athletes, as well as preventive measures. However, because such events are uncommon relative to the vast numbers of athletes participating safely in sports, it is an important concern that information about athletic field deaths should not raise undue anxiety among youthful athletes and their families and thereby inhibit participation in sports.

Ethical considerations

Within a benevolent society, responsibility exists on the part of the physician to initiate prudent efforts to identify life-threatening diseases in athletes to minimize those cardiovascular risks associated with sport and to protect the health of such individuals.[1,11,12,68,69] Specifically, there is an implicit ethical obligation on the part of educational institutions (e.g. high schools and colleges) to implement cost-effective strategies to assure that student athletes are not subject to unacceptable and unavoidable medical risks.[69] The libertarian view, held by some, that high school and college-aged athletes should be permitted to assume any specifically disclosed cardiovascular risk associated with sport as part of the overall uncertainty and risk of living is not subscribed to by most institutions and interested parties.

The extent to which preparticipation screening can be supported at any level are mitigated by cost–efficiency and practical limitations, and also by the awareness that it is not possible to achieve a zero-risk circumstance in competitive sports.[12,69] Indeed, there is often an implied acceptance of risk on the part of athletes; for example, as a society, we permit or condone many sporting activities known to have intrinsic risks that cannot be controlled absolutely, such as automobile racing and mountain climbing, as well as more traditional sports such as football, in which the possibility of serious traumatic injury exists. Despite sufficient resources, it is recognized that in professional sports the sufficient motivation to implement cardiovascular screening may not presently exist due to the economic pressures in such sports environments, where athletic participation represents a vocation and the remuneration for services is often substantial.

Legal considerations

Although educational institutions and professional teams are required to use reasonable care in conducting their athletic programs, there is currently no clear legal precedent regarding their duty to conduct preparticipation screening of athletes for the purpose of detecting medically significant cardiovascular abnormalities.[11] Indeed, at present it would appear that very few lawsuits have been brought forward alleging negligence by the failure to either perform cardiovascular screening or diagnose cardiac disease in young competitive athletes. In the absence of binding requirements established by state law or athletic governing bodies, most institutions and teams presently rely on the team physician (or other medical personnel) to determine appropriate medical screening procedures.[11]

A physician who has medically cleared an athlete to participate in competitive sports is not necessarily legally liable for an injury or death caused by an undetected cardiovascular condition. Malpractice liability for failure to discover a latent, asymptomatic cardiovascular condition requires proof that a physician deviated from customary or accepted medical practice in his (or her) specialty in performing preparticipation screening of athletes, and furthermore that the use of established diagnostic criteria and techniques would have disclosed the medical condition.

It should be emphasized that the law permits the medical profession to establish the appropriate nature and scope of preparticipation screening based on the exercise of its collective medical judgment.[69] This necessarily involves the development of reliable diagnostic procedures in light of cost–benefit and feasibility factors. Of note, the AHA recommendations for cardiovascular preparticipation screening of athletes described here[11] represent evidence of the proper medical standard of care; however, these guidelines establish the legal standard of care only if generally accepted or customarily followed by physicians and/or relied upon by courts in determining the nature and scope of the legal responsibility borne by sponsors of competitive athletes.

Analysis of customary screening practices in the USA

It is important to clearly acknowledge the limitations of the preparticipation screening process currently in place for student athletes in the USA.[69–72]

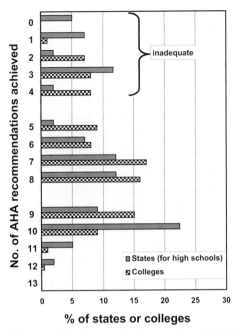

Fig. 28.9 Assessment of history and physical examination questionnaires used in 43 states for high school athletes and 879 colleges and universities, judged with respect to the American Heart Association screening recommendations.[11] Adapted from Glover and Maron (1998)[70] and Pfister *et al.* (2000);[71] reproduced with permission of the American Medical Association.

Only in this way can an informed public be created which otherwise might harbor important misconceptions regarding the principles and efficacy of athletic screening. Currently, there are no universally accepted standards for the screening of high school and college athletes, nor are there approved certification procedures for the professionals who perform such screening examinations.[70,71]

For high school athletes, some form of medical clearance by a physician or other trained health-care worker, usually consisting of a history and physical examination, presently appears to be customary. However, there is not uniform agreement among the states as to the precise format of preparticipation medical evaluations (Fig. 28.8). Indeed, 40% of all states either do not require this process, do not have recommended standard history and physical forms to serve as guides to the examiners (some only require a signature to provide medical clearance), or have approved forms that are judged inadequate[70] when evaluated against the specific screening recommendations proposed by the 1996 AHA consensus panel (Fig. 28.9).[11] These findings also emphasize that it is not possible to assume that a medical clearance for sports competition precludes the possibility of underlying and potentially lethal cardiovascular disease. In a substantial proportion of states (*n* = 21), nonphysician health-care workers (such as nurses and physician assistants) are sanctioned to perform

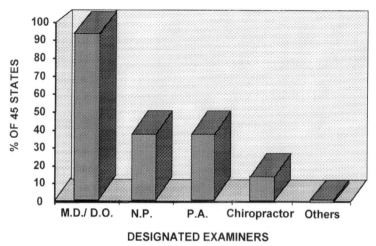

DESIGNATED EXAMINERS

Fig. 28.10 Approved examiners for preparticipation screening of athletes in US high schools. Individual states may have approved more than one category of examiner. D.O. = Doctor of Osteopathy; N.P. = nurse practitioner; P.A. = physician assistant.

preparticipation screening and 11 states specifically provide for practitioners with limited or no cardiovascular training (such as chiropractors) (Fig. 28.10).

Findings relative to screening practices in US colleges and universities are similar to those in the high schools (Fig. 28.9).[71] Of the history and physical examination screening forms analyzed from 625 institutions, only 26% had forms that contained at least nine of the recommended 12 AHA screening guidelines (and therefore were judged to be adequate), whereas 24% contained four or fewer of these parameters, and were considered to be inadequate. Relevant items that were omitted from more than 40% of the screening forms included a history of exertional chest pain, dyspnea, or fatigue; evidence of familial heart disease or premature sudden death; and physical stigmata or family history of Marfan syndrome.

Screening in Italy

While preparticipation examinations in US high schools and colleges occur largely at the discretion of the examining physician and as customary practice, a considerably different circumstance has existed in Italy since 1971 in the form of benevolent government legislation (Medical Protection of Athletic Activities Act) mandating preventive medical evaluations for all competitive athletes.[57] Unique to Italy, all citizens (aged 12–40 years) who are engaged in organized sports activities must obtain annual medical clearance from an approved physician stipulating that the athlete is free of cardiovascular abnormalities that could represent a risk for sudden death during training or competition. Since 1982, more detailed guidelines for these preparticipation examinations have been formulated and include as a minimum a history and physical examination, 12-lead ECG and exercise and pulmonary function tests. Echocardiography has been specifically required (since 1994) only in selected professional sports (soccer, boxing and cycling).

Under Italian law the examining physician is primarily responsible for the accuracy of this clinical assessment, and stands as the final arbiter of sports eligibility by issuing the official certification of medical clearance. In the event of an incorrect or incomplete medical diagnosis that leads directly to the impaired health or death of an athlete, the physician responsible for sanctioning athletic competition can be held accountable in a civil (as well as criminal) court.[55]

Expectations of screening strategies

Preparticipation screening by history and physical examination alone (without noninvasive testing) does not possess sufficient power to guarantee the detection of many critical cardiovascular abnormalities that could occur in large populations of young trained athletes in high school or college.[13,70,71] Indeed, hemodynamically significant congenital aortic valve stenosis is probably the lesion most likely to be reliably detected during routine screening due to its characteristically loud heart murmur. Detection of HCM by the standard screening history or physical examination can be unreliable because most patients characteristically express no or only a soft heart murmur, even if provoked by change in position during screening.[11,32] Furthermore, HCM is not easily detected by the preparticipation personal history since most patients with this disease do not experience syncope or have a family history of premature sudden death.[32] Also, when symptoms such as chest pain or impaired consciousness are involved, the standard personal history conveys a generally low specificity for the detection of many cardiovascular abnormalities that lead to sudden cardiac death in young athletes.

It should also be emphasized that most of the lesions being considered here as potentially responsible for sudden death in young athletes may be particularly challenging to detect, even when echocardiography, ECG or other noninvasive tests are incorporated into the standard screening process; for example, the congenital coronary anomalies. Nevertheless, despite these major limitations, standard history and physical examination screening is of potential value by virtue of its capability for identifying (or raising the suspicion of) cardiovascular abnormalities in at least some at-risk athletes. For example, genetic diseases such as HCM, Marfan syndrome and arrhythmogenic right ventricular cardiomyopathy (as well as premature atherosclerotic coronary artery disease) can possibly be suspected from the family history alone or transient symptoms from the personal history; physical examination may identify the stigmata of Marfan syndrome, systemic hypertension, and some athletes with LV outflow obstruction (aortic valvular stenosis and certain patients with HCM) by a loud heart murmur.

Prior screening efforts

While there are no prospective data available that permit a direct assessment of the efficacy of large-scale athletic screening, a recent retrospective analysis of 134 young athletes who died suddenly from a variety of cardiovascular diseases showed that only 3% of those individuals exposed to standard preparticipation screening were suspected of having cardiac disease by virtue of these examinations, and less than 1% ultimately received an accurate diagnosis (Fig. 28.11).[3] Based on these observations, the preparticipation screening process as currently structured and carried out in US high schools with only history and physical examination clearly lacks sufficient power to consistently and reliably recognize clinically important cardiovascular abnormalities in many athletes. Of note, however, preparticipation screening in Italy routinely includes a 12-lead ECG, as well as a history and physical examination. Investigators in the Veneto region report an experience in which an expected number of new HCM cases (relative to the known prevalence of HCM in the general

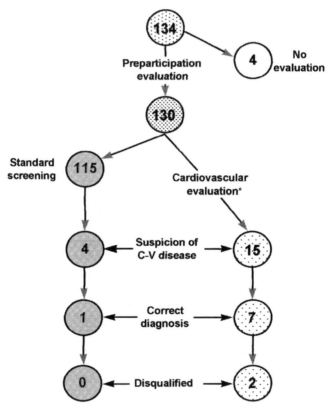

Fig. 28.11 Impact of preparticipation medical history and physical examinations on the detection of structural cardiovascular disease (and causes of sudden death). *Cardiovascular evaluation with testing (independent of standard school or institutional preparticipation screening) performed in 15 athletes because of symptoms, family history, cardiac murmur, or physical findings suggestive of heart disease. From Maron et al. (1996);[3] reproduced with permission of the American Medical Association.

population) were identified over a 7-year period among 33 000 consecutive athletes, most of whom were initially suspected of HCM due to abnormal ECG patterns.[19]

Several cardiovascular preparticipation screening efforts in large US populations have implemented noninvasive testing (i.e. conventional or limited echocardiographic examination or 12-lead ECG) in high school or collegiate athletes.[71-73] These athlete populations ranged in size from 250 to 2000 athletes, and in most the screening process was carried out over only a 1-year period. In general, these studies have reported the detection of very few definitive examples of potentially lethal cardiovascular abnormalities.

Noninvasive screening tests: echocardiography

The addition of noninvasive diagnostic tests to the screening process clearly has the potential to enhance the detection of certain cardiovascular defects in young athletes. For example, the two-dimensional echocardiogram is the principal diagnostic tool for the clinical recognition of HCM by virtue of demonstrating otherwise unexplained and asymmetric LV wall thickening.[11,30-32,39,42,43,75] Comprehensive and routine screening for HCM by genetic testing (for a variety of known disease-causing mutations) is not yet practical for application to large populations of athletes, given the substantial genetic heterogeneity of the disease and the expensive and time-intensive methodologies involved.[35,76]

Echocardiography could also be expected to detect other relevant abnormalities associated with sudden death in young athletes, such as valvular heart disease (e.g. mitral valve prolapse and aortic valvular stenosis), aortic root dilatation, and LV dysfunction (associated with myocarditis or dilated cardiomyopathy). However, even such diagnostic testing cannot guarantee recognition of all important lesions, and some relevant diseases may be beyond detection with any screening methodology. For example, identification of many congenital coronary artery anomalies usually requires sophisticated laboratory examination, including coronary arteriography, although it is possible in selected young athletes to raise a strong suspicion of important anomalies, such as left main coronary artery from the right sinus of Valsalva with echocardiography.[48,49] ARVC usually cannot be reliably diagnosed solely by echocardiography or ECG; the best available noninvasive test for this disease is probably magnetic resonance imaging (demonstrating adipose tissue replacement within the right ventricular wall), which is both expensive and not yet universally available.[53]

Cost–efficiency issues are important when assessing the feasibility of applying expensive noninvasive testing to the screening of large athletic populations.[11] In the vast majority of instances adequate financial and personnel resources are lacking for such endeavors. In those situations in which the full (i.e. unreduced) expense of testing would be the responsibility of administrative bodies (such as a school, university or team) the costs are probably prohibitive; for example, the cost of an echocardiographic study ranges from about $600 to

$2000 (the average is about $750).[77] For example, if the occurrence of HCM in a young athletic population is assumed to be 1:500,[39] even at $500 per study it would theoretically cost $250 000 to detect even one previously undiagnosed case using echocardiography as the primary screening tool.

Screening protocols incorporating noninvasive testing at greatly reduced cost have been described.[13] However, these efforts have involved unique circumstances in which echocardiographic equipment was donated and professional expenses waived for all but technician-related costs. Recently, small and lightweight (mobile) echocardiographic instruments have been introduced for high-resolution athletic field screening for cardiovascular disease.[78] While such individual initiatives are encouraged, it is also noted that public service projects based largely on volunteerism usually cannot be sustained on a consistent basis.

An important limitation of preparticipation screening with two-dimensional echocardiography is the potential for false-positive or false-negative test results. False-positive results may arise from the finding of particularly enlarged LV cavity size or the assignment of borderline values for wall thicknesses—the gray zone—which require formulation of a differential diagnosis between extreme (but normal) physiologic adaptations of athlete's heart and pathologic conditions such as HCM and other cardiomyopathies (Fig. 28.4).[22,24,27] Indeed, such clinical dilemmas (which are not always definitively resolvable in individual athletes) generate emotional, financial and medical burdens for the athlete, family, team, and institution by virtue of the requirement for additional testing and the uncertainty which is created. False-negative screening results may occur in athletes with HCM when testing by echocardiography occurs at a time of incomplete phenotypic expression during adolescence.[36,45,46,77] For example, in young athletes with HCM less than about 13–15 years of age, LV hypertrophy is often absent or mild, and therefore the phenotypic findings may not yet be diagnostic at the time of preparticipation screening with standard echocardiography.[11]

Noninvasive screening test: ECG

The 12-lead ECG has been proposed as a more practical and cost-efficient alternative to routine echocardiography for population-based screening.[19,57] Indeed, the ECG is abnormal in about 75–95% of patients with HCM[80] and will usually identify the long QT syndrome.[58,59] However, a certain proportion of genetically affected relatives in families with long QT syndrome may not show phenotypic expression on the ECG[58,59] and abnormalities on the ECG are usually absent in random recordings of patients with congenital coronary artery anomalies.[48]

As a primary screening test, the ECG does not have the power of the echocardiogram due to its lack of imaging capability for recognition of structural cardiovascular malformations. Also, the ECG has relatively low specificity as a screening test in athletic populations because of the frequency with which ECG alterations occur in association with the normal physiologic adaptations to training (athlete's heart).[25] Such false-positive ECG test results complicate the use of the 12-lead ECG as a primary screening tool in athletic populations. It can be anticipated that about 20–25% of athletes examined in the context of preparticipation screening will have ECG patterns that trigger echocardiographic study.[73] Elite athletes not infrequently demonstrate distinctly abnormal ECG patterns reminiscent of pathologic conditions such as HCM or ARVC, in the absence of structural heart disease and even without increased cardiac dimensions due to training.[25]

Eligibility considerations for athletes with known cardiovascular disease

When a cardiovascular abnormality is identified in a competitive athlete the following considerations arise: (1) the magnitude of risk for sudden cardiac death associated with continued participation in competitive sports; and (2) the criteria to be implemented for determining whether individual athletes should be withdrawn from sports competition. In this regard, the 26th Bethesda Conference sponsored by the American College of Cardiology[12] offers prospective and consensus recommendations for athletic eligibility or disqualification, taking into account the severity of the cardiovascular abnormality as well as the nature of sports training and competition.

The 26th Bethesda Conference recommendations are predicated on the likelihood that intense athletic training will increase the risk for sudden cardiac death (or disease progression) in trained athletes with clinically important underlying structural heart disease, although at present it is not possible to quantify that risk in precise terms.[12] Consequently, it is presumed that the temporary or permanent withdrawal of selected athletes from participation in certain sports is prudent and likely to be beneficial by virtue of diminishing the perceived risk. By virtue of its citation by a US Appellate Court,[81] the Bethesda Conference report can be relied upon by team physicians in formulating appropriate eligibility decisions, and also resolving future medicolegal disputes involving collegiate athletes. The intent of these conservative eligibility criteria is the maintenance of a safe athletic environment, but not to unnecessarily discourage sports participation.

References

1 Maron BJ. Sudden death in young athletes: Lessons from the Hank Gathers affair. *N Engl J Med* 1993; **329**: 55–7.

2 Burke AP, Farb V, Virmani R *et al*. Sports-related and non-sports-related sudden cardiac death in young adults. *Am Heart J* 1991; **121**: 568–75.

3 Maron BJ, Shirani J, Poliac LC *et al*. Sudden death in young competitive athletes: Clinical, demographic and pathological profiles. *JAMA* 1996; **276**: 199–204.

4 van Camp SP, Bloor CM, Mueller FO *et al*. Nontraumatic sports death in high school and college athletes. *Med Sci Sports Exerc* 1995; **27**: 641–7.

5 Maron BJ, Roberts WC, McAllister HA *et al.* Sudden death in young athletes. *Circulation* 1980; **62**: 218–29.

6 Corrado D, Thiene G, Nava A *et al.* Sudden death in young competitive athletes: Clinico-pathologic correlations in 22 cases. *Am J Med* 1990; **89**: 588–96.

7 Thiene G, Nava A, Corrado D *et al.* Right ventricular cardiomyopathy and sudden death in young people. *N Engl J Med* 1988; **318**: 129–33.

8 Maron BJ, Epstein SE, Roberts WC. Causes of sudden death in competitive athletes. *J Am Coll Cardiol* 1986; **7**: 204–14.

9 Liberthson, RR. Sudden death from cardiac causes in children and young adults. *N Engl J Med* 1996; **334**: 1039–44.

10 Maron BJ, Garson A. Arrhythmias and sudden cardiac death in elite athletes. *Cardiol Rev* 1994; **2**: 26–32.

11 Maron BJ, Thompson PD, Puffer JC *et al.* Cardiovascular preparticipation screening of competitive athletes. A Statement for Health Professionals from the Sudden Death Committee (Clinical Cardiology) and Congenital Cardiac Defects Committee (Cardiovascular Disease in the Young), American Heart Association. *Circulation* 1996; **94**: 850–6.

12 Maron BJ, Mitchell JH. 26th Bethesda Conference. Recommendations for determining eligibility for competition in athletes with cardiovascular abnormalities. *J Am Coll Cardiol* 1994; **24**: 845–99.

13 Maron BJ. Sudden death in young athletes. *N Engl J Med* 2003; **349**: 1064–75.

14 Maron BJ, Carney KP, Lever HM *et al.* Relationship of race to sudden cardiac death in competitive athletes with hypertrophic cardiomyopathy. *J Am Coll Cardiol* 2003; **41**: 974–80.

15 Maron BJ, Poliac LV, Kaplan JA *et al.* Blunt impact to the chest leading to sudden death from cardiac arrest during sports activities. *N Engl J Med* 1995; **33**: 337–42.

16 Maron BJ, Gohman TE, Kyle SB, Estes NAM, Link MS. Clinical profile and spectrum of commotio cordis. *JAMA* 2002; **287**: 1142–6.

17 Maron BJ, Gohman TE, Aeppli D. Prevalence of sudden cardiac death during competitive sports activities in Minnesota high school athletes. *J Am Coll Cardiol* 1998; **32**: 1881–4.

18 Corrado D, Basso C, Rizzoli G, Schiavon M, Thiene G. Does sport activity enhance the risk of sudden death in adolescents and young adults? A prospective population-based study. *J Am Coll Cardiol* 2003; **42**: 1959–63.

19 Corrado D, Basso C, Schiavon M *et al.* Screening for hypertrophic cardiomyopathy in young athletes. *N Engl J Med* 1998; **339**: 364–9.

20 Maron BJ. Structural features of the athlete heart as defined by echocardiography. *J Am Coll Cardiol* 1986; **7**: 190–203.

21 Huston TP, Puffer JC, Rodney WM. The athletic heart syndrome. *N Engl J Med* 1985; **313**: 24–32.

22 Pelliccia A, Maron BJ, Spataro A *et al.* The upper limit of physiologic cardiac hypertrophy in highly trained elite athletes. *N Engl J Med* 1991; **324**: 295–301.

23 Pelliccia A, Maron BJ, Culasso F *et al.* Athlete's heart in women: Echocardiographic characterization of highly trained elite female athletes. *JAMA* 1996; **276**: 211–15.

24 Pelliccia A, Culasso F, Di Paolo F *et al.* Physiologic left ventricular cavity dilatation in elite athletes. *Ann Intern Med* 1999; **130**: 23–31.

25 Pelliccia A, Maron BJ, Culasso F *et al.* Clinical significance of abnormal electrocardiographic patterns in trained athletes. *Circulation* 2000; **102**: 278–84.

26 Pluim BM, Zwinderman AH, van der Laarse A, van der Wall EE. The athlete's heart. A meta-analysis of cardiac structure and function. *Circulation* 1999; **100**: 336–44.

27 Maron BJ, Pelliccia A, Spirito P. Cardiac disease in young trained athletes: Insights into methods for distinguishing athlete's heart from structural heart disease with particular emphasis on hypertrophic cardiomyopathy. *Circulation* 1995; **91**: 1596–601.

28 Douglas PS, O'Toole ML, Katz SE, Ginsburg GS, Hiller WD, Laird RH. Left ventricular hypertrophy in athletes. *Am J Cardiol* 1997; **80**: 1384–8.

29 Wigle ED, Sasson Z, Henderson MA *et al* Hypertrophic cardiomyopathy: The importance of the site and extent of hypertrophy – a review. *Prog Cardiovasc Dis* 1985; **28**: 1–83.

30 Spirito P, Seidman CE, McKenna WJ, Maron BJ. The management of hypertrophic cardiomyopathy. *N Engl J Med* 1997; **336**: 775–85.

31 Klues HG, Schiffers A, Maron BJ. Phenotypic spectrum and patterns of left ventricular hypertrophy in hypertrophic cardiomyopathy: Morphologic observations and significance as assessed by two-dimensional echocardiography in 600 patients. *J Am Coll Cardiol* 1995; **26**: 1699–708.

32 Maron BJ. Hypertrophic cardiomyopathy: A systematic review. *JAMA* 2002; **287**: 1308–20.

33 Maron BJ, Klues HG. Surviving competitive athletics with hypertrophic cardiomyopathy. *Am J Cardiol* 1994; **73**: 1098–104.

34 Maron BJ, Olivotto I, Spirito P *et al.* Epidemiology of hypertrophic cardiomyopathy-related death. Revisited in a large non-referral-based patient population. *Circulation* 2001; **102**: 858–64.

35 Maron BJ, Moller JH, Seidman CE *et al.* Impact of laboratory molecular diagnosis on contemporary diagnostic criteria for genetically transmitted cardiovascular disease: Hypertrophic cardiomyopathy, long-QT syndrome, and Marfan syndrome. *Circulation* 1998; **98**: 1460–71.

36 Niimura H, Bachinski LL, Ganwatanaroj S *et al.* Mutations in the gene for human cardiac myosin-binding protein C and late-onset familial hypertrophic cardiomyopathy. *N Engl J Med* 1998; **338**: 1248–57.

37 Richard P, Charron P, Carrier L *et al.* Hypertrophic cardiomyopathy. Distribution of disease genes, spectrum of mutations, and implications for a molecular diagnosis strategy. *Circulation* 2003; **107**: 2227–32.

38 Seidman JG, Seidman CE. The genetic basis for cardiomyopathy: From mutation identification to mechanistic paradigms. *Cell* 2001; **104**: 557–67.

39 Maron BJ, Gardin JM, Flack JM *et al.* Assessment of the prevalence of hypertrophic cardiomyopathy in a general population of young adults: Echocardiographic analysis of 4111 subjects in the CARDIA study. *Circulation* 1995; **92**: 785–9.

40 Maron BJ, Kogan J, Proschan MA *et al.* Circadian variability in the occurrence of sudden cardiac death in patients with hypertrophic cardiomyopathy. *J Am Coll Cardiol* 1994; **23**: 1405–9.

41 Maron BJ. Hypertrophic cardiomyopathy. *Lancet* 1997; **3350**: 127–133.

42 Maron BJ, Epstein SE. Hypertrophic cardiomyopathy: A discussion of nomenclature. *Am J Cardiol* 1979; **43**: 1242–4.

43 Maron BJ, Gottdiener JS, Epstein SE. Patterns and significance of the distribution of left ventricular hypertrophy in hypertrophic cardiomyopathy: A wide-angle, two-dimensional echocardiographic study of 125 patients. *Am J Cardiol* 1981; **48**: 418–28.

44 Maron BJ, Gross BW, Stark SI. Extreme left ventricular hypertrophy. *Circulation* 1995; **92**: 2748.

45 Charron P, Dubourg O, Desnos M *et al.* Diagnostic value of electrocardiography and echocardiography for familial hypertrophic cardiomyopathy in a genotyped adult population. *Circulation* 1997; **96**: 214–19.

46 Maron BJ, Niimura H, Casey SA *et al*. Development of left ventricular hypertrophy in adults with hypertrophic cardiomyopathy caused by cardiac myosin-binding protein C mutations. *J Am Coll Cardiol* 2001; **38**: 315–21.

47 Roberts WC, Kragel AH. Anomalous origin of either the right or left main coronary artery from the aorta with subsequent coursing of the anomalously arising artery between aorta and pulmonary trunk. *Am J Cardiol* 1988; **62**: 1263–7.

48 Basso C, Maron BJ, Corrado D *et al*. Clinical profile of congenital coronary artery anomalies with origin from the wrong aortic sinus leading to sudden death in young competitive athletes. *J Am Coll Cardiol* 2000; **35**: 1493–501.

49 Maron BJ, Leon MB, Swain JA *et al*. Prospective identification by two-dimensional echocardiography of anomalous origin of the left main coronary artery from the right sinus of Valsalva. *Am J Cardiol* 1991; **68**: 140–2.

50 Cheitlin MD, De Castro CM, McAllister HA. Sudden death as a complication of anomalous left coronary origin from the anterior sinus of Valsalva, a not-so-minor congenital anomaly. *Circulation* 1974; **50**: 780–7.

51 Choi JH, Kornblum RN. Pete Maravich's incredible heart. *J Forensic Sci* 1990; **35**: 981–6.

52 Roberts WC, Glick BN. Congenital hypoplasia of both right and left circumflex coronary arteries. *Am J Cardiol* 1992; **70**: 121–3.

53 McKenna WJ, Thiene G, Nava A *et al*. Diagnosis of arrhythmogenic right ventricular dysplasia/cardiomyopathy. *Br Heart J* 1994; **71**: 215–18.

54 Corrado D, Basso C, Thiene G *et al*. Spectrum of clinicopathologic manifestations of arrhythmogenic right ventricular cardiomyopathy/dysplasia: A multicenter study. *J Am Coll Cardiol* 1997; **30**: 1512–20.

55 Rampazzo A, Nava A, Malacrida S *et al*. Mutation in human desmoplakin domain binding to plakoglobin causes a dominant form of arrhythmogenic right ventricular cardiomyopathy. *Am J Hum Genet* 2002; **71**: 1200–6.

56 Tiso N, Stephan DA, Nava A *et al*. Identification of mutations in the cardiac ryanodine receptor gene in families affected with arrhythmogenic right ventricular cardiomyopathy type 2 (ARVD2). *Hum Mol Genet* 2001; **10**: 189–94.

57 Pelliccia A, Maron BJ. Preparticipation cardiovascular evaluation of the competitive athlete: Perspectives from the 30 year Italian experience. *Am J Cardiol* 1995; **75**: 827–8.

58 Vincent GM, Timothy KW, Leppert M *et al*. The spectrum of symptoms and QT intervals in carriers of the gene for the long-QT syndrome. *N Engl J Med* 1992; **327**: 846–52.

59 Priori SG, Schwartz PJ, Napolitano C *et al*. Risk stratification in the long QT syndrome. *N Engl J Med* 2003; **348**: 1866–74.

60 Feldman AM, McNamara D. Myocarditis. *N Engl J Med* 2000; **343**: 1388–98.

61 Yetman AT, McCrindle BW, MacDonald C, Freedom RM, Gow R. Myocardial bridging in children with hypertrophic cardiomyopathy – a risk factor for sudden death. *N Engl J Med* 1998; **339**: 1201–9.

62 Schwarz ER, Klues HG, vom Dahl J *et al*. Functional, angiographic and intracoronary Doppler flow characteristics in symptomatic patients with myocardial bridging: Effect of short-term intravenous beta-blocker medication. *J Am Coll Cardiol* 1996; **27**: 1637–45.

63 Yetman AT, Bornemeier RA, McCrindle BW. Long-term outcome in patients with Marfan syndrome: Is aortic dissection the only cause of sudden death? *J Am Coll Cardiol* 2003; **41**: 329–32.

64 Lange RA, Hillis LD. Cardiovascular complications of cocaine use. *N Engl J Med* 2001; **345**: 351–8.

65 Thiene G, Pennelli N, Rossi L. Cardiac conduction system abnormalities as a possible cause of sudden death in young athletes. *Hum Pathol* 1983; **14**: 706–9.

66 Brugada P, Brugada J. Right bundle-branch block: Persistent ST segment elevation and sudden cardiac death: A distinct clinical and electrocardiographic syndrome. A multicenter report. *J Am Coll Cardiol* 1992; **20**: 1391–6.

67 Priori SG, Napolitano C, Tiso N *et al*. Mutations in the cardiac ryanodine receptor gene (hRyR2) underlie catecholaminergic polymorphic ventricular tachycardia. *Circulation* 2001; **103**: 196–200.

68 Maron BJ. Cardiovascular risks to young persons on the athletic field. *Ann Intern Med* 1998; **129**: 379–86.

69 Mitten MJ, Maron BJ. Legal considerations that affect medical eligibility for competitive athletes with cardiovascular abnormalities and acceptance of Bethesda Conference recommendations. *J Am Coll Cardiol* 1994; **24**: 861–3.

70 Glover DW, Maron BJ. Profile of preparticipation cardiovascular screening for high school athletes. *JAMA* 1998; **279**: 1817–19.

71 Pfister GC, Puffer JC, Maron BJ. Preparticipation cardiovascular screening for US collegiate student-athletes. *JAMA* 2000; **283**: 1597–9.

72 Lewis JF, Maron BJ, Diggs JA *et al*. Preparticipation echocardiographic screening for cardiovascular disease in a large, predominantly black population of collegiate athletes. *Am J Cardiol* 1989; **64**: 1029–33.

73 Maron BJ, Bodison SA, Wesley YE *et al*. Results of screening a large group of intercollegiate competitive athletes for cardiovascular disease. *J Am Coll Cardiol* 1987; **10**: 1214–21.

74 Fuller CM, McNulty CM, Spring DA *et al*. Prospective screening of 5,615 high school athletes for risk of sudden cardiac death. *Med Sci Sports Exerc* 1997; **29**: 1131–8.

75 Shapiro LM, McKenna WJ. Distribution of left ventricular hypertrophy in hypertrophic cardiomyopathy: A two-dimensional echocardiographic study. *J Am Coll Cardiol* 1983; **2**: 437–44.

76 Ackerman MJ, Van Driest SL, Ommen SR *et al*. Prevalence and age dependence of malignant mutations in the beta-myosin heavy chain and troponin T genes in hypertrophic cardiomyopathy: A comprehensive outpatient perspective. *J Am Coll Cardiol* 2002; **39**: 2042–8.

77 Corrado D, Basso C, Schiavon M *et al*. Identification of athletes with hypertrophic cardiomyopathy at risk of sudden death: Cost-effectiveness analysis of screening strategies [abstract]. *Circulation* 2002; **106** (Suppl. II): II-701.

78 Movahed MR, Ahmadi-Kashani M, Sabnis M *et al*. Left ventricular hypertrophy correlates with body surface area and body mass index in healthy teenage athletes [abstract]. *Circulation* 2002; **106**: II-352.

79 Maron BJ, Spirito P, Wesley YE *et al*. Development and progression of left ventricular hypertrophy in children with hypertrophic cardiomyopathy. *N Engl J Med* 1986; **315**: 610–14.

80 Maron BJ. The electrocardiogram as a diagnostic tool for hypertrophic cardiomyopathy: Revisited [editorial]. *Ann Noninvas Electrocardiol* 2001; **6**: 277–9.

81 Maron BJ, Mitten MJ, Quandt EK *et al*. Competitive athletes with cardiovascular disease – the case of Nicholas Knapp. *N Engl J Med* 1998; **339**: 1632–5.

Appendix

AHA recommendations for preparticipation screening

These recommendations are reproduced from Maron *et al.*, *Circulation* 1996; 94: 850–6.[11]

The 1996 American Heart Association consensus panel recommendations[11] state that some form of preparticipation cardiovascular screening for high school and college student athletes is justifiable and compelling based on ethical, legal and medical grounds. Preparticipation sports examinations are presently performed by a variety of individuals, including paid or volunteer physicians or nonphysician health-care workers with variable training and experience. Examiners may be associated with, or administratively independent of, the concerned institution, school or team.

Consequently, we strongly recommend that athletic screening be performed by an appropriately trained health-care worker with the requisite training, medical skills and background to reliably perform a detailed cardiovascular history and physical examination and to recognize heart disease. While it is preferable that such an individual be a licensed physician, this may not always be feasible, and under certain circumstances it may be acceptable for an appropriately trained registered nurse or physician-assistant to perform the screening examination. In those states in which nonphysician health-care workers (including chiropractors) are permitted to perform preparticipation screening, it will be necessary to establish a formal certification process to demonstrate expertise in performing cardiovascular examinations (the precise nature of which is presently undetermined).

Specifically, athletic screening evaluations should comprise a complete medical history and physical examination including brachial artery blood pressure measurement. This examination should be conducted in a physical environment conducive to optimal cardiac auscultation, whether performed individually in a private office or in a station format as part of a school program. The evaluation should also emphasize certain elements critical to the detection of those cardiovascular diseases known to be associated with morbidity or sudden cardiac death in athletes.

The cardiovascular history should include key questions designed to determine from the athlete: (1) prior occurrence of exertional chest pain/discomfort or syncope/near-syncope as well as excessive, unexpected and unexplained shortness of breath/fatigue associated with exercise; (2) past recognition of a heart murmur or increased systemic blood pressure; and (3) a family history of premature death (sudden or otherwise), or morbidity from cardiovascular disease in close relative(s) under the age of 50, or specific knowledge of the occurrence of certain conditions in family members (e.g. hypertrophic cardiomyopathy, dilated cardiomyopathy, long QT syndrome, Marfan syndrome or clinically important arrhythmias). These recommendations are offered recognizing that the accuracy of some responses elicited from young athletes may depend on their level of compliance and historical knowledge. Indeed, parents should be responsible for completing the history form of high school athletes.

The cardiovascular physical examination should emphasize (but not necessarily be limited to): (1) precordial auscultation in both the supine and the standing position to identify, in particular, those heart murmurs consistent with LV outflow obstruction; (2) assessment of the femoral artery pulses to exclude coarctation of the aorta; (3) recognition of the physical stigmata of Marfan syndrome; and (4) brachial blood pressure measurement in the sitting position.

As noted previously, when cardiovascular abnormalities are identified or suspected, the athlete should be referred to a cardiovascular specialist for further evaluation and/or confirmation. Definitively identified cardiovascular abnormalities should be judged with respect to the 26th Bethesda Conference consensus panel guidelines regarding the final determination of eligibility for future athletic competition.

CHAPTER 29

Sudden Death Due to Chest Blows (Commotio Cordis)

Mark S. Link, MD, N. A. Mark Estes III, MD, and Barry J. Maron, MD

Sudden death due to nonpenetrating chest wall impact in the absence of structural injury to the ribs, sternum and heart is known as commotio cordis. Although once considered to be a particularly rare event, it has recently become apparent that these events are more common than once believed. Furthermore, an important proportion of deaths on the athletic field are due to chest wall impact. The incidence of this event has been stated to be two to four deaths per annum in youth baseball,[1] but under-reporting and misclassification of deaths undoubtedly occur and the true number of deaths due to relatively mild chest wall blows is unknown. The Commotio Cordis Registry, in its 5-year existence, has documented 128 cases of commotio cordis,[2] and examples of sudden deaths initially classified as due to unknown causes are now more properly reclassified as commotio cordis.[3,4]

Definition

Commotio cordis, or cardiac concussion, is a term initially used to describe any cardiac manifestations of chest trauma in individuals, whether fatal or nonfatal and whether or not cardiac morphologic damage was present.[5,6] Initially reports were confined to adults, with trauma of generally significant magnitude, such as that caused by stone throws to the chest or falls from heights, most commonly in workplace environments.[7] More recently, sudden death due to low-energy chest wall trauma in the absence of cardiac damage (such as that seen in sporting activities such as youth baseball) have been reported; therefore, the common understanding of the term commotio cordis has been narrowed to events in which structural cardiac damage to the heart and chest wall is absent.[8–16] The first well-documented case of death due to a blunt chest blow in baseball was in 1978, involving a 7-year-old boy struck in the chest by a baseball during a T-ball game.[8] In the 1980s and 1990s, case reports documented several other occurrences of sudden death due to chest impact, not only in baseball[11,14] but also in hockey,[15] lacrosse,[13] and softball,[9,10] as well as fist blows to the chest.[11]

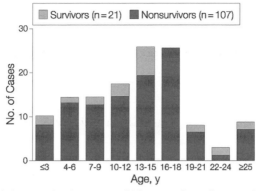

Fig. 29.1 Bar graph documenting the ages at which commotio cordis events have occurred in the Commotio Cordis Registry. Reproduced with permission from Maron *et al*. Clinical profile and spectrum of commotio cordis. *JAMA* 2002; **287**: 1142–6.

In 1984 the United States Consumer Product Safety Commission reported 23 deaths due to baseball chest impact, and found that there were more deaths in baseball from such blows than from head impact.[12] In 1995, Maron and colleagues provided the first comprehensive analysis of the commotio cordis phenomenon.[16] Subsequently, reports from the Commotio Cordis Registry[2,17] and the development of an experimental model of sudden death with low-energy chest wall impact[18] have contributed to a more complete understanding of the mechanisms and prevention of sudden death due to largely unintentional chest blows.

Human observations

Demographics

Commotio cordis appears to predominantly affect young individuals. In the Commotio Cordis Registry, with 128 individuals, the mean age of events is 14 years, 78% of them occurring at less than 18 years of age (Fig. 29.1).[2,17] The oldest individual reported to date is a 43-year-old cricket player.[4] It is thought that young athletes are at particular risk because of their more pliable chest wall, which facilitates the transmission of chest impact energy to the myocardium. With age, the thoracic cage stiffens and the chest wall absorbs more of the impact energy. However, there may be other variables that explain this predilection for young people, such as (the experimental finding) that impacts of lower energy, such as are more frequently encountered with youthful participants, may actually increase the likelihood of sudden death.[19]

The overwhelming majority of the victims are male, and only 5% are females.[2,17] The reason for this gender predominance is not clear. It is possibly due to the higher frequency of male sports participants or largely undefined biologic differences between the genders relevant to commotio cordis, such as differences in repolarization, hormonal influences, or chest wall anatomy.

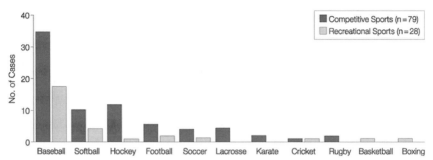

Fig. 29.2 Bar graph showing the frequency of sports (and ratio of competitive to recreational play) during which commotio cordis events occurred. More than one-half of the deaths have been due to baseball impacts. Reproduced with permission from Maron *et al.* Clinical profile and spectrum of commotio cordis. *JAMA* 2002; **287**: 1142–6.

Commotio cordis has most commonly been reported in baseball ($n = 53$), softball ($n = 14$), ice hockey ($n = 12$), football ($n = 8$) and lacrosse ($n = 5$) (Fig. 29.2). In addition, cases have been reported occasionally in a variety of other sports, including karate and soccer, as well as nonsports-related contact with a body part, usually the hand, foot, or elbow.[2]

In the Commotio Cordis Registry, competitive sporting activities account for about 60% of the cases, while victims were involved in recreational sports in 20%, and nonsports-related activities in the remaining 20%. These commotio cordis events unrelated to sports are generally due to innocent-appearing chest wall strikes with fists or hands in acts such as shadow-boxing, as a remedy for hiccups, or child discipline. A few of these cases have even resulted in criminal convictions for murder or manslaughter.[2]

Implements

In most commotio victims, the impact object is an implement of the game, i.e. a relatively hard object such as a baseball, hockey puck or lacrosse ball. However, more recent data from the Commotio Cordis Registry demonstrates that even softer projectiles (such as plastic hollow bats and soccer balls) and broader surface blows (by falls to the ground, chest wall collisions, or from football helmets) can cause sudden death. For example, of the 53 events due to baseballs, 50 have been with standard baseballs, while three occurred with softer-than-standard or 'safety' baseballs.

Protection

Standard, commercially available chest wall protection was worn by about 30% of the commotio cordis victims in organized sports.[2] Some chest wall barriers did not adequately cover the left chest wall and precordium; this was the case for at least 8 of 13 hockey players in whom chest protection was flawed or inadequate, either due to the angulation of the shot or by the raising of the arms, causing displacement of the protector and subsequent direct impact to the precordium. In addition, five football players were wearing standard shoulder/chest pads that did not cover the precordium and thus experienced direct trauma to the critical area of the chest overlying the heart. However, in others (including three lacrosse goalkeepers, two baseball catchers, and two hockey goalkeepers) the chest wall protector covered the heart and the projectile struck the chest protector; nonetheless, a commotio cordis event occurred.[2]

Characterization of blows

Although the energy or force of chest blows in victims of commotio cordis cannot be quantified in precise terms, in the vast majority of cases it appears as if the energy level of impact (velocity of the impact object) is not of unusual force for the sport or activity involved. For example, most of the victims died while playing with their peers, and much less commonly with older and stronger individuals.

In youth baseball, the most common sport in which commotio cordis has been reported, a pitched baseball can generally achieve a velocity of up to about 50 m.p.h. and, in the exceptional pitcher, 70 m.p.h.[20] However, in youth baseball, only 25% of the deaths were secondary to pitched baseballs; many more occurred with batted balls or balls thrown from one player to another. In these cases the velocity of the baseball is more difficult to estimate. In 3 of the 53 baseball-related commotio cordis events reported to the Registry, the impact object was a softer-than-standard (safety) ball. Furthermore, sudden cardiac death has been reported with a chest impact that was as seemingly minor as with a hollow plastic bat and a circular plastic sledding saucer.[2] By definition, none of the reported cases of commotio cordis had chest wall or cardiac damage to explain death, in contrast to the cases of death reported with motor vehicular accidents, in which myocardial contusion or severe cardiac and thoracic damage occurs.[21]

In commotio cordis victims, the chest blows strike the left chest directly over the cardiac silhouette (Fig. 29.3); however, the exact location of the chest wall strike cannot always be determined with precision since a precordial bruise is evident at autopsy in only about one-third of the cases.[16]

Circumstances of collapse

Instantaneous collapse occurs in approximately one-half of the victims. In the others, collapse follows a brief period of consciousness that is often marked by extreme lightheadedness, during which physical activity may occur.[16] When a cardiac rhythm can be documented after the event, it is most commonly ventricular fibrillation (VF).[8,14,15,22–24] Recent data from the Commotio Cordis Registry show a high frequency of asystole, especially after prolonged events.[2] Following resuscitation, the 12-lead ECG occasionally shows marked ST segment elevation, especially in the anterior leads (Fig. 29.4).[23] However, the ECG manifestations of commotio cordis generally resolve with time, without the development of Q-waves, or elevation of myocardial enzymes.[23]

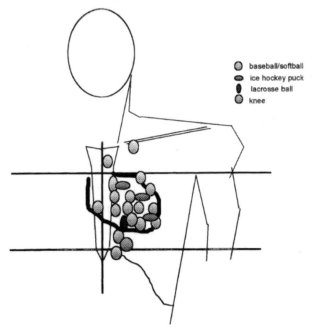

baseball/softball
ice hockey puck
lacrosse ball
knee

Fig. 29.3 Location of chest wall impacts that caused commotio cordis in the original series of 25 individuals ascertained by contact bruises. Note that impacts clustered over the cardiac silhouette. From Maron *et al.* Blunt impact to the chest leading to sudden death from cardiac arrest during sports activities. *N Engl J Med* 1995; **333**: 337–42. © 1995 Massachusetts Medical Society. All rights reserved. Adapted with permission, 2003.

Survival

Although commotio cordis initially was reported to be almost invariably fatal, survival now appears to approach 15%, including some cases of spontaneous resolution of hemodynamic collapse, which are judged to be aborted events.[2] It is also possible that many of these spontaneously resolved events occur with greater frequency as such cases are rarely reported to the Registry. As with other causes of VF, the most important determinant of survival is early resuscitation. Of those events in which resuscitation was begun within 3 minutes, 25% of individuals survived compared with only 3% when resuscitation was delayed for more than 3 minutes.[2]

Experimental models of chest wall trauma

The entity of sudden death with low-energy chest wall impact was not generally appreciated until 20 years ago. Therefore, early experimental efforts focused on severe chest wall trauma, such as that typically encountered in manual laborers, victims of motor vehicular accidents, falls from heights, and bomb blasts. These models are therefore limited in their relevance to commo-

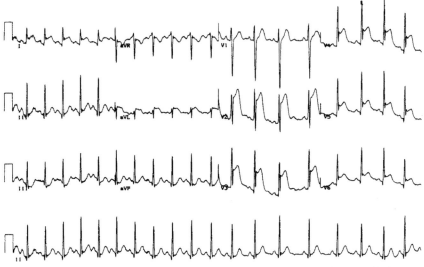

Fig. 29.4 Electrocardiogram from a 14-year-old boy obtained 35 minutes after resuscitation from ventricular fibrillation caused by a knee blow to the chest during a game of football. Note the marked ST segment elevation in the anterior leads. This patient underwent immediate cardiac catheterization, which documented normal coronary arteries. A myocardial infarction was excluded and the ST segment elevation normalized over several days without the development of Q-waves. Reproduced with permission from Link *et al.* Commotio cordis: cardiovascular manifestations of a rare survivor. *Chest* 1998; **114**: 326–8.

tio cordis by the severity of the cardiac damage resulting from substantial and traumatic impact energies.

Animal models of chest wall trauma date from 1879.[6,25] Riedinger distinguished between 'contusion', in which morphologic damage was present, and 'commotion', in which damage was absent, although he commented that he had observed only two cases of true 'commotion'.[25] In these early models, sudden death was occasionally ascribed to heightened vagal stimulation. In Schlomka's experiments with hammer blows to the chest of various animals, frequent ECG changes (ST segment abnormalities) were reported and occasionally VF.[26,27] In these experiments, the impact was not gated to the cardiac cycle and the force of the blow was quantified only subjectively; most blows were of sufficient strength to cause readily evident cardiac damage. Severing or blocking the vagus nerve had no effect on the ECG or survival. Schlomka and colleagues[26,27] surmised that the immediate ECG and arrhythmic changes and the long-term pathologic abnormalities (60% of animals followed for more than 80 days had permanent heart damage) were due to either coronary spasm or trauma-related myocardial damage. Similarly, Bright and Beck,[28] in their experiments with open-chest, direct cardiac blows, ascribed the ECG changes to myocardial contusion and hemorrhage.

In the first experiments using graded force, ventricular arrhythmias frequently resulted from marked impact energies.[29–31] However, most animals that died were found to have severe cardiac damage that could account for their death, and thus these were experimental studies of cardiac contusion rather than true commotio cordis. One experiment gated the chest impact to the cardiac cycle; although VF was more commonly triggered by T-wave impacts, the substantial energies of the blows (on average, equivalent to a 123 m.p.h. baseball) caused severe chest wall trauma in most of the animals (i.e. swine).[31] In the early 1990s a swine model of chest wall impact was developed using baseballs propelled at 95 m.p.h.[32] In this experiment, bradyarrhythmias and ventricular tachyarrhythmias were observed, but with no correlation to the cardiac cycle, and nearly all animals suffered cardiac contusions.

We concluded that the aforementioned models did not truly reflect the mechanisms of commotio cordis because they used high-energy projectiles with resultant chest wall and cardiac damage. Therefore, to study the pathophysiology of commotio cordis, we have developed a model in which low-energy chest wall blows were gated to the cardiac cycle. In this model we used wooden spheres (subsequently actual baseballs) mounted on an aluminum shaft to deliver chest blows to 8–12 kg swine at 30 m.p.h.[18] Juvenile swine were

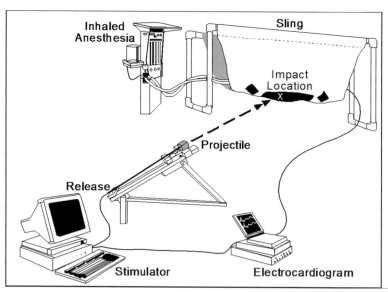

Fig. 29.5 Experimental commotio cordis showing the pronated juvenile swine in a sling attached to a standard six-lead electrocardiogram. Chest impact is directed by transthoracic echocardiography to the precordium directly over the papillary muscles. The baseball is affixed to an aluminum shaft propelled by a spring. With a known flight time of 130 ms and the release adjusted in accordance with the cardiac cycle, the impact can be delivered at any time in the cardiac cycle. Reproduced with permission from Link *et al.* Selective activation of the K+ATP channel is a mechanism by which sudden death is produced by low-energy chest-wall impact (commotio cordis). *Circulation* 1999; **100**: 413–18.

anesthetized with ketamine and isoflurane and suspended in a sling in order to approximate physiological cardiac anatomy and function (Fig. 29.5). The impact was directed to the center of the left ventricle using transthoracic echocardiographic guidance, and gated to the cardiac cycle with an electrophysiological stimulator. In addition to quantifying the electrophysiologic effects of low-energy chest wall trauma, wall motion abnormalities were assessed with transthoracic echocardiography, and myocardial blood flow was measured by technetium-99m sestamibi imaging and coronary angiography.

We found the consequences of such chest wall blows to be largely dependent on the portion of the cardiac cycle in which the impact occurred (Table 29.1). Impacts occurring during repolarization at the vulnerable portion of the T-wave (10–30 ms prior to the T-wave peak) triggered VF instantaneously and reproducibly (Fig. 29.6). Blows during other portions of the cardiac cycle did not produce VF but often caused ST-segment elevations and transient complete heart block. Segmental, transient wall motion abnormalities were observed in the apex of the heart, a region distant from the area of precordial impact. In addition, mild apical perfusion defects in one-fourth of the animals were noted on sestamibi imaging, in the absence of epicardial coronary artery abnormalities.[18]

In subsequent experiments, other variables relevant to the risk of VF with chest wall blows were examined. First, the incidence of VF was directly correlated with the hardness of the impact object (Fig. 29.7); firmer objects were more likely to trigger VF.[18] With 30 m.p.h. impacts, standard baseballs caused VF in 35% of the blows compared with 8% with safety baseballs (marketed for T-ball use). Impact object hardness correlated with the induction of VF not only at 30 m.p.h. but also at 40 m.p.h., a velocity more relevant to that causing commotio cordis in youth baseball.[33]

Secondly, we found that the energy level at impact represents a major determinant of whether commotio cordis will occur in the animal model and best fits a Gaussian curve. In these experiments, blows at 20 m.p.h. did not cause VF (lower limit of vulnerability for commotio cordis).[19] As impact velocity increased, the risk of VF increased, up to almost 70% at 40 m.p.h. At velocities of 50 m.p.h. or greater, however, the likelihood of VF decreased (i.e. the upper limit of vulnerability) and cardiac structural damage more commonly

Table 29.1 Incidence of ventricular fibrillation with impacts during different segments of the cardiac cycle. Ventricular fibrillation (VF) was only produced with impact on the upslope of the T wave, the vulnerable area of repolarization

	QRS	ST	−40 to −31 ms to T peak	−30 to −21 ms to T peak	−20 to −10 ms to T peak	−9 to −1 ms to T peak	T downslope
Total impacts (no.)	59	89	46	287	196	17	34
VF induced	0	0	2	77	65	2	0
% VF	**0%**	**0%**	**4%**	**27%**	**33%**	**11%**	**0%**

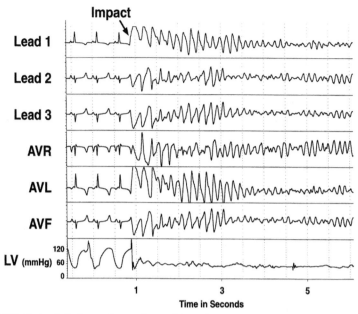

Fig. 29.6 Six-lead electrocardiogram from a 9 kg swine experiencing chest wall impact with a 30 m.p.h. object the shape and weight of a standard baseball. Ventricular fibrillation occurs immediately following chest impact within the vulnerable zone of repolarization (10–30 ms prior to the T peak). From Link *et al.* An experimental model of sudden death due to low energy chest wall impact (commotio cordis). *N Engl J Med* 1998; **338**: 1805–11, © 1998 Massachusetts Medical Society. All rights reserved. Reproduced with permission.

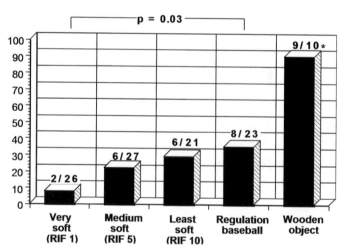

Fig. 29.7 Incidence of ventricular fibrillation with chest wall impacts at 30 m.p.h. with a regulation baseball compared with softer-than-standard (safety) baseballs of three grades of hardness. From Link *et al.* An experimental model of sudden death due to low energy chest wall impact (commotio cordis). *N Engl J Med* 1998; **338**: 1805–11. © 1998 Massachusetts Medical Society. All rights reserved. Adapted with permission, 2003.

occurred (i.e. left ventricular rupture and papillary muscle tears), indicating that at these velocities the electrophysiologic abnormalities are often due to structural damage (contusio cordis). These findings are similar to those obtained with the induction of VF using electrical shocks, which also exhibit a Gaussian curve, the lowest or highest energies failing to induce VF.[34–36] The mechanism for decreased vulnerability for commotio cordis at higher impact velocities is unresolved.

Finally, the precise region of impact on the chest wall proved to be crucial for determining whether a commotio cordis event would result from a chest blow. The area with the highest predilection was the precordium over the center of the cardiac silhouette (i.e. over the anterolateral papillary muscle).[37] Impacts at sites that did not overlie the cardiac silhouette did not cause VF. However, differences in VF incidence were also observed between sites within the cardiac silhouette. For example, blows directly over the center of the heart more frequently triggered VF (30%) compared with those over the base of left ventricle (13%) or at the apex (4%) (Fig. 29.8).

Mechanisms of commotio cordis

Based on the findings in humans and the experimental data, VF would appear to be the cause of death associated with low-energy chest wall blows. Since human victims collapse either virtually instantaneously or shortly after impact and the VF produced in our model is also instantaneous, commotio cordis

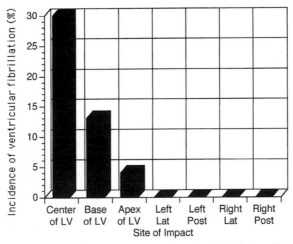

Fig. 29.8 Bar graph demonstrating the occurrence of ventricular fibrillation with 30 m.p.h. baseball impacts with respect to different sites on the chest wall in the experimental swine model of commotio cordis. Ventricular fibrillation was produced only by impacts directly over the cardiac silhouette, with the highest incidence evident at the center of the left ventricle (LV). Ventricular fibrillation did not occur with blows to the right and left lateral (Lat) or the right and left posterior (Post) chest wall sites. Reprinted with permission from the American College of Cardiology (*J Am Coll Cardiol* 2001; **37**: 649–54).

is likely a primary electrical event rather than secondary to heart block, or myocardial ischemia or hemorrhage. Therefore, we considered the possibility that specific ion channels are activated by the mechanical impact of commotio cordis blows. A likely candidate is the K^+_{ATP} channel, given that it is probably responsible for ST-segment elevation and contributes to the risk of VF in the presence of myocardial ischemia.[38-44] This channel is normally inactivated by physiologic concentrations of ATP; when ATP is reduced and ADP increases (as occurs with myocardial ischemia), the channel is opened and potassium exits the cell. Increased extracellular potassium will lead to ST-segment elevation and increased risk for VF. Because of similarities in ECG changes and arrhythmias observed in commotio cordis and with myocardial ischemia, we hypothesized that the K^+_{ATP} channel may play an important role in the generation of the consequences of chest blows in our commotio cordis model. Indeed, we found that glibenclamide, a specific blocker of the K^+_{ATP} channel reduced the magnitude of ST-segment elevation and the incidence of VF following experimental chest blows (Fig. 29.9).[45] Whether activation of other ion channels play a role in commotio cordis is unknown.

Also, there are data to suggest that instantaneous left ventricular pressure rise concomitant with the blow may mediate the electrophysiologic consequences of commotio cordis. In experiments designed to define both the site of impact[37] and the energy levels of impact,[46] the left ventricular pressure rise created by the chest wall blow correlated with the risk of VF. A threshold peak

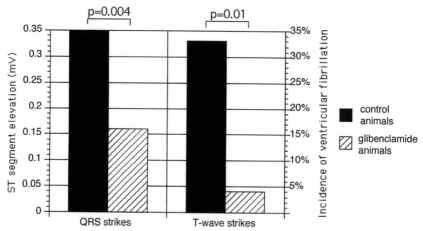

Fig. 29.9 Magnitude of ST-segment elevation and the incidence of ventricular fibrillation induced by 30 m.p.h. chest wall impacts by a spherical object the size and weight of a regulation baseball in the experimental swine model of commotio cordis. Significant differences between the control animals and animals given glibenclamide (a selective blocker of the K^+_{ATP} channel) were observed with respect to the magnitude of ST-segment elevation with QRS strikes and the incidence of ventricular fibrillation with T-wave strikes. Reprinted with permission from Link *et al.* Selective activation of the K+ATP channel is a mechanism by which sudden death is produced by low-energy chest-wall impact (commotio cordis). *Circulation* 1999; **100**: 413–18.

left ventricular pressure for initiation of VF was about 250 mm Hg. These observations suggest that it may be the rapid pressure rise immediately following the chest blow that causes the VF, possibly mediated by stretch-activated channels. The K^+_{ATP}[47] and other channels[48–50] may be activated by myocardial stretch, and in this way underlie the genesis of ventricular arrhythmias following chest blows.

Treatment of commotio cordis

Only about 15% of human commotio cordis victims are successfully resuscitated. As with other sudden death events, the major determinant of survival would appear to be rapid resuscitation, and in particular early defibrillation. In the Commotio Cordis Registry there was 25% survival when cardiopulmonary resuscitation was begun within 3 minutes compared with only 3% when resuscitation was delayed for more than 3 minutes ($P = 0.03$).

In our animal model of commotio cordis, early defibrillation with an automated external defibrillator (AED) was found to be critical for survival,[51] and survival was inversely related to the duration in VF ($P < 0.0001$). After 1 and 2 minutes of VF, 96% of animals survived with defibrillation. However, after 4 minutes of VF, only 46% survived, and at 6 minutes just 25% survived.

Currently the AED is only approved for use in individuals aged at least 8 years because of concerns for appropriate arrhythmia recognition and potentially adverse consequences emanating from adult defibrillation energy levels. We have also evaluated the accuracy of the AED algorithms for the detection of VF in our experimental model.[51] The sensitivity of the AED for the recognition of VF was 98%, and the specificity for nonshockable rhythms was 100%. Therefore, an important implication of these data is that coaches and other sports personnel (including parents) should be trained in basic life support, and consideration should be given to obtaining ready public access to AEDs.

Prevention of commotio cordis

Since resuscitation is so seldom successful in commotio cordis, the primary prevention of these catastrophic events should be stressed. Based on experimental data, softer-than-standard (safety) baseballs appear to diminish the risk of commotio cordis.[18,52] In one laboratory using a 95 m.p.h. baseball impact with swine, minor reductions in fatalities were reported when a softer-than-standard baseball was used in combination with commercially available chest wall protectors.[53] In another publication from the same group evaluating the risk of cardiac injury with 40–60 m.p.h. impacts, safety baseballs were compared with regulation baseballs using dummy models;[54] 78% of the safety balls tested had significantly lower impact force than the standard baseball at one or more of the velocities tested. In a three-rib dummy model, only 20% of the commercially available chest protectors tested were found to statistically lower the impact force with baseballs at 40 m.p.h.; at velocities of 50–70 m.p.h., 80% of the chest wall protectors decreased the impact force.[55]

Our experiments with baseball chest blows in a juvenile swine model showed a statistically significant reduction in the risk of fatal ventricular arrhythmias with safety baseballs at both 30 m.p.h. and 40 m.p.h. (Fig. 29.7).[18,52] The softest ball [Reduced Injury Factor (RIF) 1®; Worth Inc., Tullahoma, Tennessee, USA], marketed for T-ball use in youths aged 5–7 years, had an incidence of VF of 8% at both 30 m.p.h. and 40 m.p.h. The incidence of VF increased linearly with the hardness of the ball and reached a peak of almost 70% with standard baseballs propelled at 40 m.p.h. The differences between our experiment and others[53–55] is likely related to the absolute velocity of the impact object. At 95 m.p.h., a safety baseball may not offer much protection. However, baseball velocities of 95 m.p.h. are extremely unlikely in youth baseball, where the average velocity of a pitched ball is in the range of 30–50 m.p.h. Thus, at lower velocities, such as those more applicable to youth baseball, it appears that safety balls will reduce the risk of cardiac injury and sudden death.

Conclusions

Commotio cordis is an unusual but devastating event occurring in young people during sports-related or routine daily activities. Its prevalence is likely to be underestimated, and self-limited cases due to nonsustained arrhythmias may be much more common than currently believed. Critical variables that determine the likelihood of VF resulting from a chest blow include the precise timing of the impact to a narrow 20 ms window on the upslope of the T-wave, greater hardness of the impact object, precordial impact location of the blow, and the energy of the impact. Successful cardiopulmonary resuscitation is uncommon, but early defibrillation is critical for saving the lives of these young people. The experimental model described herein simulates the human scenario of commotio cordis, offers specific insights into its mechanism and helps to explain why commotio cordis is a relatively rare event.

References

1 Adler P, Monticone RCJ. Injuries and deaths related to baseball. In: Kyle SB, ed. *Youth Baseball Protective Equipment Project Final Report*. Washington, DC: United States Consumer Product Safety Commission, 1996: 1–43.

2 Maron BJ, Gohman TE, Kyle SB, Estes NAM III, Link MS. Clinical profile and spectrum of commotio cordis. *JAMA* 2002; **287**: 1142–6.

3 Link MS. Commotio cordis, sudden death due to chest wall impact in sports. *Heart* 1999; **81**: 109–10.

4 Haq CL. Sudden death due to low-energy chest-wall impact (commotio cordis). *N Engl J Med* 1998; **339**: 1399.

5 Nelaton A. *Elements de Pathologie Chirurgicale*. Paris: Librairie Germer Bateliere, 1876.

6 Meola F. La commozione toracica. *G Internaz Sci Med* 1879; **1**: 923–37.

7 Nesbitt AD, Cooper PJ, Kohl P. Rediscovering commotio cordis. *Lancet* 2001; **357**: 1195–7.

8 Dickman GL, Hassan A, Luckstead EF. Ventricular fibrillation following baseball injury. *Phys Sport Med* 1978; **6**: 85–6.

9 Froede RC, Lindsey D, Steinbronn K. Sudden unexpected death from cardiac concussion (commotio cordis) with unusual legal complications. *J Forensic Sci* 1979; **24**: 752–6.

10 Green ED, Simson LR, Kellerman HH, Horowitz RN. Cardiac concussion following softball blow to the chest. *Ann Emerg Med* 1980; **9**: 155–7.

11 Frazer M, Mirchandani H. Commotio cordis, revisited. *Am J Forensic Med Pathol* 1984; **5**: 249–51.

12 Rutherford GW, Kennedy J, McGhee L. Baseball and softball related injuries to children 5–14 years of age. Washington DC: United States Consumer Product Safety Commission, 1984.

13 Edlich RF, Mayer NE, Fariss BL *et al.* Commotio cordis in a lacrosse goalie. *J Emerg Med* 1987; **5**: 181–4.

14 Abrunzo TJ. Commotio cordis, the single, most common cause of traumatic death in youth baseball. *Am J Dis Child* 1991; **145**: 1279–82.

15 Kaplan JA, Karofsky PS, Volturo GA. Commotio cordis in two amateur ice hockey players despite the use of commercial chest protectors: Case reports. *J Trauma* 1993; **34**: 151–3.

16 Maron BJ, Poliac LC, Kaplan JA, Mueller FO. Blunt impact to the chest leading to sudden death from cardiac arrest during sports activities. *N Engl J Med* 1995; **333**: 337–42.

17 Maron BJ, Link MS, Wang PJ, Estes NAM III. Clinical profile of commotio cordis: An under-appreciated cause of sudden death in the young during sports and other activities. *J Cardiovasc Electrophysiol* 1999; **10**: 114–20.

18 Link MS, Wang PJ, Pandian NG *et al.* An experimental model of sudden death due to low energy chest wall impact (commotio cordis). *N Engl J Med* 1998; **338**: 1805–11.

19 Link MS, Wang PJ, Pandian NG *et al.* Upper and lower energy limits of vulnerability to sudden death with chest wall impact (commotio cordis) [abstract]. *Circulation* 1998; **98**: I-51.

20 Seefeldt VD, Brown EW, Wilson DJ, Anderson D, Walk S, Wisner D. Influence of low-compression versus traditional baseballs on injuries in youth baseball. East Lansing, MI: Institute for the Study of Youth Sport, 1993: 1–32.

21 Tenzer ML. The spectrum of myocardial contusion: A review. *J Trauma* 1985; **25**: 620–7.

22 Maron BJ, Strasburger JF, Kugler JD, Bell BM, Brodkey FD, Poliac LC. Survival following blunt chest impact induced cardiac arrest during sports activities in young athletes. *Am J Cardiol* 1997; **79**: 840–1.

23 Link MS, Ginsburg SH, Wang PJ, Kirchhoffer JB, Estes NAM III, Parris YM. Commotio cordis: Cardiovascular manifestations of a rare survivor. *Chest* 1998; **114**: 326–8.

24 Van Amerongen R, Rosen M, Winnik G, Horwitz J. Ventricular fibrillation following blunt chest trauma from a baseball. *Pediatr Emerg Care* 1997; **13**: 107–10.

25 Riedinger F. Die Verletzungen und Erkrankungen des Thoraz und seines Inhaltes. In: von Bergman E, von Bruns P, eds. *Handbuch der Praktischen Chirurgie.* Stuttgart: Ferd. Enke, 1903: 373–456.

26 Schlomka G, Schmitz M. Experimentelle Untersuchungen uber den Einfluss stumpfer Brustkorbtraumen auf das Electrokardiogramm. *S Ges Exp Med* 1932; **85**: 171–90.

27 Schlomka G. Commotio Cordis und ihre Folgen. Die Einwirkung stumpfer Brustwandtraumen auf das Herz. *Ergebn Inn Med Kinderheilk* 1934; **47**: 1–91.

28 Bright EF, Beck CS. Nonpenetrating wounds of the heart. A clinical and experimental study. *Am Heart J* 1935; **10**: 293–321.

29 Liedtke AJ, Gault JH, Demuth WE. Electrocardiographic and hemodynamic changes following nonpenetrating chest trauma in the experimental animal. *Am J Physiol* 1974; **226**: 377–82.

30 Viano DC, Artinion CG. Myocardial conducting system dysfunctions from thoracic impact. *J Trauma* 1978; **18**: 452–9.

31 Cooper GJ, Pearce BP, Stainer MC, Maynard RL. The biomechanical response of the thorax to nonpenetrating impact with particular reference to cardiac injuries. *J Trauma* 1982; **22**: 994–1008.

32 Viano DC, Andrzejak DV, Polley TZ, King AI. Mechanism of fatal chest injury by baseball impact: Development of an experimental model. *Clin J Sport Med* 1992; **2**: 166–71.

33 Link MS, Wang PJ, VanderBrink BA, Maron BJ, Estes NAM III. Reduced risk of death with safety balls in an experimental model of commotio cordis: Sudden death from low energy chest wall impact [abstract]. *J Am Coll Cardiol* 1999; **33**: 534.

34 Chen P-S, Shibata N, Dixon EG, Martin RO, Ideker RE. Comparison of the defibrillation threshold and the upper limit of ventricular vulnerability. *Circulation* 1986; **73**: 1022–8.

35 Fabritz CL, Kirchhof PF, Behrens S, Zabel M, Franz MR. Myocardial vulnerability to T wave shocks: Relation to shock strength, shock coupling interval, and dispersion of ventricular repolarization. *J Cardiovasc Electrophysiol* 1996; **7**: 231–42.

36 Swerdlow CD, Peter CT, Kass RM *et al.* Programming of implantable cardioverter-defibrillators on the basis of the upper limit of vulnerability. *Circulation* 1997; **95**: 1497–504.

37 Link MS, Maron BJ, VanderBrink BA *et al.* Impact directly over the cardiac silhouette is necessary to produce ventricular fibrillation in an experimental model of commotio cordis. *J Am Coll Cardiol* 2001; **37**: 649–54.

38 Bekheit S-S, Restivo M, Boutjdir M *et al.* Effects of glyburide on ischemia-induced changes in extracellular potassium and local myocardial activation: A potential new approach to the management of ischemia-induced malignant ventricular arrhythmias. *Am Heart J* 1990; **119**: 1025–33.

39 Kubota I, Yamaki M, Shibata T, Ikeno E, Hosoya Y, Tomoike H. Role of ATP-sensitive K^+ channel on ECG ST segment elevation during a bout of myocardial ischemia. *Circulation* 1993; **88**: 1845–51.

40 Kondo T, Kubota I, Tachibana H, Yamaki M, Tomoike H. Glibenclamide attenuates peaked T wave in early phase of myocardial ischemia. *Cardiovasc Res* 1996; **31**: 683–7.

41 Hiraoka M. Pathophysiological functions of ATP-sensitive K channels in myocardial ischemia. *Jpn Heart J* 1997; **38**: 297–315.

42 Isomoto S, Kurachi Y. Function, regulation, pharmacology, and molecular structure of ATP-sensitive K^+ channels in the cardiovascular system. *J Cardiovasc Electrophysiol* 1997; **8**: 1431–46.

43 Lepran I, Baczko I, Varro A, Papp JG. ATP-sensitive potassium channel modulators: Both pinacidil and glibenclamide produce antiarrhythmic activity during acute myocardial infarction in conscious rats. *J Pharmacol Exp Ther* 1996; **277**: 1215–20.

44 Billman GE, Avendano CE, Halliwill JR, Burroughs JM. The effects of the ATP-dependent potassium channel antagonist, glyburide, on coronary blood flow and susceptibility to ventricular fibrillation in unanesthetized dogs. *J Cardiovasc Pharmacol* 1993; **21**: 197–204.

45 Link MS, Wang PJ, VanderBrink BA *et al.* Selective activation of the K+ ATP channel is a mechanism by which sudden death is produced by low-energy chest-wall impact (commotio cordis). *Circulation* 1999; **100**: 413–18.

46 Link MS, Maron BJ, VanderBrink BA *et al.* Upper and lower energy limits of vulnerability to sudden death with chest wall impact (commotio cordis). *J Am Coll Cardiol* 2001; **37**: 135A.

47 Van Wagoner DR. Mechanosensitive gating of atrial ATP-sensitive potassium channels. *Circ Res* 1993; **72**: 973–83.

48 Yang X-C, Sachs F. Block of stretch-activated ion channels in *Xenopus* oocytes by gadolinium and calcium ions. *Science* 1989; **243**: 1068–71.

49 Hu H, Sachs F. Stretch-activated ion channels in the heart. *J Mol Cell Cardiol* 1997; **29**: 1511–23.

50 Kohl P, Hunter P, Noble D. Stretch-induced changes in heart rate and rhythm: Clinical observations, experiments and mathematical models. *Prog Biophys Mol Biol* 1999; **71**: 91–138.

51 Link MS, Maron BJ, Stickney RE *et al.* Automated external defibrillator arrhythmia detection in a model of cardiac arrest due to commotio cordis: Importance and efficacy of early defibrillation. *J Cardiovasc Electrophysiol* 2003; **14**: 83–7.

52 Link MS, Maron BJ, Wang PJ, Pandian NG, VanderBrink BA, Estes NAM III. Reduced risk of sudden death from chest wall blows (commotio cordis) with safety baseballs. *Pediatrics* 2002; **109**: 873–7.

53 Janda DH, Viano DC, Andrzejak DV, Hensinger RN. An analysis of preventive methods for baseball-induced chest impact injuries. *Clin J Sport Med* 1992; **2**: 172–9.

54 Janda DH, Bir CA, Viano DC, Cassatta SJ. Blunt chest impacts: Assessing the relative risk of fatal cardiac injury from various baseballs. *J Trauma* 1998; **44**: 298–303.

55 Viano DC, Bir CA, Chaney AK, Janda DH. Prevention of commotio cordis in baseball: An evaluation of chest wall protectors. *J Trauma* 2000; **49**: 1023–30.

CHAPTER 30

Naturally Occurring Animal Models of Cardiovascular Disease Causing Premature Death

Philip R. Fox, DVM

A number of spontaneously occurring animal models of cardiovascular diseases occur in the domestic dog and cat.[1-6] These are characterized by structural and functional abnormalities that are remarkably similar to their respective human conditions. The natural history of these cardiovascular diseases ranges from asymptomatic status to heart failure, syncope, tachyarrhythmias, and sudden death. Of particular interest are primary myocardial diseases. Hypertrophic cardiomyopathy in felines[7-18] is associated with diastolic heart failure, thromboembolism, and occasionally sudden death. Idiopathic dilated cardiomyopathy often occurs in large, purebred dogs and is associated with myocardial failure, atrial fibrillation, ventricular tachyarrhythmias, and sudden death.[1,2,6,19-24] Arrhythmogenic right ventricular cardiomyopathy in felines is noted for the clinical prevalence of heart failure and arrhythmias.[25] In Boxer dogs this condition is clinically characterized by ventricular arrhythmias and sudden death.[26,27] Inherited ventricular tachyarrhythmias in German Shepherd dogs is a notable model of sudden death in which autonomic imbalance underlies arrhythmogenesis.[28-36] Additional breed-specific inherited arrhythmias include atrial standstill in English Springer Spaniels,[37] Duchenne cardiomyopathy in the dog (notably the Golden Retriever),[38-40] and sick sinus syndrome in miniature Schnauzer dogs.[41]

Hypertrophic cardiomyopathy

Hypertrophic cardiomyopathy (HCM) is a primary myocardial disease characterized by increased left ventricular wall thickness and myocardial mass. It is associated with a diverse range phenotypic and functional characteristics in man[42-44] and domestic cats.[8-18]

Hypertrophic cardiomyopathy in the feline
Prevalence and demographics
Feline HCM is commonly encountered in veterinary practice. Liu recorded a 5.2% incidence of HCM based upon 4933 consecutive feline necropsies at the Animal Medical Center (1962–1976).[7] A 1.6% prevalence of HCM was reported

from a retrospective clinical study conducted between 1985 and 1989.[16] Left ventricular hypertrophy (predominantly idiopathic HCM), was diagnosed in 27–64% of the cats examined by echocardiography for suspected heart disease at the Animal Medical Center between 1985 and 1998.[1] Ages of affected animals vary from 3 months to 17 years[1,2,9,11,12,17] (mean age, 4.8–7 years). HCM is most frequently diagnosed in the domestic short-hair cat, which represents the most common feline breed.

Etiology

A heritable form of HCM has been identified in a highly interrelated colony of Maine Coon cats that is compatible with autosomal dominance with 100% penetrance.[12] Familial transmission suggestive of an autosomal dominant pattern has also been noted in related American short-hair cats with systolic anterior motion of the mitral valve and/or HCM,[18] and in an inbred colony of Persian cats with left ventricular hypertrophy.[17] There is a tendency for male predominance. Disruption of sarcomere assembly and myofibrillar organization due to mutant β-myosin heavy-chain protein with the Arg403Gln mutation has been reported.[47] While polymorphisms have been described on the cardiac troponin T and β-myosin heavy-chain genes of felines with HCM,[48,49] specific mutations have not yet been identified.

Clinical presentation

As in human patients, the majority of affected cats are asymptomatic. However, heart failure manifested by acute pulmonary edema is common. Systemic embolization is a well-documented sequela of advanced disease and is thought to be associated with blood stasis from severe left atrial enlargement, endocardial pathology, hyperhomocysteinemia, and other factors. Syncope occurs less commonly, but generally accompanies severe, dynamic, left ventricular outflow tract obstruction. Sudden death without congestive heart failure (CHF) has been reported in approximately 5% of cases,[50] particularly with sudden stress, activity or Valsalva maneuvers (defecation or urination).[1,2,11,12]

At physical examination the left precordial apex beat may be palpably normal or hyperdynamic. Auscultation may reveal a soft, systolic murmur (I to III/VI), heard loudest over the mitral and/or tricuspid valve areas, or over the sternum. A diastolic gallop rhythm (usually S_4) is common. Rales, arrhythmias and femoral arterial pulse deficits frequently accompany CHF. Heart and lung sounds will be muffled if large pleural or pericardial effusion is present. Paresis and absence of femoral arterial pulses accompany distal aortic thromboembolism. Ascites and cachexia attend chronic, end-stage disease.

Radiography

The ventrodorsal or dorsoventral view is the most sensitive radiographic position to demonstrate auricular enlargement. In symptomatic cats with pulmonary edema, interstitial and/or alveolar pulmonary densities, pulmonary venous distention (congestion) with or without pulmonary arterial congestion, and occasionally, mild pleural effusion may be present. Pulmonary edema may be diffuse, patchy, or focal in location and often involves the right caudal lung lobe. With chronic or advanced HCM, generalized cardiomegaly and severe biventricular failure can occur. Characteristic angiographic features include left ventricular free wall hypertrophy; pronounced left ventricular chamber reduction (which often appears slit-like); extremely hypertrophied papillary muscles; moderate to severe left atrium enlargement with variable right atrium enlargement; distended pulmonary veins; and left atrial or left ventricular thrombi.[1,11,12,14–16]

Electrocardiography

The ECG recordings are generally nonspecific. Ventricular and supraventricular tachyarrhythmias are common, but hemodynamically important tachycardia is infrequent.[1–3,11,12] Supraventricular arrhythmias are most pronounced in cats whose atria have marked structural abnormalities (myocytolysis, fibrosis, myocyte hypertrophy, thickened basement membrane).[3] Left axis deviation compatible with left anterior fascicular block may be recorded in up to one-third of cats with severe hypertrophy. Other ECG changes reflect left atrium enlargement (P-wave duration greater than 40 ms) and left ventricular enlargement (R_{II} greater than 0.8 mV; QRS duration greater than 40 ms).

Echocardiography

HCM is a heterogeneous disease with a wide phenotypic array of left ventricular hypertrophy. This ranges from localized and relatively mild wall thickening involving an individual wall segment to diffuse and pronounced hypertrophy of all portions of the left ventricle.[11,12,15,51] Pathologic hypertrophy is present when the thickness of the ventricular septum or the left ventricular posterior (free) wall measured at end-diastole exceeds 6 mm. No single pattern of hypertrophy can be considered pathognomonic of the disease.

In breeding studies to determine the phenotypic expression in Maine Coon cats,[12] when affected cats were bred with unaffected cats HCM was not present before 6 months of age. Papillary enlargement, usually accompanied by systolic anterior motion, developed first, typically between 9 and 21 months of age. When affected cats were bred to affected cats, phenotypic evidence of HCM occurred before 6 months of age and severe heart failure occurred during young adulthood.

In a study assessing the distribution of left ventricular hypertrophy in 46 HCM cats, four patterns of left ventricular hypertrophy were identified.[11] When viewed from the short axis, hypertrophy was most often diffuse (31 cats, 67%) and substantial, involving portions of the ventricular septum as well as contiguous anterolateral and posterior free wall. Fifteen of these 31 showed a concentric distribution of hypertrophy of all segments; 16 of these 31 had involvement of the anterior portion of the septum as well as the anterolateral and posterior free wall (but not posterior septum). Less often (in the remaining 15 of the 46 cats, 33%), segmental patterns of hypertrophy were recorded: in 13 of these 15, wall thickness was confined to only one left ventricular segment (anterior septum in 12 cats and posterior free wall in one cat). In 2 of the 15 cats wall thickening involved noncontiguous segments of the left ventricle; i.e. the anterior septum or posterior free wall. When viewed from the longitudinal axis, 26 of the 46 cats (56%) showed greater wall thickening of the basal than of the apical portion of left ventricle. Some had proximal septal thickening which protruded into the left ventricular outflow tract. The other 20 cats had diffuse thickening involving basal and apical left ventricle. Additional findings included left atrium and often right atrium enlargement; decreased left ventricular internal dimensions with hypertrophied papillary muscles; normal to elevated left ventricular fractional shortening; mild hypertrophy of the right ventricle wall and mild to moderate hypertrophy of the right ventricle outflow tract; right ventricular dilatation (late in the disease course of some cases); and pericardial effusion. Systolic anterior motion of the mitral valve was present in 31 (67%) of the 46 animals (Fig. 30.1). The anterior leaflet was observed in most animals to make a sharp angled bend and mid-systolic contact with the ventricular septum, as viewed during two-dimensional imaging. Mitral–septal contact was mild (2+) in 23% of the 31, moderate (3+) in 29% of the 31, and prolonged (4+) in 48% of the 31. Continuous wave Doppler assessment of left ventricular outflow tract velocities (and estimate of outflow gradient) displayed velocities ranging from 2.6 to 6.7 m/s, with estimated subaortic

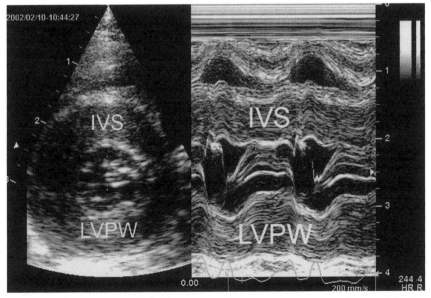

Fig. 30.1 Two-dimensional guided M-mode echocardiogram through the basal left ventricle of a cat with idiopathic hypertrophic obstructive cardiomyopathy. The anterior mitral valve leaflet moves anterior during systole (i.e. systolic anterior motion, SAM) and makes prolonged contact with the interventricular septum (IVS). LVPW = left ventricular posterior wall.

gradients of 27–179 mm Hg. Cats with and without systolic anterior motion appear not to differ with respect to maximal mean left ventricular septal wall thickness, or mean left ventricular free wall thickness. Cats with prolonged (3+ to 4+) systolic anterior motion tend to have the most extensive patterns of left ventricular hypertrophy. In cases of dynamic left ventricular outflow tract obstruction, there is typically a narrowed left ventricular outflow tract, a fibrous plaque on the basal ventricular septum corresponding to the point of systolic anterior mitral valve contact, and thickening of the anterior mitral valve leaflet.

Mitral regurgitation is common in HCM cats and regurgitant jets can be imaged with color-flow Doppler echocardiography in almost all cases. The degree of regurgitation is generally mild. Cats with systolic anterior motion usually have eccentric mitral regurgitation jets oriented toward the posterolateral wall and result from systolic disruption of the mitral valve apparatus. Tricuspid regurgitation is less common. With dynamic left ventricular outflow tract obstruction, the maximal left ventricular outflow tract velocity is increased. Mitral inflow Doppler waveforms may be normal or indicate a relaxation abnormality indicative of diastolic dysfunction (Fig. 30.2). Systolic abnormalities are not limited to the left ventricle. Dynamic right ventricular outflow tract gradients have been recorded from cats with HCM[52] and most gradients are relatively mild (less than 25 mm Hg).

Gross findings

Left ventricular hypertrophy exhibits a broad morphologic spectrum (Figs 30.3 and 30.4).[2,4,7–13,51] Most cats have a diffuse but asymmetric distribution of left

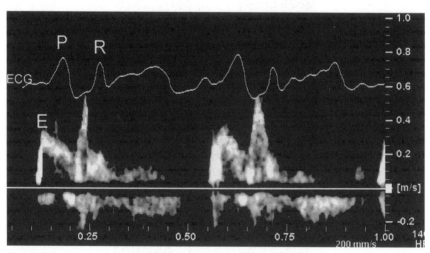

Fig. 30.2 Pulse-wave Doppler echocardiographic recording from a cat with hypertrophic cardiomyopathy. This transmitral filling profile suggests a relaxation abnormality and is characterized by E/A-wave inversion and prolonged E-wave deceleration time. E = E wave; ECG = electrocardiogram; P = P wave; R = R wave.

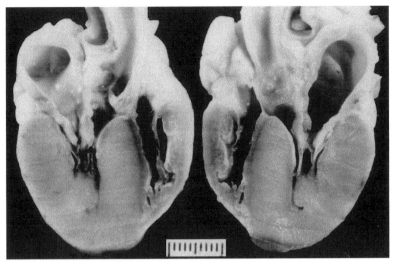

Fig. 30.3 Gross heart from a cat with idiopathic hypertrophic obstructive cardiomyopathy. There is concentric left ventricular hypertrophy and fibrous endocardial contact scar in the left ventricular (LV) outflow tract in close proximity to the anterior mitral valve leaflet. This animal had dynamic LV outflow tract obstruction (systolic anterior motion, SAM). The LV cavity is small. From Fox. Feline cardiomyopathies. In: Ettinger SJ, Feldman EC, eds. *Textbook of Veterinary Internal Medicine*, 5th edn. Philadelphia: WB Saunders, 2000: 896–923, with permission.

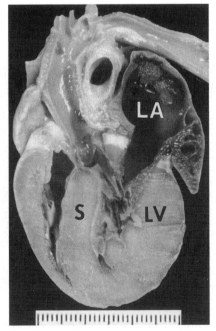

Fig. 30.4 Gross heart from a cat with idiopathic hypertrophic cardiomyopathy. Thickening is more pronounced in the left ventricular posterior free wall (LV). The left atrium (LA) is markedly enlarged and the left ventricular cavity is small. S = interventricular septum.

ventricular hypertrophy. Segmental patterns of hypertrophy occur less commonly. Heart weights range from 19 to 40 g (normal, less than 19 g). The ratio of heart weight to body weight ranges from 5 to 8.6 (normal, less than 3.9). Generally, anterior interventricular wall thickness ranges from 7 to 14 mm and posterior left ventricular free wall thickness from 7 to 12 mm. Biatrial enlargement is common, and mild to moderate right ventricular hypertrophy is often present. In cases of dynamic left ventricular outflow obstruction, the anterior mitral valve leaflet is thickened. A mural, endocardial fibrous plaque is generally present on the basal ventricular septum in apposition to the anterior mitral leaflet. Pulmonary congestion or edema may occur and, less commonly, pericardial, pleural, or abdominal effusions are present. Systemic thromboembolism is common, especially involving the renal arteries and distal aorta. Thrombi are often detected in the left atrium or left ventricle.

Histopathology

Histopathologic changes are often marked.[1,2,4,7–9, 10–12] The hallmark lesion is left ventricular myofiber disarray (cellular disorientation in more than 5% of the tissue section) (Fig. 30.5). Myocytes may be hypertrophied and frequently display varying degrees of myocytolysis and necrosis. Other common findings include coronary microcirculation remodeling (arteriosclerosis or small vessel disease) and matrix changes. Thickening of intramural coronary arterioles is due to medial and intimal proliferation associated with increased connective tissue elements and, less commonly, smooth muscle cells (Fig. 30.6). Matrix

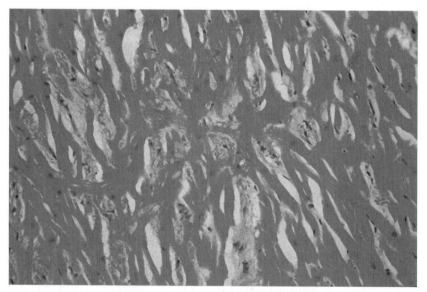

Fig. 30.5 Photomicrograph from a section of basilar interventricular septum of a cat with idiopathic hypertrophic cardiomyopathy. Myofiber disarray is evident. Hematoxylin and eosin stain; magnification ×100.

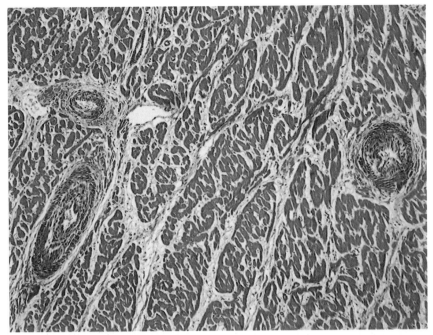

Fig. 30.6 Photomicrograph of a section of ventricular septum from a cat with idiopathic hypertrophic cardiomyopathy. There are three intramural coronary arterioles. The two larger vessels display severe wall thickening (arteriosclerosis, small vessel disease) and are surrounded by fibrous connective tissue. There is increased interstitial fibrosis. Masson trichrome stain; magnification ×100.

changes range from mild interstitial fibrosis to severe replacement fibrosis. This is often present in proximity to thickened intramural coronary arterioles. In a series of 51 cats, ventricular septal myofiber disorganization was recorded in 30%; septal disorganization constituting at least 5% of the relevant tissue sections was present in 27%, whereas extensive myocyte disarray (at least 25%) was present in 14%. Cellular disorganization was predominantly of the type I pattern, comprising small foci of adjacent myocardial cells. Interstitial fibrosis or severe replacement fibrosis was present in half of the cats.[9]

Clinical outcome

The clinical course and outcome are variable owing to the wide variation in disease expression.[1,9–12,16,50] Many HCM cats achieve adulthood without clinical signs and have a normal life expectancy. Some who present with heart failure, particularly pulmonary edema, stabilize with drug therapy and then remain asymptomatic. Others experience recurrent heart failure and ultimately die, or occasionally experience sudden death. In a highly inbred colony of Maine Coon cats with familial HCM,[12] when affected cats were bred to nonaffected cats heart failure was first noted at 33 ± 10 months and the age of death (sudden or due to heart failure) was 32 ± 12 months. When affected cats were bred with affected cats, heart failure occurred at 20 ± 3 months and death occurred at 23 ± 4 months of age. Clinical disease developed earlier in males. Five of 16 affected cats in this study died suddenly. Other investigators reported a family of cats with asymptomatic HCM that developed hypodynamic left ventricular systolic function and relative left ventricular chamber dilation over the course of 13 years.[51]

The morbidity and mortality of HCM have been reported from three veterinary medical centers.[11,16,50] In a series of 46 HCM cats in which 43 were followed for up to 49 months,[11] nonsurvivors showed a significantly greater magnitude and extent of left ventricular hypertrophy (maximum wall thickness, 8.1 ± 1.5 mm) than survivors (7.3 ± 0.9 mm); nonsurvivors had a significantly larger left atrium (20.1 ± 4.6 mm) than survivors (16.8 ± 3.4 mm). In addition, systolic anterior motion was more common in survivors [16 of 18 cats (89)%] than in nonsurvivors [10 of 21 cats (48%)]. This finding, subsequently reported in another series of cats,[50] contrasts with outcomes in human patients, who experience greater morbidity and mortality with the obstructive compared with the nonobstructive form of HCM.[46]

Median survival in a series of 61 HCM cats was 732 days.[16] Longevity was not affected by age, breed, gender, or body weight. Cats without clinical signs lived longer (median survival was longer than 1830 days) than those with clinical signs (heart failure patients survived a median of 92 days and cats with arterial embolism survived a median of 61 days). Six months after diagnosis, all cats with systemic embolism and 60% of cats with heart failure were dead. Cats with heart rates less than 200 beats/min at initial examination survived significantly longer than those with heart rates greater than 200 beats/min.

Median survival in a series of 260 HCM cats was 709 days for all cats that survived longer than 24 hours. Cats that were asymptomatic at the time of initial examination had a median survival of 1129 days. Subgroup analysis reported median survival for cats with syncope (654 days), heart failure (563 days), and arterial thromboembolism (184 days).[50]

Hypertrophic cardiomyopathy in the canine

In canines HCM is a rare condition. It has been identified in a variety of large- and small-breed dogs and most of the reported cases have been males.[5,6,9,53–56] An apparent familial form of HCM, suspected to have a polygenic or autosomal recessive pattern of inheritance, has been reported in pointer dogs.[56] Most dogs with HCM are asymptomatic and diagnosis is made incidentally at necropsy, or when identification of heart murmur or arrhythmia during routine physical examination prompts echocardiographic evaluation. In some cases syncope occurs. Sudden death is a well recognized feature of this disease, generally occurring during or immediately following exertion. Physical examination may be unremarkable. In cases with dynamic left ventricular outflow tract obstruction, a left basilar systolic ejection heart murmur is present. These cases may also have a systolic left apical murmur associated with mitral insufficiency caused by systolic anterior motion of the mitral valve.

Radiography is usually unremarkable or left atrial enlargement may be evident. Electrocardiography may indicate left ventricular enlargement (high-amplitude R waves in left precordial chest leads) or be unremarkable. Reported arrhythmias include atrial and ventricular extrasystoles, ventricular tachycardia, and first- and third-degree atrioventricular block. Echocardiography reveals left ventricular hypertrophy, which tends to be symmetric. Dynamic left ventricular outflow tract obstruction is a common feature. It may be evident at rest or be latent, requiring provocative interventions.

Pathologic changes are usually prominent. In one study comparing morphologic findings in spontaneously occurring HCM in humans, cats, and dogs,[9] left ventricular hypertrophy was most commonly asymmetric. Marked septal disorganization (5% of the tissue section) was present in 20% of dogs affected with HCM. Moderate to severe septal fibrosis was identified more commonly in humans (39%) compared with animals (21%). Abnormal intramural coronary arteries (small vessel disease, caused by hyperplasia of the intima and media) were detected in 60% of the dogs, most commonly within or at the margins of areas of fibrous tissue. In cases where dynamic left ventricular outflow tract obstruction was present, the anterior mitral valve leaflet was thickened and corresponding basilar septal fibrotic plaque was evident in the left ventricular outflow tract. Myocyte hypertrophy, focal myocytolysis and necrosis, and dystrophic calcification are additional features. Clinical outcome is variable. Affected dogs may remain asymptomatic or experience sudden death. Owing to the infrequent nature of this disease, survival data are lacking.

Arrhythmogenic right ventricular cardiomyopathy

Arrhythmogenic right ventricular cardiomyopathy (ARVC) is an uncommon but important primary myocardial disease. It is responsible for substantial cardiovascular morbidity in humans[57–62] and is a largely unappreciated cause of sudden death in the young.[61,62] Right ventricular cardiomyopathy has been reported sporadically in mammals.[63–66] A naturally occurring cardiomyopathy that closely resembles ARVC in man has been described in domestic cats[25] and the Boxer dog.[26,27]

Arrhythmogenic right ventricular cardiomyopathy in the feline
Prevalence and demographics
The clinical features of ARVC have been recorded in a wide age range of cats from 1 to 20 years old (mean 7.3 ± 5.2 years). Breeds included domestic shorthair, Burmese, and Burman ($n = 2$). Approximately equal numbers of males and females have been recorded.[25]

Etiology
The etiology is unresolved. A familial tendency has been observed in the Burman breed.

Clinical presentation
Right-sided CHF with tachypnea, jugular venous distention, abdominal effusion, or hepatosplenomegaly has been recorded in about two-thirds of advanced cases.[25] It is uncertain whether the predominance of heart failure reflects the true clinical profile of feline ARVC or whether there is over-representation in this series due to patient selection. A soft, pansystolic heart murmur is usually detected along the right sternal border, consistent with tricuspid regurgitation. Syncope may occur but is uncommon. Asymptomatic cases may be detected during evaluation for other conditions.

Radiography
Thoracic radiographs show enlargement of the cardiac silhouette compatible with right atrial and right ventricular dilatation. Additional radiographic changes compatible with right-sided congestive heart failure, including pleural effusion, ascites, pericardial effusion, and posterior vena caval dilatation, may be evident. Left atrial enlargement may be present in some animals.

Electrocardiography
A variety of arrhythmias have been described, including ventricular tachycardia, atrial fibrillation, supraventricular tachycardia, premature ventricular complexes (of right and left ventricular origin), right bundle branch block, and first-degree atrioventricular block (Fig. 30.7).[25] Most of the cats studied to date have not had precordial chest leads evaluated, so it is uncertain whether T-wave inversion and epsilon waves, characteristic of some human patients with ARVC, also occur in cats. Moreover, the dampening effects of pleural effusion may have hindered identification of subtle depolarization abnormalities.

Echocardiography
Marked right atrial and right ventricular enlargement is readily evident by transthoracic echocardiography in advanced cases (Figs 30.8 and 30.9). Additional abnormalities include paradoxic septal motion, abnormal muscular trabecular patterns, particularly in the apical right ventricular cavity, and images consistent with localized right ventricular aneurysm formation (i.e. akinetic or dyskinetic areas with diastolic outward bulging) in the apical or subtricuspid region. Doppler color-flow imaging demonstrates tricuspid regurgitation.[25]

Gross pathology
Morphologic abnormalities in affected cats[25] are striking and consistent with those previously described in human ARVC patients.[57,61] Moderate to severe right ventricular dilatation is present. Right ventricular wall thinning is ei-

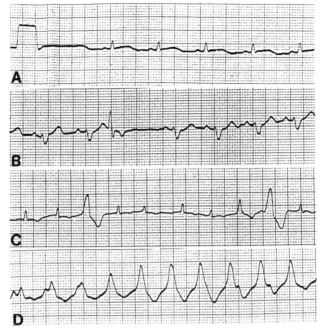

Fig. 30.7 Lead II rhythm strips from cats with arrhythmogenic right ventricular cardiomyopathy. Paper speed, 50 mm/s; 1 cm = 1 mv. (**A**) Normal control, sinus rhythm. (**B**) Atrial fibrillation with right bundle branch block morphology. (**C**) Atrial fibrillation with ventricular premature beats with left bundle branch block morphology. (**D**) Ventricular tachycardia with right bundle branch block configuration. From Fox *et al*. Spontaneously occurring arrhythmogenic right ventricular cardiomyopathy in the domestic cat. A new animal model similar to the human disease. *Circulation* 2000; **102**: 1863–70, with permission.

ther diffuse or segmental and associated with a flattened appearance of the right ventricular wall trabeculae; right ventricular septoparietal bands appear prominent. Right ventricular wall thickness in ARVC cats is reduced (1.4 ± 0.3 mm) compared with normal controls (2.3 ± 0.1 mm). Aneurysms are present (apical, subtricuspid, and infundibular regions of the right ventricle) in approximately half of cats and severity varies from focal aneurysms (with external bulging) to larger translucent aneurysms. Right atrial cavity dilation is present and portions of the right atrial walls are markedly thinned, facilitating transillumination (Fig. 30.10). Left atrial dilatation is present in about one-third of the cases. Mural thrombosis is occasionally observed.

Histopathology

Histopathologic lesions in affected cats[25] closely resembled those of human patients with ARVC.[57,61] Most prominent is myocardial right ventricular atrophy with myocytes replaced by adipose or fibrous tissue in two patterns: fibro-fatty (75%) (Fig. 30.11) and fatty (25%) (Fig. 30.12). The fibro-fatty pattern

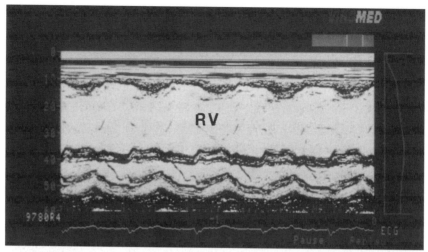

Fig. 30.8 M-mode echocardiogram from a cat with arrhythmogenic right ventricular cardiomyopathy. Note the severe right ventricular dilatation. From Fox *et al*. Spontaneously occurring arrhythmogenic right ventricular cardiomyopathy in the domestic cat. A new animal model similar to the human disease. *Circulation* 2000; **102**: 1863–70, with permission.

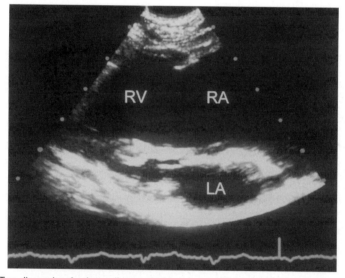

Fig. 30.9 Two-dimensional echocardiogram (right parasternal four-chamber view) of a cat with arrhythmogenic right ventricular cardiomyopathy. Note severe enlargement of the right ventricle (RV) and right atrium (RA). LA = left atrium.

consists of focal or diffuse myocardial atrophy associated with adipose tissue and replacement-type fibrosis and extending from the epicardium toward the endocardium. The fatty pattern within the right ventricle wall and trabeculae is characterized by multifocal areas of adipose cell infiltration with only scant

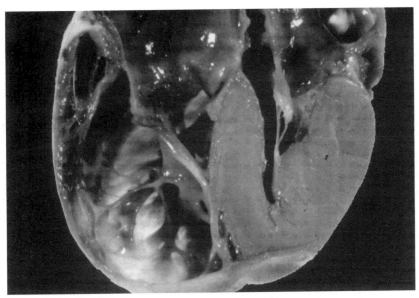

Fig. 30.10 Heart from a cat with arrhythmogenic right ventricular cardiomyopathy. There is severe enlargement of the right ventricle and thinned, translucent right ventricle walls associated with trabecular flattening. Septoparietal bands appear prominent. From Fox *et al.* Spontaneously occurring arrhythmogenic right ventricular cardiomyopathy in the domestic cat. A new animal model similar to the human disease. *Circulation* 2000; **102**: 1863–70, with permission.

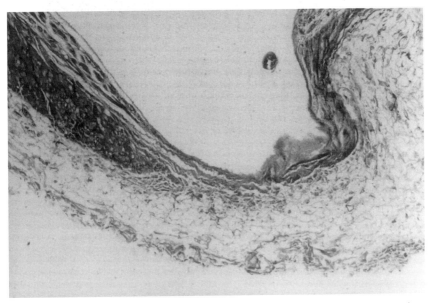

Fig. 30.11 Photomicrograph of apical right ventricle aneurysm from a cat with arrhythmogenic right ventricular cardiomyopathy. There is severe transmural fibro-fatty replacement with organized mural thrombosis. Heidenhain trichrome stain; magnification ×100. From Fox *et al.* Spontaneously occurring arrhythmogenic right ventricular cardiomyopathy in the domestic cat. A new animal model similar to the human disease. *Circulation* 2000; **102**: 1863–70, with permission.

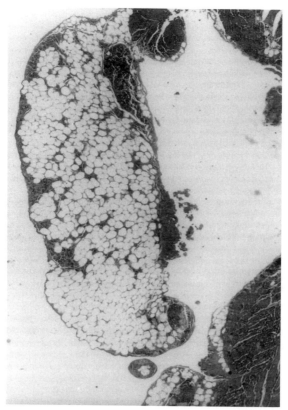

Fig. 30.12 Photomicrograph of right ventricle from a cat with the fatty variant of arrhythmogenic right ventricular cardiomyopathy. There is fatty replacement of the right ventricle myocardium. Heidenhain trichrome stain; magnification ×80. From Fox *et al*. Spontaneously occurring arrhythmogenic right ventricular cardiomyopathy in the domestic cat. A new animal model similar to the human disease. *Circulation* 2000; **102**: 1863–70, with permission.

interstitial fibrosis. In both morphologic forms, residual surviving myocytes are usually scattered within the areas of fibrosis or fat. Focal or multifocal right ventricular myocarditis is common, particularly with the fibro-fatty pattern (Fig. 30.13). Inflammatory infiltrates, mostly of T lymphocytes, are associated with myocyte cell death and mild to severe fibrous tissue deposition. Similar findings, consistent with patchy inflammatory myocardial injury and fibro-fatty repair, are usually present in the left and right atrial walls, the left ventricular free wall and the ventricular septum. Fatty infiltration is occasionally present in the left ventricular free wall. The epicardium frequently shows tiny areas of fibrous thickening in the fibro-fatty cases associated with focal mononuclear infiltrates, mostly at the atrial level.

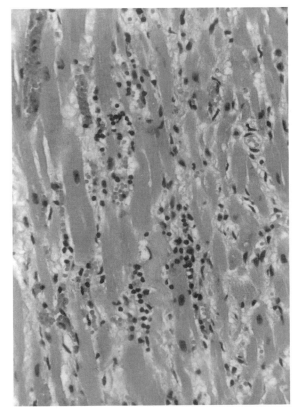

Fig. 30.13 Section of right ventricle from cat with arrhythmogenic right ventricular cardiomyopathy. Round cell inflammatory infiltrates associated with myocyte death are evident. Hematoxylin and eosin stain; magnification ×80. From Fox *et al.* Spontaneously occurring arrhythmogenic right ventricular cardiomyopathy in the domestic cat. A new animal model similar to the human disease. *Circulation* 2000; **102**: 1863–70, with permission.

Apoptosis
Apoptotic myocytes have been identified in three-quarters of affected cats with ARVC.

Clinical outcome
Most cats with advanced CHF die within 3 months of clinical presentation. In absence of CHF, cats with arrhythmias may be managed with appropriate anti-arrhythmic drugs. Sudden death may occur.

Arrhythmogenic right ventricular cardiomyopathy in the canine
Prevalence and demographics
Several sporadic cases of ARVC have been reported in dogs.[63–65] A form of myocardial disease in the Boxer breed, termed 'Boxer cardiomyopathy',[26] was

observed with clinical signs that included syncope, sudden death, ventricular arrhythmias, and CHF. Recently, this disease has been characterized in detail in Boxer dogs[27] and has been demonstrated to be very similar to ARVC in human patients. Affected dogs range from 4 to 15 years of age and show approximately equal sex prevalence.

Etiology

Familial ventricular arrhythmias have been reported in Boxer dogs and appear to be inherited as an autosomal dominant trait.[67] Although this study did not include pathologic characterization of affected animals, it is highly likely that the underlying disease was ARVC. Moreover, ventricular arrhythmias of right ventricular origin are clinically regarded as a surrogate marker for the underlying substrate representing ARVC, in the absence of other congenital or acquired heart disease.

Clinical presentation

Data from a cohort of 23 Boxer dogs[27] documented sudden death in 39%, syncope in 52%, ventricular arrhythmias of right ventricular origin in 78%, and right heart failure in 9%. These clinical signs have been previously noted in the Boxer breed.[26]

Radiography, MRI

Radiographs may be unremarkable or show right ventricular enlargement. Some cases have left heart enlargement or extracardiac signs of heart failure. *In vitro* magnetic resonance imaging reveals diffuse, bright signals in the right ventricular anterolateral and/or infundibular walls in most affected Boxer dogs.[27]

Electrocardiography

Ventricular tachycardia typically displays a left bundle branch block configuration. Paroxysmal ventricular tachycardia has been recorded in a high percentage of affected Boxer dogs (Fig. 30.14).[27] A variety of arrhythmias including atrial fibrillation and conduction disturbances may also occur.

Pathology

From examination of 23 affected Boxer dogs, 35% had right ventricle chamber dilatation and 13% had right ventricular aneurysms.[27] There was no evidence of increased heart weight, mural thrombosis, or wall thinning. Right ventricular histomorphometry revealed a mean fatty tissue area of approximately 45% and correspondingly reduced residual myocardium area in ARVC dogs. Significant replacement fibrosis was also present in one-quarter of ARVC hearts. Moreover, mild lymphocyte infiltrates were detected in 61% and apoptotic myocytes in 39%.

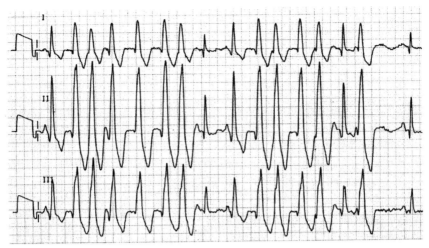

Fig. 30.14 Simultaneous lead I, II and III recordings from a 4-year-old Boxer dog with syncope. There is paroxysmal ventricular tachycardia with left bundle branch configuration. The dog died suddenly during exercise. Paper speed, 50 mm/s; 1 cm = 1 mV.

Clinical outcome

There is a high incidence of sudden death in affected dogs.[26,27] A smaller percentage develop CHF. Pharmacologic therapies for ventricular tachycardia have been recently investigated. Treatment with mexiletine–atenolol or sotalol was efficacious in one trial to reduce the number of VPCs, severity of arrhythmia, and heart rate.[68]

Dilated cardiomyopathy in the canine

Dilated cardiomyopathy (DCM) is the second most common acquired heart disease in the dog (valvular myxomatous degeneration resulting in volume overload is the most frequent cause of cardiac morbidity and mortality).[5,6,69] While cardiac dilation and systolic dysfunction define this condition, substantial differences occur between breeds relative to clinical characteristics, morbidity and mortality.

Prevalence and demographics

Prevalence has been estimated at 0.5%,[5] although this figure is subject to referral institutional bias. This condition occurs almost exclusively in large and giant purebred dogs that are young to middle-aged,[6] and the Doberman Pinscher breed is the most frequently afflicted breed in North America. Males are over-represented. Juvenile forms of DCM have been reported in the Doberman Pinscher[70] and Portuguese Water Spaniel breeds.[71] DCM is rare in dogs of small breeds (less than 12 kg) but may occur in certain medium-sized breeds, including the English and American Cocker Spaniels and the Dalmatian.

Etiology

Secondary DCM is occasionally detected and can be caused by dietary deficiency of taurine,[72] L-carnitine abnormalities, [73] or myocarditis. The cause of DCM in most cases is unknown, although the disease appears to be familial in many breeds. DCM may be an X-linked recessive trait in Great Danes[74] and has been suggested to be an autosomal recessive trait in the Portuguese Water Spaniel.[71] Familial occurrence of DCM in Doberman Pinscher dogs is common.

Clinical presentation

Clinical signs associated with congestive heart failure include exercise intolerance, tachypnea, dyspnea, coughing, weight loss and syncope. Dogs with occult DCM are increasingly detected.

Radiography

Generalized cardiomegaly is generally present. Pulmonary edema is more common in the Doberman Pinscher and Boxer breeds, whereas right-sided (pericardial, pleura, abdominal effusions) or biventricular failure are more common in giant breed dogs.

Electrocardiography

The ECG is generally abnormal. Changes often include increased R-wave amplitude, increased QRS complex duration, and/or widened P waves. There is a high prevalence of arrhythmias. Atrial fibrillation is the most prevalent supraventricular tachyarrhythmia. Ventricular arrhythmias have been recorded in up to 80% of selected cohorts.[19,20] The presence or development of ventricular arrhythmias is a strong predictive indicator for development of DCM in Doberman Pinscher dogs with equivocal echocardiographic evidence of dilated cardiomyopathy.[21] Thus, 24-hour ambulatory ECG can help identify overtly healthy Doberman Pinschers with cardiomyopathy.[22]

Echocardiography

Characteristic findings include dilatation of all cardiac chambers, normal or slightly reduced left ventricular wall thickness, left ventricular hypokinesis and marked left ventricular dysfunction. Mild atrioventricular valvular regurgitation is usually present.

Pathology

Marked dilatation of all four cardiac chambers with eccentric hypertrophy is a hallmark finding. A characteristic histolopathologic lesion is the presence of attenuated wavy myocardial fibers.[23] Mild interstitial fibrosis and patchy areas of myocytolysis and necrosis are usually present.

Clinical outcome

Congestive heart failure and related morbidity and mortality is the most common outcome.[24] Doberman Pinscher dogs suffer high morbidity and sudden death compared with other breeds.

Inherited ventricular arrhythmias and sudden death in German Shepherd dogs

Key features of this model are ventricular arrhythmias (Fig. 30.15) and sudden death. Selected breeding and pedigree analysis have determined that the disorder is inherited, but the mode of inheritance is unresolved.[28–30] Physical examination, routine electrocardiography, thoracic radiography, and necropsy are unremarkable and arrhythmia is the sole abnormality.[29] Sudden death usually occurs between 4 and 18 months of age. The overall incidence of sudden death in affected dogs is 15–20%. However, the incidence of sudden death varies between litters and ranges from none to all dogs in an individual litter. Arrhythmias are dependent upon behavior, age, and heart rate.[29,31,32] Except for the most severely affected dogs, arrhythmia diagnosis requires Holter monitoring for diagnosis.

Ventricular tachycardia is usually polymorphic, nonsustained, preceded by a pause, and at times appears similar (although not identical) to torsade de pointes. The rate is usually very rapid and may approach up to 500 beats/min in the most severely affected animals.[29,32] In addition, supraventricular arrhythmias occur in up to 20% of affected dogs.

Arrhythmias are age-dependent in that affected dogs do not generally manifest arrhythmias before 12 weeks of age.[29] Thereafter, arrhythmias progressively increase, with peak activity between 24 and 30 weeks of age. Subsequently, the natural history of arrhythmia is variable, some dogs remaining static and others experiencing sudden death. An important influence of heart rate on arrhythmias was noted in that a pause precedes each episode of ven-

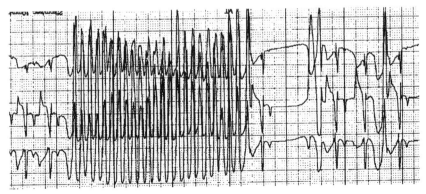

Fig. 30.15 Ambulatory ECG recording (X, Y, Z leads) from a German Shepherd puppy with inherited ventricular tachycardia demonstrating paroxysms of rapid ventricular tachycardia. The dog subsequently experienced sudden death. Paper speed, 25 mm/s. Courtesy of Dr N. Sydney Moïse, College of Veterinary Medicine, Cornell University.

tricular tachycardia.[29,30,32] Thus, arrhythmia is most severe and common in the setting of sinus arrhythmia, and high heart rate is associated with reduced arrhythmia frequency and severity. Arrhythmias are infrequent during ambulatory periods and are prevalent during rest or rapid eye movement sleep.[32]

Abnormal sympathetic innervation to the heart is apparently important in the genesis of these arrhythmias.[33] Abnormal sympathetic innervation has been documented, particularly involving the anterior interventricular septum and left ventricular free wall.[31] Delayed afterdepolarization-induced triggered activity originating in the ventricular myocardium is a mechanism for some age-dependent inherited ventricular tachycardias.[29-32]

Abnormal ventricular repolarization is implicated in the cardiac arrhythmias, and I(Ks) may be involved.[34] Isoproterenol effects the action potential and triggered activity through β_1-adrenoreceptor-mediated signaling that is subject to β_2-adrenergic modulation.[35] Altered density and inactivation of I(to) has been shown to be associated with severe ventricular tachycardia in affected dogs.[36]

References

1 Fox PR, Sisson DD, Moise NS, eds. *Textbook of Canine and Feline Cardiology: Principles and Clinical Practice*, 2nd edn. Philadelphia: WB Saunders, 1999.

2 Van Vleet JF, Ferrans V. Myocardial diseases of animals. *Am J Pathol* 1986; **124**: 98–178.

3 Boyden PA, Tilley LP, Albala A *et al*. Mechanisms for atrial arrhythmias associated with cardiomyopathy: A study of feline hearts with primary myocardial disease. *Circulation* 1984; **69**: 1036–47.

4 Liu SK, Fox PR. Cardiovascular pathology. In: Fox PR, Sisson DD, Moise NS, eds. *Textbook of Canine and Feline Cardiology: Principles and Clinical Practice*, 2nd edn. Philadelphia: WB Saunders, 1999: 817–44.

5 Sisson D, Thomas WP. Myocardial diseases of dogs and cats. In: Ettinger SJ, ed. *Textbook of Veterinary Internal Medicine*, 4th edn. Philadelphia: WB Saunders, 1995: 995–1032.

6 Sisson DD, Thomas WP, Keene BW. Myocardial disease in the dog. In: Ettinger SJ, Feldman EC, eds. *Textbook of Veterinary Internal Medicine*, 5th edn. Philadelphia: WB Saunders, 2000: 874–95.

7 Liu SK. Pathology of feline heart disease. *Vet Clin North Am* 1977; **7**: 323–39.

8 Tilley LP, Liu SK, Gilbertson SR *et al*. Primary myocardial disease in the cat: A model for human cardiomyopathy. *Am J Pathol* 1977; **87**: 493–522.

9 Liu SK, Roberts WC, Maron BJ. Comparison of morphologic findings in spontaneously occurring hypertrophic cardiomyopathy in humans, cats and dogs. *Am J Cardiol* 1993; **72**: 944–51.

10 Liu SK, Maron, BJ, Tilley LP. Feline hypertrophic cardiomyopathy: Gross anatomic and quantitative histologic features. *Am J Pathol* 1981; **102**: 388–95.

11 Fox PR, Liu SK, Maron BJ. Echocardiographic assessment of spontaneously occurring feline hypertrophic cardiomyopathy. An animal model of human disease. *Circulation* 1995; **92**: 2645–51.

12 Kittleson MD, Meurs KM, Liu S-K *et al*. Familial hypertrophic cardiomyopathy in Maine coon cats An animal model of human disease. *Circulation* 1999; **99**: 3172–80.

13 Van Vleet J, Ferrans VJ, Weirich WE. Pathologic alterations in hypertrophic and congestive cardiomyopathy of cats. *Am J Vet Res* 1980; **41**: 2037–48.

14 Bright JM, Golden AL, Daniel GB. Feline hypertrophic cardiomyopathy: Variations on a theme. *J Small Anim Pract* 1992; **33**: 266–74.

15 Peterson EN, Moise NS, Brown CA *et al.* Heterogeneity of hypertrophy in feline hypertrophic heart disease. *J Vet Intern Med* 1993; **7**: 183–9.

16 Atkins CE, Gallo AM, Kurzman ID *et al.* Risk factors, clinical signs, and survival in cats with a clinical diagnosis of idiopathic hypertrophic cardiomyopathy: 74 cases (1985–1989). *J Am Vet Med Assoc* 1992; **201**: 613–18.

17 Martin L, VandeWoude S, Boon J *et al.* Left ventricular hypertrophy in a closed colony of Persian cats [abstract]. *J Vet Intern Med* 1994; **8**: 143.

18 Meurs K, Kittleson MD, Towbin J *et al.* Familial systolic anterior motion of the mitral valve and/or hypertrophic cardiomyopathy is apparently inherited as an autosomal dominant trait in a family of American shorthair cats [abstract]. *J Vet Intern Med* 1997; **11**: 138.

19 Calvert CA, Hall G, Jacobs G *et al.* Clinical and pathologic findings in Doberman pinschers with occult cardiomyopathy that died suddenly or developed congestive heart failure: 54 cases (1984–1991). *J Am Vet Med Assoc* 1997; **210**: 505–11.

20 Calvert CA, Jacobs GJ, Smith DD *et al.* Association between results of ambulatory electrocardiography and development of cardiomyopathy during long-term follow-up of Doberman pinschers. *J Am Vet Med Assoc* 2000; **16**: 34–9.

21 Calvert CA, Wall M. Results of ambulatory electrocardiography in overtly healthy Doberman Pinschers with equivocal echocardiographic evidence of dilated cardiomyopathy. *J Am Vet Med Assoc* 2001; **219**: 782–4.

22 Calvert CA, Jacobs G, Pickus CW *et al.* Results of ambulatory electrocardiography in overtly healthy Doberman Pinschers with echocardiographic abnormalities. *J Am Vet Med Assoc* 2000; **217**: 1328–32.

23 Tidholm A, Haggstrom J, Jonsson L. Prevalence of attenuated wavy fibers in myocardium of dogs with dilated cardiomyopathy. *J Am Vet Med Assoc* 1998; **212**: 1732–4.

24 Tidholm A, Svensson H, Sylven C. Survival and prognostic factors in 189 dogs with dilated cardiomyopathy. *J Am Anim Hosp Assoc* 1997; **33**: 364–8.

25 Fox PR, Maron BJ, Basso C *et al.* Spontaneously occurring arrhythmogenic right ventricular cardiomyopathy in the domestic cat. A new animal model similar to the human disease. *Circulation* 2000; **102**: 1863–70.

26 Harpster NK. Boxer cardiomyopathy. A review of the long-term benefits of antiarrhythmic therapy. *Vet Clin North Am Small Anim Pract* 1991; **21**: 989–1004.

27 Basso C, Fox P, Meurs K *et al.* Arrhythmogenic right ventricular cardiomyopathy causing sudden cardiac death in Boxer dogs: A new animal model of human disease. *Circulation* 2003. (In press.)

28 Moise NS, Gilmour RF Jr, Riccio ML *et al.* Diagnosis of inherited ventricular tachycardia in German shepherd dogs. *J Am Vet Med Assoc* 1997; **210**: 403–10.

29 Moise NS, Meyers-Wallen V, Flahive WJ *et al.* Inherited ventricular arrhythmias and sudden death in German shepherd dogs. *J Am Vet Med Assoc* 1994; **24**: 233–43.

30 Moise NS, Moon PF, Flahive WJ *et al.* Phenylephrine induced ventricular arrhythmias in German shepherd dogs with inherited sudden death. *J Cardiovasc Electrophysiol* 1996; **7**: 217–30.

31 Gilmour RF Jr, Moise NS. Triggered activity as a mechanism for inherited ventricular arrhythmias in German shepherd dogs. *J Am Coll Cardiol* 1995; **27**: 1526–33.

32 Moise NS, Dugger DA, Brittain D *et al.* Relationship of ventricular tachycardia to sleep/wakefulness in a model of sudden cardiac death. *Pediatr Res* 1996; **40**: 344–50.

33 Dae MW, Lee RJ, Chin MC *et al.* Heterogeneous sympathetic innervation in German shepherd dogs with inherited ventricular arrhythmia and sudden cardiac death. *Circulation* 1997; **96**: 1337–42.

34 Merlot J, Probst V, Debailleul M *et al.* Electropharmacological characterization of cardiac repolarization in German shepherd dogs with an inherited syndrome of sudden death: Abnormal response to potassium channel blockers. *J Am Coll Cardiol* 2000; **36**: 939–47.

35 Sosunov EA, Gainullin RZ, Moise NS *et al.* Beta(1) and beta(2)-adrenergic receptor subtype effects in German shepherd dogs with inherited lethal ventricular arrhythmias. *Cardiovasc Res* 2000; **48**: 211–19.

36 Freeman LC, Pacioretty LM, Moise NS *et al.* Decreased density of Ito in left ventricular myocytes from German shepherd dogs with inherited arrhythmias. *J Cardiovasc Electrophysiol* 1997; **8**: 872–83.

37 Holland CT, Canfield PJ, Watson ADJ *et al.* Dyserythropoiesis, polymyopathy, and cardiac disease in three related English springer spaniels. *J Vet Intern Med* 1991; **5**: 151–9.

38 Cooper BJ, Winand NJ, Stedman H *et al.* The homologue of the Duchenne locus is defective in X-linked muscular dystrophy of dogs. *Nature* 1988; **334**: 154–6.

39 Valentine BA, Cummings JF, Cooper BJ. Development of Duchenne-type cardiomyopathy: Morphologic studies in a canine model. *Am J Pathol* 1989; **135**: 671–8.

40 Moïse NS, Valentine BA, Brown CA *et al.* Duchenne's cardiomyopathy in a canine model: Electrocardiographic and echocardiographic studies. *J Am Coll Cardiol* 1991; **17**: 812–20.

41 Hamlin RL, Smetzer DL, Breznock EM. Sinoatrial syncope in miniature Schnauzers. *J Am Vet Med Assoc* 1972; **161**: 1022–8.

42 Maron BJ, Bonow RO, Cannon RO III *et al.* Hypertrophic cardiomyopathy. Interrelations of clinical manifestations, pathophysiology, and therapy (first of two parts). *N Engl J Med* 1987; **316**: 844–52.

43 Maron BJ, Spirito P, Green KJ *et al.* Noninvasive assessment of left ventricular diastolic function by pulsed Doppler echocardiography in patients with hypertrophic cardiomyopathy. *J Am Coll Cardiol* 1987; **10**: 733–42.

44 Wigle ED, Rakowski H, Kimball BP *et al.* Hypertrophic cardiomyopathy: Clinical spectrum and treatment. *Circulation* 1995; **92**: 1680–92.

45 Seidman CE, Seidman JG. Gene mutations that cause familial hypertrophic cardiomyopathy. In: Haber E, ed. *Scientific American Molecular Cardiovascular Medicine*. New York: Scientific American, 1995: 193.

46 Maron MS, Olivotto I, Betocchi S *et al.* Effect of left ventricular outflow tract obstruction on clinical outcome in hypertrophic cardiomyopathy. *N Engl J Med* 2003; **348**: 295–303.

47 Marian AJ, Yu Q-T, Mann FL *et al.* Expression of a mutation causing hypertrophic cardiomyopathy disrupts sarcomere assembly in adult feline cardiac myocytes. *Circ Res* 1995; **77**: 98–106.

48 Meurs KM, Kittleson M, Spangler E *et al.* Nine polymorphisms within the head and hinge region of the feline cardiac beta-myosin heavy gene. *Anim Genet* 2000; **31**: 231.

49 Magnon AL, Meurs KM, Kittleson MD *et al.* A highly polymorphic marker identified in intron 15 of the feline cardiac troponin T gene by SSCP analysis. *Anim Genet* 2000; **31**: 236–7.

50 Rush JE, Freeman LM, Fenollosa NK *et al.* Population and survival characteristics of cats with hypertrophic cardiomyopathy: 260 cases (1990–1999). *J Am Vet Med Assoc* 2002; **220**: 202–7.

51 Baty CJ, Malarkey DE, Atkins CE *et al.* Natural history of hypertrophic cardiomyopathy and aortic thromboembolism in a family of domestic shorthair cats. *J Vet Intern Med* 2001; **15**: 595–9.

52 Rishniw M, Thomas WP. Dynamic right ventricular outflow obstruction: A new cause of systolic murmurs in cats. *J Vet Intern Med* 2002; **16**: 547–52.

53 Liu S-K, Maron BJ, Tilley LP *et al.* Canine hypertrophic cardiomyopathy. *J Am Vet Med Assoc* 1979; **174**: 708–13.

54 Liu S-K, Maron BJ, Tilley LP *et al.* Hypertrophic cardiomyopathy in the dog. *Am J Pathol* 1979; **94**: 497–507.

55 Thomas WP, Mathewson JF, Suter PF *et al.* Hypertrophic obstructive cardiomyopathy in a dog: Clinical, hemodynamic, angiographic, and pathologic studies. *J Am Anim Hosp Assoc* 1984; **20**: 253–60.

56 Sisson DD. Heritability of idiopathic myocardial hypertrophy and dynamic subaortic stenosis in pointer dogs [abstract]. *J Vet Intern Med* 1990; **4**: 118.

57 Basso C, Thiene G, Corrado D *et al.* Arrhythmogenic right ventricular cardiomyopathy. Dysplasia, dystrophy, or myocarditis? *Circulation* 1996; **94**: 983–91.

58. Fontaine G, Fontaliran F, Frank R. Arrhythmogenic right ventricular cardiomyopathies. Clinical forms and main differential diagnoses. *Circulation* 1998; **97**: 1532–5.

59 Nava A, Rossi L, Thiene G. *Arrhythmogenic Right Ventricular Cardiomyopathy-dysplasia.* Amsterdam: Elsevier, 1997.

60 Marcus FI, Fontaine G, Guiraudon G *et al.* Right ventricular dysplasia. A report of 24 adult cases. *Circulation* 1982; **65**: 384–98.

61 Thiene G, Nava A, Corrado D *et al.* Right ventricular cardiomyopathy and sudden death in young people. *N Engl J Med* 1988; **318**: 129–33.

62 Corrado D, Thiene G, Nava A *et al.* Sudden death in young competitive athletes: Clinico-pathologic correlations in 22 cases. *Am J Med* 1990; **89**: 588–96.

63 Bright JM, McEntee M. Isolated right ventricular cardiomyopathy in a dog. *J Am Vet Med Assoc* 1995; **207**: 64–6.

64 Simpson KW, Bonagura JD, Eaton KA. Right ventricular cardiomyopathy in a dog. *J Vet Intern Med* 1994; **8**: 306–9.

65 Fernandez Del Palacio MJ, Bernal LJ, Bayon A *et al.* Arrhythmogenic right ventricular dysplasia/cardiomyopathy in a Siberian husky. *J Small Anim Pract* 2001; **42**: 137–42.

66 Ishikawa S, Zu Rhein GM, Gilbert EF. Uhl's anomaly in the mink: Partial absence of the right atrial and ventricular myocardium. *Arch Pathol Lab Med* 1977; **101**: 388–90.

67 Meurs KM, Spier AW, Miller MW *et al.* Familial ventricular arrhythmias in boxers. *J Vet Intern Med* 1999; **13**: 437–9.

68 Meurs KM, Spier AW, Wright NA *et al.* Comparison of the effects of four antiarrhythmic treatments for familial ventricular arrhythmias in Boxers. *J Am Vet Med Assoc* 2002; **221**: 522–7.

69 Buchanan JW. Prevalence of cardiovascular disorders. In: Fox PR, Sisson DD, Moise NS, eds. *Textbook of Canine and Feline Cardiology: Principles and Clinical Practice*, 2nd edn. Philadelphia: WB Saunders, 1999: 457–70.

70 Vollmar A, Fox PR, Meurs K *et al.* Dilated cardiomyopathy in juvenile Doberman pinschers. *J Vet Cardiol* 2003; **5**: 23–7.

71 Alroy J, Rush JE, Freeman L *et al.* Inherited infantile dilated cardiomyopathy in dogs: Genetic, clinical, biochemical, and morphologic findings. *Am J Med Genet* 2000; **95**: 57–66.

72 Kramer GA, Kittleson MD, Fox PR *et al.* Plasma taurine concentrations in normal dogs and in dogs with heart disease. *J Vet Intern Med* 1995; **9**: 253–8.

73 Keene BW, Panciera DP, Atkins CE. Myocardial L-carnitine deficiency in a family of dogs with dilated cardiomyopathy. *J Am Vet Med Assoc* 1991; **198**: 647–50.

74 Meurs KM, Miller MW, Wright NA. Clinical features of dilated cardiomyopathy in Great Danes and results of a pedigree analysis: 17 cases (1990–2000). *J Am Vet Med Assoc* 200; **218**: 729–32.

CHAPTER 31

The Role of the Internet and Patient Support Groups for Those Living with Hypertrophic Cardiomyopathy

Lisa Salberg

Hypertrophic cardiomyopathy (HCM) is an uncommon genetic disease with a wide variety of clinical manifestations. Few cardiology practices evaluate more than a few patients affected with HCM, thus limiting clinician experience and interest in this condition. HCM has a prevalence of up to 1 in 500 in the general population. Based on these figures, the average cardiologist would have between one and four patients in their practice with HCM, thus leading to a significant lack of experience with a disease that is complex and extremely variable.

Considering the prevalence of HCM, it is highly unlikely that a patient would randomly know any other person with the condition, with the exception of a family member. Patients with HCM have long suffered isolation, fear, lack of adequate information regarding available treatment options and, in too many cases, years of misinformation or even misdiagnosis. In the experience of the Hypertrophic Cardiomyopathy Association (HCMA), the time from first consultation with a health-care provider to diagnosis and treatment of their HCM is over 2 years. During this time the anxiety of not knowing what is wrong can lead to loss of employment, difficulties in relationships, depression and various other social and economic problems.

The diagnosis of HCM often presents unique issues for physicians. HCM can offer challenges in meeting the needs of patients for risk stratification, family screening and recognition. The diagnosis of HCM changes not only the life of that patient, but also that of the entire family. In an overwhelming number of cases, the patient who 'seems fine' leaves the physician's office with knowledge that he or she has a profound diagnosis and a disability. Great difficulty is encountered in explaining this new condition to family, friends and employers. At that juncture, patients may feel the need to gather information about their disease, and they increasingly use the Internet for this purpose.

The Internet

The Internet is a tool with incredible power, and when used properly can yield a wealth of valuable factual information quickly. In this respect, the Internet has found an important application in understanding relatively uncommon genetic diseases such as HCM, both for patients and physicians. Many search engines will lead to hundreds of sites containing pertinent information. For example, a recent search for 'hypertrophic cardiomyopathy' yielded 23 400 web matches on the search engine 'Yahoo,' and 48 498 web matches on 'Lycos'.

Internet terminology

• *Match*. Simply refers to the location of the item searched for, although it may not be precisely what you are looking for. For example, if you search for 'hypertrophic cardiomyopathy,' some of the matches may be for 'dilated cardiomyopathy,' thus causing confusion to a patient who may now be under the impression that these are the same condition.

• *Domain name*. Refers to the formal name of the web site. In many cases it is the Internet 'address'. For example, the domain name of the Hypertrophic Cardiomyopathy Association is www.4HCM.org.

• *Web site*. An entire site devoted to a given topic. A site is typically multiple pages long.

• *Web page*. Would refer to one page within a web site.

• *Article*. Normally refers to any mention of the word on web pages or in the media.

• *Webmaster*. This is normally the person responsible for the maintenance of the site.

• *Chat room*. This is a real-time conversation device allowing free and open dialog. A variation of a chat room is a closed chat room; for this you must pre-register with the controlling party to participate.

• *Moderator*. The individual responsible for monitoring the dialog and who also has authority to dismiss unwanted parties from a closed chat room.

• *Address*. The World Wide Web address for a web site. The address of the HCMA is www.4HCM.org.

• *Bulletin/message board*. An open forum that enables you to leave messages that are available for all to read.

Each search engine has its own criteria for defining a 'match'. Searches will prioritize results by listing them in the order most frequently visited by people who have previously done a similar search. The data contained in these matches often are not monitored, edited, peer-reviewed or guided by the medical community. This issue has led to apprehension in the medical community, with good reason. The Internet has given rise to patients turning up at their doctor's appointments all over the world armed with reams of Internet-based information, which is often contradictory. Therefore we must ask ourselves, how do we harness the power of the Internet to help patients adjust to and live with a chronic condition such as HCM?

To begin with we must learn to navigate the Internet for quality information. Choosing search engines is primarily a matter of personal preference. The mainstream search engines provide excellent service and enable you to be very selective in your search. Yahoo, Lycos, Iwon, and Google are examples that are simple to use (all search engines require you to enter a proper World Wide Web address/domain name, such as www.yahoo.com).

Investigation is the most important aspect of seeking information on the Internet, yet it is often overlooked. The prevalent assumption of accuracy of information may lead to a pitfall in using the Internet. Here are some quick tips for confirming the quality of Internet information for conditions such as HCM.

• Look for contact information. If the site contains a phone number, address or email, use it. Contact the Webmaster or call the contact person directly and ask them about the site. If a web site lacks contact information or only will allow email contacts, this should raise concern that it may contain information of poor quality.

• In the case of a medical site, question who actually reviews the information on the site. Is the information based on one person's views or on a compilation of data, and what is the Webmaster's involvement and/or what additional sites are recommended? These questions (and their answers) offer a better idea of the intentions of the creator or keeper of the site. Some web sites are profit-driven while others are not. If someone has a financial interest in the web site, it should be disclosed. During the investigation process it may be confusing to see a variety of suffixes on the addresses. A suffix of '.com' refers to any domain name purchased in the private sector, while '.org' was created to indicate organizations other than commercial businesses. The suffix '.gov' refers to government organizations and '.edu' to educational organizations. In addition, various countries have added an abbreviation of their country name to denote the origin of their site. When reviewing medical information, the country of origin is of relevance, as the standard of care varies around the world, and some medications are known under different names, thereby potentially adding to the confusion for patients. The web site www.networksolutions.com will allow the owner to search for any domain name or purchase a site. However, simply knowing who maintains ownership of the site will not necessarily yield insight about quality or content, as many sites are owned by communications companies on behalf of a client.

• Verify the information found on the web site. Many people build web sites to further their own business interest or opinions. While such a site may look attractive and seem reasonable, one would be well advised to confirm the data elsewhere. Search further on the Internet; contact your health-care provider, instructor or colleague to confirm the accuracy of the data. References or endorsements can be found on the Internet without asking. Simply see how many web sites 'link' to the page you are trusting for information. In the case of HCM, the HCMA web site is a link on the web sites of physicians specializing in HCM. These links would suggest that the physicians find the content to be of high quality and the organization credible.

Given these considerations, use the Internet and access the quality of information available.

Patient support groups

Support groups take a variety of forms, the most important being the family unit and close friends. Individual patients, however, often find the need to discuss unique issues and problems or find the answers to complex questions that family or friends simply cannot provide. Such has been the rationale for support or advocacy groups focused on specific but often uncommon medical conditions, such as HCM. Previously, such support/advocacy groups were largely located in a particular geographical area or community so that people could gather to discuss common problems and new ideas, and share insights. This format allows each person to seek the support of others affected by similar life circumstances, but has often been limited to major metropolitan areas, which are not easily accessible to those unable to travel or residing in some regions of the country.

Many physicians also understand the need for, and benefits of, support/advocacy groups. Moreover, recent studies have shown that a positive attitude on the part of patients has a direct relationship to expected quality of life.[1-8]

Support/advocacy groups offer patients and families the information, support and education needed to cope more effectively with their medical condition, which in some cases may represent a familial disease. The understanding gained from the support group may also aid the patient in communicating more effectively and accurately with his or her physician. This, in itself, is time-saving and helpful to all because it clearly identifies serious medical issues in a timely fashion. The support/advocacy groups help to fill voids that may have existed between patient and family, as well as between patient and physician.

For those living with HCM, specific areas of concern often begin prior to definitive diagnosis, as misdiagnosis is so frequent in this condition. Indeed, it has been the observation of the HCMA that nearly one-half of our membership was misdiagnosed for a period ranging from 3 weeks to more than 30 years.

Finally, while HCM may be a serious disease with important risks for some, many patients live a relatively normal lifespan without significant disability or major therapeutic interventions. In many ways, patients simply need support, but in other instances it is more important that the patient has a strong advocate. For example, after diagnosis or progression of symptoms, patients may find themselves in need of assistance to retain their jobs. Although the Family Medical Leave Act has been in effect since 1993 and the Americans with Disabilities Act since 1990, patients, employers and physicians alike may not be familiar with the law and protections available. The most difficult aspect of enacting a patient's rights under these statutes is simply to determine what the law truly protects. Patients rarely seek such legal advice, as it is costly and intimidating. In too many cases, a skilled worker (with HCM) may leave a good paying job with benefits for a lower-paying position without health coverage due to the need for a position that is less demanding physically or emotionally. In many cases, patients do not know that an employer (one with more than 15 employees in the case of Americans with Disabilities Act and 50 employees in the case of the Family Medical Leave Act) cannot hold the disability against them for any time absent from the job for the purpose of treating a serious medical condition (up to 12–26 weeks, depending on the state of residence). Furthermore, patients may be unaware that their employer is required to provide for them (at no cost), reasonable accommodations to allow them to perform their job, including staggered work hours, moving their office to a space requiring less walking, a mid-afternoon rest period, or anything deemed medically necessary by the employee's health-care provider. In the case of the Family Medical Leave Act, leave and accommodations must also be made available for an employee to deal with the serious medical condition of a spouse, child or adult in their care.

Another significant role of a patient support/advocacy group is to help educate patients regarding the importance of research. Such groups form alliances and cooperative relationships with other organizations having similar interests and concerns. In the case of human subjects research, support/advocacy groups can provide a central repository of opinions concerning national and international authorities in the field. One such organization is the National Bioethics Advisory Committee (www.bioethics.gov). They suggest patients have the following questions answered prior to participation in clinical research.

• What exactly are you planning to do to me? Step-by-step, day-by-day?
• How many people have you done this to before, and what happened to them?
• What happened in animal studies researching this drug or technique?
• What do you suspect might happen to me based on all the other research that's gone on before?
• What sort of things might make this project more dangerous than usual?
• How hard will it be to discontinue the medication (or use of device)?
• What would be my alternatives in a non-research setting?

Furthermore, the HCMA suggests to all potential research participants that they retain a copy of the entire protocol and consent form, and review it carefully with a trusted physician unconnected with the center conducting the research.

True informed consent is imperative for the patient and researcher alike. If the center or researcher will not provide such documentation (or answer questions) or if the patient is in any way uncomfortable, then they should decline participation in the research protocol.

HCM support groups

Over the past 10 years, patients with HCM from all over the world have made substantial progress in building partnerships with the medical community. The early mark of success in this effort came from a woman with HCM (Carolyn Biro) who herself had endured misinformation about the disease. Her efforts in establishing the Cardiomyopathy Association of the United Kingdom (www.CardiomyopathyAssociation.uk) have helped countless patients with HCM.

It was Carolyn Biro who assisted me in the creation of the Hypertrophic Cardiomyopathy Association—USA (www.4HCM.org) in 1996. In the past 7 years we have also seen the creation of Canadian, Australian, and Israeli support groups. While it is true that many of these organizations were initially formed due to tragic circumstances, they have all grown into pillars of hope, friendship and a feeling that patients with HCM are far from alone. Although all these groups operate in somewhat different ways, the organizational objectives are remarkably similar.

The HCMA

Almost 80% of our HCMA membership initially locates us on-line; 10% come from physician referral, 5% from the media and the remainder are referred from friends or family. The HCMA comprises two branches: patient/family support and medical community relations. In the area of medical community relations, the HCMA regularly participates at annual scientific sessions, such as those of the American Heart Association, the American College of Cardiology, and the North American Society of Pacing and Electrophysiology. At these events, information is distributed in the form of educational materials, such as posters, journal articles and newsletters. This allows prompt reporting of all advances in the field of HCM to our membership.

There are four specific steps taken by the HCMA when a patient or family member makes an initial inquiry. The first step is to provide educational material through our web site, newsletter, medical journal articles and graphics. The second is a conversation, either by email or telephone, to ensure that the person is aware of all available treatment options and the importance of family screening in this genetic disease. Thirdly, we ensure that patients and family members are aware of all information disseminated by the HCMA, which consists of a compilation of data collected from various journals, medical centers and experts in the field of HCM and reviewed by our medical advisors. Finally, and most importantly, the HCMA makes it clear to its membership that we are not medical professionals (i.e. physicians or nurses) and that all information provided by the HCMA must be discussed with their medical provider.

Since HCM is uncommon, the opportunity for a patient to speak to someone who has 'been there' is of great comfort and can dispel many fears. The HCMA also provides a 'Network Enrollment Form' to all members, who may opt to be available to speak to others on an ongoing basis. The availability of the book written specifically for patients, *Hypertrophic Cardiomyopathy: For Patients, Their Families, and Interested Physicians*,[9] available through the HCMA, has proven to be of great value in this regard.

Conclusions

Patient support/advocacy groups and the advent of the Internet have had an incredible impact on the lives of patients with HCM and other chronic diseases. Strong ties between the medical community and such support groups may help to ensure informed participation in research, the prompt dissemination of new data, and well-informed patients and families. Strong ties between patients improve the psychological well-being of patients and families with HCM.

References

1 Seaward TH. Stressful life events, personality, and health: An inquiry into hardiness. *J Pers Soc Psychol* 1992: **37**: 1–11.

2 Cousins N. *Anatomy of an Illness as Perceived by the Patient.* New York: Bantam Books, 1979: 126–89.

3 Hirsch J, Hofer M, Holland J. Toward a biology of grieving. In: Osterweis M, Solomon F, Green M, eds. *Bereavement Reactions, Consequences and Care.* Washington, DC: National Academy Press, 1984: 236–312.

4 Steen KF. A comprehensive approach to bereavement. *Nurse Pract* 1998; **23**: 54–68.

5 Richman J. The lifesaving function of humor with the depressed and suicidal elderly. *Gerontologist* 1995; **35**: 271–3.

6 Averill J. Autonomic response patterns during sadness and mirth. *Psychophysiology* 1996; **5**: 339–414.

7 Schieifer SJ, Keller SE, Camerino M *et al.* Suppression of lymphocyte stimulation following bereavement. *JAMA* 1983; **250**: 374–7.

8 Ware JE, Karmos A. *Ware Health Perceptions Questionnaire. Development and validation of scales to measure perceived health and patient role propensity. Volume II.* Carbondale, IL: Southern Illinois University School of Medicine, 1984.

9 Maron BJ, Salberg LF. *Hypertrophic Cardiomyopathy: For Patients, Their Families, and Interested Physicians.* Futura/Blackwell Publishing, 2001: 96 pp.

Afterword

The following is a speech delivered by Dr Robert Jon Pensack, a physician and psychiatrist, and a patient with hypertrophic cardiomyopathy (HCM), to the 6th annual meeting of the Hypertrophic Cardiomyopathy Association (HCMA) in Morristown, New Jersey on June 12, 2003. The text is published here as the afterword because of its obvious relevance to HCM and the patients who are afflicted, which is the subject of this book. Dr Pensack is also the author of *Raising Lazarus*, an autobiographical memoir of his life with HCM, published by GP Putnam's Sons in 1994 and critically acclaimed by the New York Times Book Review.

My earliest memories begin at age 4 with the traumatic loss of my 31-year-old mother. My older brother Richard was 7 years old at the time. Our mother died of what was then a mysterious, poorly understood disease which destroyed the muscle of her heart … and which we now understand to be HCM. Her death painted a dark landscape for me to survive and develop in. Certainly, it reshaped my entire life. I remember the feelings of alienation, abandonment, and yes, hopelessness. But time and resilience, which children have plenty of, allowed me to heal and carry on.

Unfortunately, both my brother and I were also diagnosed in our early teens at approximately age 14 with IHSS, now called HCM, the same disease that had killed our mother. We became chronic heart patients at The National Institutes of Health (NIH). As most of you know, this is one of the largest federally funded research medical facilities in the world. There, we underwent a litany of both invasive and noninvasive medical procedures which were repeated seemingly endless times throughout our young lives. Since our treatment was often experimental, it often felt like we were white rats … albeit very well cared for white rats.

This was my first exposure to the world of medical research. I also psychologically perceived it as the answer to my frightening new problems. I was confident that, no matter what was wrong with my brother's and my hearts, those well-meaning, intelligent doctors and scientists would certainly correct it. They gave me immediate hope merely by the fact that they existed.

With the onset of our illness and the traumatic procedures we endured, came a new definition of who we were. We were no longer Richard and Bob. Our definition of self now became our illness. We were different from our peers, our friends, and our loved ones. We couldn't participate in all of the sports we would have liked to. We hid our true darkest fears from others. We began to fear death at the ripe old age of 15. This was our secret, and we developed coping mechanisms to keep it that way. Humor played a big part in allowing me to cope. Despite our realities, we still had our hopes and aspirations for our futures.

I certainly had my dreams. I wanted to survive my illness. I wanted to become a physician and help others. I also wanted to fall in love and have a family. I fantasized about how I would achieve all of these. I dreamed that I might someday live high in the Rocky Mountains in a beautiful little town. I set about achieving these goals with great tenacity and determination.

Soon after entering college, in the fall of 1968 at the University of Colorado in Boulder, my hopes and dreams became gravely threatened. My disease and fate had a much different course planned for me. I began to experience severe dizzy spells and breathlessness upon mild exertion. I returned to the NIH for more heart catheterizations. I was treated with medications and told to refrain from all competitive athletics. My symptoms worsened, and I began to have outright fainting spells. We increased my medication.

In 1967, the year prior to my entering college, Dr Christian Barnard had performed the world's first human heart transplant on a 59-year-old man named Louis Weshlansky. He died 18 days later of overwhelming infection and pneumonia. Barnard transplanted several more patients, but the immune suppressants used left them all vulnerable to infection. Many patients died, and his longest surviving cardiac transplant patient lived only 18 months. Barnard's detractors were many. As one of his harshest critics said at the time of his death in 2001, 'so successful was Barnard, that others tried to emulate him with the same miserable failures.' So much so that Britain banned heart transplants in the 1970s. One writer, in a scathing article written at the time of Barnard's death, declared 'those who are well informed will not mourn the loss of Barnard, but the animals and patients who died at his hands.'

I was acutely aware of Barnard's clinical experiments with patients that were performed far too early and without the scientific understanding that should have preceded such a heroic effort at preserving human life. However, these first efforts at heart transplantation, in spite of their miserable failures, still affected me in a positive way emotionally, because I felt, even at that young age in college, that the procedure might someday be used to save my own life. I followed the clinical history of transplantation from then on, beginning in 1969 when I began to have more of my own serious symptoms. Simply knowing that the quest for the eventual success of this miraculous surgical and immunological treatment would still continue gave me hope for my own future.

It should be obvious to all of us that scientists and clinical researchers must proceed cautiously when crossing the line between animal research and human trials. But the point that I want to make is that scientific research represents hope for all of us who suffer from life-threatening illness.

In 1972, I decided to attempt to get a job doing medical research at the University of Colorado School of Medicine. I did not have a specific area of interest. I simply wanted to be involved in some aspect of medicine. Whether it was divine intervention, or simply a stroke of uncanny coincidence, I was hired by the Chief of Surgery to work in his animal research lab on liver transplantation experiments and to help produce a new immunosuppressive drug called ALG, anti-lymphocyte globulin, which he was developing. Now called anti-thymocyte globulin, it is still used today for immune suppression induction in new transplant patients. I had no idea at the time, but this drug, that I had helped work on, along with this brilliant and driven Chief of Surgery himself, would both play a very large part in my own survival some 20 years later. This physician was someone very special. He never seemed to sleep, and his endless energy astounded me. Surgeons from countries around the world were flying to Denver to work in his animal transplant lab in order to learn his surgical techniques for liver and kidney transplantation.

In the fall of 1974, I entered medical school while suffering from increasing symptoms of shortness of breath on mild exercise, as well as syncopal and pre-syncopal episodes. At the completion of my first year of medical school, I was told I would need open-heart surgery in the next year. At age 24, I had to drop out of medical school to undergo this surgery. My brother Richard, who had become extremely religious, eventually underwent the same heart surgery 2 years later. We both went on to have several near-death experiences.

Several weeks after the surgery, I had a cardiac arrest and was resuscitated. The first of what would be nine pacemakers was implanted at that time. I went on to complete medical school, but my disease continued to deteriorate. I was faced with more surgeries, more fear, and at times hopelessness. I became my own best doctor and made sure that the best that medical science had to offer was always available to me. New pacemaker-device technologies were becoming available in the 1980s, which had the multiple capabilities of increasing a patient's cardiac output with increased exercise demand as well as terminating any life-threatening arrhythmias when necessary. Pacemakers also allowed patients like me to become more active as a result of their ability to mimic a normal heart's response to exercise. The biomedical engineers who developed these devices worked closely with me, as I became one of the first patients to ever receive what is now called a dual-chamber pacemaker. These pacemakers are now used routinely by thousands of cardiac patients. The biomedical advances lagged just slightly behind my clinical status, but always seemed to catch up to me in time to improve my quality of life. As a result, I continued to have hope for my long-term survival.

Throughout all of these years, I continued to watch with more than a curious eye the research that was occurring in transplantation. In 1974, a medical researcher discovered cyclosporin, a new immunosuppressant which would change the entire face of modern organ transplantation. The earliest pioneer to do the clinical trials with cyclosporin was Dr Thomas Starzl. Earlier, back in 1967, he performed the world's first successful human liver transplant at the University of Colorado School of Medicine. He is widely thought of as the Father of Liver Transplantation, and an argument could (and should be made) that he is the man most responsible for the success of all human organ transplantation. He is, in case you haven't figured it out by now, the Chief of Surgery who hired me in 1972 to work in his transplant lab after I finished college. In 1980, he moved on to the University of Pittsburgh Medical Center, which he built into the finest organ transplant center in the world.

In 1980, I married my wife Abbe. She stood by me through thick and thin. After becoming a general practitioner and emergency room physician for several years, I returned to residency and specialized in Psychiatry. In July of 1989, my wife gave birth to an 8½ lb baby boy named Max. I delivered him. One month later, the three of us moved to Steamboat Springs where I set up a practice in psychiatry. We were very happy. But within a year, I was suffering from increasing congestive heart failure. In October of 1990, my brother Richard underwent successful heart transplantation in San Francisco.

On May 9, 1991, my wife gave birth to our beautiful daughter Miriam Rose whom I also delivered. In November of 1991, I had to stop work because of severe heart failure. I could barely walk up the stairs to my office or negotiate the stairs in my own home. I was told I had less than 18 months to live unless I received a new heart. I was placed on the transplant list at the University of Colorado Health Sciences Center. On October 26th, 1992, I received the gift of life that I had so anxiously waited for. I underwent a 12-hour heart transplant operation, and despite near devastating complications, I survived. Three weeks later, my right femoral artery unexpectedly ruptured in my apartment near the hospital. I controlled the hemorrhaging the best I could until the paramedics arrived. I arrived at the emergency room unconscious, having nearly bled to death. I was transfused and taken to the operating room where my artery was reconstructed in a 3-hour operation.

Over the last 10 years, I have learned to live with another man's heart inside my chest. At times, it has been very difficult, as I have had recurrent bouts of organ rejection, which were all diagnosed via cardiac biopsies, a procedure that I have now endured on more than 80 different occasions. These episodes of tissue rejection have been treated with increasing doses of prednisone, a drug that as you know has many undesirable side effects. In 1995, more than 2 years after my heart transplant, I was continuing to suffer from serious bouts of tissue rejection, each of which was eating away at the precious function of my new heart. I had read about a new drug, still called by its experimental name FK-506, now known as tacrolimus or Prograf, that my old friend Dr Starzl was using in Pittsburgh to successfully rescue people from organ rejection. He arranged for me to make a trip there, and after the switch was made, I was once again free of rejection. He and his astounding career of cutting-edge medical research always has represented continual hope for me. As patients and families of patients, we all realize that scientists and researchers represent this same hope to us and to the unfortunate victims of all humanity's most devastating diseases. Recently, my 12-year-old daughter Miriam, began to manifest symptoms of our family's genetic heart disease ... HCM. The genetic flaw has also been passed on to both of my nephews.

Medical research has already significantly improved the treatment of HCM with much improved early diagnosis, medical management, and technological therapies in the form of small implantable cardiac defibrillators to prevent the occurrence of sudden death in this population. Most of us with HCM will have normal life expectancy. However, some of us will go on to develop crippling symptoms of degenerative heart disease. The quality of many of our lives will be greatly compromised. I do not want to see this happen to my daughter.

Molecular genetics has the potential to someday modify the phenotypic expression and severity of our disease. Ultimately, there will be a cure for HCM. It may sound far fetched, but no more so than the idea that I could be standing here in front of you with a deceased man's heart that was given to me over 10 years ago.

My past hopes have all come to fruition. I have two beautiful children and a wife, all of whom I cherish. I live in a beautiful mountain town called Steamboat Springs located high in the Rocky Mountains. I am called upon regularly to help others with their own struggles in life. Sure, I had my moments of desperation and temptation to surrender to feelings of hopelessness, but I always somehow found a reason to go on. What I learned from all of this is that survival is instinctual and life is worth living and that it is very, very precious.

Robert Jon Pensack, MD
Steamboat Springs
Colorado

Index